Unilateral Biportal Endoscopy of the Spine

Foreword

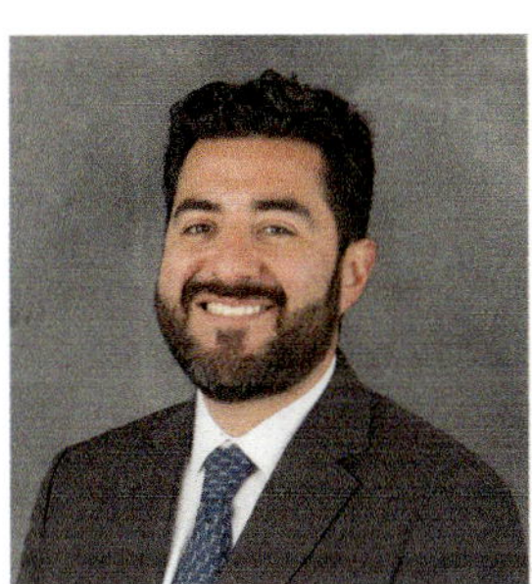

Dr. Javier Quillo-Olvera is a neurosurgeon/spine surgeon, constantly innovating and reinventing himself and his clinical practice with the only goal of improving patient outcomes. It was during this quest that, after finishing neurosurgery training, Javier decided to follow further MIS training under the mentorship of Dr. "Luke" Kim in Korea. After a few years of practice on his own, Dr. Quillo became an expert in the endoscopic field. To date, he and his group are one of the leading spine endoscopic practitioners in the world.

On the other hand, endoscopic spine surgery is one of the most innovative branches of MIS spine surgery. It has evolved at an accelerated pace over the last couple of decades. However, modern spine surgery progress comes with technological development plus and/or in parallel to keen minds pushing the boundaries of regular clinical practice. In this book, Dr. Quillo and his group have put an extraordinary effort into understanding, mastering, and promoting the use of biportal endoscopic techniques to treat spinal pathologies.

Unilateral biportal endoscopic surgery is a technique that was only available for orthopedic "knee" surgeons until a few years ago. The fact that this book is written/edited by an expert endoscopist neurosurgeon means that Dr. Quillo's process required surgical skills and a comprehensive understanding of the hardware, adapted anatomy, pitfalls, complications, success tips, etc. I am thrilled about what this book offers. This book is a full "biportal endoscopic guide" for any spine surgery enthusiast, from the spine surgeons in training to the expert spine orthopedic surgeons and neurosurgeons looking to expand their scope of practice.

This book is divided into six parts: Part I, "why and how," where the authors go through the history and evidence-based reasoning behind these techniques to the current technology available in the market; Part II, "Foundation": basic instruments, infrastructure, anesthesia, and anatomy; Part III, "the learning process" for UBE; Part IV, "UBE bread and butter": disc herniations, decompressions, revision, CSF leak management, and navigation; Part V, "UBE cervical special cases"; and Part VI, "experts only, future of biportal surgery, and lessons learned." I have no doubt that this book will become a basic tool in the armamentarium for any spine surgeon interested in endoscopic spine surgery.

"If you want to learn, improve, or master your UBE technique, read this book."

New York-Presbyterian,
Weill Cornell Medical College
New York, NY, USA

Rodrigo Navarro-Ramirez

Preface

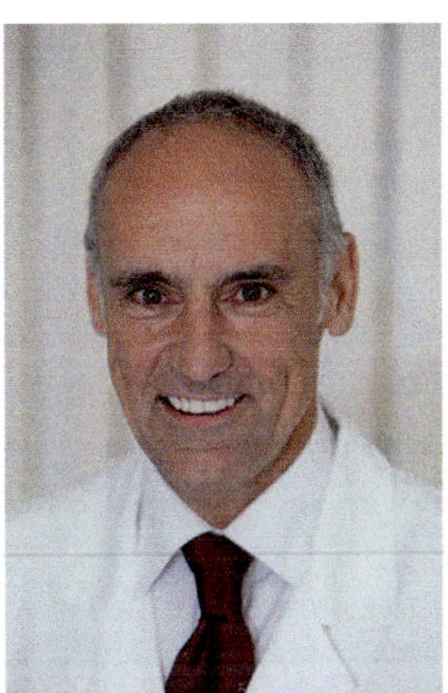

Degenerative disorders of the cervical and lumbar spine constitute a significant burden of nearly all healthcare systems in industrialized countries. Even though conservative treatment plays a predominant role in treating such disorders, a considerable number of patients need surgical treatment. Since the first half of the last century, efforts have been made to adequately treat degenerative conditions such as disc herniations, spinal stenosis, or degenerative segmental instabilities. However, until the early 70s of the last century, such operations were characterized by a (nowadays unacceptable) surgical collateral damage to tissues surrounding the target areas (spinal canal, disc).

It was the merit of Wolfhard Caspar and Gazi Yasargil who have introduced microsurgical access techniques in the second half of the 1970s. These techniques have triggered the development of less invasive procedures in the last five decades. It took a long time until microsurgical techniques became a gold standard in the spine world, but technical progress did not stop. In 1975, 2 years before Caspar and Yasargil published their first clinical experiences, Hijikata, a Japanese spine surgeon, first published a new technique called "percutaneous nucleotomy."

This was the start of the development of endoscopic techniques, which took place in a parallel timeline to microsurgical techniques. However, it was less successful in the first three decades mainly because of technical problems and because many spine surgeons who had just shifted from conventional to microsurgical approaches were not motivated to change their surgical strategy again. Moreover, the early results of full-endoscopic procedures were not really promising.

It took until the beginning of this century when a technical detail completely changed the world of endoscopic surgery. This was the use of continuous irrigation during surgery, as well known from other arthroscopic procedures such as knee or hip arthroscopy.

Working "underwater" decreased the problem of venous bleeding and its management, and it also allowed a more clear vision of the target area.

In the last 20 years, full-endoscopic techniques for the treatment of disc herniations, decompression of the spinal canal, and removal of synovial cysts in the lumbar and the cervical spine have become a standard in most countries around the world. The tremendous scientific and technical work, mainly of colleagues from South Korea and the People's Republic of China, and extensive case series "boosted" the development and acceptance of full-endoscopic spine surgery.

It was a logical consequence that with more experience and routine in these techniques, there was a trend to use these techniques for more complex indications or anatomical situations such as problems in the thoracic spine, surgical revision cases, and even fusion techniques.

Soon, the surgeons realized that full-endoscopic uniportal approaches have their limitations in this respect. This was the birth of unilateral biportal endoscopic procedures (UBE) or biportal endoscopic spine surgery (BESS).

Interestingly, UBE is the technical return of surgical triangulation applied in most other endoscopic techniques such as arthroscopy, laparoscopy, or thoracoscopy. UBE is a new principle in endoscopic spine surgery. Therefore, it is a great pleasure for me to present this book, which contains a comprehensive survey of the current UBE knowledge.

The first three parts deal with historical aspects and then describe basic principles, including the use of radiation, the transition process, and the learning curve that surgeons have to go through when shifting from conventional or full-endoscopic or microsurgical approaches to UBE.

In Part IV, all current UBE techniques are described in detail, including challenging cases such as revisions or complication management and use of navigation technology to perform interbody fusions. The same is valid for Parts V and VI, which deal with cervical and thoracic applications.

I have to congratulate and thank all the authors for sharing their tremendous experiences and achievements. A special thank goes to the initiator and editor of this book, my good friend Javier Quillo-Olvera, for giving me the honor to be a co-editor and for succeeding in gathering such a prestigious and renowned group of key opinion leaders in this field to contribute chapters to this book. I would also like to thank Springer Nature for having agreed to publish this and for their help in editing and finalizing this work. I believe and hope that this book will be a standard textbook for the coming years and will be a tremendous help to all young surgeons who wish to learn and practice this technique.

Muenchen, Germany Michael Mayer

Preface

Minimally invasive surgery (MIS) has emerged as a highly effective and safe option in all surgical areas of medicine, and spine surgery is no exception. The "minimally invasive" concept includes various elements: the in-depth analysis of each case, allowing planning the surgical treatment for each patient. Among the critical information that must be known to plan is the correct identification of the anatomical structure that generates the pathology, which leads to the most important advantage of MIS in spinal surgery, the ability to be highly precise and targeted to the pathology avoiding the procedure-related damage to normal anatomy. Therefore, accuracy is a distinctive quality of MIS, especially in spinal surgery.

The way to be more precise in MIS to avoid iatrogenic damage motivates the evolution in surgical techniques. This defines MIS spine surgery as a set of procedures applied to different pathologies that depend on the development of skills by the surgeon and the use of various technologies to resolve the disease with the least possible impact on the patient's anatomy, with minimal repercussions on the daily life of each person requiring care. This means a quicker and more tolerable return to physical activity.

Endoscopic spine surgery is based on a target-addressed concept that determines its ability to be highly accurate. This book will focus on one particular spinal endoscopic technique, the biportal endoscopic spine surgery (BESS) or unilateral biportal endoscopy (UBE).

Focusing on the human being as an essential part of all medical care processes defines us as ethical professionals, and if, in addition, we are constantly evolving, developing new skills and knowledge to be applied to patients to improve those care processes defines us as good surgeons in search of the well-being of each person who needs it.

These efforts to improve patients' quality of life crystallized when our group comprising Dr. Javier Quillo Reséndiz, my father; Dr. Diego Quillo Olvera, my brother; and I, Javier Quillo Olvera, decided to look further into our training as spinal neurosurgeons, defining our medical practice as spinal neurosurgeons with high experience in minimally invasive techniques, of which biportal endoscopic surgery stands out.

UBE is one more tool in the spine surgeon's armamentarium to offer what we have described before, highly accurate and functional procedures that favor each patient from a less aggressive perspective, that is, a minimally invasive procedure.

In this book, we have tried to detail the experience obtained from our patients and professors on the most recent biportal spinal endoscopic techniques for various degenerative pathologies of the spine so that any spine surgery enthusiast can consult.

The entire book is the result of the efforts of not only the editors (Fig. 1) but also all the authors who have participated by sharing their experience in UBE. All the authors are opinion leaders in their respective countries and healthcare centers in the field of biportal endoscopic surgery. Our most sincere thanks to them for their outstanding work throughout each chapter.

Biportal endoscopic surgery is part of a phenomenon in the field of spine surgery that is currently happening, and that aims to leave less impact on the lives of patients

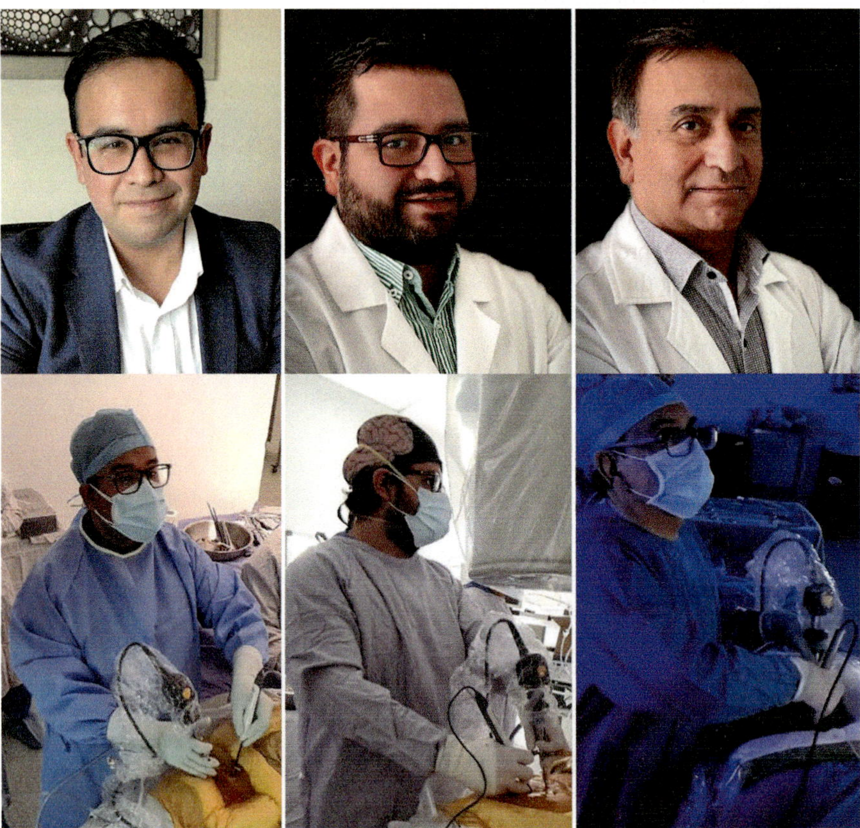

Fig. 1 From left to right. Dr. Javier Quillo-Olvera, Dr. Diego Quillo Olvera, and Dr. Javier Quillo-Reséndiz

by reducing the collateral effect of spine surgery, but under the same standards that are required for each surgical decision made regardless of whether it is MIS or conventional.

Current biportal endoscopic surgical techniques are the result of the efforts of pioneers such as Eum Jin Hwa, Cheol Woong Park, Heo Dong Hwa, and San Kyu Son, whom we must personally thank for their motivation and teaching and for devoting their time to share with us the necessary knowledge to establish an acceptable practice in our country, Mexico.

As we mentioned, this book has been the product of all the experiences acquired from our patients who benefited from various biportal endoscopic techniques, which will be a source of education for surgeons who use what they have learned in this book as a basis. To them, our most sincere thanks, every doctor we owe to our patients.

The realization of this book was possible thanks to the people who encouraged the idea of sharing our knowledge and experience in biportal endoscopic surgery, especially Alicia Olvera Sánchez, our beautiful mother and a wonderful wife, who has always emphasized that the essential thing in expertise is the application for the benefit of every human being.

Finally, thanks go to our dear Professor Jin-Sung Kim, who has been a pioneer and a constant promoter of minimally invasive spine surgery in the world; who has been a true friend and supporter in every personal and academic decision, not only of our medical group, but also on a personal level; and who has dedicated most of his time to teaching and sharing.

We conclude this preface wishing you enjoy this book, which was made for you readers, hoping that the seed of knowledge will spread and that this first edition of "Unilateral Biportal Endoscopy of the Spine: An Atlas of Surgical Techniques" will only be the beginning of a long way of learning and development of biportal endoscopic surgery in favor of our patients.

Querétaro, Mexico Javier Quillo-Olvera
Querétaro, Mexico Diego Quillo-Olvera
Querétaro, Mexico Javier Quillo-Reséndiz

Acknowledgments

This book is particularly dedicated to Alicia Olvera Sanchez. Her unconditional support in each process allowed this project to be completed. The effort, dedication, and faith you share inspire and motivate us to do incredible things. Thank you for being so much exceptional and essential in our lives—this book is for you (Fig. 2).

We acknowledge Michelle Barrera-Arreola, M.D., for her support in research and reviewing each chapter of this book (Fig. 3).

Our gratitude goes to Olivia Zuñiga-Tenorio and Juan-Carlos Tejeda-Olvera for unconditionally assisting each patient in our practice (Fig. 4).

Thanks go to our patients for putting their faith in our hands. They not only are the axis of our work but also enrich our lives with experiences, allowing our growth as doctors and humans.

Finally, gratitude goes to our professors, who introduced the UBE technique in our lives, Professors Dong-Hwa Heo, Sang-Kyu Son, and Jin-Sung Kim; this book is their legacy.

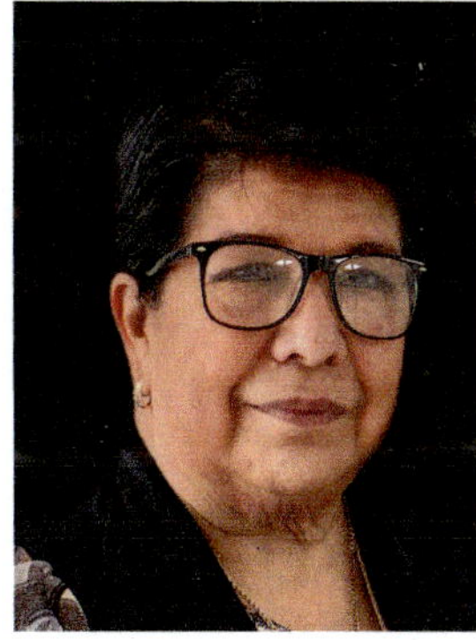

Fig. 2 Alicia Olvera Sanchez

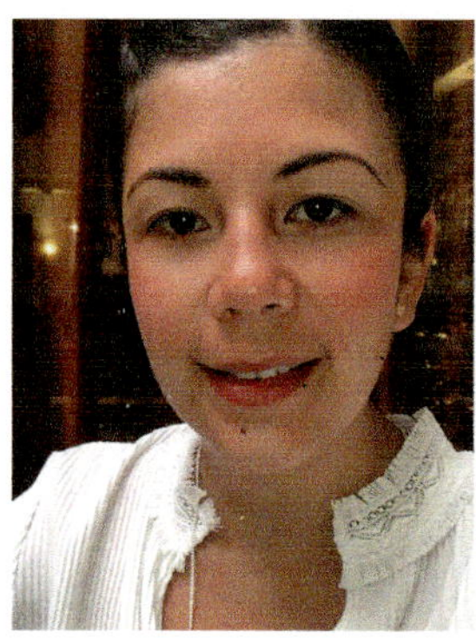

Fig. 3 Michelle Barrera-Arreola, M.D.

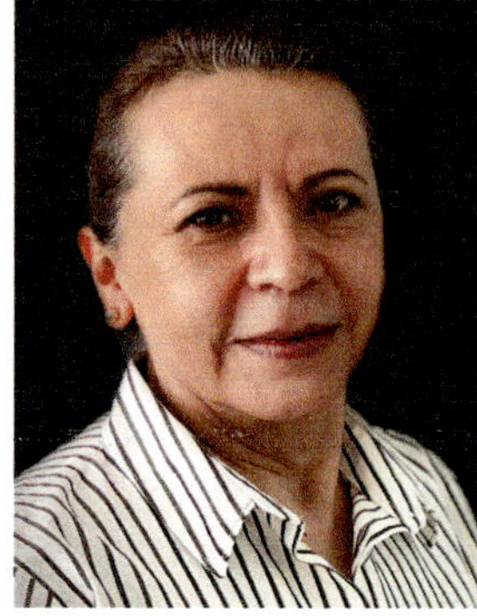

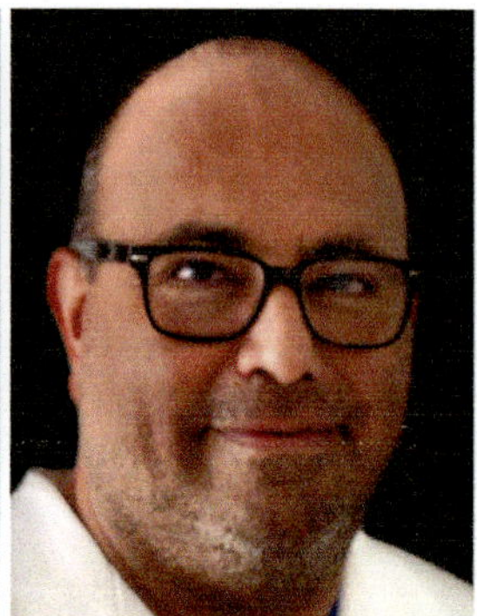

Fig. 4 Administrative and clerical team at the Brain and Spine Care, Minimally Invasive Spine Surgery Group. (Left) Olivia Zuñiga-Tenorio. (Right) Juan-Carlos Tejeda-Olvera

Contents

Part I
Generalities

Chapter 1
The Unilateral Biportal Endoscopic Spine Surgery Concept: An Overview

Javier Quillo-Olvera, Diego Quillo-Olvera, Javier Quillo-Reséndiz, and Michelle Barrera-Arreola

Abbreviations

EQ-5D	European Quality of Life—5 dimensions
ODI	Oswestry Disability Index
PROs	Patient-reported outcomes
RF	Radiofrequency
SAP	Superior articular process
UBE	Unilateral biportal endoscopy
UBE-TLIF	Unilateral biportal endoscopic transforaminal lumbar interbody fusion
ULBD	Unilateral laminotomy bilateral decompression
VAS	Visual analogue scale

Introduction

"Primum non nocere," or "first, not harm," is a principle that has prevailed over time in medicine, and in spinal surgery, it has directed its evolution and development. In other words, the surgeon tries to do when he or she faces a disease to find the way that least impacts the patient life.

Supplementary Information The online version contains supplementary material available at [https://doi.org/10.1007/978-3-031-14736-4_1].

J. Quillo-Olvera (✉) · D. Quillo-Olvera · J. Quillo-Reséndiz · M. Barrera-Arreola
The Brain and Spine Care, Minimally Invasive Spine Surgery Group, Hospital H+ Querétaro, Spine Clinic, Querétaro, México
e-mail: neuroqomd@gmail.com; drquilloolvera86@gmail.com; kitnoz@hotmail.com; michelle.barrera@anahuac.mx

J. Quillo-Olvera et al. (eds.), *Unilateral Biportal Endoscopy of the Spine*,
https://doi.org/10.1007/978-3-031-14736-4_1

For example, when a surgeon performs a lumbar decompression, the first thing to do is think about the minor procedure-related collateral damage. Or, when it is necessary to correct a sagittal or coronal imbalance because of degenerative processes, the chosen technique is based not only on fixing the X-rays that made our decision but also on relieving the symptoms of the disease.

For this reason, the "Primum non nocere or non-maleficence principle" is a bioethical concept and a medical one that implies the knowledge and surgical skills of the surgeon applied through proper judgments based on variables that make up a patient an individual entity.

Given this situation, surgical techniques have evolved, and one of the reasons why spinal surgery has transcended is to visualize the anatomical structure that generates the disease to be more specific and decrease the collateral damage in patients.

Spinal surgery has had to adopt different modalities to visualize the pathology. A historical milestone was the microscopic assistance procedures [1, 2]. This event made it possible to significantly reduce the collateral damage of procedures such as total laminectomy for disc herniation, established as a standard. Over time, its traumatic and iatrogenic potentials were observed [3].

Knowledge and technology from other medical specialties redefined spinal surgery, incorporating cameras to visualize and magnify anatomical structures [4].

Hijikata and Parviz Kambin conducted spinal surgery to another step: percutaneous procedures addressed to the intervertebral disc anatomically, observing bony and connective structures to allow safer and less aggressive access to the disc, using lenses or endoscopes [5–9].

However, the simple use of lenses and cameras in the spine would not define the least invasiveness procedure nature assisted by these technologies. The continuous irrigation of saline solution allowed the boom that we know at this time of water-based spinal endoscopy [10].

Then, the rationale of water-based spinal endoscopy we currently know is the direct visualization of structures, the magnification of the anatomy, and the proper illumination of the surgical field, which leads to complying with the principle that we mentioned at the beginning, "Primum non nocere," or trying to mitigate the collateral effect related to the procedure. Spinal endoscopy is transforming the way of treating spinal diseases surgically since more and more indications for its use are accepted as effective treatments.

The main advantage of current spinal endoscopy over other surgical options is simple, more minor damage to vertebral and paravertebral tissues [11]. In addition, the high effectiveness in decompressing the neural elements after overcoming the learning curve has made it possible to relate current endoscopic techniques with good results in the short and medium terms, mainly used in degenerative diseases [10].

Water-based spinal endoscopy can be divided into two major variants, uniportal techniques, of which multiple texts have been published, and unilateral biportal endoscopy (UBE), which is the focus of this book.

The UBE technique was reported for the first time in 1994 by Dr. Daniel Julio De Antoni, and several texts after that were published demonstrating the effectiveness [12]. The earliest indications consisted of epidural pathology related to the intervertebral disc. Contraindications that exceeded the technique at that time were:

- Multilevel degenerative spinal disease
- Posterior vertebral osteophytes
- Degenerative foraminal stenosis
- Bilateral lumbar segment disease
- Far-lateral disc herniations
- Infections
- Patients with spinal tumors
- Revision surgery

Twenty-eight years later, this technique can be used in most diseases for which it was not indicated at that time, except in spinal tumors yet [13–18].

The procedure described by De Antoni evolved thanks to updates that the technique underwent, especially in South Korea. Expert surgeons such as Jin Hwa Eum, who in 2016 for the first time reported encouraging results similar to those obtained through microsurgical technique in 75 patients with herniated discs and lumbar stenosis, treated with UBE and bilateral decompressions through a unilateral laminotomy (UBE-ULBD) [19]. And Professor Cheol Woong Park, the current President of the World UBE Society.

San Kyu Son developed cervical and thoracic decompression procedures through biportal endoscopy, and Dong Hwa Heo has been a key promoter of biportal endoscopic surgery describing various techniques, including biportal endoscopic lumbar interbody fusion and lumbar segmental, multifocal decompressions [20, 21].

An Overview of the UBE Technique

The UBE technique consists of a correct triangulation of two vectors addressed to a site under the guidance of intraoperative fluoroscopy. The vectors are used as ports, one for the endoscope and the other to introduce the surgical tools (Fig. 1.1). This is a true water-based endoscopic technique. The endoscopic system irrigates 0.9%

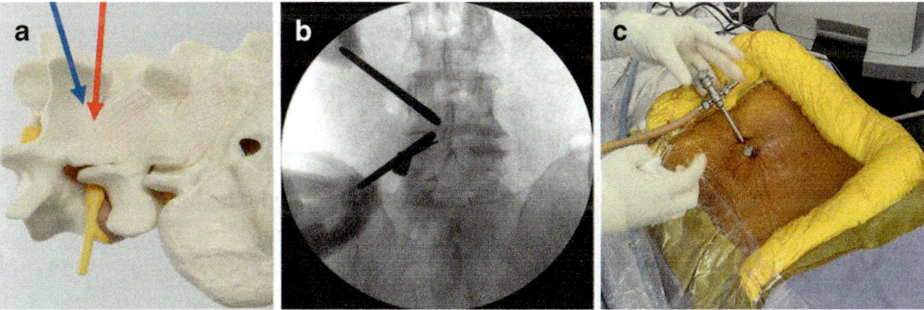

Fig. 1.1 (**a**) Lumbar spine with two trajectories (blue and red arrows). The blue arrow represents the endoscopic port and the red one the working channel. (**b**) Intraoperative AP view of C-arm showing proper triangulation during a paramedian biportal lumbar approach. (**c**) Right paramedian UBE lumbar approach

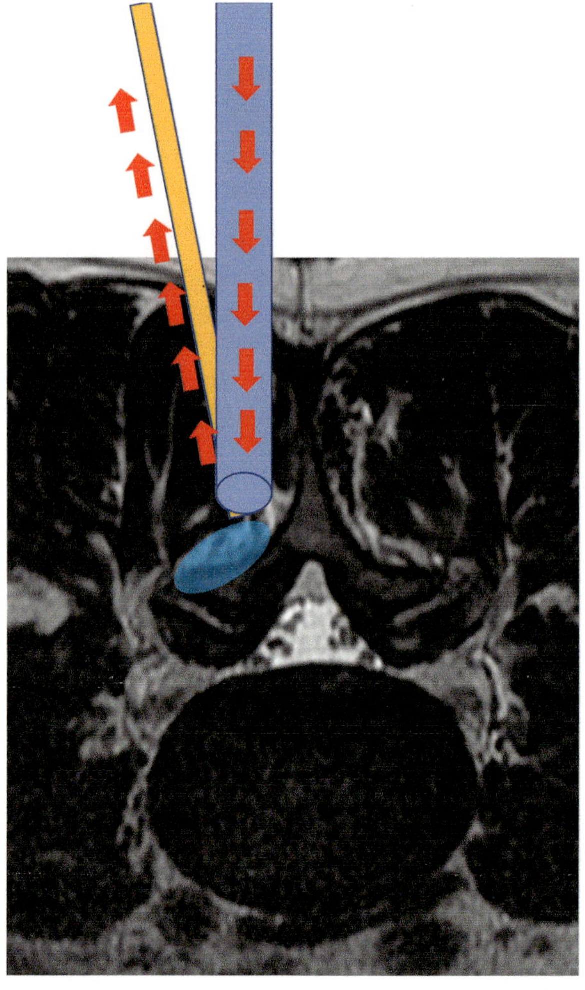

Fig. 1.2 Inflow-outflow system. The red arrows represent the continuous flow of saline irrigated by the endoscopic system and exit through the working channel (orange bar)

saline throughout the procedure, and the outflow exits directly through a semi-tubular working cannula placed independently as the second channel (Fig. 1.2).

Then, the spine surgeon must be patient in learning first how to co-locate the instruments with the endoscope through a correct unilateral biportal approach. Subsequently, the surgeon must locate specific anatomical landmarks that will serve as a guide to orient himself or herself and adequately conclude the planned procedure (Video 1.1).

The author's suggestion is to respect this learning process. Therefore, the UBE technique can be systematically divided into the following steps:

- Correct triangulation of the ports.
- Co-locate the surgical instruments with the endoscope.
- Confirm a proper inflow-outflow system of saline.

- Observe and recognize the bone landmarks.
- Complete the procedure previously planned.
- Develop skills based on the repetition of cases.
- Expand the indications of the technique.

Unilateral biportal endoscopic surgery (UBE), as it is currently known, works through a water-based medium, which means that the endoscopic system continuously irrigates saline solution at a recommended pressure of between 4.41 and 31.00 cmH_2O [22].

The saline irrigated by the endoscope aims to:

- Create a positive hydrostatic pressure to maintain a permeable space below the back muscles.
- Keep the surgical field clean, without particles from the procedure. The cleaning field is obtained through a continuous inflow-outflow of the saline from the endoscope to the working channel.
- Act as a less aggressive hemostatic medium, allowing the bleeding site to be accurately located.
- Allow a clear, magnified, and illuminated visualization of an anatomical structure.

The visualization system used in the UBE consists of rigid rod lens of 4.0 mm shaft diameter and 175 mm of length. The optical features of the arthroscope depend on the diameter, angle of inclination, and field of view. The angle of inclination is the angle between the arthroscope axis and a perpendicular line to the surface of the lens. The angle of inclination used in UBE oscillates between 0° and 30° (Fig. 1.3).

The field of view refers to the viewing angle encompassed by the lens and varies according to the type of arthroscope. For example, the 4.0 mm scope has a 115° field of view. On the other hand, rotation of a 30° arthroscope produces a larger field of view compared with 0°, which is of help in ipsilateral subarticular decompression or craniocaudal viewing of the contralateral foramen (Fig. 1.4). The 0° scope is helpful in central stenosis decompression.

The scope is attached to a light source and a camera to display the spine's image on a video monitor so that the surgeon can observe the procedure.

The arthroscope should always be inserted into a sheath. In UBE, different brands have developed special ones for the spine, completely different from others used in peripheral joints. The sheath is used to maintain the scope into the portal ensuring visual clarity and providing continuous flow into the surgical site. Besides, the arthroscope sheath protects the lens against the drill or shaver.

Arthroscopic sheath is composed of different elements (Fig. 1.5).

- A coupler lets to fix the obturator and lens with the sheath.
- The sheath barrel protects the lens. Different beveled-ended tip barrels have been developed for only use in the spine.
- The spigot plane is equipped with valves to manage the fluid inflow. Commonly, it can rotate to avoid tubing twisting during the procedure.

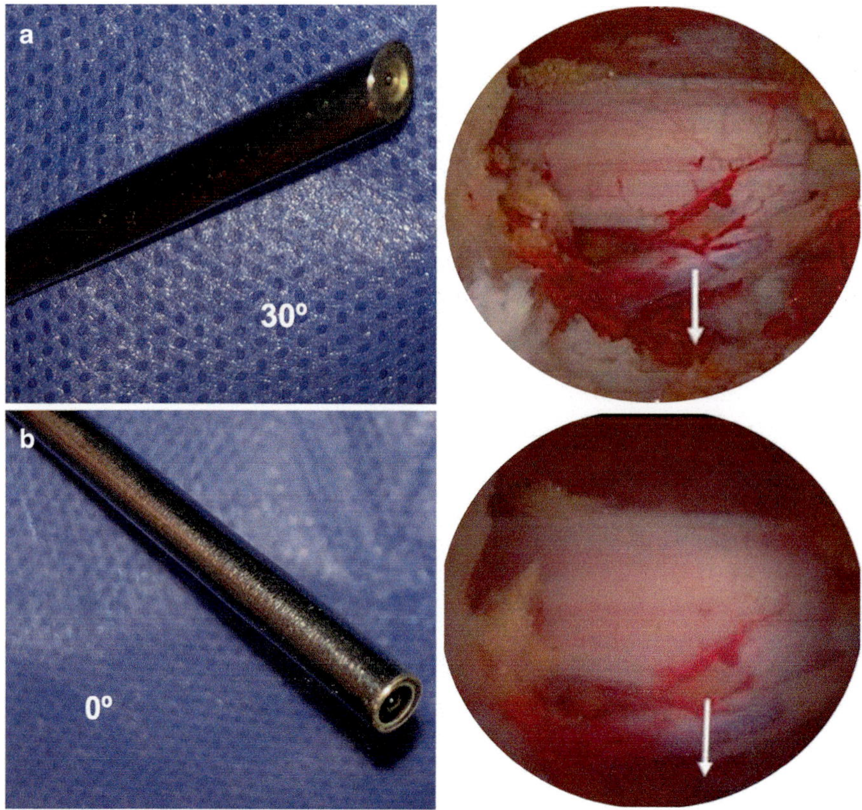

Fig. 1.3 The angle of inclination. (**a**) 0° and (**b**) 30°

The sheath should always be inserted in the spine coupled with a blunt obturator. Then, the obturator is removed, and the scope is inserted.

As we mentioned before, irrigation is essential to clean the surgical field. In UBE, the inflow passes directly through the arthroscopic sheath and the outflow through the other portal employing a semi-tubular cannula. The second portal is for the surgical instruments with independence (Video 1.2). When a pump for irrigation is unavailable, the hydrostatic pressure increases by elevating the 3 L 0.9% saline bag. For each foot of elevation of the solution bag above the joint level, approximately 30 cmH_2O of pressure is produced.

In UBE, the surgeon freely handles the surgical tools with the dominant hand, and the nondominant hand holds the endoscope, which follows the instruments throughout the procedure (Video 1.2).

An essential tool used in UBE is the radiofrequency (RF) probe. The RF plasma can ablate, coagulate, and allow hemostasis of the target tissue at a relatively low temperature (Video 1.1). Thus, the surgeon should avoid a nerve heat injury in

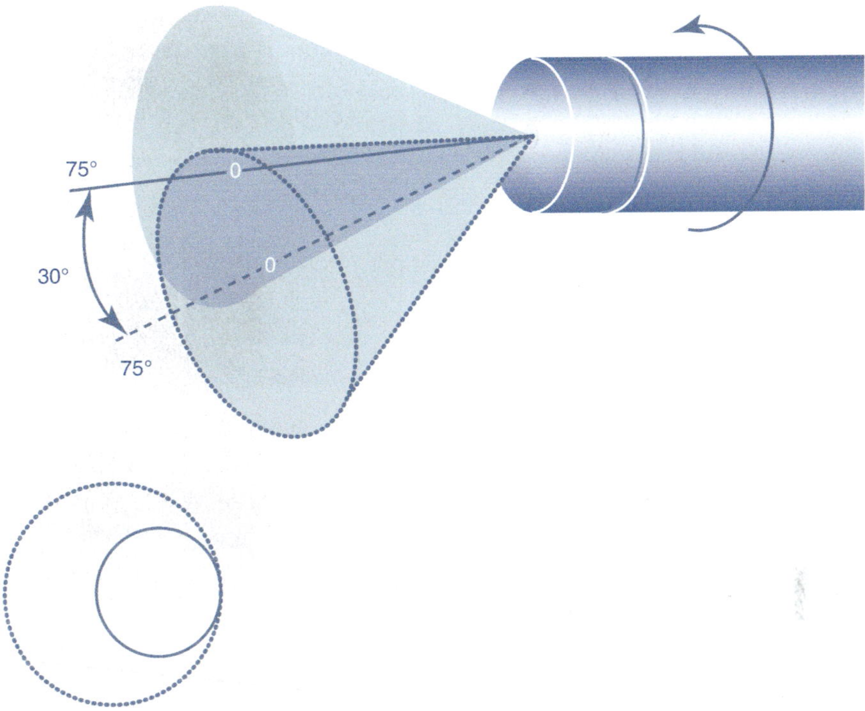

Fig. 1.4 Field of view of a 30° arthroscope

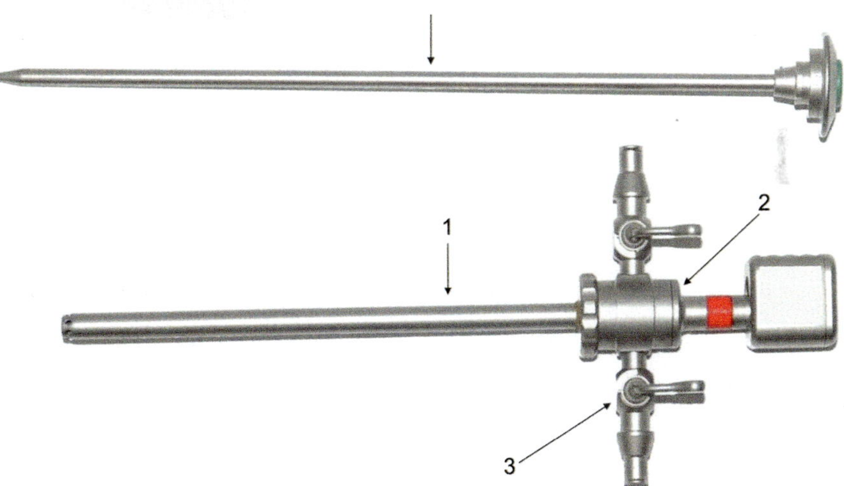

Fig. 1.5 Arthroscopic sheath and obturator. 0. Blunt-tip obturator, 1. sheath barrel, 2. coupler, 3. spigot plane

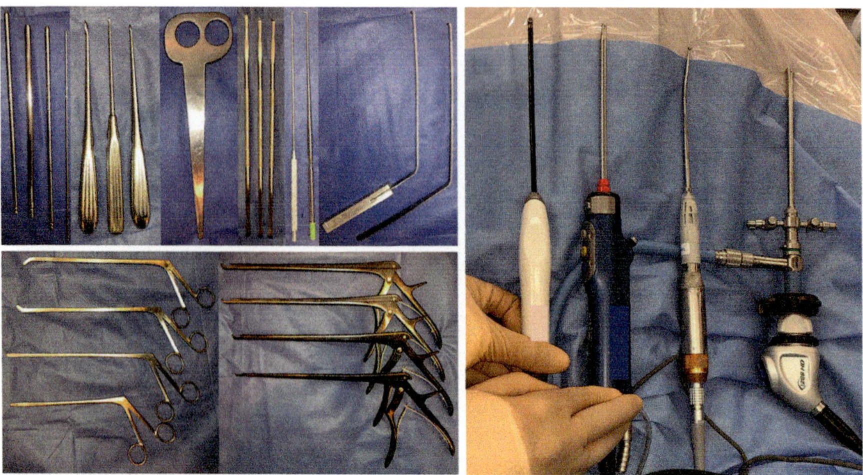

Fig. 1.6 Different surgical tools are commonly employed in UBE

spinal procedures at maximum. Currently, low-energy RF probes for UBE use are specially designed by different brands.

Other surgical tools like special-designed water-based high-speed drill systems with different ball tips to undercutting the bone are commonly used in UBE. Different tip measures and angulations of Kerrison rotary punches, pituitary grasps, dissectors, and nerve hooks are also used to perform the procedure. In general, this technique introduces working tools commonly used in spinal microsurgery, which is quite familiar to the surgeon (Fig. 1.6).

Generalities of UBE

The UBE technique has been gaining popularity. In Western countries, it is increasingly common to observe the interest of young surgeons in different endoscopic procedures that derive from the oriental experience (South Korea, China, and Japan).

In social networks, a medium that has been exploited from the COVID-19 pandemic, there is more information concerning UBE; for example, on FACEBOOK (https://www.facebook.com/), we can find the following groups where expert surgeons share clinical cases and multimedia about their experiences with the biportal endoscopy.

Here are the following groups with their electronic address:

1. UBE, Society of Unilateral Biportal Endoscopy—https://www.facebook.com/groups/586843421514791
2. Korea UBE—https://www.facebook.com/groups/166265787324002

3. UBE Spine Foundation India—https://www.facebook.com/groups/3428968007128468
4. World UBE Society—http://ubeworld.com/default/

In addition, different authors have reported encouraging results in various pathologies treated by biportal endoscopy, mainly in degenerative spinal diseases [23, 24]. A systematic review reported a reduction in the overall VAS and ODI scores at the final follow-up compared with preoperative scores in 11 studies included. Therefore, it meant an improvement in function and disability with satisfying results. The study also measured the satisfaction of patients who underwent UBE technique only for lumbar degenerative pathology finding 84.3% (range, 75.35–95%) from 7 of 11 studies analyzed. However, this study threw 6.7% (range 0–13.8%) of complications reported in 10 of 11 studies analyzed, with the dural tear as the most common complication [24].

There are three particular advantages of UBE:

1. UBE is a minimally invasive technique associated with minimal collateral damage, allowing reduced surgical trauma, less intraoperative bleeding than other conventional methods, rapid discharge from the hospital, and early return to activities.
2. UBE allows some freedom in using the endoscope and surgical instruments, unlike the restrictions observed through the tubular retractor or the uniportal endoscopy.
3. The familiarity of the posterior approaches for any spine surgeon reduces the learning curve compared to uniportal endoscopy.

Several authors have reported their results regarding UBE for lumbar disc herniation (LDH). For example, Soliman in 2013 carried out a prospective study including 43 patients with a diagnosis of noncontained LDH treated with the biportal endoscopic technique, reporting an average hospitalization time of 8 h, a range of complications of 11.6% that included 2 cases of dural tears, 1 case of transient urinary retention, 1 case of recurrence, and 1 case of persistent severe lower back pain. In addition, the clinical results showed improved postoperative VAS and ODI scores compared to the preoperative ones and 95% satisfaction after surgery [25]. Other studies have reported the association of reduced surgical time and the number of cases completed; the more cases, the shorter the surgical time [19, 25, 26].

On the other hand, Park et al. found no clinical inferiority between the UBE technique and microsurgery in treating patients with lumbar spinal stenosis through patient-reported outcomes (PROs) using ODI, VAS, and EQ-5D at 3-, 6-, and 12-month follow-up, in 30 patients allocated in the microscopy group and 29 in the biportal endoscopic group. Therefore, the authors suggested that UBE is a suitable alternative for patients with symptomatic lumbar spinal stenosis through the results of this randomized control trial [17]. In another study published by Kim et al., the outcomes of 105 patients who underwent lumbar decompression surgery by UBE were reported. The mean age of the patients was 71.2 years (range, 52–86 years), and they were followed up for an average of 14 months. The authors reported an average surgical time of 53 min per decompressed level. The postoperative satisfaction results based on the Macnab criteria were also encouraging since 88 patients rated their postoperative results as excellent and 12 as good. In addition, the VAS and ODI scores improved significantly after surgery compared to the preoperative scores. However, there were complications reported in this study; however, these were only 2.9% (3/105); two patients presented a dural tear treated with conservative measures, and 1 patient presented a postoperative epidural hematoma evacuated utilizing UBE [27].

Another degenerative pathology treated by UBE is lumbar foraminal stenosis. This technique aims to remove the tip of SAP through a paraspinal approach or through a contralateral inter- or translaminar approach to decompress the foraminal area of stenosis [28]. These techniques are not usually associated with a high risk of instability since decompression is limited to the most cranial part of the SAP, respecting the joint capsule and other stabilizing ligaments and structures of the spine. In addition to preserving the movement and stability of different segments through minimal collateral damage to other spinal and paraspinal structures, the need for lumbar fusion in many of these degenerative cases is reduced [29].

Ahn et al. reported results obtained in 21 patients with foraminal stenosis treated with UBE. The authors included 11 cases of foraminal stenosis, 9 cases with a herniated disc, and 1 case associated with the disease of the adjacent segment. The mean surgical time reported was 96.7 min per level, and the mean follow-up was 14.8 months. The complication rate was 4.8% (1/21), of which 1 was a dural tear. However, postoperative satisfaction was excellent and good in 80.9% (17/21) [30].

Recently, the indications for unilateral biportal endoscopy have expanded. Currently, it is possible to perform biportal endoscopic fusions through transforaminal approaches (UBE-TLIF), which has been discussed in various articles concluding that the early radiological and clinical results of these procedures are favorable [16]. Heo et al. reported results of 69 patients who underwent single-level UBE-TLIF. One of the advantages observed through the UBE-TLIF technique is the adequate preparation of the endplates under direct endoscopic vision. The authors reported an average of 85.5 mL of bleeding and an approximate surgical time of 165.8 min. The incidence of complications was 7.2% (5/69), 2 cases of dural tear, and 3 cases of postoperative epidural hematoma; all the patients overcame their complications with conservative measures [31].

Lastly, an attempt has been made to measure the collateral effect related to a UBE procedure. Choi et al. compared the inflammatory response from various decompression procedures (MD, transforaminal PELD, interlaminar PELD, and UBE) by measuring biological markers such as creatine phosphokinase and C-reactive protein. Both endoscopic techniques (uniportal and biportal) were characterized by lower increasing values of these inflammatory markers after surgery than MD. The muscular area involved in the approach was also delimited and recognized as a zone of hyperintensity in the cross-sectional area of paraspinal muscles. The largest hyperintense muscle zone was observed in the MD group, the smallest in the PELD group, and in the middle, the UBE group [32].

The above has only been a glimpse of the unilateral biportal endoscopic (UBE) technique. However, throughout this book, essential aspects will be highlighted to be taken into account for the surgeon interested in UBE.

Conclusion

Unilateral biportal endoscopy (UBE) is a set of techniques based on two ports independent of each other, used to introduce the endoscope and surgical tools. Despite using an arthroscopic type lens and having adopted specific visualization technology used in other peripheral joint surgeries, the UBE technique is specific for spinal surgery, with significant differences such as the type of solution to irrigate throughout the procedure, the irrigation pressure suggested in spinal procedures, the use and intensity of energies to coagulate or for hemostasis, and the surgical instruments, among others. Thus, the biportal endoscopic technique has been adapted to the needs of the spine surgeon. In this book, different techniques derived from UBE will be described.

References

1. Yasargil MG. Microsurgical operation of herniated lumbar disc. In: Lumbar disc adult hydrocephalus, Advances in neurosurgery, vol. 4. Berlin: Springer; 1977. p. 81.
2. Caspar W. A new surgical procedure for lumbar disc herniation causing less tissue damage through a microsurgical approach. In: Lumbar disc adult hydrocephalus, Advances in neurosurgery, vol. 4. Berlin: Springer; 1977. p. 74–80.
3. Mixter W, Barr J. Rupture of the intervertebral disc with involvement of the spinal canal. N Engl J Med. 1934;211:210–5.
4. Simpson AK, Lightsey HM 4th, Xiong GX, Crawford AM, Minamide A, Schoenfeld AJ. Spinal endoscopy: evidence, techniques, global trends, and future projections [published online ahead of print, 2021 Jul 13]. Spine J. 2021. pii: S1529-9430(21)00819-6.
5. Hijikata S. A method of percutaneous nuclear extraction. J Toden Hosp. 1975;5:39–42.
6. Kambin P, Sampson S. Posterolateral percutaneous suction-excision of herniated lumbar intervertebral discs. Report of interim results. Clin Orthop Relat Res. 1986;(207):37–43.
7. Kambin P, Brager MD. Percutaneous posterolateral discectomy. Anatomy and mechanism. Clin Orthop Relat Res. 1987;(223):145–54.
8. Kambin P, Nixon JE, Chait A, Schaffer JL. Annular protrusion: pathophysiology and roentgenographic appearance. Spine (Phila Pa 1976). 1988;13(6):671–5.
9. Kambin P, Schaffer JL. Percutaneous lumbar discectomy. Review of 100 patients and current practice. Clin Orthop Relat Res. 1989;(238):24–34.
10. Mayer HM. A history of endoscopic lumbar spine surgery: what have we learnt? Biomed Res Int. 2019;2019:4583943. Published 2019 Apr 3. https://doi.org/10.1155/2019/4583943.
11. Kim HS, Wu PH, Jang IT. Rationale of endoscopic spine surgery: a new paradigm shift in spine surgery from patient's benefits to public interest in this new era of pandemic. J Minim Invasive Spine Surg Tech. 2021;6(Suppl 1):S77–80. https://doi.org/10.21182/jmisst.2021.00031.
12. De Antoni D, Claro ML. Cirugia artroscopica del disco lumbar. Rev Arg de Artr. 1994;1:81–5.
13. De Antoni DJ, Claro ML, Poehling GG, Hughes SS. Translaminar lumbar epidural endoscopy: anatomy, technique, and indications. Arthroscopy. 1996;12(3):330–4.

14. DeAntoni DJ, Claro ML, Poehling GG, Hughes SS. Translaminar lumbar epidural endoscopy: technique and clinical results. J South Orthop Assoc. 1998;7(1):6–12.
15. Pairuchvej S, Muljadi JA, Ho JC, Arirachakaran A, Kongtharvonskul J. Full-endoscopic (bi-portal or uni-portal) versus microscopic lumbar decompression laminectomy in patients with spinal stenosis: systematic review and meta-analysis. Eur J Orthop Surg Traumatol. 2020;30(4):595–611.
16. Heo DH, Lee DC, Kim HS, Park CK, Chung H. Clinical results and complications of endoscopic lumbar interbody fusion for lumbar degenerative disease: a meta-analysis. World Neurosurg. 2021;145:396–404.
17. Park SM, Park J, Jang HS, et al. Biportal endoscopic versus microscopic lumbar decompressive laminectomy in patients with spinal stenosis: a randomized controlled trial. Spine J. 2020;20(2):156–65.
18. Pranata R, Lim MA, Vania R, July J. Biportal endoscopic spinal surgery versus microscopic decompression for lumbar spinal stenosis: a systematic review and meta-analysis. World Neurosurg. 2020;138:e450–8.
19. Eun SS, Eum JH, Lee SH, Sabal LA. Biportal endoscopic lumbar decompression for lumbar disk herniation and spinal canal stenosis: a technical note. J Neurol Surg A Cent Eur Neurosurg. 2017;78(4):390–6.
20. Kim HS, Raorane HD, Heo DH, Yi YJ, Jang IT. Endoscopic spine surgery in Republic of Korea. J Spine Surg. 2020;6(Suppl 1):S40–4.
21. Kim JY, Heo DH. Contralateral sublaminar approach for decompression of the combined lateral recess, foraminal, and extraforaminal lesions using biportal endoscopy: a technical report [published online ahead of print, 2021 Aug 26]. Acta Neurochir (Wien). 2021. https://doi.org/10.1007/s00701-021-04978-x.
22. Hong YH, Kim SK, Hwang J, et al. Water dynamics in unilateral biportal endoscopic spine surgery and its related factors: an in vivo proportional regression and proficiency-matched study. World Neurosurg. 2021;149:e836–43.
23. Park CK. Uniportal and bi-portal techniques in endoscopic lumbar spine surgery: their reciprocal relations. J Minim Invasive Spine Surg Tech. 2021;6(Suppl 1):S75–6.
24. Lin GX, Huang P, Kotheeranurak V, et al. A systematic review of unilateral biportal endoscopic spinal surgery: preliminary clinical results and complications. World Neurosurg. 2019;125:425–32.
25. Soliman HM. Irrigation endoscopic discectomy: a novel percutaneous approach for lumbar disc prolapse. Eur Spine J. 2013;22:1037–44.
26. Choi DJ, Choi CM, Jung JT, Lee SJ, Kim YS. Learning curve associated with complications in biportal endoscopic spinal surgery: challenges and strategies. Asian Spine J. 2016;10:624–9.
27. Kim JE, Choi DJ. Unilateral biportal endoscopic decompression by 30 endoscopy in lumbar spinal stenosis: technical note and preliminary report. J Orthop. 2018;15:366–71.
28. Lee CK, Rauschning W, Glenn W. Lateral lumbar spinal canal stenosis: classification, pathologic anatomy and surgical decompression. Spine (Phila Pa 1976). 1988;13(3):313–20.
29. Yang HS, Lee N, Park JY. Current status of biportal endoscopic decompression for lumbar foraminal stenosis: endoscopic partial facetectomy and outcome factors. J Minim Invasive Spine Surg Tech. 2021;6(Suppl 1):S157–63.
30. Ahn JS, Lee HJ, Choi DJ, Lee KY, Hwang SJ. Extraforaminal approach of biportal endoscopic spinal surgery: a new endoscopic technique for transforaminal decompression and discectomy. J Neurosurg Spine. 2018;28:492–8.
31. Heo DH, Son SK, Eum JH, Park CK. Fully endoscopic lumbar interbody fusion using a percutaneous unilateral biportal endoscopic technique: technical note and preliminary clinical results. Neurosurg Focus. 2017;43:E8.
32. Choi KC, Shim HK, Hwang JS, et al. Comparison of surgical invasiveness between microdiscectomy and 3 different endoscopic discectomy techniques for lumbar disc herniation. World Neurosurg. 2018;116:e750–8.

Chapter 2
Brief History Review of Unilateral Biportal Spinal Endoscopy

Diego Quillo-Olvera, Javier Quillo-Reséndiz, Alexa Borbolla-Ruiz, Michelle Barrera-Arreola, and Javier Quillo-Olvera

Abbreviations

KOLs Key opinion leaders
MISS Minimally invasive spine surgery
UBE Unilateral biportal endoscopy

Introduction

Spine surgeons have developed minimally invasive techniques to decrease the procedure-related collateral effect on the patients leading to a faster return to their normal activities. However, a deep analysis case basis includes an accurate diagnosis to determine the anatomical pathology generator, a key feature of any spinal procedure. Unilateral biportal endoscopy (UBE) is an option among the broad spectrum of minimally invasive techniques with some advantages like familiarity for the surgeon, a shorter learning curve than uniportal endoscopy, and the capacity to have a certain degree of freedom with the surgical tool independent from the endoscope. Nevertheless, everything begins, and this chapter describes a brief history of UBE.

D. Quillo-Olvera (✉) · J. Quillo-Reséndiz · M. Barrera-Arreola · J. Quillo-Olvera
The Brain and Spine Care, Minimally Invasive Spine Surgery Group, Hospital H+ Querétaro, Spine Clinic, Querétaro, México
e-mail: drquilloolvera86@gmail.com; kitnoz@hotmail.com; michelle.barrera@anahuac.mx; neuroqomd@gmail.com

A. Borbolla-Ruiz
Anáhuac University, School of Medicine, Querétaro, México
e-mail: alexaborbolla@gmail.com

J. Quillo-Olvera et al. (eds.), *Unilateral Biportal Endoscopy of the Spine*, https://doi.org/10.1007/978-3-031-14736-4_2

Important Milestones for the Development of UBE

In 1918, Professor Kenji Takagi started the concept of examining knee joints in patients suffering from tuberculosis with the use of a cystoscope. In 1920, he utilized his first arthroscope, which Dr. Watanabe improved. However, Burman (1931) and Stern (1936) were the first surgeons to perform cadaver lumbar spine dissections under endoscopic visualization. Other pathfinders like Pool (1938) and Ooi (1967) conducted myeloscopy. These graphical probes of their work demonstrated an evolution in anatomical visualization [1, 2].

In 1970, an arthroscope of 2 mm diameter was introduced. It was the first ultrathin fiber-optic endoscope. Arthroscopic surgery supported the development of uni- and biportal endoscopy of the spine [1, 2].

Kambin and Casey et al. performed posterolateral lumbar approaches using two working ports. The authors used a 70° arthroscope and a working tool port in the triangular foraminal safety zone to remove a large central or paramedian subligamentous and extra ligament herniated disc, reporting encouraging clinical outcomes [3, 4] (Fig. 2.1).

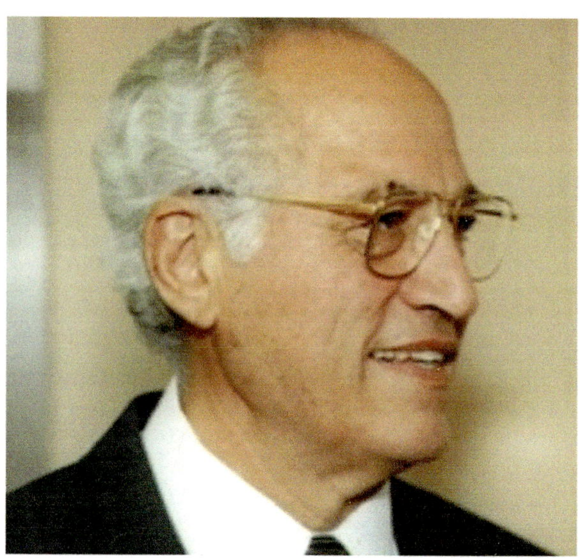

Fig. 2.1 Parviz Kambin

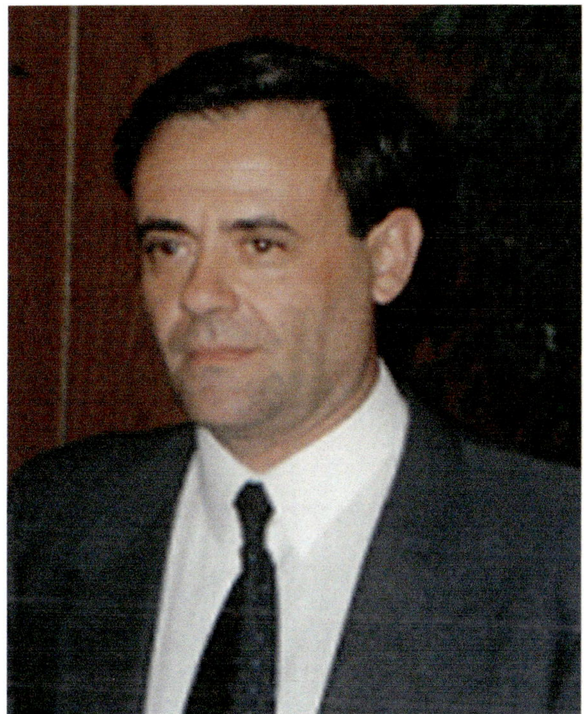

Fig. 2.2 Daniel Julio De Antoni

Dr. Daniel Julio De Antoni in 1994 reported for the first time in a publication titled Cirugía artroscópica del disco lumbar the first trial with biportal endoscopic spinal surgery [5] (Fig. 2.2). The following surgical instruments used in this technique were arthroscopes of 0° and 30°, a water pump with regulated pressure, working cannulas, curettes, dissectors, basket arthroscopy scissors, shaver drill, Kerrison rongeur, and pituitary forceps. For this purpose, Dr. De Antoni employed the surgical technique in 5 specimens, and he performed it in 14 patients who underwent different types of anesthesia (local, epidural, and general). For the first description of his technique, he used a lateral position with the operating table flexed at the patient's hips. As a result, he found a complete visualization of the neural structures, which decreases the risk of injury, and handling the instrument independently from the endoscope allows free motion within the surgical field. Dr. De Anotni's following reports [6, 7] included more indications for the aforementioned biportal endoscopy.

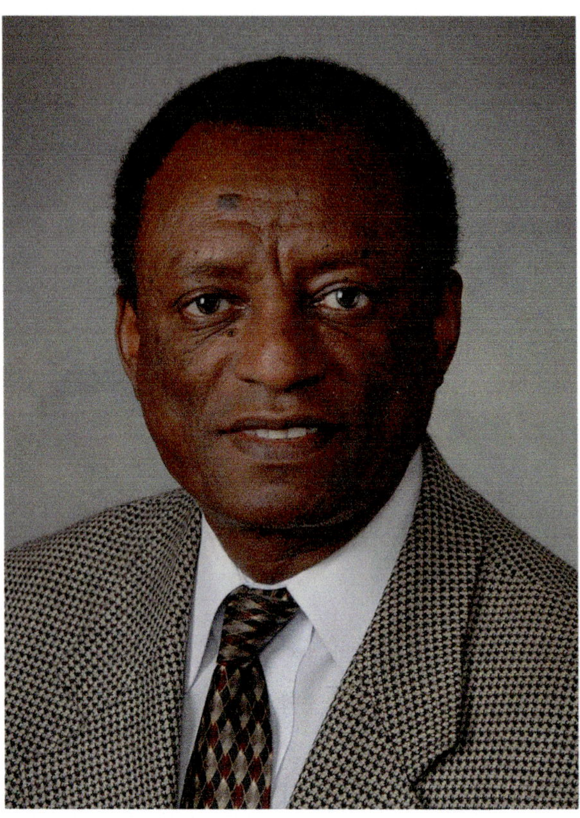

Fig. 2.3 Said G. Osman

Osman [8], in 2012, described a thoracic discectomy with interbody fusion using a biportal posterolateral arthroscopic approach. He performed the technique in 15 patients between 1995 and 1998 (Fig. 2.3).

Eum et al. [9], in 2017, published a case series including 17 patients who underwent unilateral biportal endoscopy (UBE) for lumbar stenosis decompression and disc herniation. It was the first time that the biportal arthroscopic technique was called UBE (Fig. 2.4).

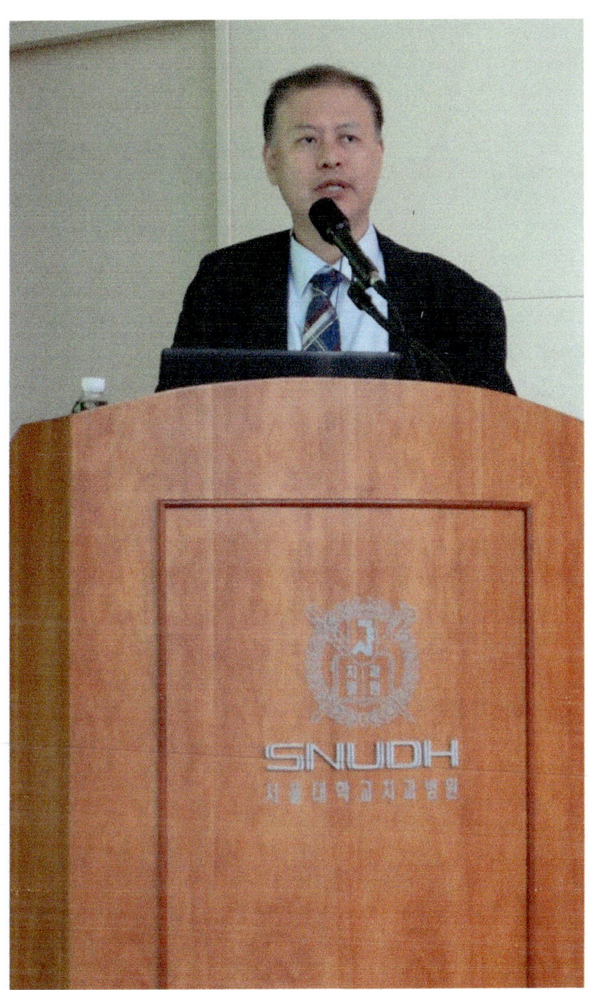

Fig. 2.4 Jin Hwa Eum

Discussion

The historical timeline of spine surgery contains numerous notable names of individuals who made significant contributions to the development of spine surgery as we know it today.

Krause and Oppenheim described the first lumbar discectomy in 1909 [10]. Goldthwait and Middleton identified for the first time a herniation of the nucleus pulposus as a cause of radicular pain or sciatic pain [11, 12]. In 1934, Mixter and Barr reported the first series of successful discectomies with total laminectomies and transdural approaches but with potential complications [13].

Love (1939) described the interlaminar approach for lumbar disc herniation [14], and Lyman Smith [15], in 1964, reported that the percutaneous chemonucleolysis technique for enzymatic dissolution of the nucleus reached an intradiscal decompression.

However, Hijikata [16], in 1970, used a posterolateral percutaneous approach for discectomy. This event changed the way to reach the disc. Parvis Kambin [17] in 1980 gave us the knowledge of a safe area to approach the lumbar disc, the Kambin triangle. So then, history has changed the way to approach the intervertebral disc, but with time, the technology also evolved, and surgeons developed different skills to treat more spinal pathologies under direct visualization with better technology.

The evolution of spinal endoscopy should include names that changed our understanding of identifying the landmarks, pain generators, and how to treat them through an endoscope. Most of these milestones were done for uniportal endoscopy. However, the current indications and applications of biportal endoscopy are due to these achievements. Both techniques have an intrinsic relationship since both are water-based endoscopic procedures.

For example, Tony Yeung (Fig. 2.5), during the 90s, moved forward using transforaminal endoscopic discectomy under continuous irrigation. His experience was shared with spinal surgeons worldwide, even the industry focused on that, and the endoscopy changed to water-based endoscopy [18, 19].

Fig. 2.5 Antony T. Yeung

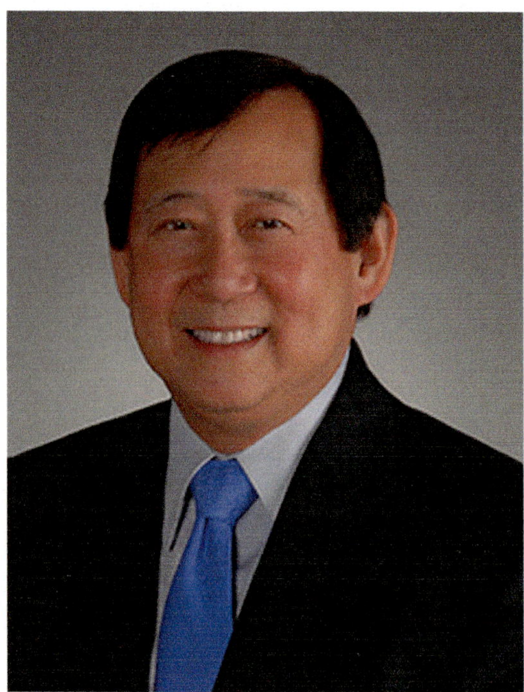

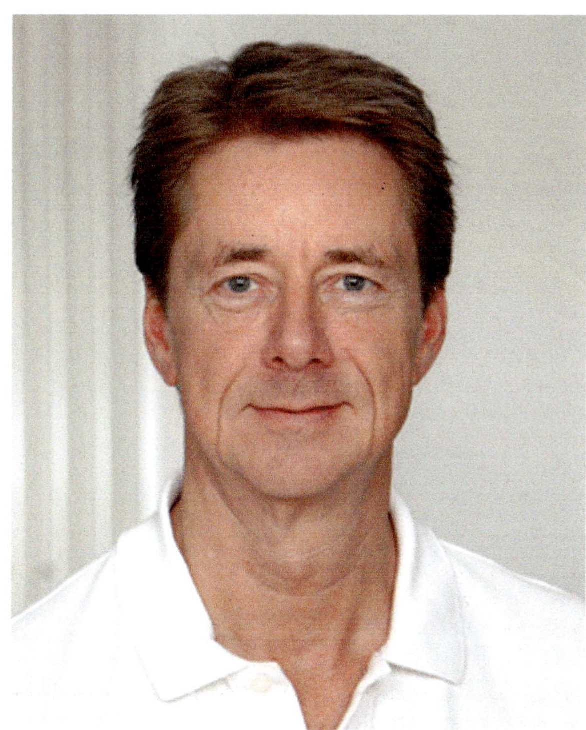

Fig. 2.6 Sebastian Ruetten

Sebastian Ruetten (Fig. 2.6) was another pioneer who applied water-based uniportal endoscopy to interlaminar approaches in the early 2000s [20–22]. Both pathfinders have spread the concept of full endoscopy of the spine abroad.

However, biportal endoscopy emerged as an alternative to uniportal endoscopy, for so many differences, such as a shorter learning curve for basic approaches, easier handling of the endoscope, and surgical tools, since in biportal endoscopy, the surgeon can use the lens and the surgical instruments independently, and finally the feasibility of the UBE technique.

The feasibility of the UBE technique depends on several factors, such as the evolution of different approaches adapted for other spinal regions and pathologies, expanding indications, and costs, which is a significant feature of UBE. Uniportal endoscopy requires expensive and highly specialized devices for performing procedures. The biportal endoscopy requires a 0° or 30° arthroscope and standard spinal surgery instruments.

This historical overview cannot be concluded without mentioning the scientific hub on endoscopy worldwide, South Korea. South Korean surgeons have contributed significantly to the development of minimally invasive spine surgery (MISS). They have evolved spinal endoscopic techniques, including biportal endoscopy.

Surgeons like Jin Hwa Eum (Fig. 2.4), Dong Hwa Heo (Fig. 2.7), Sang Kyu Son (Fig. 2.8), and Cheol Woong Park (Fig. 2.9) have contributed to the advance of biportal endoscopic surgery during the last years. They have reported most biportal endoscopic techniques and trained many spine surgeons abroad, spreading the modern concept of biportal spinal endoscopy. In addition, they have evolved biportal endoscopic surgery making it feasible for all spine regions [9, 23–29].

Fig. 2.7 Dong Hwa Heo

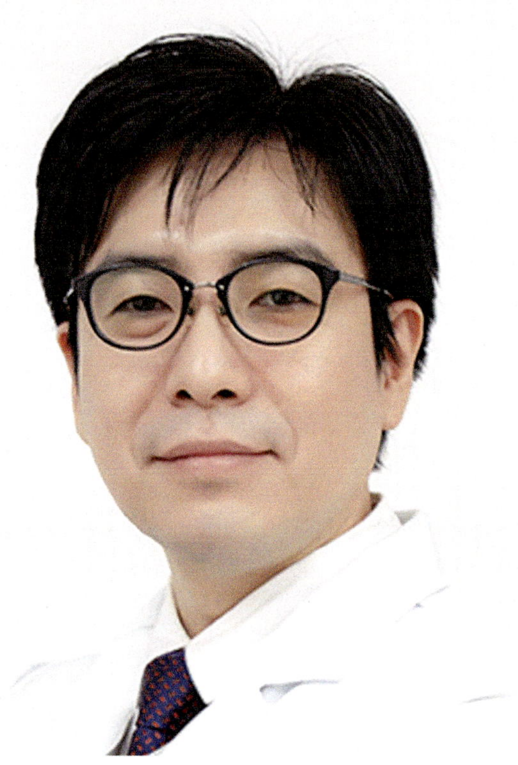

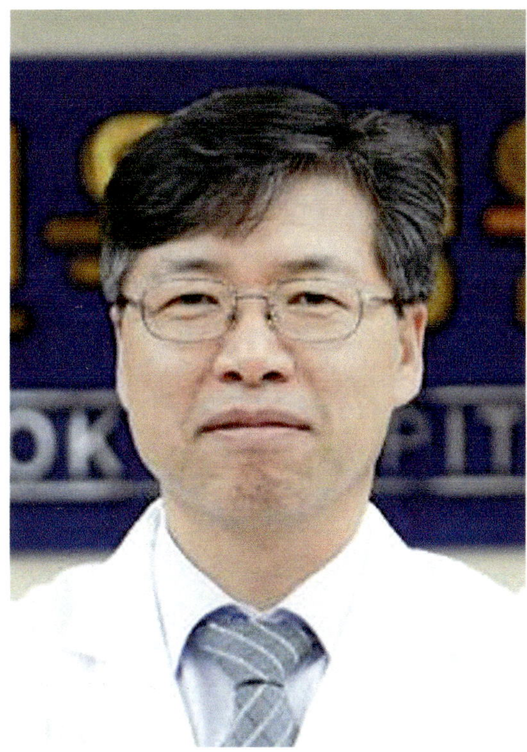

Fig. 2.8 Sang Kyu Son

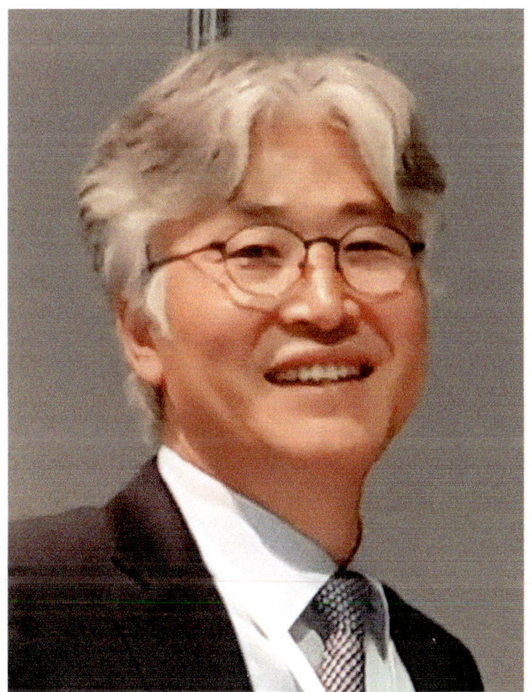

Fig. 2.9 Cheol Woong Park

Conclusion

The concept of unilateral biportal endoscopy (UBE) evolved since Dr. Daniel Julio De Antoni reported the first description of the technique. That evolution has been possible thanks to the efforts of key opinion leaders (KOLs), especially from South Korea, who have taken this technique to the next step. However, the evolution and advancement of endoscopic spinal surgery continue. Right now, this is only a glimpse of the historic milestones for achieving our glorious present full of options to treat spinal pathologies.

References

1. Jackson RW. A history of arthroscopy. Arthroscopy. 2010;26(1):91–103.
2. Forst R, Hausmann B. Nucleoscopy—a new examination technique. Arch Orthop Trauma Surg. 1983;101(3):219–21.
3. Kambin P, O'Brien E, Zhou L, Schaffer JL. Arthroscopic microdiscectomy and selective fragmentectomy. Clin Orthop Relat Res. 1998;347:150–67.
4. Casey KF, Chang MK, O'Brien ED, et al. Arthroscopic microdiscectomy: comparison of preoperative and postoperative imaging studies. Arthroscopy. 1997;13(4):438–45.
5. De Antoni DJ, Claro ML, Jañez RR. Cirugía artroscópica del disco lumbar. Artroscopia. 1994;1(2):81–5.
6. De Antoni DJ, Claro ML, Poehling GG, Hughes SS. Translaminar lumbar epidural endoscopy: anatomy, technique, and indications. Arthroscopy. 1996;12(3):330–4.
7. De Antoni DJ, Claro ML. Translaminar epidural lumbar endoscopy in hernias occupying over 50% of the radicular canal and decompression in lateral spinal stenosis. Arthroskopie. 1999;12:79–84.
8. Osman SG, Schwartz JA, Marsolais EB. Arthroscopic discectomy and interbody fusion of the thoracic spine: A report of ipsilateral 2-portal approach. Int J Spine Surg. 2012;6:103–9.
9. Eun SS, Eum JH, Lee SH, Sabal LA. Biportal endoscopic lumbar decompression for lumbar disk herniation and spinal canal stenosis: a technical note. J Neurol Surg A Cent Eur Neurosurg. 2017;78(4):390–6.
10. Oppenheim H, Krause F. Ueber Einklemmung bzw. Stran- gulation der Cauda equina. Deutsche Medizinische Wochen- schrift. 1909;35(16):697–700.
11. Goldthwait JE. The lumbosacral articulation: an explanation of many cases of lumbago, sciatica, and paraplegia. N Engl J Med. 1911;164(11):365–72.
12. Middleton GS, Teacher JH. Injury of the spinal cord due to rupture of the intervertebral disc during muscular effort. Glasgow Med J. 1911;76:1–6.
13. Mixter WJ, Barr JS. Rupture of the intervertebral disc with involvement of the spinal canal. N Engl J Med. 1934;211(5):210–4.
14. Love JG. Removal of the protruded interlaminar discs without laminectomy. Mayo Clin Proc. 1939;14:800.
15. Smith L. Enzyme dissolution of the nucleus pulposus in humans. J Am Med Assoc. 1964;187(2):137–40.
16. Hijikata S. A method of percutaneous nuclear extraction. J Toden Hosp. 1975;5:39–42.
17. Kambin P, Sampson S. Posterolateral percutaneous suction-excision of herniated lumbar intervertebral discs. Report of interim results. Clin Orthop Relat Res. 1986;(207):37–43.

18. Tsou PM, Yeung AT. Transforaminal endoscopic decompression for radiculopathy secondary to intracanal noncontained lumbar disc herniations: outcome and technique. Spine J. 2002;2(1):41–8.
19. Yeung AT, Yeung CA. Advances in endoscopic disc and spine surgery: foraminal approach. Surg Technol Int. 2003;11:255–63.
20. Ruetten S, Komp M, Merk H, Godolias G. Surgical treatment for lumbar lateral recess stenosis with the full-endoscopic interlaminar approach versus conventional microsurgical technique: a prospective, randomized, controlled study. J Neurosurg Spine. 2009;10(5):476–85.
21. Ruetten S, Komp M, Merk H, Godolias G. Use of newly developed instruments and endoscopes: full-endoscopic resection of lumbar disc herniations via the interlaminar and lateral transforaminal approach. J Neurosurg Spine. 2007;6(6):521–30.
22. Ruetten S, Komp M, Godolias G. A new full-endoscopic technique for the interlaminar operation of lumbar disc herniations using 6-mm endoscopes: prospective 2-year results of 331 patients. Minim Invasive Neurosurg. 2006;49(2):80–7.
23. Heo DH, Lee DC, Park CK. Comparative analysis of three types of minimally invasive decompressive surgery for lumbar central stenosis: biportal endoscopy, uniportal endoscopy, and microsurgery. Neurosurg Focus. 2019;46(5):E9.
24. Heo DH, Ha JS, Lee DC, Kim HS, Chung HJ. Repair of incidental durotomy using sutureless nonpenetrating clips via biportal endoscopic surgery [published online ahead of print, 2020 Nov 5]. Global Spine J. 2020:2192568220956606.
25. Heo DH, Son SK, Eum JH, Park CK. Fully endoscopic lumbar interbody fusion using a percutaneous unilateral biportal endoscopic technique: technical note and preliminary clinical results. Neurosurg Focus. 2017;43(2):E8.
26. Park MK, Park SA, Son SK, Park WW, Choi SH. Clinical and radiological outcomes of unilateral biportal endoscopic lumbar interbody fusion (ULIF) compared with conventional posterior lumbar interbody fusion (PLIF): 1-year follow-up. Neurosurg Rev. 2019;42(3):753–61.
27. Park JH, Jang JW, Park WM, Park CW. Contralateral keyhole biportal endoscopic surgery for ruptured lumbar herniated disc: a technical feasibility and early clinical outcomes. Neurospine. 2020;17(Suppl 1):S110–9.
28. Akbary K, Kim JS, Park CW, Jun SG, Hwang JH. Biportal endoscopic decompression of exiting and traversing nerve roots through a single interlaminar window using a contralateral approach: technical feasibilities and morphometric changes of the lumbar canal and foramen. World Neurosurg. 2018;117:153–61.
29. Heo DH, Lee N, Park CW, Kim HS, Chung HJ. Endoscopic unilateral laminotomy with bilateral discectomy using biportal endoscopic approach: technical report and preliminary clinical results. World Neurosurg. 2020;137:31–7.

Chapter 3
Unilateral Biportal Endoscopic Spinal Surgery Evidence-Based Outcome

Tsz-King Suen, Sheung-Tung Ho, and Yip-Kan Yeung

Abbreviations

CK	Creatine kinase
CRP	C-reactive protein
CSA	Cross-sectional area
ERAS	Enhanced recovery after surgery
ODI	Oswestry Disability Index
PCF	Posterior cervical foraminotomy
PSEH	Postoperative spinal epidural hematoma
RCT	Randomized controlled trial
TLIF	Transforaminal lumbar interbody fusion
UBE	Unilateral biportal endoscopy
ULBD	Unilateral laminotomy for bilateral decompression
VAS	Visual analog scale

T.-K. Suen (✉)
Hong Kong Baptist Hospital, Hong Kong SAR, China
e-mail: aarsuen@gmail.com

S.-T. Ho · Y.-K. Yeung
Department of Orthopaedics and Traumatology, Caritas Medical Centre, Hong Kong SAR, China
e-mail: drhosheungtung@gmail.com; yyk028@ha.org.hk

J. Quillo-Olvera et al. (eds.), *Unilateral Biportal Endoscopy of the Spine*,
https://doi.org/10.1007/978-3-031-14736-4_3

Introduction

Unilateral biportal endoscopy (UBE) was first reported in 1996 by Dr. De Antoni [1]. However, it did not gain popularity until 2010. Most of the clinical trials and researches are published by Korean surgeons. UBE combines the advantages of open surgery and endoscopic spine surgery. It allows similar approach as standard microscopic decompression and allows ipsilateral and contralateral decompression under high magnification. Due to lack of requirement of specialized instrument, experienced spine surgeon and hospital can incorporate this technique quickly. Nowadays, it is most widely used in lumbar decompression for spinal stenosis and discectomy. This technique was extended to perform transforaminal lumbar interbody fusion (TLIF) in some high-volume centers. It has also been used in posterior cervical foraminotomy (PCF) and management of complications after microscopic surgeries. Evidence-based outcome was emerging in the last decade and had been promising. Enhanced recovery after surgery (ERAS) was also applied to UBE to improve the clinical outcome and shorten hospital stay [2].

Laminectomy for Spinal Stenosis and Disc Herniation

Clinical Outcomes

The clinical outcomes after UBE decompression for spinal stenosis and disc herniation were mostly published as case series studies. Lin et al. [3] reviewed 11 case series including 556 patients and 679 operated levels with a mean follow-up of 15.2 months and overall complication rate of 6.7%. The mean visual analog scale (VAS) score for leg decreased from preoperative 7.9 to 1.9 at the final follow-up visit and the mean back pain VAS scores decreased from 5.7 to 1.8. The mean Oswestry Disability Index (ODI) significantly improved from preoperative 63.7 to 18.6 at the final follow-up. The average satisfied outcome (excellent/good: based on the Macnab criteria was 84.3%). The results between UBE in lumbar disc herniation and stenosis in terms of operative time, length of hospital stay, complications, and satisfaction rate were similar. Up to date, there were only 2 randomized controlled trials (RCTs) comparing UBE with microscopic decompression for spinal stenosis [4, 5]. Kang et al. [4] included 36 patients with spinal stenosis operated with UBE, and 34 patients were operated under microscopy. He concluded that the VAS scores and ODI scores between the two groups did not differ significantly at immediate postoperative period and 1, 3, and 6 months. Park et al. included 64 patients with lumbar spinal stenosis with VAS score >4 and definite central stenosis of Schizas grade ≥B on magnetic resonance imaging in 1:1 ratio. There were no significant differences between the two groups in the mean ODI score, effect in back and leg pain, disability, quality of life, and neuropathic pain at 1 year. The non-inferiority of UBE laminectomy was confirmed by the modified intention-to-treat strategy and per-protocol analysis. A meta-analysis included these two RCTs, and four non-RCTs confirmed a similar finding [6].

UBE outcomes were also compared to those with micro-endoscopy. A retrospective analysis [7] of 181 patients showed that there was no significant difference between two groups in terms of VAS back score, VAS leg score, and ODI and EuroQol5-Dimension questionnaire.

Learning Curve

The learning curve for ULBD by an experienced microscopic orthopedic surgeon was studied using a learning curve cumulative summation test [8]. They defined procedure time less than 75 min as procedure success. 22 out of the first 30 patients were over 75 min, while only 6 out of the later 30 cases were over 75 min. They concluded that a surgeon can achieve adequate performance at 58 cases.

Operative Time, Opioid Use, and Hospital Stay

Kang's trial [4], which includes 70 patients, compared via UBE against microscopic decompression showed that UBE had significant operative time 36 ± 11 min vs. 54 ± 9 min and is associated with significant less drain output (25.5 ± 15.8 mL vs. 53.2 ± 32.1 mL), less opioid usage, and shorter hospital stay (1.2 ± 0.3 days vs. 3.5 ± 0.8 days). In Park's trial [5], it showed similar findings of significant less amount of fentanyl use in UBE group (6.6 μg/kg vs. 10.4 μg/kg) and shorter hospital stay (45.6 h vs. 58.4 h). However, there were no significant differences in terms of operative time (67.2 min vs. 70.2 min). The drainage output was significantly higher in UBE group. This could be explained by the use of irrigation saline during the operation and its leak through the drain after surgery. Lin et al. [3] did a systematic review of UBE spine surgery, which included 134 patients with lumbar disc herniation and 333 patients with spinal stenosis. The average operative time was 79.2 min for disc herniation and 74.2 min for spinal stenosis. The mean hospital stay was 3.5 days for disc herniation and 4.6 days for spinal stenosis.

Dural Expansion, Facet Preservation, and Secondary Instability

The amount of improvement of cross-sectional area (CSA) in spinal stenosis can be used to assess the extent of surgical decompression, while the facet joint preservation percentage assessed future risk of iatrogenic instability [9]. A retrospective analysis [10] of 81 patients showed that the CSA of dura was significantly increased from 71.4 ± 36.5 to 177.3 ± 59.2 mm^2 corresponding to 201.9%. The percentage of facet preservation was 84.2% on the approach side and 92.9% on the contralateral side. Another retrospective study [11] with 30 patients showed that the spinal canal CSA increased from 99.34 ± 34.01 to 186.83 ± 41.41 mm^2, while facet joint CSA decreased from 231.37 ± 62.53 to 194.96 ± 50.56 mm^2. Ito et al. [7] showed that the facet preservation rates were significantly better in UBE compared to micro-endoscopy with the advancing side 85% in UBE and 78% in micro-endoscopy while the contralateral side being 94% vs. 86%.

Kim et al. [12] compared the preoperative and postoperative horizontal displacement of the operated level on standing flexion/extension X-rays in UBE group and microscopic group. The percentage of displacement was significantly less in UBE group 0.28 ± 0.27% vs. 2.92 ± 1.82%.

Kim and Choi [13] reported no significant progress of slippage and lumbar instability 2 years after UBE ULBD in terms of dynamic intervertebral angle, slippage percentage, and dynamic slippage percentage. However, there was significant change in intervertebral angle from 6.26° to 5.58° ($p = 0.027$) and in intervertebral distance from 10.43 to 10 mm ($p = 0.00$). Their patients were also compared to microscopic ULBD, which showed no significant difference in radiological outcomes [14].

Muscle Damage

Serum creatine kinase (CK) and C-reactive protein (CRP) were found to lower in UBE patients compared to microscopic decompression for spinal stenosis (CK: 130.87 ± 51.49 vs. 331.4 ± 118.09, CRP 2.36 ± 1.09 vs. 2.92 ± 1.34) [12]. CRP changes at postoperative day 2 were also compared between UBE, microscopic decompression, and instrumented fusion in another case series [15], which were 0.32, 6.53, and 6. However, there were no significant differences between these groups at postoperative 2 weeks. This could mean that the tissue destruction was much less in UBE procedure and possible inflammatory debris was washed away during the procedure.

Safety

The fundamental difference between microscopic and endoscopic surgery is the use of irrigation fluid. Endoscopic surgery requires continuous inflow and outflow of irrigation with creation of water pressure to obtain a clear operative view. The use of percutaneous endoscopic lumbar discectomy has been reported with the risk of increasing intracerebral pressure, which could lead to potential neurological complications, for example, seizure [16]. However, up to date, there were no reported cases of seizure or change in consciousness after biportal lumbar decompression. This could be due to the use of a separate viewing and working channels in biportal surgery, which prevents the buildup of irrigation pressure. Cervical epidural pressure during lumbar discectomy via biportal endoscopy was measured [17, 18]. The pressure was not significantly increased unless the outflow was clogged. This may prove the safety of UBE, and usage of semicircular tube in the working portal was helpful to maintain adequate outflow.

Complications

The complication rate in the systematic review and meta-analysis for UBE decompression was reported to be ranging from 5.9% to 6.7% [3, 6]. There was no statistically significant difference in the complication rates compared to those in the microscopic method. The risk of dural tear is one of the common complications, being 3.9–4.1% [19]. The most frequent site of dural injury was at the center part of dura. As the center part was attached to ligamentum flavum by a few lines of fibrous tissues, the water pressure could compress on either side of dura causing the infolding of dura. Kerrison punch under the epidural fat at midline could cause dural tear. Small dural tear was successfully treated with patch technique. For large dural tear >1 cm; the use of clipping suture with patch compression had been suggested. Patients were then managed with 2 days of bed rest. If this process fails, proceed to open repair. The use of nerve retractor and knot pusher had also been suggested for watertight suture [20]. The second complication was postoperative epidural hematoma (POSEH). It could result in paraplegia and cauda equine syndrome. The severity of POSEH was defined clinically and radiologically. Kim et al. [21] reported that the risk factors for POSEH in UBE include female sex, old age, preoperative anticoagulation medications, and use of intraoperative saline pump. The chance of hematoma was higher in bilateral laminectomy than that in unilateral laminectomy [22]. The incidence of symptomatic POSEH (8.4%) was higher than that in conventional spine surgery (1.4%) in a study of a total of 237 patients [22]. It would be due to the masking of epidural venous bleeding by saline pressure. To prevent complication, it was recommended to control any bleeding point during the procedure and insertion of drainage catheter epidural space after decompression. The use of Floseal may reduce the incidence of postoperative radiological POSEH (26.4% vs. 13.6%) and improve clinical outcomes in terms of ODI and VAS leg [23]. Another complication of direct nerve injury was uncommon, probably because of superior visualization under endoscope.

Lumbar Spinal Interbody Fusion

Transforaminal lumbar spinal interbody fusion (TLIF) via UBE is more technically demanding as compared to conventional microscopic technique. Several hurdles have to be achieved for a successful outcome. Adequate decompression of neural structures and meticulous preparation of fusion site without violation of bony endplate were the first steps. The use of endoscopy can allow excellent direct visualization of the junction between cartilaginous endplate and bony endplate [24]. The next step is the packing of bone graft into the prepared fusion bed. The intraoperative saline flow may interfere with the bone packing. The use of specialized funnel may be helpful in bone packing. During the insertion of cage, there is a chance of nerve root injury, and specialized retractor could be used to overcome this [25]. Compared to full endoscopic technique, the size of cage was not limited by the working cannula and large TLIF cage or two cages were feasible [24]. The techniques of UBE-TLIF are well described in multiple technical reports [26–30].

Clinical Outcomes

Up to the end of July 2021, there are 8 reports published on the results of UBE-TLIF in 290 patients. Of these reports, 4 were case series [26–28, 31] and 4 were case-control studies [2, 25, 32, 33]. There were also two review articles on the results of UBE-TLIF [34, 35]. There are so far no randomized controlled trials comparing full endoscopic, biportal endoscopic, and conventional microscopic TLIF. The reports are summarized in Table 3.1. The common indications for TLIF were low-grade degenerative spondylolisthesis, isthmic spondylolisthesis, instability, central stenosis with instability, foraminal stenosis, end-stage degenerative disc disease, and herniated lumbar disc. Of the 6 studies from Korea, the mean age of a patient was 68.4, while the mean patient age was only 46 in the series from Mexico [28]. Of the 290 cases reported, 265 cases were single-level TLIF, while 25 cases had two-level TLIF [31, 33]. The mean operative time was 165.4 min. Five studies reported estimated intraoperative blood loss; the mean was 138.2 mL (range: 70–190 mL) [2, 25–27, 31–33].

Table 3.1 Reports on clinical outcomes of UBE-TLIF

	n	Age (yr)	Minimal FU (m)	Operative time (min)	Blood loss (mL)	Length of stay (day)
Case series						
Heo (2017) [26]	39	71.2 ± 7.8	12	165.8 ± 25.5	85.5 ± 19.4	n/a
Kim (2018) [27]	14	68.7 ± 8.5	2	169 ± 10	74 ± 9	n/a
Kim (2020) [31]	57	68.5 ± 9.4	12	171.7 ± 35.1	n/a	7.1 ± 3.3
Quillo-Olvera (2020) [28]	7	46 ± 7.5	9	167.1 ± 19.3	70 ± 18.3	n/a
Case-control						
Heo (2019) vs. MIS TLIF [2]	23 46	61.4 ± 9.4	12	452.4 ± 9.6122.4 ± 13.1	190.3 ± 31 289 ± 58.5	n/a
Park (2019) vs. open PLIF [25]	71 70	68 ± 8	12	158.2 ± 26.7136.6 ± 21.5	0% transfusion 18.6% transfusion	n/a
Kim (2020) vs. MIS TLIF [32]	32 55	70.5 ± 8.3	12	169.5 ± 24.9173 ± 47.1	n/a	6 ± 3.1 9.1 ± 2.9
Kang (2021) vs. MT TLIF [33]	47 32	66.9 ± 10.4	12	170.5 ± 34.8 135.7 ± 42.9	185.7 ± 172.5 395.3 ± 180.4	14.5 ± 4 12.6 ± 4.5

n: patient number, yr: year, FU: follow-up, m: month, min: minutes, n/a: not available

Table 3.2 Outcomes of UBE-TLIF

			Preoperative-postoperative difference				
Series	*n*	Time (m)	ODI	VAS leg	VAS back	Complication rate: number (%)	Radiographic fusion rate (%)
Heo 2017 [26]	39	12	30.24	n/a	n/a	7.2% (5/39)	n/a
Kim 2018 [27]	14	2	n/a	n/a	n/a	14.3% (2/14)	n/a
Heo 2019 [2]	23	12	36	5.6	n/a	4.3% (1/23)	73.8%
Park 2019 [25]	71	12	31.2	3	2.9	7% (5/71)	95.1%
Kim 2020 [32]	32	12	52.5	6.3	4.5	3.1% (1/32)	93.7%
Quillo-Olvera 2020 [28]	7	9	43.2	6.2	6	0% (0/7)	n/a
Kim 2020 [31]	57	12	48.9	6.5	4.3	5.3% (3/57)	n/a
Kang 2021 [33]	47	12	24	4	3.8	12.8% (6/47)	87.7%
Overall			**36.7**	**5**	**3.8**	**7.9% (23/290)**	**88.7%**

n: patient number, m: month, n/a: not available

Only three studies reported the length of stay; the average was 6.7 days (range: 6–7.1 days) reported by Kim et al. [31, 32] and 14.5 days reported by Kang et al. [33].

Most series reported the Oswestry Disability Index (ODI) score and visual analogue scale (VAS) scores of leg and back. One study [27] with only 2 months' FU was excluded in the synthesis of clinical outcomes. All reported significant improvement in ODI and VAS of leg and back (Table 3.2). The average difference of preoperative and postoperative ODI score was 36.7. The average improvement of VAS after operation was 5 and 3.8 for leg and back, respectively. The improvement in ODI and VAS scores was well above the reference minimal clinically important difference (MCID) of 15 points for ODI and 3 points for VAS [36].

Compared with Minimally Invasive TLIF or PLIF

There are four case-control studies comparing UBE-TLIF with minimally invasive TLIF [2, 32, 33] or open posterior lumbar interbody fusion (PLIF) [25]. UBE group had significantly less intraoperative blood loss [2, 33]. None of the patients in the UBE-TLIF group required blood transfusion, whereas 18.6% of patients in open PLIF group required blood transfusion [25]. In another comparative study, blood transfusion was required in 8.5% in UBE group versus 15.6% in tubular microscopic group [33]. UBE-TLIF gave significant less back pain on days 1–2 [2], at 1 week [25], at 2 weeks [32], and at 1 month [33] after surgery. There was a significant reduction in the time to ambulation: 13.8 h in UBE group versus 18.8 h in minimally invasive group [32]. However, there was no significant difference between groups for ODI and VAS back and leg scores [2, 25, 32, 33]. Furthermore, there was no significant difference in the radiographic fusion rate and complication rate between UBE-TLIF and other MIS TLIF [2, 25, 32, 33].

Fusion Rate

Four studies reported the radiographic fusion rate at 12 months; the average was 88.7% (range: 78.3–95.1%) [2, 25, 32, 33].

Complications

The average reported complication rate was 7.9% (23/290), range: 0–14.3%. Complications included 10 dural tears, 7 postoperative epidural hematoma, 3 nerve injury (2 transient paralysis), 1 infection, 1 cage subsidence, and 1 incomplete decompression [2, 25–28, 31–33].

Learning Curve

A study of a single surgeon's learning curve [25] suggested that a stable point could be achieved after 400th day and 34 cases. Mean operative time was 193 min against 139 min, and time to ambulation was 13.7 h against 9.9 h before and after the stable point. The overall VAS and ODI scores did not differ between the two groups.

Lumbar Foraminal Stenosis

Foraminal stenosis is a more heterogenous group of pathologies. Lee et al. [37] defined locations of pathologies in three zones (entry, middle, and exit). The pathologies could be foraminal disc, hypertrophic facet, and decrease in foraminal height. The clinical outcomes were also affected by the presence of spinal instability, scoliosis, lumbar lordosis, and posterior intervertebral disc height [38]. Moreover, the degree of foraminal stenosis in imaging may not correlate with clinical symptoms [39]. This may be the reason why there are so far no series merely reporting on the outcomes of decompression of lumbar foraminal stenosis. The techniques of decompression of foraminal stenosis via UBE had been described via two main approaches. One is via the interlaminar window where both the contralateral traversing and exiting nerve roots could be decompressed [11, 40]. The other approach is by floating technique similar to Wiltse approach [41]. Combined approach could also be performed if necessary. Kim [41] reported on 31 patients (including 18 patients with lumbar foraminal stenosis alone and 13 patients with lumbosacral foraminal stenosis). The mean VAS for back improved from 5.13 to 2.61 at 3 months and 1.5 at 1 year. The VAS leg improved from 7.87 to 2.55 at 3 months and 1.45 at 1 year. ODI improved from 66.81 to 24.14 at 3 months and 17.39 at 1 year.

Extraforaminal Decompression at Lumbosacral Lesion

The lumbosacral compression was considered as a separate entity as the anatomical approach and compressive lesions were different. Heo et al. [42] presented 14 patients with lumbosacral lesion operated by UBE. VAS leg score improved from 8.4 to 2.8, and ODI score improved from 60.2 to 22.1 with a mean follow-up of 11 months. However, two patients complained of abdominal pain immediately after surgery, and one of them was found to have retroperitoneal fluid collection in an abdominal CT scan. The authors thus suggested that the decompression around the pseudoarthrosis should be completed within 30 min to avoid such complications. Another retrospective case series [43] also reported on 44 patients treated with this technique, and they also suggested that the penetration beyond the transverse process to psoas muscle layer could result in hydroperitoneum.

Cervical Foraminotomy

Cervical foraminotomy and discectomy were effective in treating cervical radiculopathy with long-lasting relief [44]. It preserves spinal motion and avoids graft-related complications as compared to anterior spinal fusion. However, it was reported that age >60 years and presence of preoperative cervical lordosis of <10° appeared to have higher risk of worsening of deformity. Utilization of uniportal endoscopy in decompression can avoid dissection of paraspinal muscle; however, the working instruments were limited by the endoscopic port and hemostasis was difficult. Biportal technique allows better maneuverability of instruments like pituitary forceps, bendable drills, and angled chisel and curette. Park et al. [45] reported the use of UBE in cervical foraminotomy and discectomy in 13 patients with a mean follow-up of 14.8 months. Neck disability index decreased from 27 to 6.8 and VAS score for the neck and upper limb 6.2 to 2.4 and 7 to 2.2, respectively. Another case series [46] reported seven cases of biportal endoscopic cervical foraminotomy using an inclinatory approach in which the surgeon stands over the opposite of the lesion. This approach allowed decompression to be achieved by undercutting with less facetectomy. Under endoscopy, the authors could locate the perineural fat on the axilla of the exiting root easily and decompression of the distal part of the root by tunnel-shaped foraminotomy without the need to directly unroof the facet for decompression. VAS and NDI scores improved from 7.71 to 0.85 and 26.85 to 10.57. There was one case of dural tear treated with Gelfoam and TachoSil without consequences. However, this technique is more technically demanding. The authors suggested that prior abundant experience in UBE surgery was required.

Cervical Spinal Stenosis

Up to date, there are only case reports for decompression using UBE in case of cervical spinal stenosis with myelopathy. Kim et al. [47] described the surgical techniques for a two-level UBE-ULBD. Three portals were used, and additional foraminotomy was performed in the same approach. More studies are required to evaluate its safety and efficacy.

Conclusion

The published clinical outcomes of UBE on various spinal pathologies were positive. However, the good clinical outcomes could be based on the previous experience in open surgeries, microscopic and uniportal endoscopy. The potential risks and complications of UBE should not be overlooked. The setup of a good UBE clinical service will be discussed in the following chapter.

References

1. De Antoni DJ, Clara ML. Arthroscopy of the spine. In: Chow JCY, editor. Advanced arthroscopy. New York, Springer; 2001. p. 683–701.
2. Heo DH, Park CK. Clinical results of percutaneous biportal endoscopic lumbar interbody fusion with application of enhanced recovery after surgery. Neurosurg Focus. 2019;46(4):E18.
3. Lin GX, Huang P, Kotheeranurak V, Park CW, Heo DH, Park CK, et al. A systematic review of unilateral biportal endoscopic spinal surgery: preliminary clinical results and complications. World Neurosurg. 2019;125:425–32.
4. Kang T, Park SY, Kang CH, Lee SH, Park JH, Suh SW. Is biportal technique/endoscopic spinal surgery satisfactory for lumbar spinal stenosis patients? A prospective randomized comparative study. Medicine (Baltimore). 2019;98(18):e15451.
5. Park SM, Park J, Jang HS, Heo YW, Han H, Kim HJ, et al. Biportal endoscopic versus microscopic lumbar decompressive laminectomy in patients with spinal stenosis: a randomized controlled trial. Spine J. 2020;20(2):156–65.
6. Chen T, Zhou G, Chen Z, Yao X, Liu D. Biportal endoscopic decompression vs. microscopic decompression for lumbar canal stenosis: a systematic review and meta-analysis. Exp Ther Med. 2020;20(3):2743–51.
7. Ito Z, Shibayama M, Nakamura S, Yamada M, Kawai M, Takeuchi M, et al. Clinical comparison of unilateral biportal endoscopic laminectomy versus microendoscopic laminectomy for single-level laminectomy: a single-center, retrospective analysis. World Neurosurg. 2021;148:e581–8.
8. Park SM, Kim HJ, Kim GU, et al. Learning curve for lumbar decompressive laminectomy in biportal endoscopic spinal surgery using the cumulative summation test for learning curve. World Neurosurg. 2019;122:e1007–13.
9. Abumi K, Panjabi MM, Kramer KM, Duranceau J, Oxland T, Crisco JJ. Biomechanical evaluation of lumbar spinal stability after graded facetectomies. Spine (Phila Pa 1976). 1990;15(11):1142–7.
10. Pao JL, Lin SM, Chen WC, Chang CH. Unilateral biportal endoscopic decompression for degenerative lumbar canal stenosis. J Spine Surg. 2020;6(2):438–46.
11. Akbary K, Kim JS, Park CW, Jun SG, Hwang JH. Biportal endoscopic decompression of exiting and traversing nerve roots through a single interlaminar window using a contralateral approach: technical feasibilities and morphometric changes of the lumbar canal and foramen. World Neurosurg. 2018;117:153–61.
12. Kim HS, Choi SH, Shim DM, Lee IS, Oh YK, Woo YH. Advantages of new endoscopic unilateral laminectomy for bilateral decompression (ULBD) over conventional microscopic ULBD. Clin Orthop Surg. 2020;12(3):330–6.
13. Kim JE, Choi DJ. Clinical and radiological outcomes of unilateral biportal endoscopic decompression by 30 degrees arthroscopy in lumbar spinal stenosis: minimum 2-year follow-up. Clin Orthop Surg. 2018;10(3):328–36.
14. Min WK, Kim JE, Choi DJ, Park EJ, Heo J. Clinical and radiological outcomes between biportal endoscopic decompression and microscopic decompression in lumbar spinal stenosis. J Orthop Sci. 2020;25(3):371–8.
15. Choi DJ, Kim JE. Efficacy of biportal endoscopic spine surgery for lumbar spinal stenosis. Clin Orthop Surg. 2019;11(1):82–8.

16. Choi G, Kang HY, Modi HN, Prada N, Nicolau RJ, Joh JY, Pan WJ, Lee SH. Risk of developing seizure after percutaneous endoscopic lumbar discectomy. J Spinal Disord Tech. 2011;24(2):83–92.
17. Kang MS, Park HJ, Hwang JH, Kim JE, Choi DJ, Chung HJ. Safety evaluation of biportal endoscopic lumbar discectomy: assessment of cervical epidural pressure during surgery. Spine (Phila Pa 1976). 2020;45(20):E1349–E56.
18. Kang T, Park SY, Lee SH, Park JH, Suh SW. Assessing changes in cervical epidural pressure during biportal endoscopic lumbar discectomy. J Neurosurg Spine. 2020:1–7. https://doi.org/10.3171/2020.6.SPINE20586.
19. Kim JE, Choi DJ, Park EJ. Risk factors and options of management for an incidental dural tear in biportal endoscopic spine surgery. Asian Spine J. 2020;14(6):790–800.
20. Hong YH, Kim SK, Suh DW, Lee SC. Novel instruments for percutaneous biportal endoscopic spine surgery for full decompression and dural management: a comparative analysis. Brain Sci. 2020;10(8):516.
21. Kim JE, Choi DJ, Kim MC, et al. Risk factors of postoperative spinal epidural hematoma after biportal endoscopic spinal surgery. World Neurosurg. 2019;129:e324–9.
22. Ahn DK, Lee JS, Shin WS, Kim S, Jung J. Postoperative spinal epidural hematoma in a biportal endoscopic spine surgery. Medicine (Baltimore). 2021;100(6):e24685.
23. Kim JE, Yoo HS, Choi DJ, Park EJ, Hwang JH, Suh JD, et al. Effectiveness of gelatin-thrombin matrix sealants (Floseal(R)) on postoperative spinal epidural hematoma during single-level lumbar decompression using biportal endoscopic spine surgery: clinical and magnetic resonance image study. Biomed Res Int. 2020;2020:4801641.
24. Heo DH, Hong YH, Lee DC, Chung HJ, Park CK. Technique of biportal endoscopic transforaminal lumbar interbody fusion. Neurospine. 2020;17(Suppl 1):S129–37. https://doi.org/10.14245/ns.2040178.089.
25. Park MK, Park SA, Son SK, Park WW, Choi SH. Clinical and radiological outcomes of unilateral biportal endoscopic lumbar interbody fusion (ULIF) compared with conventional posterior lumbar interbody fusion (PLIF): 1-year follow-up. Neurosurg Rev. 2019;42(3):753–61. https://doi.org/10.1007/s10143-019-01114-3.
26. Heo DH, Son SK, Eum JH, Park CK. Fully endoscopic lumbar interbody fusion using a percutaneous unilateral biportal endoscopic technique: technical note and preliminary clinical results. Neurosurg Focus. 2017;43(2):E8.
27. Kim JE, Choi DJ. Biportal endoscopic transforaminal lumbar interbody fusion with arthroscopy. Clin Orthop Surg. 2018;10(2):248–52.
28. Quillo-Olvera J, Quillo-Reséndiz J, Quillo-Olvera D, Barrera-Arreola M, Kim JS. Ten-step biportal endoscopic transforaminal lumbar interbody fusion under computed tomography-based intraoperative navigation: technical report and preliminary outcomes in Mexico. Oper Neurosurg (Hagerstown). 2020;19(5):608–18.
29. Heo DH, Eum JH, Jo JY, Chung HT. Modified far lateral endoscopic transforaminal lumbar interbody fusion using a biportal endoscopic approach: technical report and preliminary results. Acta Neurochir. 2021;163(4):1205–9.
30. Kang MS, Chung HJ, Jung HJ, Park HJ. How I do it? Extraforaminal lumbar interbody fusion assisted with biportal endoscopic technique. Acta Neurochir. 2021;163(1):295–9. https://doi.org/10.1007/s00701-020-04435-1.
31. Kim JE, Yoo HS, Choi DJ, Hwang JH, Park E, Chung S. Learning curve and clinical outcome of biportal endoscopic-assisted lumbar interbody fusion. Biomed Res Int. 2020;2020:8815432. https://doi.org/10.1155/2020/8815432.
32. Kim JE, Yoo HS, Choi DJ, Park EJ, Joe SM. Comparison of minimally invasive versus biportal endoscopic transforaminal lumbar interbody fusion for single level lumbar disease. Clin Spine Surg. 2021;34(2):E64–71.
33. Kang MS, You KH, Choi JY, Heo DH, Chung HJ, Park HJ. Minimally invasive transforaminal lumbar interbody fusion using the biportal endoscopic techniques versus microscopic

tubular technique. Spine J. 2021. pii: S1529-9430(21)00777-4; https://doi.org/10.1016/j.spinee.2021.06.013.
34. Heo DH, Lee DC, Kim HS, Park CK, Chung H. Clinical results and complications of endoscopic lumbar interbody fusion for lumbar degenerative disease: a meta-analysis. World Neurosurg. 2021;145:396–404.
35. Park MK, Son SK. Biportal endoscopic lumbar interbody fusion: review of current evidence and the literature. J Minim Invasive Spine Surg Tech. 2021;6:S171–8.
36. Lee C, Chung CK, Jang J, et al. Effectiveness of deformity-correction surgery for primary degenerative sagittal imbalance: a meta-analysis. J Neurosurg Spine. 2017;27:540–51.
37. Lee CK, Rauschning W, Glenn W. Lateral lumbar spinal canal stenosis: classification, pathologic anatomy and surgical decompression. Spine (Phila Pa 1976). 1988;13(3):313–20.
38. Yang H-S, Lee N, Park J-Y. Current status of biportal endoscopic decompression for lumbar foraminal stenosis: endoscopic partial facetectomy and outcome factors. J Minim Invasive Spine Surg Tech. 2021;6(Suppl 1):S157–63.
39. Hasegawa T, An HS, Haughton VM, Nowicki BH. Lumbar foraminal stenosis: critical heights of the intervertebral discs and foramina. A cryomicrotome study in cadavera. J Bone Joint Surg Am. 1995;77(1):32–8.
40. Song KS, Lee CW, Moon JG. Biportal endoscopic spinal surgery for bilateral lumbar foraminal decompression by switching surgeon's position and primary 2 portals: a report of 2 cases with technical note. Neurospine. 2019;16(1):138–47.
41. Kim JE, Choi DJ, Park EJ. Clinical and radiological outcomes of foraminal decompression using unilateral biportal endoscopic spine surgery for lumbar foraminal stenosis. Clin Orthop Surg. 2018;10(4):439–47.
42. Heo DH, Sharma S, Park CK. Endoscopic treatment of extraforaminal entrapment of L5 nerve root (far out syndrome) by unilateral biportal endoscopic approach: technical report and preliminary clinical results. Neurospine. 2019;16(1):130–7.
43. Choi DJ, Kim JE, Jung JT, Kim YS, Jang HJ, Yoo B, et al. Biportal endoscopic spine surgery for various foraminal lesions at the lumbosacral lesion. Asian Spine J. 2018;12(3):569–73.
44. Jagannathan J, Sherman JH, Szabo T, Shaffrey CI, Jane JA. The posterior cervical foraminotomy in the treatment of cervical disc/osteophyte disease: a single-surgeon experience with a minimum of 5 years' clinical and radiographic follow-up: clinical article. J Neurosurg Spine. 2009;10(4):347–56.
45. Park JH, Jun SG, Jung JT, Lee SJ. Posterior percutaneous endoscopic cervical foraminotomy and diskectomy with unilateral biportal endoscopy. Orthopedics. 2017;40(5):e779–83.
46. Song KS, Lee CW. The biportal endoscopic posterior cervical inclinatory foraminotomy for cervical radiculopathy: technical report and preliminary results. Neurospine. 2020;17(Suppl 1):S145–53.
47. Kim J, Heo DH, Lee DC, Chung HT. Biportal endoscopic unilateral laminotomy with bilateral decompression for the treatment of cervical spondylotic myelopathy. Acta Neurochir. 2021;163(9):2537–43.

Chapter 4
Current Technology Available for Unilateral Biportal Endoscopic Spinal Surgery

Diego Quillo-Olvera, Javier Quillo-Reséndiz, Isaac Morán Morales, Michelle Barrera-Arreola, and Javier Quillo-Olvera

Abbreviations

BESS	Biportal endoscopic spinal surgery
CCU	Camera control unit
LED	Light-emitting diode
RF	Radiofrequency
RPM	Revolutions per minute
UBE	Unilateral biportal endoscopy
UHD	Ultrahigh-definition

Introduction

Technology is an essential support for spinal surgery. It allows us to be more accurate to avoid unnecessary damage in spinal and extraspinal tissues. In addition, it can shorten the learning curve of a given surgical procedure and enables safer surgeries to be offered. And when technology is used correctly, it can reduce human error. Therefore, it is worthy of having a comprehensive suite of technological

D. Quillo-Olvera (✉) · J. Quillo-Reséndiz · M. Barrera-Arreola · J. Quillo-Olvera
The Brain and Spine Care, Minimally Invasive Spine Surgery Group, Hospital H+ Querétaro, Spine Clinic, Querétaro, México
e-mail: drquilloolvera86@gmail.com; kitnoz@hotmail.com; michelle.barrera@anahuac.mx; neuroqomd@gmail.com

I. M. Morales
Anáhuac University, School of Medicine, Querétaro, México
e-mail: isaacmoran9090@gmail.com

J. Quillo-Olvera et al. (eds.), *Unilateral Biportal Endoscopy of the Spine*,
https://doi.org/10.1007/978-3-031-14736-4_4

possibilities as advanced as possible to favor any patient. However, there are drawbacks to implementing technology in spinal surgery. Limited access because of particular health regulations of each country, the costs of highly specialized devices, the correct use of technology, and the proper decision-making of the surgeon when applying it are factors that can limit their use. Precisely, endoscopic spine surgery requires visualization devices or lenses that allow us to directly observe the anatomical structures, which will lead to all the known advantages. In addition, these lenses should work in a water environment to obtain the maximum benefit in terms of visualization. But not all that is required in spinal endoscopy is optical devices. Other tools will allow manipulating the tissues to obtain retraction, hemostasis, dissection, etc. This chapter summarizes the technology required to properly perform unilateral biportal endoscopic (UBE) spinal surgery.

Brief Summary of UBE in the Market

Recently and due to the boom that biportal endoscopy is having in the world, different companies have launched biportal endoscopic systems that include complete sets for surgery. However, despite offering particular advantages associated with their quality systems, they all provide at least the basic requirements to perform the unilateral biportal endoscopic (UBE) technique.

EndoSpineMax (Suyeong-ro, Suyeong-gu, Busan, Republic of Korea) has in its portfolio surgical tools for decompression and working cannulas to create endoscopic ports, in addition to having an excellent academic activity teaching foreign doctors from all over the world.

Endovision Co. (Geumcheon-gu, Seoul, Republic of Korea) is another Korean company that offers a standard kit of tools specially designed for biportal endoscopy, which also has radiofrequency (RF) and shaver with different burrs and blades, specially designed for biportal endoscopy and compatible with other drilling systems.

A German company recognized worldwide for its uniportal endoscopy technology has recently joined the biportal endoscopic surgery industry. MaxMoreSpine (Hoogland Spine Products GmbH, Unterföhring, Germany) has launched a biportal endoscopic spine surgery (BESS) set, which includes working cannulas, special Kerrison punches, and pituitary forceps, among other tools.

Another company called Amplify Surgical (Irvine, CA, USA) has ventured into developing a biportal endoscopic system called dualPortal (Amplify Surgical, Irvine, CA, USA). Still, the most exciting thing about this proposal is that they also developed other devices for spinal surgery, among which the expanding interbody fusion system stands out, which can be placed with its biportal system under development.

Technology for UBE

Arthroscopic Lenses

Curiosity to know how the body looks inside motivated the development of different optical systems in medicine. In 1920, Professor Kenji Takagi became a pioneer in developing arthroscopes [1]. However, in 1958, Watanabe modified and improved arthroscopy and in 1967 incorporated a fiber light for illumination, which brought arthroscopy into the modern era [1].

The arthroscope is a rigid viewfinder composed of thin lenses that vary in diameter. It comprises three parts:

1. Mechanical axis
2. Fiberglass bundles for light illumination
3. Optic system

Arthroscopes can be found from 1 to 6 mm on outer diameter and 4 to 18 cm in length, depending on the surgeon's need. Viewing angles from 0°, 30°, and 70° allow different observational perspectives. For example, more panoramic views could be obtained with 0° lenses, while more extended or profound perception is getting with 30° and 70°. The length of arthroscopes commonly used in unilateral biportal endoscopy (UBE) is 18 cm with angles of view of 0° and 30° and an outer diameter of 4 mm [2–10] (Fig. 4.1).

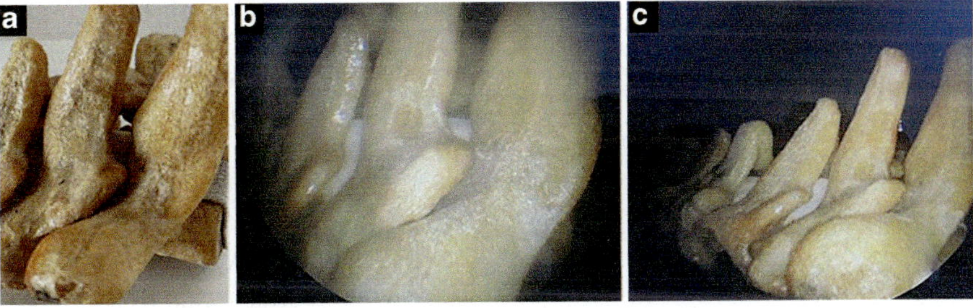

Fig. 4.1 An anatomical model of the cervical spine observed through different angles of view (0° and 30°). (**a**) Image of an anatomical model. (**b**) View with a 0° lens. (**c**) View with the 30° lens

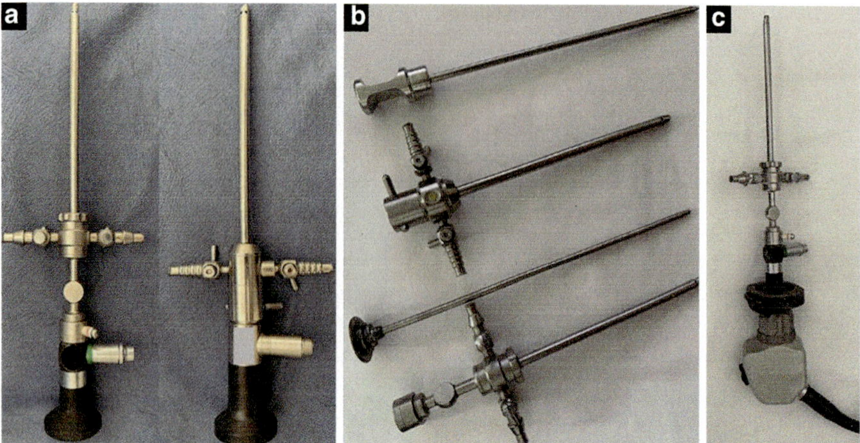

Fig. 4.2 (**a**) Arthroscopes attached to the sheath. (**b**) Sheaths and obturators. (**c**) Arthroscope and sheath connected to the camera

Arthroscopy Sheath

The arthroscope sheath protects the lens, and its spigot plane includes two valves to favor the fluid inflow. Standard sheaths usually give a larger outer diameter, approximately 1–2 mm more than the outer diameter of the arthroscope. An obturator should be introduced through the sheath, and both fixed with a coupler. Then, the sheath with the obturator is inserted in the spine to create the endoscopic port in the UBE technique. The mentioned brands have developed different barrels to protect the lens; barrels with different ending-tip shapes have also been designed for retracting the neural tissue with the endoscope during UBE procedures (Fig. 4.2).

Light Sources

Arthroscopy for UBE requires high-quality surgical lighting. The powerful white light is transmitted along a fiber-optic cable from a light source. For several decades, xenon bulbs have been used for endoscopy systems. Xenon's features like brightness, broadband output, and uniformity over a large spectrum make it ideal for deep-cavity surgical illumination. However, a light-emitting diode (LED) can also produce high-quality lighting. This technology offers high energy efficiency and durability, and the heat generation from the light source is less. In addition, an optical fiber for surgical lighting is used in UBE. It allows high-intensity light to improve visualization through the arthroscope, avoiding eyestrain during the procedure with a clear surgical field (Fig. 4.3).

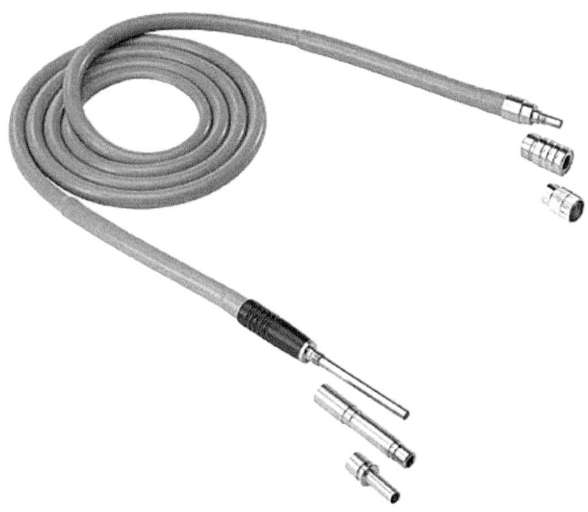

Fig. 4.3 Fiber-optic cable with different attachments

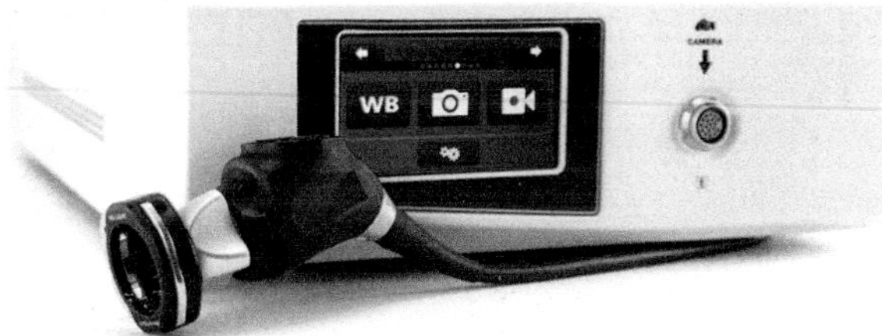

Fig. 4.4 Camera and camera control unit

Cameras

High-definition endoscopic camera systems are used in UBE to produce and record video images from the surgical field during the procedure. The system is sensitive in the visible and infrared spectrum. The imaging is transferred from the surgical field to the camera head by the arthroscope attached to the camera head. The system consists of a camera control unit (CCU) and a camera head with an integral cable that connects to the CCU (Fig. 4.4).

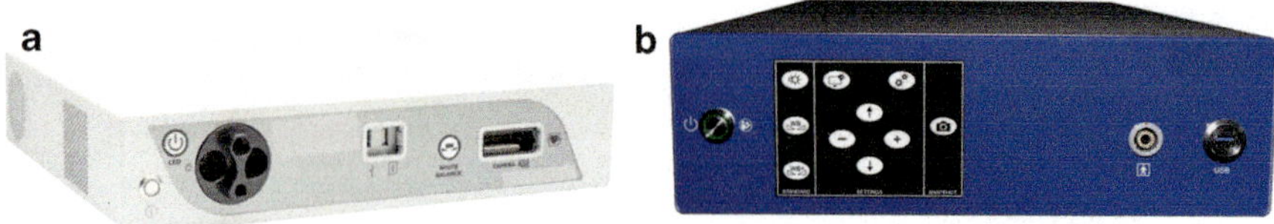

Fig. 4.5 (**a**) Synergy UHD4 (Arthrex, Inc., Naples, Florida, USA) and (**b**) Camsource LED (Joimax, GmbH, Karlsruhe, Germany)

Advanced Imaging Platforms Available for UBE

Some brands have introduced intelligent platforms to handle high-definition images during arthroscopic or endoscopic spinal procedures. Synergy UHD4 (Arthrex, Inc., Naples, Florida, USA) is an ultrahigh-definition (UHD) 4K video imaging, high-output LED light source, image management system, and integration in a single unit controlled from a tablet. Joimax (GmbH, Karlsruhe, Germany) has developed a fully integrated documentation and command system for multiple usages in one single device. The visual integration system or Vitegra Docu + Command (Joimax, GmbH, Karlsruhe, Germany) is an intelligent visual integration system for recording in the operating room. The integration system has several video inputs for different signal sources such as an endoscopic camera, X-ray, ultrasound, microscope, and OR camera. And the Camsource LED (Joimax, GmbH, Karlsruhe, Germany) provides extremely brilliant images (Fig. 4.5).

Radiofrequency

Since the 1990s, radiofrequency (RF) has been used in various medical fields such as orthopedics, oncology, cardiology, proctology, and neurology; its application is based on thermal energy at temperatures between 40 and 70 °C. The RF creates a controlled plasma field by generating thermal energy through monopolar and bipolar electrodes, resulting in the denaturalization of proteins, breaking of cell junctions, tissue dissolving, and creating of a uniform circumscribed scar. As a

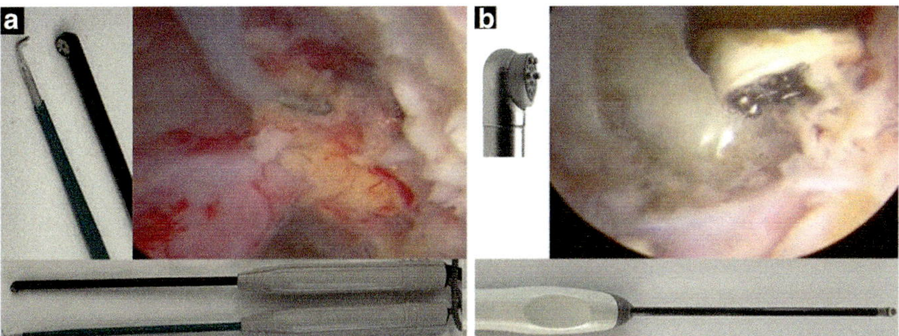

Fig. 4.6 Different RF probes used in UBE. (**a**) A more accurate coagulation or hemostasis can be achieved through a fine-ending-tip probe. The authors use a 90° hook-type ending-tip RF. In the intraoperative image, the RF hook type is used for more precise coagulation. (**b**) The broad 90° ending-tip RF can be used for ablation of outer layer tissues over the bone surfaces or for creating the working space as is shown in the intraoperative image

result, surrounding tissues are preserved, and uncontrolled inflammatory cytokine production is prevented [11–14]. The central console has cutting and coagulation modalities that can be used with the probe (Fig. 4.6).

High-Speed Drill, Shaver, and Burrs

Rotating motorized instruments that debride soft tissue and bone comprise a central console that controls the engine speed (usually between 3000 and 9000 RPM), a pedal, and a handpiece with an incorporated speed control, suction, and irrigation system. However, high-speed drills and shavers used in UBE require work in a water-based medium. These instruments are attached to a tip that may vary in diameter (usually 4 or 5 mm), a rotating blade, and a diamond or coarse bur located at the distal end.

Since radiofrequency is used for soft tissues (fat, muscle, fibrous scar, ligaments, intervertebral disc, blood vessels) as a less aggressive approach due to the result being a regular surface tissue, the primary use of high-speed drills and burrs is the drilling and undercutting of the bone structures (Fig. 4.7) [13].

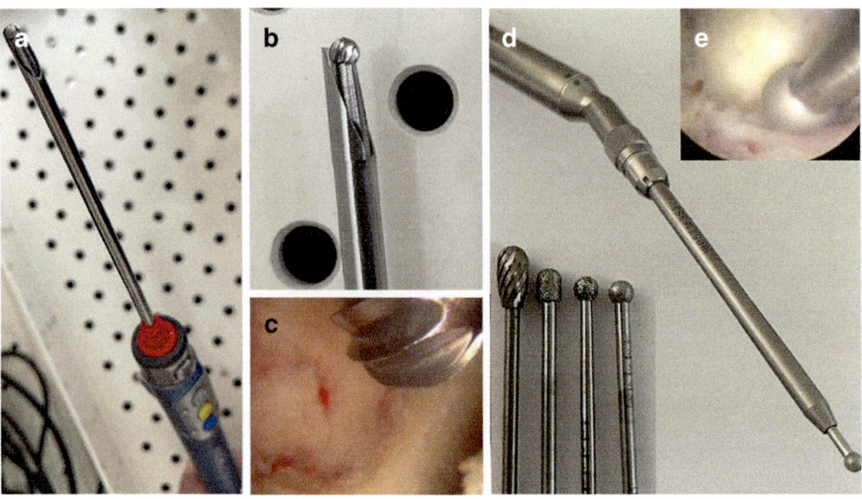

Fig. 4.7 Shaver and high-speed drill systems for UBE. (**a**) Shaver. (**b**) Shaping of the bone is determined by the type of blade, either fast or smooth. It includes a protective piece that will prevent contact with other tissues in order to avoid injuries by the blade. (**c**) Intraoperative view through the endoscope showing a cutting blade tip for bone removal. (**d**) High-speed drill with different burrs. (**e**) Endoscopic view showing the diamond burr drilling the middle part of facet joint close to the yellow ligament

Water Pumps

Water pumps were invented in Sweden in the 1970s to maintain the surgical field clean in arthroscopy. In addition, the fluid pressure produced by the pump helps keep the working space in UBE [15].

Two methods create pressure during UBE surgery:

1. Gravity: Placing the fluid bag over the patient. The bag is connected to a system of pipes attached to the endoscope sheath, allowing an inflow with a pressure dependent on the bag's height. A constant raising or lowering of the fluid bag height is needed to modify the inflow pressure.
2. Automatic pressure control pump system: The pressure generated by the water pump system is regulated by a console. The irrigation tube passes through the pump controlling the pressure of the fluid bag. That allows the surgeon to increase or decrease the pressure as required [15, 16].

The hydrostatic pressure to fulfill the expected objectives in other arthroscopic procedures is 30–60 mmHg [16]. Nonetheless, in UBE, most authors agree to set the pump on 25–30 mmHg or place the fluid bag 50–60 cm above the patient (Fig. 4.8) [4–7, 17].

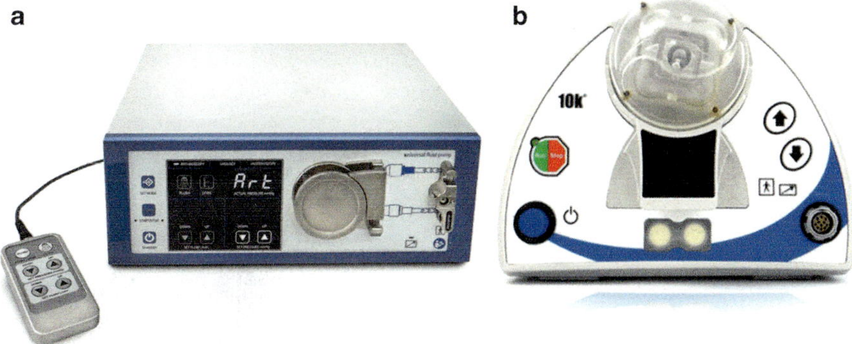

Fig. 4.8 Examples of different water pump brands. (**a**) Vimex Sp. (Z o.o. Gliwice, Poland) universal water pump. (**b**) Conmed (Utica, New York, USA) water pump for arthroscopy

Intraoperative Navigation-Assisted UBE

Intraoperative navigation improves accuracy, anatomical orientation, and safety for the patient and the medical team. In addition, this technology has instruments that locate and register images in real time, reducing exposure to intraoperative radiation. Literature has demonstrated the benefits of using this technology in spinal surgery [18].

Optical and electromagnetic technology for navigation is available. Optical navigators work by scanning 360° and providing 2D or 3D spine images. A camera registers the surgical tools, enabling the instrument's location in real time [18].

Electromagnetic navigation does not require registering the surgical tools with an infrared camera. Instead, it uses an electromagnetic sensor that, unlike optical navigation, can be used with a small workspace by using a calibrated instrument or probe, resulting in acquiring images of the spine and meeting the objectives of intraoperative navigation [19, 20].

Intraoperative navigation can be linked to UBE. It can contribute to a correct arrangement of the surgical plan. Intraoperative navigation-assisted UBE could be useful for different procedures, for example, fusion procedures [21], spinal stabilization, implant placement, and decompression of neural structures in severe cases of degenerative diseases.

Other Technologies

Biportal endoscopic surgery is versatile and easily adaptable to different technologies to favor the visualization obtained through the arthroscope. We can obtain better visualization of the surgical field through specialized 3D endoscopes that give the surgeon a better perception of depth, e.g., IMAGE1 S 3D (Karl Storz SE & Co. KG, Tuttlingen, Germany).

Navigation through augmented reality and its clinical application may include biportal endoscopy. Augmented reality systems such as BRAINLAB AG (Munich, Germany) will allow us to perform more accurate biportal endoscopic approaches and depend less on intraoperative fluoroscopic devices. Other technologies such as robotics, expanding intersomatic devices for fusion, and constant evolution and innovation supported by the industry will allow unilateral biportal endoscopic spinal surgery advancement.

Conclusion

The technology that currently allows biportal endoscopic surgery (UBE) is commonly used and easily accessible, which gives UBE an advantage over other spinal techniques that require highly specialized and expensive devices. However, advancement, development, and innovation follow an established course, and biportal endoscopic spine surgery cannot be excluded. As a result, different brands that only contemplated uniportal spinal endoscopy are turning to look at biportal endoscopic techniques. That will allow the evolution of this technique by creating more and better tools and devices specially designed for the UBE technique.

References

1. Jackson RW. A history of arthroscopy. Arthroscopy. 2010;26(1):91–103.
2. Mariani PP. The 45 degrees arthroscope: a forgotten scope in knee surgery. Orthop Traumatol Surg Res. 2019;105(4):691–5.
3. Stornebrink T, Altink JN, Appelt D, Wijdicks CA, Stufkens SAS, Kerkhoffs GMMJ. Two-millimetre diameter operative arthroscopy of the ankle is safe and effective. Knee Surg Sports Traumatol Arthrosc. 2020;28(10):3080–6.
4. Choi DJ, Kim JE, Jung JT, et al. Biportal endoscopic spine surgery for various foraminal lesions at the lumbosacral lesion. Asian Spine J. 2018;12(3):569–73.
5. Ahn JS, Lee HJ, Choi DJ, Lee KY, Hwang SJ. Extraforaminal approach of biportal endoscopic spinal surgery: a new endoscopic technique for transforaminal decompression and discectomy. J Neurosurg Spine. 2018;28(5):492–8.
6. Kang T, Park SY, Park GW, Lee SH, Park JH, Suh SW. Biportal endoscopic discectomy for high-grade migrated lumbar disc herniation [published online ahead of print, 2020 May 15]. J Neurosurg Spine. 2020:1–6. https://doi.org/10.3171/2020.2.SPINE191452.
7. Kang T, Park SY, Kang CH, Lee SH, Park JH, Suh SW. Is biportal technique/endoscopic spinal surgery satisfactory for lumbar spinal stenosis patients? A prospective randomized comparative study. Medicine (Baltimore). 2019;98(18):e15451.
8. Eun SS, Eum JH, Lee SH, Sabal LA. Biportal endoscopic lumbar decompression for lumbar disk herniation and spinal canal stenosis: a technical note. J Neurol Surg A Cent Eur Neurosurg. 2017;78(4):390–6.
9. Ahn JS, Lee HJ, Park EJ, et al. Multifidus muscle changes after biportal endoscopic spinal surgery: magnetic resonance imaging evaluation. World Neurosurg. 2019;130:e525–34.
10. Kim JE, Choi DJ. Bi-portal arthroscopic spinal surgery (BASS) with 30° arthroscopy for far lateral approach of L5-S1—technical note. J Orthop. 2018;15(2):354–8.

11. Spaner SJ, Warnock GL. A brief history of endoscopy, laparoscopy, and laparoscopic surgery. J Laparoendosc Adv Surg Tech A. 1997;7(6):369–73.
12. Anderson SR, Faucett SC, Flanigan DC, Gmabardella RA, Amin NH. The history of radiofrequency energy and Coblation in arthroscopy: a current concepts review of its application in chondroplasty of the knee. J Exp Orthop. 2019;6(1):1.
13. Rocco P, Lorenzo DB, Guglielmo T, Michele P, Nicola M, Vincenzo D. Radiofrequency energy in the arthroscopic treatment of knee chondral lesions: a systematic review [published correction appears in Br Med Bull. 2017 May 19:1]. Br Med Bull. 2016;117(1):149–56.
14. Lu Y, Edwards RB 3rd, Cole BJ, Markel MD. Thermal chondroplasty with radiofrequency energy. An in vitro comparison of bipolar and monopolar radiofrequency devices. Am J Sports Med. 2001;29(1):42–9.
15. Hsiao MS, Kusnezov N, Sieg RN, Owens BD, Herzog JP. Use of an irrigation pump system in arthroscopic procedures. Orthopedics. 2016;39(3):e474–8.
16. Bomberg BC, Hurley PE, Clark CA, McLaughlin CS. Complications associated with the use of an infusion pump during knee arthroscopy. Arthroscopy. 1992;8(2):224–8.
17. Kang MS, Park HJ, Hwang JH, Kim JE, Choi DJ, Chung HJ. Safety evaluation of biportal endoscopic lumbar discectomy: assessment of cervical epidural pressure during surgery. Spine (Phila Pa 1976). 2020;45(20):E1349–56.
18. Virk S, Qureshi S. Navigation in minimally invasive spine surgery. J Spine Surg. 2019;5(Suppl 1):S25–30.
19. Fraser JF, Von Jako R, Carrino JA, Härtl R. Electromagnetic navigation in minimally invasive spine surgery: results of a cadaveric study to evaluate percutaneous pedicle screw insertion. SAS J. 2008;2(1):43–7.
20. von Jako R, Finn MA, Yonemura KS, et al. Minimally invasive percutaneous transpedicular screw fixation: increased accuracy and reduced radiation exposure by means of a novel electromagnetic navigation system. Acta Neurochir. 2011;153(3):589–96.
21. Quillo-Olvera J, Quillo-Reséndiz J, Quillo-Olvera D, Barrera-Arreola M, Kim JS. Ten-step biportal endoscopic transforaminal lumbar interbody fusion under computed tomography-based intraoperative navigation: technical report and preliminary outcomes in Mexico. Oper Neurosurg (Hagerstown). 2020;19(5):608–18.

Part II
Basic Principles

Chapter 5
Basic Principles of Unilateral Biportal Endoscopic Spinal Surgery: Operative Room Setup, Anesthesia, and Patient Positioning

Javier Quillo-Reséndiz, Diego Quillo-Olvera, Alexa Borbolla Ruiz, Michelle Barrera-Arreola, and Javier Quillo-Olvera

Abbreviations

IONM	Intraoperative neuromonitoring
LED	Light-emitted diode
OR	Operating room
TJC	The Joint Commission
UBE	Unilateral biportal endoscopy
USA	The United States
WHO	World Health Organization

Introduction

The operating room (OR) must be a controlled space where the interaction between the human and technological components must aim to improve the results for the patient. That is achieved by creating routines to ensure patient safety in the face of the proposed surgical treatment. For example, The Joint Commission (TJC) is the largest and oldest organization in the USA that accredits hospital quality and safety

J. Quillo-Reséndiz (✉) · D. Quillo-Olvera · M. Barrera-Arreola · J. Quillo-Olvera
The Brain and Spine Care, Minimally Invasive Spine Surgery Group, Hospital H+ Querétaro, Spine Clinic, Querétaro, México
e-mail: kitnoz@hotmail.com; drquilloolvera86@gmail.com; michelle.barrera@anahuac.mx; neuroqomd@gmail.com

A. B. Ruiz
Anáhuac University, School of Medicine, Querétaro, México
e-mail: alexaborbolla@gmail.com

J. Quillo-Olvera et al. (eds.), *Unilateral Biportal Endoscopy of the Spine*,
https://doi.org/10.1007/978-3-031-14736-4_5

processes. In 2003, it implemented a time-out within its security processes to confirm or reconsider the proposed plan and thus avoid any failure just before starting the surgery. A similar protocol was launched by the WHO called the "Safe Surgery Checklist" in 2008 [1].

Biportal endoscopic surgery, like any other surgical procedure, must be performed under the strictest safety standards to guarantee an optimal result for the patient, and this must be based on the guidelines mentioned above. Although this chapter does not strictly discuss the items that make up the checklist of any surgery, we will descript the essential technical requirements for a correct configuration of the OR in biportal endoscopy procedures.

The OR setting must be done in a specific order. It will provide patient safety and efficiency during the surgical procedure. The medical team, technicians, and assistants must ensure the correct working of all technological devices required during the procedure preoperatively. The checklist should include operative room lighting, operative table, C-arm, other intraoperative imaging devices, anesthesia machine, and for sure the endoscopic tower (Fig. 5.1).

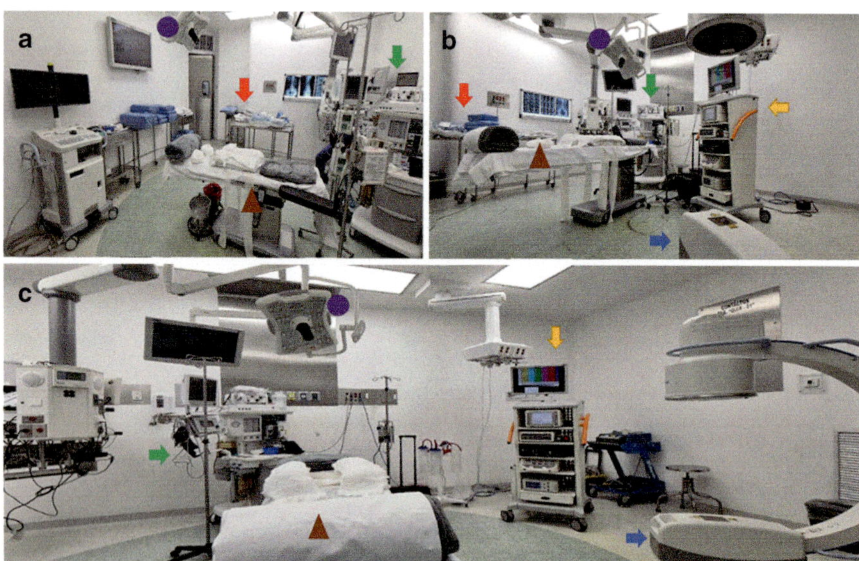

Fig. 5.1 Operative room setup. (**a**–**c**) The operating table (brown triangle) with soft lateral pads or abdominal support frame can be used. All the bone eminences and joints should be protected by covering with soft pads. The operative room lights (purple circle) are essential during the surgical approach before introducing the endoscope. The anesthesia machine (green arrow) is placed at the head of the operative table. The endoscopic tower (yellow arrow), the C-arm (blue arrow), and the surgical nurse table (red arrow) are also pointed

Operative Room Setup

Operating Table

The operating table, located in the center of the room, must be fixed on the floor to avoid movements during the procedure. It should be set for the patient size, with different adjustable settings for the surgeon's ergonomics. Especially in biportal endoscopy, the height of the surgical table must be sufficient to avoid excessive shoulder strain. The specific configuration of the surgical table should include a frame to support the abdominal wall and a pad for elevating the legs to favor the venous return. Soft cushions, cotton, or any other material covering the bony eminences and joints supporting the patient's weight throughout the procedure is recommended. This will reduce the patient's pain-related position after surgery. The surgical table for spinal procedures should work with the C-arm to avoid imaging bias during the surgery.

Lighting Equipment

The operating room lighting should be addressed to the surgical table and prepared before beginning the surgery. Different halogen or light-emitting diode (LED) types are available, fixed in the ceiling. They have an adjustable light intensity that will enable the surgeon to have a clear and visible surgical field. In addition, some light devices include a complete high-definition camera system that can record surgical approaches for descriptive purposes.

Anesthesiology Machine

The anesthesiology machine is a high-precision medical device that controls the patient's level of consciousness during the surgery by administering a mixture of anesthetic gases to the patient and monitoring the correct pressure and continuous flow. This machine monitors the vital signs; vaporizers, pneumatic systems, and valves create a gas control circuit that will regulate the ventilatory parameters, ensuring an optimal respiratory function during surgery. This machine is placed for ergonomics at the head of the patient. This machine is managed and controlled by the anesthetist throughout the procedure.

Intraoperative Fluoroscopy

The C-arm or intraoperative fluoroscopic arch is an X-ray machine consisting of a generator tube and an image intensifier that generates images and transfers to a monitor. It is attached to an arm that encircles the operating table by 180° and can perform rotary and tilting movements to produce 2D images in real time. C-arm is placed on the side of the surgical table and in front of the surgeon. With this device, the surgeon will plan the entries, confirm the triangular approach, and get oriented during most UBE procedures (Fig. 5.2) [2].

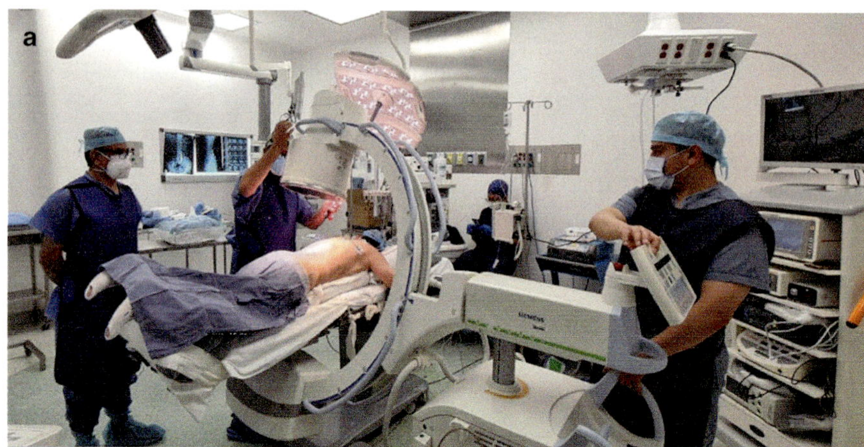

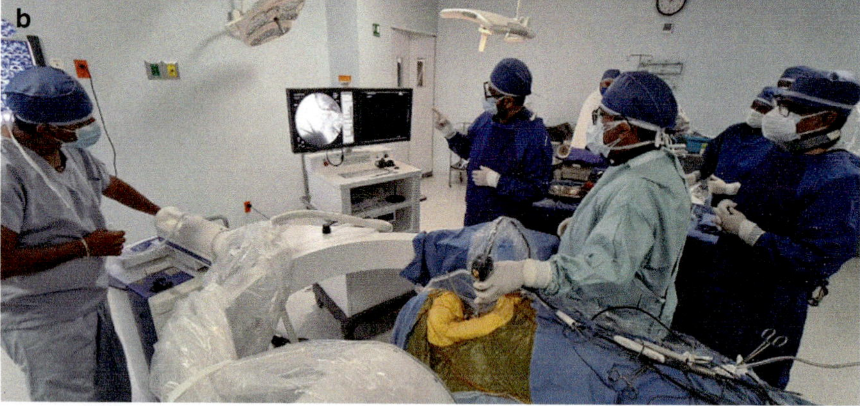

Fig. 5.2 C-arm use in the operative room. (**a**) Imaging acquisition through the C-arm for planning the UBE procedure. (**b**) Intraoperative fluoroscopy use in UBE cervical procedure

Endoscopy Tower

The endoscopy tower is placed in front of the surgeon, on the opposite side of the surgical approach. The tower generally includes:

- A display
- A video recorder system with a camera
- A light source
- A water pump
- Radiofrequency generator
- The drilling system

The height of the display should be at the surgeon's viewing field to avoid neck extension and fatigue. In addition, along with an appropriate operating table height, continued abduction of the surgeon's shoulders during the procedure should be prevented. Therefore, ergonomics is essential to avoid strain during surgery (Fig. 5.3). Prior to surgery, the medical staff and technician should review the proper working of the tower. Emphasize the camera, light source, and video recording. If a water pump is not available for the procedure, a tripod next to the side of the viewing portal is placed for holding the irrigation bags. However, if a water pump is used, the initial pressure should be 25–30 mmHg [3]. The radiofrequency generator should be set on the less coagulation and ablation intensity mode when the epidural space is exposed.

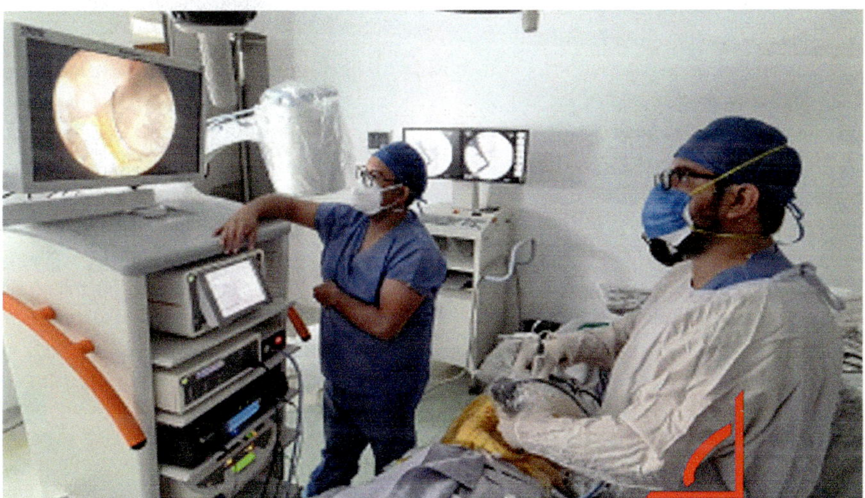

Fig. 5.3 Endoscopic tower disposition during a UBE procedure. The tower is placed in front of the surgeon on the opposite side of the approach. The surgeon observes the display directly without forced neck postures, and the shoulders are not elevated or abducted for handling the instruments. It is highlighted with a red angle

Anesthesia

The objective of anesthesia during the UBE procedure is to avoid pain and a traumatic experience for the patient related to the procedure. Also, if the patient moves during the surgery, it could be dangerous. Therefore, general anesthesia and conscious sedation are commonly used for UBE. In addition, epidural and total intravenous anesthesia are excellent options, especially in the lumbar spine. Communication with the anesthesia team includes comments if intraoperative neuromonitoring (IONM) will be used. Medications such as midazolam, remifentanil, propofol, and dexmedetomidine can be used in UBE procedures for different types of anesthesia.

Patient Positioning

In UBE, the prone position is commonly used. The patient's head can rest comfortably on a pillow if conscious sedation is chosen, and an anesthesia air cushion mask could be used to control the airway. A face-cradle prone support system can be used if general anesthesia is used for the UBE surgery. There are some considerations for the prone position and the head. The first one is complete control of the airway, and the second one is to avoid excessive neck extension to prevent any spinal cord damage in a setting of severe cervical spondylosis. The third one is to protect always and pay attention to the face, especially the eyes; ocular compression injury could happen if the eyes are not covered and protected during prolonged surgical times. The arms should be abducted cautiously to avoid damage to the shoulder joints or cervical plexus traction. The venous return should be favored with the position. An abdominal support frame or lateral soft pads can be used. The goal is to avoid compression of the abdomen to prevent indirect epidural venous plexus hypertension that results in intraoperative bleeding. A slight flexion is made to reduce lumbar lordosis, and opening the interlaminar space may be beneficial. The knees can be slightly flexed and elevated to decrease venous stasis in the legs. All the bone eminences should be protected and rested over soft pads (Fig. 5.4).

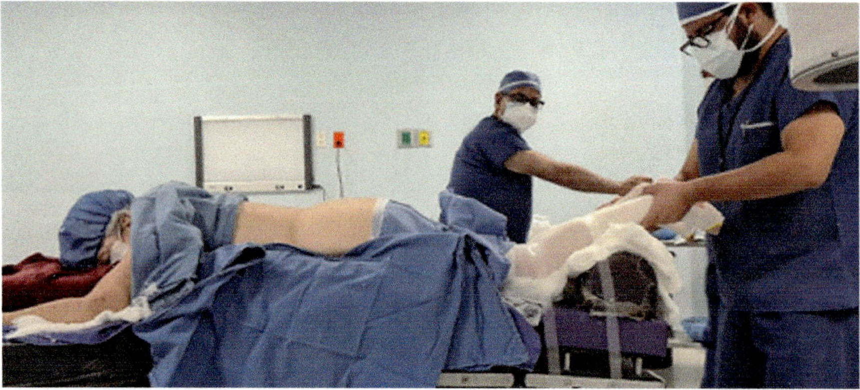

Fig. 5.4 Prone position for a lumbar UBE procedure with a patient under conscious sedation

Surgical Area Preparation

The surgical field is cleaned and prepared with antiseptic solutions. Finally, the patient is draped with an antimicrobial incise drape. For water-based endoscopic procedures, including biportal endoscopy, a waterproof adhesive sheet with a fluid collection pouch is required (Fig. 5.5).

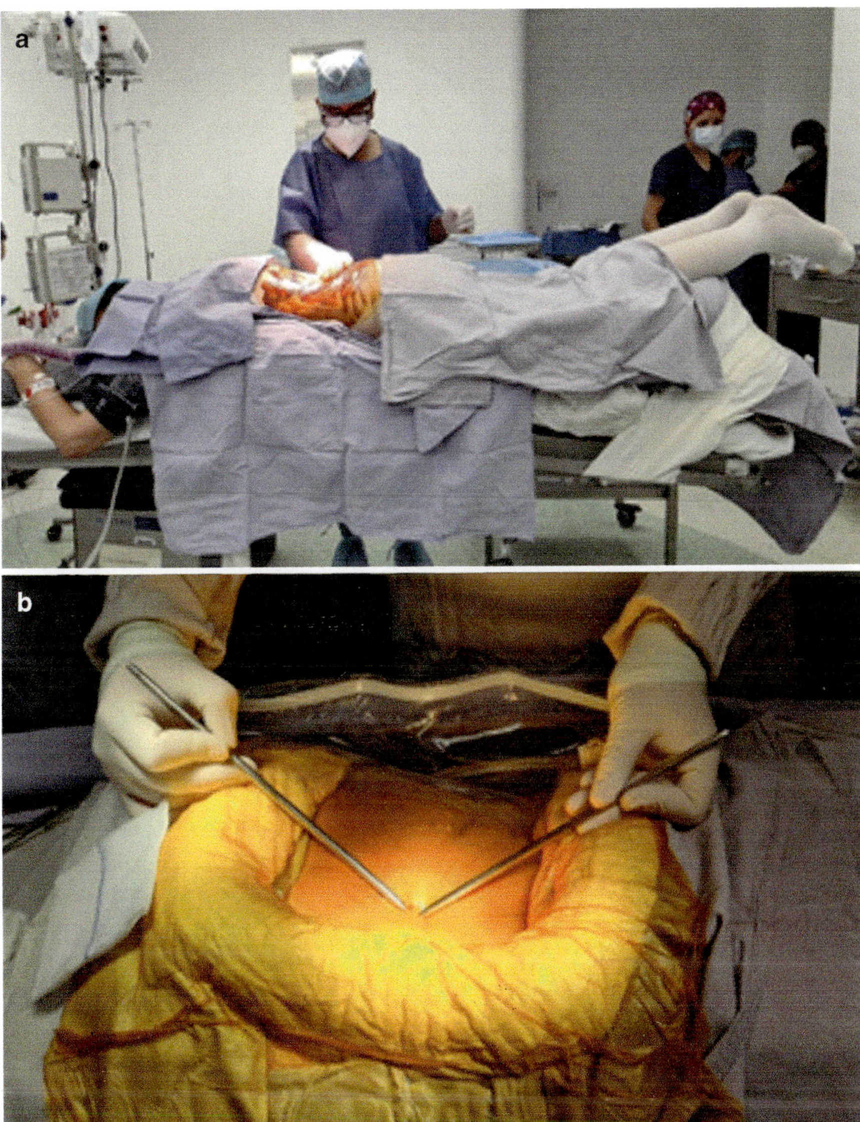

Fig. 5.5 Patient preparation. (**a**) The surgical field is cleaned. (**b**) Surgical field drapes

Surgical Instruments

The surgical nurse or the assistant should organize the required materials for UBE surgery (Fig. 5.6), including instruments from a standard spine surgery set such as:

- A scalpel with blade numbers 15 and 20
- 1 and 3 mm Kerrison punches with ending tip of 90° and 130°
- 2 mm straight and angled pituitary forceps
- Microdissectors
- Straight and angled curettes
- Tubular progressive dilators
- Nerve hook
- Semi-tubular customized working cannula
- Arthroscopic surgery tools
- Radiofrequency probes
- 0° and 30° endoscope lenses
- Arthroscope trocar
- Optical fiber
- Different-sized osteotomes
- Hammer
- Shaver and high-speed drill specially for the water environment

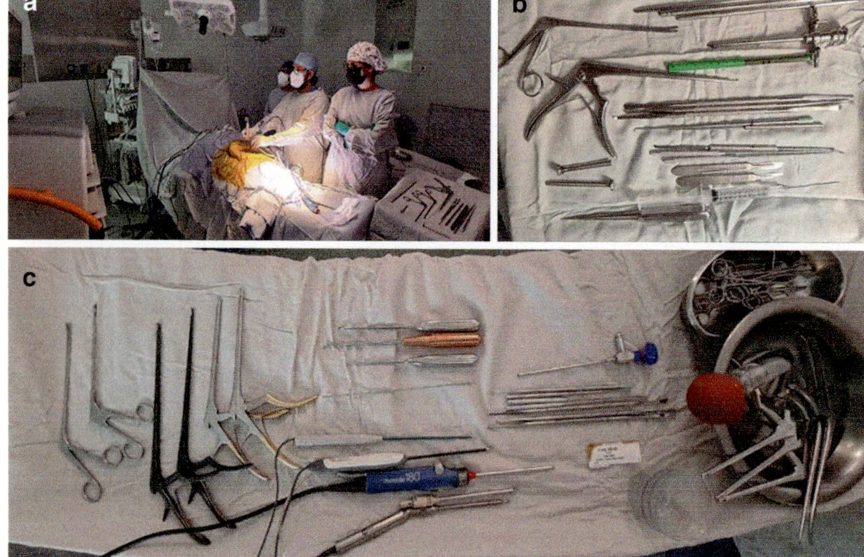

Fig. 5.6 Surgical tools used in a UBE surgery. (**a**) Disposition of the operative theater. The assistant or scrub nurse is next to the surgeon. (**b**) Disposition of the surgical tools in the Mayo stand. (**c**) Back table with additional instruments required during a UBE procedure

Discussion

The requirements commented in this chapter to configure the operating room (OR) for a biportal endoscopy surgical procedure aim to offer safe and efficient surgery. The most important component of efficiency is patient safety. Setting up the OR and preparing the patient for the surgical procedure are some concerns discussed in this chapter, and the fundamentals must always be patient safety and comfort.

The key to efficiency is the staff: technicians, nurses, assistants, anesthetists, and surgeons, everybody is important in the OR, and each has a reason for being. So, the best surgeons should know that technical skills are just a part of achieving efficiency, and all the staff efforts should focus only on the patient.

Therefore, efficiency in the operating room could reduce delays in operative procedures and consequently hospital costs for the patient [4]. So then, this chapter is not only a guide that mentions the basic requirements for performing a UBE procedure. This chapter aims to demonstrate reproducible conduct that the authors always follow to achieve fluid workflow beneficial for the patient.

The preparation and organization of the OR are essential when a UBE procedure is considered for a patient. Therefore, the setup of the OR needs to be planned according to the needs of the procedure. The other point is that as a minimally invasive spinal procedure, UBE enhances patient safety through different manners.

For example, the personnel required in the surgical field is reduced in the biportal endoscopic surgery since the surgeon can use endoscopic retractors specially designed for these procedures, avoiding the help of an extra surgical assistant. This process reduces the risk of contamination of the instruments or the surgical field.

Also, as mentioned in the type of anesthesia required, many biportal endoscopic lumbar procedures can be performed with conscious sedation. It reduces anesthesia-related hospital costs and the risk of requiring postoperative airway care or the use of a ventilator or postanesthetic care in the ICU.

In addition, the extent of the soft-tissue damage related to the procedure impacts the patient outcome, first due to the risk of infection of the surgical wound. In biportal endoscopic procedures, a pair of 6–8 mm skin incisions is sufficient for surgical access. Therefore, there is less exposure to deep tissues and a reduced risk of intraoperative contamination. The other situation is that continuous fluid irrigation throughout the procedure reduces the risk of infections due to constant washing of the surgical field.

Finally, biportal access is associated with less muscle and deep tissue damage. It is also associated with less postoperative analgesic consumption, zero postoperative opioid consumption, and earlier out-of-bed mobilization.

The aforementioned has a direct relationship with the correct planning of the procedure, with the proper operating room setting, adequate cleaning of the surgical field, positioning of the patient on the surgical table, and excellent communication with the anesthesiologist.

Therefore, the operating room setup is not a technical activity only before a surgical procedure but is an essential step of the patient care process that allows efficiency during the surgery and will provide safety for the patient. It will positively affect patient outcomes.

Conclusion

To achieve the best possible postoperative outcome, the staff involved in the UBE procedure must be appropriately organized and knowledgeable. It will allow a fluid workflow during the procedure and efficiency in the perioperative care process, ensuring safety for the patient, high-quality care, and good outcomes.

References

1. Papadakis M, Meiwandi A, Grzybowski A. The WHO safer surgery checklist time out procedure revisited: strategies to optimise compliance and safety. Int J Surg. 2019;69:19–22.
2. Kim JE, Choi DJ, Park EJJ, et al. Biportal endoscopic spinal surgery for lumbar spinal stenosis. Asian Spine J. 2019;13(2):334–42.
3. Choi CM, Chung JT, Lee SJ, Choi DJ. How I do it? Biportal endoscopic spinal surgery (BESS) for treatment of lumbar spinal stenosis. Acta Neurochir. 2016;158(3):459–63.
4. Nundy S, Mukherjee A, Sexton JB, et al. Impact of preoperative briefings on operating room delays: a preliminary report. Arch Surg. 2008;143(11):1068–72.

Chapter 6
Basic Principles of Unilateral Biportal Endoscopic Spinal Surgery: Technical Considerations Before Starting

Iakiv Fishchenko and Claudia-Angelica Covarrubias-Rosas

Abbreviations

AP	Anteroposterior
OR	Operating room
RF	Radiofrequency
UBE	Unilateral biportal endoscopy

Introduction

The unilateral biportal endoscopy (UBE) technique is a minimally invasive procedure for treating degenerative diseases of the lumbar spine. Compared to uniportal endoscopy, one of the significant advantages of this method is that it does not require an expensive, fragile, and specialized toolkit. In most cases, arthroscopic and standard instrumentation for spinal surgery is sufficient. The basic principles of the UBE are the following: triangulation, adjustment of fluid irrigation, and workspace creation. The combination of two portals provides clear video control over the procedure and the formation of correct liquid circulation. The absence of a natural cavity, as in a joint, slightly complicates the surgery. That is why creating a workspace is an essential component of UBE surgery. The operation is facilitated with the routine observance of these principles, and the likelihood of serious complications is reduced.

I. Fishchenko (✉)
Institute of Traumatology and Orthopedics of Ukraine, Kyiv, Ukraine
e-mail: fishchenko@gmail.com

C.-A. Covarrubias-Rosas
Department of Experimental Surgery, McGill University, Montreal, QC, Canada
e-mail: claudia.covarrubias@mcgill.ca

J. Quillo-Olvera et al. (eds.), *Unilateral Biportal Endoscopy of the Spine*,
https://doi.org/10.1007/978-3-031-14736-4_6

Organization of the Working Space in the Surgery Room

Prior to initiating the surgical procedure, it is necessary to properly equip the operating room (OR) (Fig. 6.1). The surgical team should include a surgeon, an assistant (optional), and a scrub nurse. The rest of the required equipment is presented in Table 6.1.

The following are the surgical instruments required for a routine UBE procedure:

Special UBE set (optional) (Fig. 6.2), dilators, curettes, pituitary forceps, Kerrison rongeurs, Indian knife, osteotome, and a mallet (Fig. 6.3). Also, nerve retractors and a drilling system for use in water are needed (Fig. 6.4).

Although some authors underlined that no special instruments are required for the UBE, several unique sets of tools, currently available on the market, facilitate the procedure (Fig. 6.2). Most often, they include instrumentation that enables access (such as telescopic dilators), tubular systems to improve saline outflow, various retractors to protect neural structures, as well as a set of curettes and osteotomes.

Finally, a radiofrequency (RF) generator and probes are used for coagulation. A 5 mm headed RF probe is helpful for debridement and coagulation outside of the spinal canal (Fig. 6.5a). A 1.5 mm headed, curved RF probe is useful for small bleeds within the spinal canal (Fig. 6.5b).

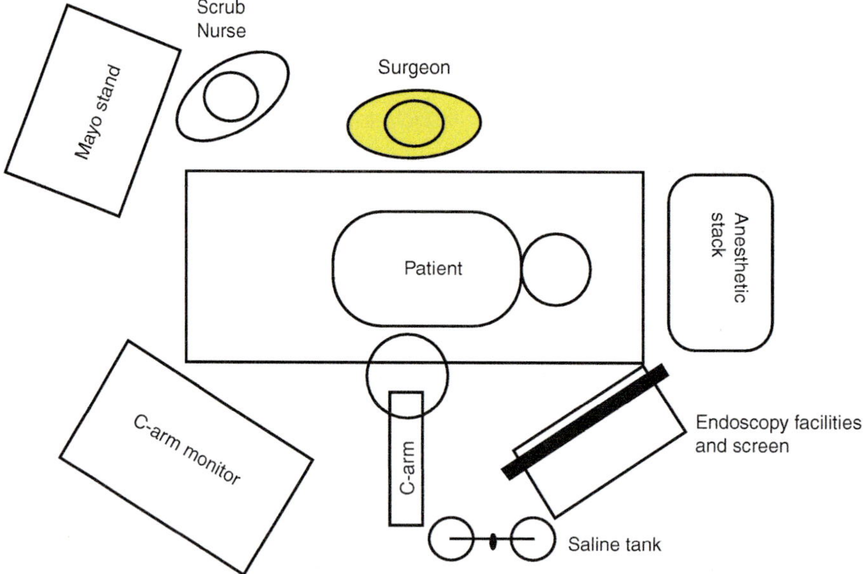

Fig. 6.1 Schematic location of personnel and equipment in the surgery room

Table 6.1 List of the required equipment

X-ray operating table	
Wilson spine frame	
C-arm	
Arthroscopic system	Monitor
	Camera system
	Light source, light cable
	Arthroscopy pump (optional)
	Shaver Console and handpiece 0° arthroscope 30° arthroscope (optional)
Radiofrequency	Generator
	5 mm headed RF electrode
	1.5 mm headed RF electrode
Aspiration system	

RF radiofrequency

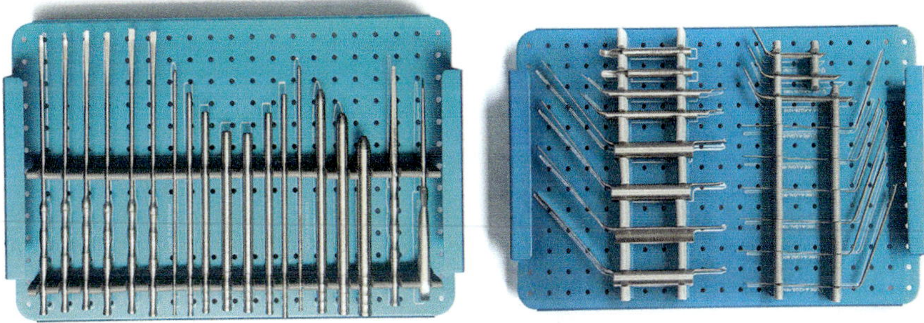

Fig. 6.2 Special UBE set

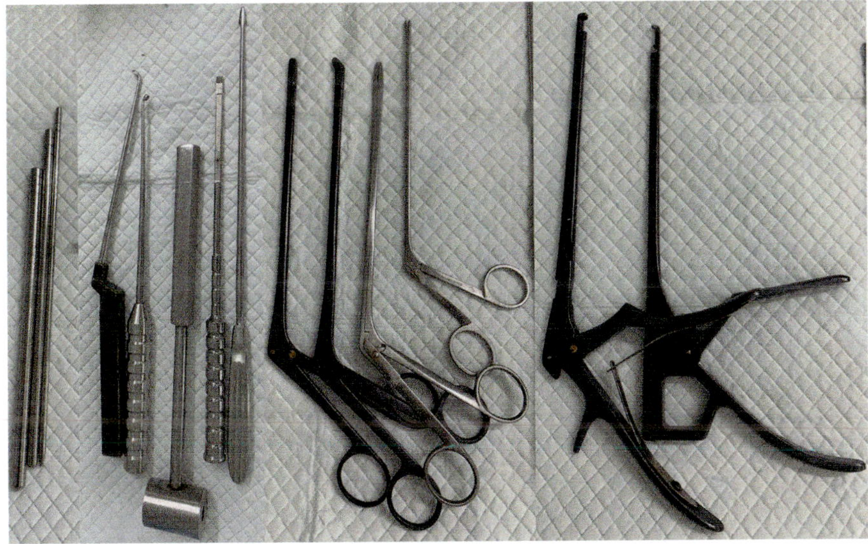

Fig. 6.3 Surgical tools employed in a UBE procedure

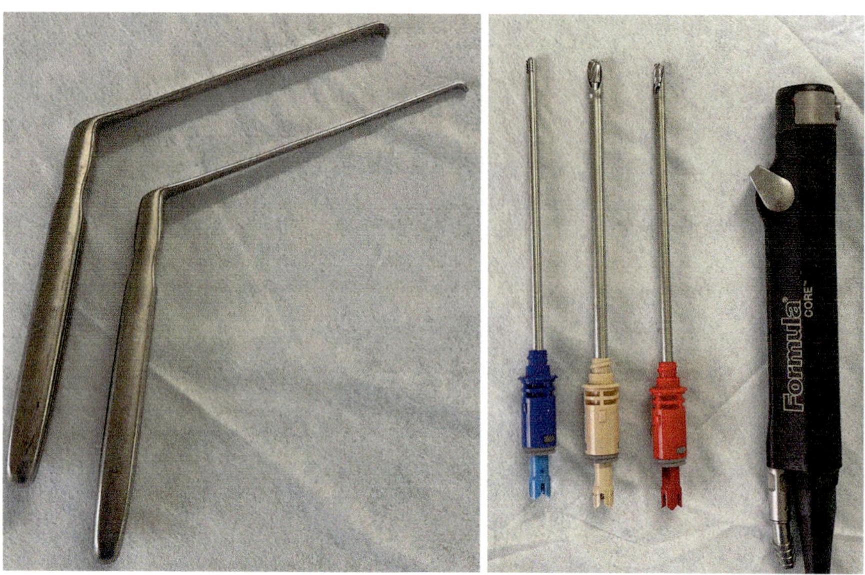

Fig. 6.4 Nerve retractors and drilling system

Fig. 6.5 (**a**, **b**) Different RF probes

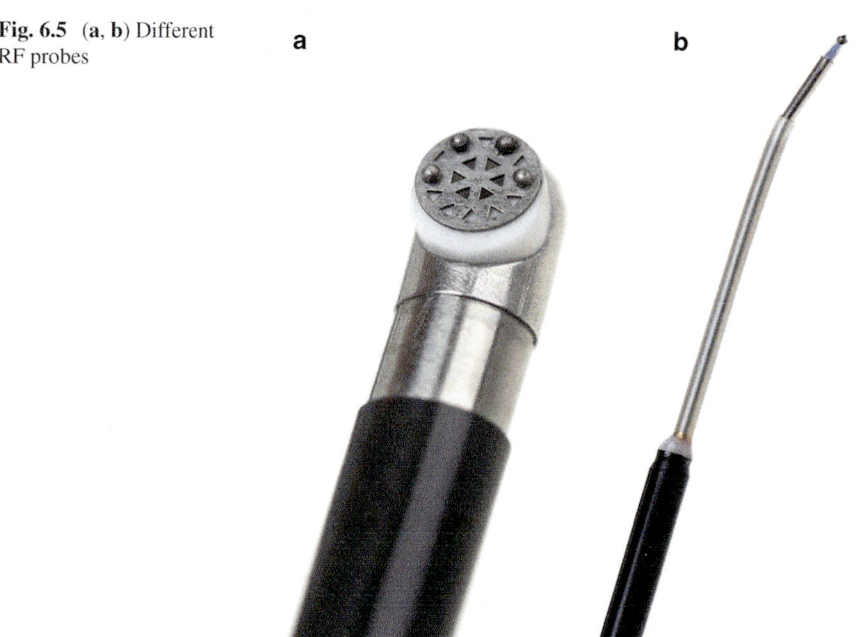

Patient Positioning

The patient is placed prone on a radiolucent table over a Wilson frame to achieve flexion in the lumbar spine. The maximum increase in the interspinous gap is achieved in this position, which is essential for reducing unnecessary bone resection (Fig. 6.6). The head and thoracic spine of the patient must be at the lumbar spine height or below it for normal blood flow. To reduce blood loss and for ease of use, it is necessary to maintain systolic blood pressure no greater than 100 mmHg. It is recommended to place soft pillows under the knees and shins.

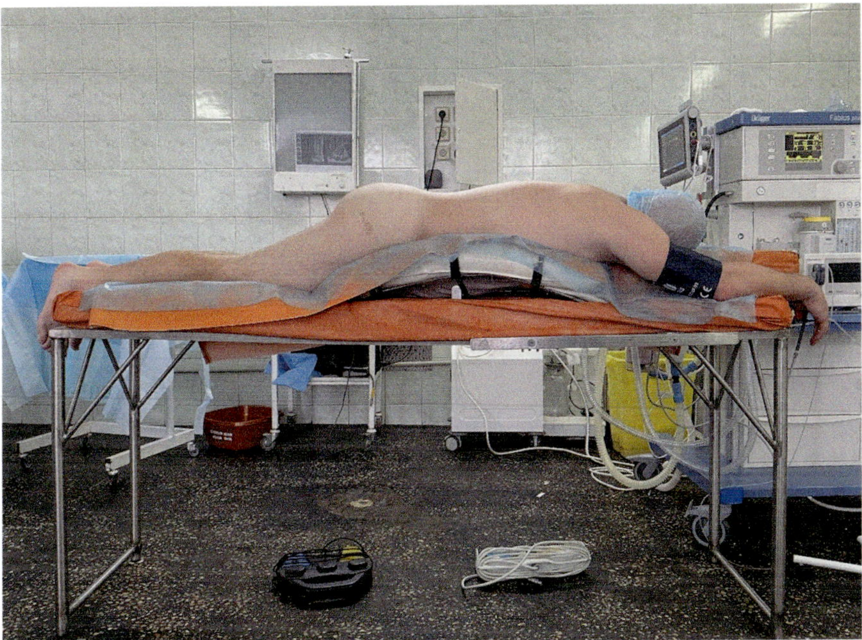

Fig. 6.6 Patient positioning

Fluid Irrigation

The correct circulation of saline is essential to keep the surgical field clear. If the flow is insufficient, the visual field may become blurred due to bleeding from various sources: muscles, cortical and cancellous bone, and epidural vessels. There are two options for fluid supply, which include using an arthroscopic pump and natural gravity. Using an arthroscopic pump, the optimal fluid pressure of 25–30 mmHg warrants a clean working field. It also prevents the development of severe complications arising from an increase in intracranial pressure in patients secondary to the flow of saline through the spinal canal.

Working under the natural gravity of the fluid is carried out by hanging the saline bags on a tripod (Fig. 6.7). The optimal height for placing saline bags is 160–170 cm. Furthermore, the pressure of the supplied fluid can be controlled by adjusting the height of the tripod.

For bleeding reduction, saline bags should never be hung too high if the saline outflow is poorly adjusted. Do not proceed if a good flow is not observed. Smooth drainage should be achieved rather than high-pressure over-infusion of saline.

Fig. 6.7 Tripod with saline bags

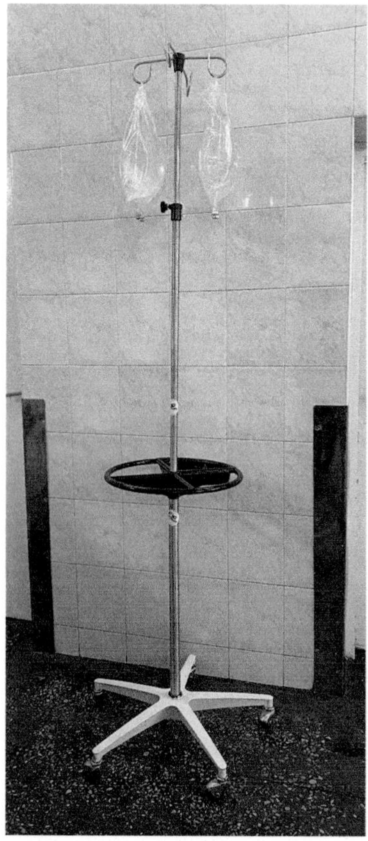

The outflow of saline can be compromised in the following cases: a small incision in the skin and muscle fascia, insufficient muscle relaxation, and thick subcutaneous adipose tissue. Optimal access incisions should be 7–10 mm. This is sufficient to ensure fluid drainage. In addition to dissecting the skin and subcutaneous adipose tissue, it is necessary to make a crosswise cut of the thoracolumbar fascia. Its insufficient dissection leads to improper outflow of fluid. Subcutaneous adipose tissue can accumulate a significant amount of effluent fluid and prevent its outflow. Never attempt to improve the circulation of saline by increasing the pressure or raising the height of the saline bags.

Radiological Landmarks for Access

The radiological landmarks for access will depend on the approach chosen. However, the spinous process, cranial lamina, and superior-inferior pedicles are the landmarks that the surgeon needs to identify in a lumbar anteroposterior (AP) view of the C-arm. These anatomical considerations will guide the entries' location in a paramedian approach (Fig. 6.8).

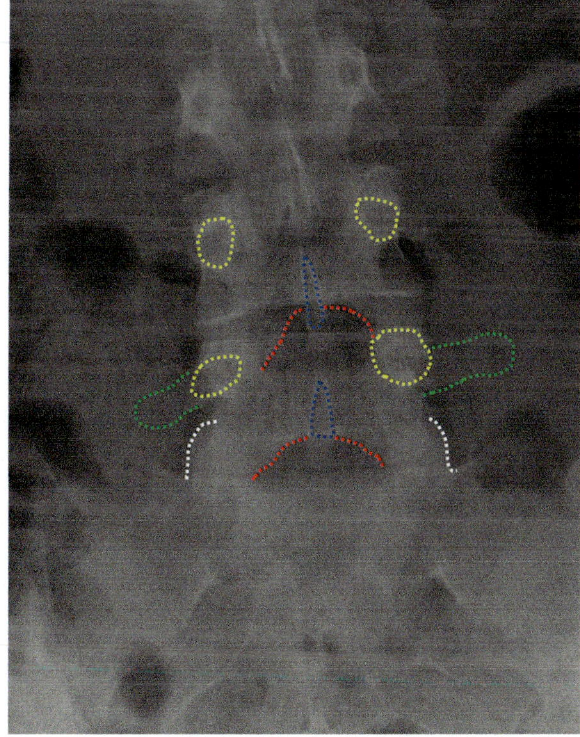

Fig. 6.8 Lumbar AP view of the C-arm. The references that usually guide the surgeon for a posterior paramedian approach are the following: the spinous process is lined in blue dots, the pedicles are lined in yellow spots, and the inferior margin of the cranial lamina is lined in red dots. The transverse process lined in green spots and the lateral surface of the SAP lined in white dots are landmarks of the paraspinal approach

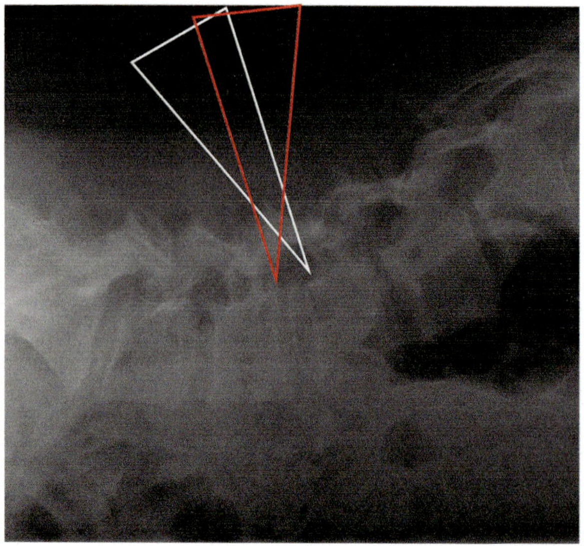

Fig. 6.9 Lumbar lateral view of the C-arm. The triangles represent a biportal approach targeted to the superior (white triangle) or inferior (red triangle) part of the foramen

When a paraspinal approach is planned, the surgeon needs to identify the superior transverse process and the lateral margin of the facet joint (Fig. 6.8). In addition, the lumbar lateral view is essential to confirm where the approach is addressed. For example, when a contralateral sublaminar approach for proximal foraminal decompression is planned, it is required to target the procedure for a specific part of the foramen (Fig. 6.9).

Discussion

The feasibility of using a standard set of spine surgery tools is an advantage seen in biportal endoscopy. In addition, unlike other water-based endoscopic procedures, in biportal endoscopy, the surgeon is familiar with the instruments, and the technique is not expensive compared with uniportal endoscopy.

Eum et al. [1] introduced the modern way to perform UBE for neural decompression of the lumbar spine. The first works mainly described the technical features of the surgical intervention. They stated that only an arthroscopic and a standard set of spinal instruments were required to perform the surgical intervention [1–3].

Liu et al. [3] described the stepwise procedure of biportal endoscopy for decompression of lateral stenosis. In his publication, the authors mentioned an arthroscope and Kerrison punches of 1–3 mm to carry out the technique.

Another interesting technical description was made by Hong et al. [4]. The authors designed special retractors to protect the nerve structures attached to the endoscope and a pusher for endoscopic suturing in case of injuries to the dural membrane. They found the customized surgical tools helpful in shortening the operative time, protecting the nerves during discectomy, and protecting the dural sac when they crossed the midline to the contralateral side.

Heo et al. [5] proposed using a titanium vascular anastomotic clip system for suturing dural tears. They repaired the dural tear completely using titanium vascular anastomotic clips without converting the surgery to an open technique.

The authors noted that the clipping method might be an effective alternative method of dural repair for incidental durotomy.

Regarding fluid irrigation, stable saline dynamics during biportal endoscopy improve the surgeon's comfort and patient outcomes. Hong et al. [6] aimed to measure the fluid dynamics during UBE procedures and identify the factors that facilitate stable dynamics. They suggest maintaining saline pressure between 4.41 cmH_2O (2.41 mmHg) and 31.00 cmH_2O (22.83 mmHg). In addition, placement of the working cannula with an appropriate length was found to be an essential factor influencing fluid dynamics.

Conclusion

With careful preoperative planning, which includes setting up the operative room, proper surgical tools, and performing in a meticulous stepwise fashion, the UBE procedure will warrant acceptable outcomes for the patient.

References

1. Eum JH, Heo DH, Son SK, Park CK. Percutaneous biportal endoscopic decompression for lumbar spinal stenosis: a technical note and preliminary clinical results. J Neurosurg Spine. 2016;24(4):602–7.
2. Choi CM, Chung JT, Lee SJ, Choi DJ. How I do it? Biportal endoscopic spinal surgery (BESS) for treatment of lumbar spinal stenosis. Acta Neurochir. 2016;158(3):459–63.
3. Liu X. A novel biportal full endoscopy technique for lumbar lateral recess stenosis: technical report. Clin Spine Surg. 2019;32(2):51–6.
4. Hong YH, Kim SK, Suh DW, Lee SC. Novel instruments for percutaneous biportal endoscopic spine surgery for full decompression and dural management: a comparative analysis. Brain Sci. 2020;10(8):516.
5. Heo DH, Ha JS, Lee DC, Kim HS, Chung HJ. Repair of incidental durotomy using sutureless nonpenetrating clips via biportal endoscopic surgery. Global Spine J. 2020; https://doi.org/10.1177/2192568220956606.
6. Hong YH, Kim SK, Hwang J, Eum JH, Heo DH, Suh DW, Lee SC. Water dynamics in unilateral biportal endoscopic spine surgery and its related factors: an in vivo proportional regression and proficiency-matched study. World Neurosurg. 2021;149:e836–43.

Chapter 7
Basic Principles of Unilateral Biportal Endoscopic Spinal Surgery: Anatomical Considerations of Elementary Approaches

Javier Quillo-Olvera, Diego Quillo-Olvera, Javier Quillo-Reséndiz, and Michelle Barrera-Arreola

Abbreviations

AP	Anteroposterior
Cau	Caudal
Cra	Cranial
CSM	Cervical spondylotic myelopathy
CT	Computed tomography
DS	Dural sac
IAP	Inferior articular process
ILS	Interlaminar space
L	Lamina
LF	Ligamentum flavum
PDM	Peridural membrane
PLL	Posterior longitudinal ligament
SAP	Superior articular process
SP	Spinous process

Supplementary Information The online version contains supplementary material available at [https://doi.org/10.1007/978-3-031-14736-4_7].

J. Quillo-Olvera (✉) · D. Quillo-Olvera · J. Quillo-Reséndiz · M. Barrera-Arreola
The Brain and Spine Care, Minimally Invasive Spine Surgery Group, Hospital H+ Querétaro, Spine Clinic, Querétaro, México
e-mail: neuroqomd@gmail.com; drquilloolvera86@gmail.com; kitnoz@hotmail.com; michelle.barrera@anahuac.mx

J. Quillo-Olvera et al. (eds.), *Unilateral Biportal Endoscopy of the Spine*, https://doi.org/10.1007/978-3-031-14736-4_7

TP Transverse process
UBE Unilateral biportal endoscopy
ULBD Unilateral laminotomy for bilateral decompression

Introduction

The unilateral biportal endoscopic (UBE) technique has evolved and adapted to the needs of the surgeon and the challenges that spinal pathology requires. This chapter discusses the aspects from planning the incisions to the relevant anatomy observed through the endoscope. UBE surgery works through two ports, which have a specific purpose. The ports are placed ipsilaterally with an angled trajectory. Both ports will join at the planned anatomical landmark (Fig. 7.1).

Therefore, the technique could be divided as follows:

(a) The two ports' placement in a determined region of the spine (unilateral biportal approach)
(b) The biportal endoscopic technique elected to address a specific spinal pathology

Both stages will be planned according to the spinal region, trajectory, and maneuvers required to reach the target.

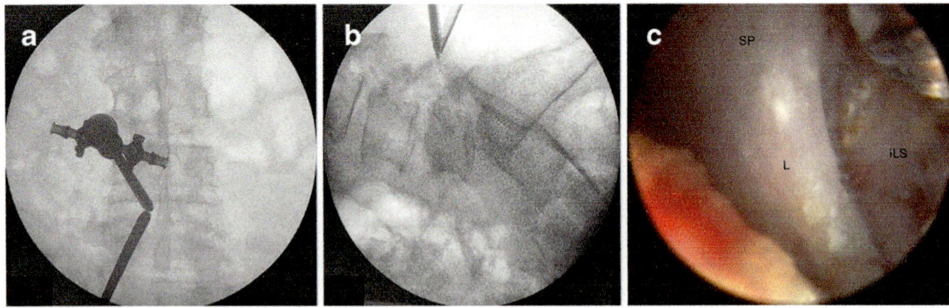

Fig. 7.1 Paramedian approach addressed to the left spinolaminar junction. (**a**) AP view of C-arm showing how two vectors (both ports) are triangled. (**b**) Lateral view of C-arm: the triangulation determines the specific point where the ports join. (**c**) Spinolaminar junction seen through the endoscope. *AP* anteroposterior, *SP* spinous process, *L* lamina, *ILS* interlaminar space

Unilateral Biportal Endoscopic Cervical Approaches

Cervical spondylosis can present with radiculopathy, myelopathy, or cervical pain, concerning the affected anatomical site, such as the intervertebral foramen, the spinal canal, and the intervertebral disc or facet joints [1]. In cases where compression of neural structures is confirmed, the UBE may be an option for its treatment. For example, bilateral decompression through a unilateral laminotomy (ULBD) to resolve central pathologies such as cervical spondylotic myelopathy (CSM), laminoforaminotomy in patients with asymmetric stenosis and foraminotomy for specific radiculopathies are procedures that are usually performed by a surgeon familiarized with the UBE.

Because one of the advantages of UBE is the direct visualization of anatomical structures, the surgeon must be familiar with the following:

1. The deep cervical muscles before reaching the bone elements
2. The bone landmarks to get access and orientation during the endoscopic biportal procedure, those that will appear as a part of the compressive pathology
3. The dorsal and ventral epidural space and how it could be addressed to achieve a successful decompression

Deep Cervical Muscles

The muscles with which the surgeon who intends to perform cervical biportal endoscopy must become familiar are those of the cervical region considered cervical extensors. Particularly, the deep layer of cervical extensor muscles is recognized during any posterior endoscopic biportal approach. These muscles are known as the transversospinalis group, of which rotator and multifidus muscles act as segmental stabilizers, providing posterior support of the cervical lordosis in synergy with the deep flexor muscles, preventing forward head position. These muscles are innervated by the dorsal rami of cervical spinal nerve roots [2]. Therefore, the surgeon must take advantage of the multifidus anatomical characteristics to access the most profound bone elements, preserving the maximum of this muscle.

The multifidus muscle has a superomedial and oblique trajectory and is attached from the spinous process to the transverse process. This can be short or long, depending on how many vertebral bodies its length is, between 2 and 4, respectively (Fig. 7.2a).

However, during the biportal approach, the surgeon addresses the bone elements through a space medial to the multifidus. This space is an interfascicular window filled with fat that gives access to the multifidus's medial and inferior plane, with connective tissue and fat adhered to the periosteum, better known as the epiperiosteal space (Video 7.1). The entry to the epiperiosteal space applies to the thoracic region where the multifidus is more developed and in the lumbar region where the medial window to the multifidus is more extensive (Fig. 7.2b, c).

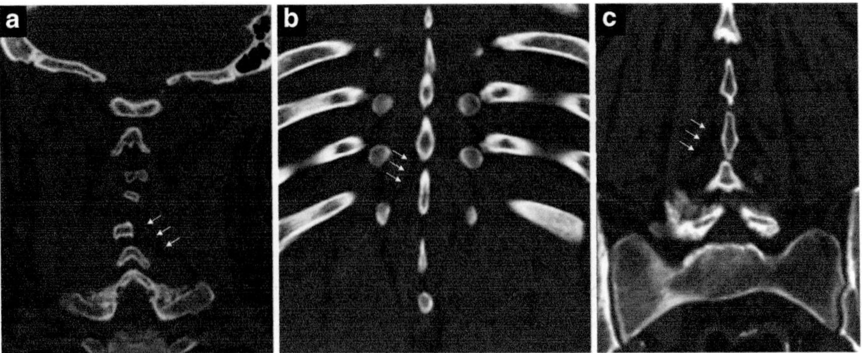

Fig. 7.2 CT coronal views of cervical (**a**), thoracic (**b**), and lumbar (**c**) spine. The white arrows point to the superomedial and oblique trajectory of the multifidus muscle in the different regions. Also, they show the window located medial to the multifidus, through which the biportal approach is performed. *CT* computed tomography

Bony Elements

The spine surgeon widely uses cervical decompression procedures such as foraminotomy, laminoforaminotomy, and laminectomy [1]. However, excessive manipulation of the neural elements in the cervical spine can lead to catastrophic complications [3, 4]. In 2019, Wu et al. analyzed the complications derived from endoscopic and microsurgical foraminotomies of the cervical spine through a systematic review and meta-analysis. The neural injury turned out to be the most common between both groups. In the endoscopic foraminotomy group, transient root palsy accounted for 79.8% of all complications, while in the microsurgical group, dural injury and transient root palsy accounted for 42.6% and 21.3%, respectively. The above indicates that direct anatomy visibility is essential [4].

Therefore, identifying bone structures results in orientation during the UBE procedure and allows successful results with the maximum possible safety. In the cervical spine, this is crucial since the spaces to work are highly reduced compared with the lumbar spine.

The bone landmark most used in UBE of the cervical spine is the V-point, formed by the bony intersection between the lower margin of the cranial lamina and the superior margin of the caudal lamina (Fig. 7.3). However, a more ventral dissection exposes the junction between the ascending portion of the SAP and the descending portion of the IAP (Fig. 7.4).

Identifying these bone structures will allow the surgeon to orient himself or herself and avoid injury to the exiting nerve root or excessive decompression associated with iatrogenic instability since segmental hypermobility after more than 50% of facet joint removed during cervical foraminotomy could result [5, 6].

In cases of central canal stenosis and cervical spondylotic myelopathy, UBE can achieve bilateral decompression. Bilateral extended laminotomy through unilateral access (ULBD) is a standard procedure performed through different minimally invasive techniques such as microsurgical tubular surgery or uniportal endoscopy [7, 8].

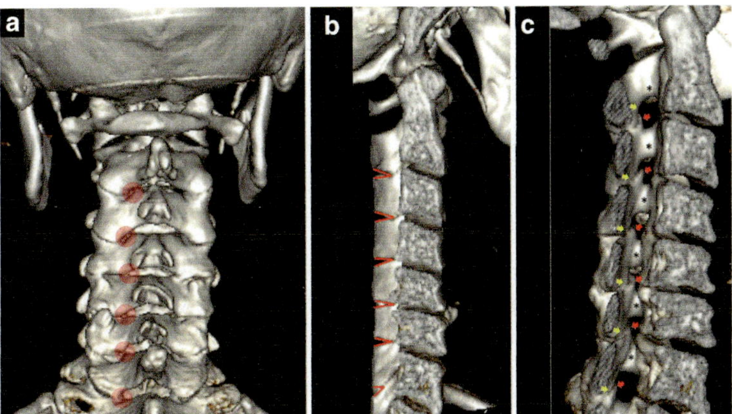

Fig. 7.3 3D CT surface reconstruction of the cervical spine. (**a**) Anteroposterior view of the cervical spine, the left-sided V-point on each segment is circled in red. (**b**) Paraspinous sagittal view of the cervical spine. The laminae are observed from inside of the cervical spinal canal. The red angles are delineating the intersection of cranial and caudal laminae. (**c**) Sagittal view of the cervical spine. The yellow arrows are showing the descendent part of the inferior articular process. The red arrows are pointing out the ventral and ascendent portion of the superior articular process. Asterisks represent the pedicles. *CT* computed tomography

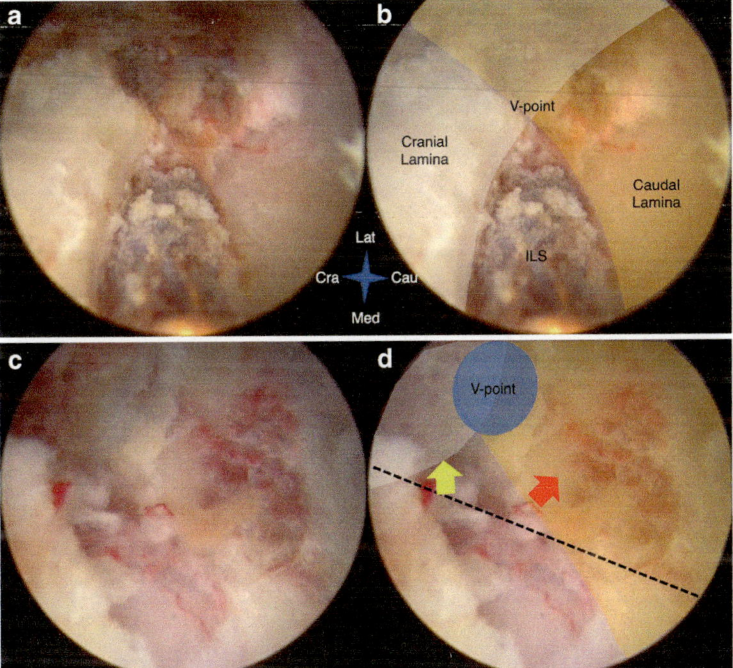

Fig. 7.4 Intraoperative views through the endoscope during a C5–C6 right biportal inclinatory foraminotomy. (**a**) The bone elements that shape the V-point are exposed. (**b**) Representation of anatomical landmarks. (**c**) Left-sided view after drilling through the V-point. (**d**) The dotted black line represents the lateral edge of the thecal sac. The yellow arrow points to the inferior articular process and the red one to the superior articular process. *Cra* cranial, *Cau* caudal, *Lat* lateral, *Med* medial, *ILS* interlaminar space

The bony landmarks identified for the proper execution of cervical UBE-ULBD are the following:

1. V-point, which we have described in detail in previous paragraphs
2. Cranial and caudal laminae
3. Base of the spinous process
4. Contralateral cranial and caudal lamina, observed through the endoscope from a shallower angle

Identifying these bone structures allows an orderly circumferential bone removal along with the attachments of the ligamentum flavum (Fig. 7.5).

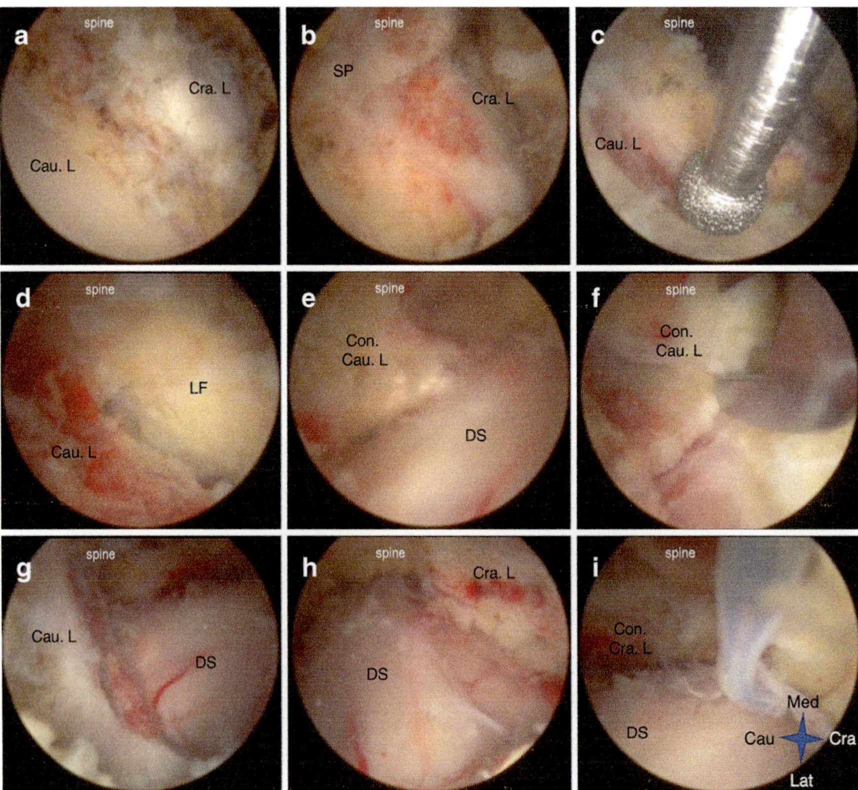

Fig. 7.5 Images from a C4–C5 biportal endoscopic ULBD. (**a**) Cranial and caudal laminae are exposed. (**b**) The ipsilateral cranial lamina and the base of the spinous process were drilled out. (**c**) The ipsilateral caudal lamina is undercut. (**d**) Inferior attachment of ligamentum flavum is exposed. (**e**) The most lateral part of caudal lamina is revealed. (**f**) Undercutting of the contralateral caudal lamina is completed. (**g**) Dural sac exposed after flavectomy. (**h**) Ipsilateral cranial lamina and base of the spinous process undercut. (**i**) Contralateral cranial lamina undercut. *Cra* cranial, *Cau* caudal, *Lat* lateral, *Med* medial, *ULBD* unilateral laminotomy bilateral decompression, *Cra. L* cranial lamina, *Cau. L* caudal lamina, *SP* spinous process, *LF* ligamentum flavum, *Con. Cau. L* contralateral caudal lamina, *Con. Cra. L* contralateral cranial lamina, *DS* dural sac

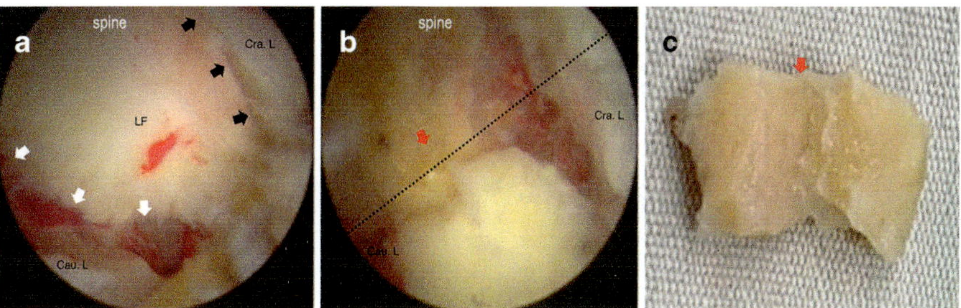

Fig. 7.6 Ligamentum flavum of the cervical spine. (**a**) Endoscopic view of the C4–C5 ipsilateral interlaminar space enlarged. The white arrows point to the caudal detachment of the flavum. The black arrows indicate the cranial attachment of flavum to the upper lamina. (**b**) Endoscopic panoramic view of a cervical interlaminar space. The black dotted line represents the midline, and the red arrow points to the midline cleft. (**c**) Peace of ligamentum flavum removed in block after cervical UBE-ULBD. The red arrow points to the midline cleft. *Cra. L* cranial lamina, *Cau. L* caudal lamina, *LF* ligamentum flavum, *UBE-ULBD* unilateral biportal endoscopic unilateral laminotomy for bilateral decompression

Ligamentum Flavum

The ligamentum flavum protects the dural sac and the exiting nerve root in its most proximal segment within the cervical spinal canal. It is a bilateral connective structure attached in the lower half of the cranial lamina's ventral aspect and the caudal lamina's superior ventral border, which is relevant since further bone remodeling may be necessary to detach it cranially (Fig. 7.6a). The ligamentum flavum fibers are arranged longitudinally in a sagittal direction with a cleft formed by lack of fusion in the midline (Fig. 7.6b, c). These findings can guide the surgeon during bilateral flavectomy since this cleft may indicate the contralateral side. The ligamentum flavum blends in the interspinous ligament and extends laterally, no further than the medial aspect of the pedicle and the SAP. Therefore, it does not enter the cervical intervertebral foramen [9–11]. Thus, during biportal endoscopic foraminotomy, the surgeon should avoid damage to the exiting nerve root with the instruments since no flavum ligament protects it in the intraforaminal segment.

The Epidural Space Through Biportal Endoscopy

The knowledge about epidural space will allow the surgeon to perform endoscopic dissections through the biportal technique safely. After bone removal, the ligamentum flavum is a barrier that must be removed in severe degenerative cases in which it is hypertrophic and directly compresses the neural elements. However, overconfidence using surgical instruments such as Kerrison punches or pituitary forceps could cause damage to the dura or the nerves during the procedure. Traction of the ligamentum flavum with tight adhesions to the dura also increases the risk of a dural tear with well-known consequences. In the same way, injury to perivertebral vascular plexuses without proper coagulation can lead to difficult-to-control bleeding or execution of risky maneuvers to achieve appropriate hemostasis.

The risk of presenting these types of adverse events during biportal endoscopic surgery may decrease if we perform a meticulous endoscopic dissection by planes, and for this, it is necessary to know which structures are found below the flavum beyond the neural elements.

Peridural Membrane

The peridural membrane (PDM) is a well-innervated structure between the dura and the wall of the spinal canal, extending into the intervertebral foramen to form the peri-radicular sheath [12]. This tubelike structure has been described in the cervical, thoracic, and lumbar regions. PDM lines the wall of the spinal canal, including the neuroforamen in which are wrapped the nerve root and the dorsal root ganglion. Then, the PDM continues as a thin peri-radicular sheath containing the exiting nerve. This membrane also contains the epidural vessels in the dorsal and ventral epidural space. It goes deep to the PLL and along with it, and the external PLL attaches to the borders of the disk-annulus complex [13]. The PDM protects neural tissues, preventing the dural tube collapse and avoiding the nerve root strain (Fig. 7.7 and Video 7.2). However, PDM can also provoke radicular symptoms due to disturbance of the nerve root mobility in severe spondylosis, peri-radicular fibrosis after any surgery, or postlaminoplastic tethering effect on the nerve root [14]. Miyauchi et al. described two types of pathological peridural membrane at the cervical spine. Type 1 is a band-like or a membranous constricting structure around the thecal sac,

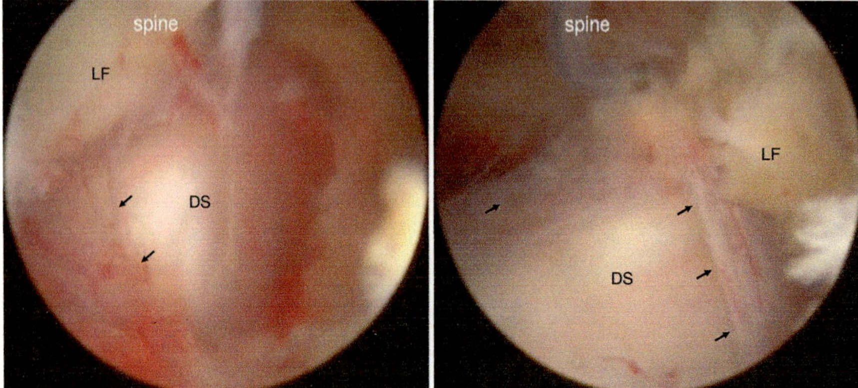

Fig. 7.7 Intraoperative endoscopic view. Both images show the PDM (black arrows) below the ligamentum flavum, lining the dural sac. *DS* dural sac, *LF* ligamentum flavum, *PDM* peridural membrane

avoiding dural expansion even after direct decompression. Type 2 maintains fixed nerve root, inducing radicular symptoms [14].

The former is relevant in the sense that an adequate dissection through the biportal endoscopic technique and the sequential release of the neural elements that may be trapped or anchoring in this pathológical epidural membrane could help to achieve the goals of direct decompression sought, for example, in cases of decompression due to cervical spondylotic myeloradiculopathy. Conversely, this membrane's aggressive release of neural elements can lead to manipulative injury, traction, or inadvertent epidural hemorrhage.

Meningovertebral Ligaments

Different texts have suggested fibrous connective tissue between the dural sac with surrounding structures throughout the spinal epidural space. Luyendijk described a dorsomedial fold of the dural sac caused by attachments of the dural sac to the lamina. However, through an anatomical study of the lumbar epidural space, Blomberg demonstrated that this fold is due to a band of connective tissue between the dural sac with the flavum ligament in the midline [15, 16]. In addition, Hofmann reported membranous bands between the PLL and the ventral dural sac called Hofmann's or meningovertebral ligaments [17].

Knowing the anatomy of these connective tissue bands can improve surgical results derived from direct decompressive procedures or dissections in the epidural space such as those performed through endoscopic techniques, reducing the risk of dural lacerations (Fig. 7.8).

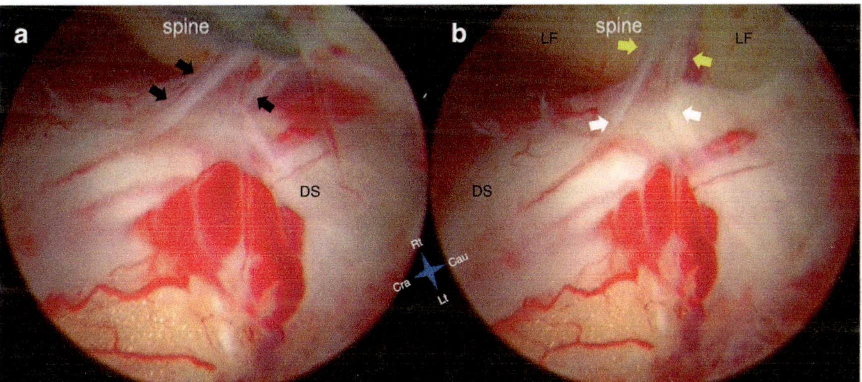

Fig. 7.8 UBE-ULBD C4–C5 procedure, endoscopic view. (**a**) Flavum retracted dorsally, and tight bands (black arrows) between the dural sac and ligamentum flavum are centered in the image. (**b**) The white arrows point to the meningovertebral ligament's dural attachments. The yellow arrows point to the meningovertebral ligament's ligamentum flavum attachments. *Cra* cranial, *Cau* caudal, *Rt* right, *Lt* left, *DS* dural sac, *LF* ligamentum flavum, *UBE-ULBD* biportal endoscopic unilateral laminotomy bilateral decompression

Shi et al. reported thick and tight dorsal meningovertebral ligaments between the dura and ligamentum flavum from C1 to C6. The authors in this study observed spaces between these ligaments filled with loose fat and areolar connective tissue, as well as venous plexuses. The orientation of these cervical dorsal meningovertebral ligaments is craniocaudal, and their location is central and paramedian. The authors also divided four types according to their appearance: strip type, cord type, grid type, and thin slice type. The meningovertebral ligaments are attached to the dorsal dura, so their attachment point in the dura is vulnerable to rupture [18].

Meningovertebral ligaments not only have been observed in the cervical region but have also been found in the thoracic and lumbar spine in ventral, lateral, and dorsal locations regarding the dural sac [19–21]. The anatomical features of the lumbar meningovertebral ligaments are similar to those of the cervical region (Fig. 7.9). In the epidural space of L5–S1, they have been found in greater quantity than other lumbar levels. They have even been classified according to their morphology into five types: strip type, cord type, "Y"-shaped type, grid type, and thin slice type. Some ligaments can have considerable dimensions (length 17.20 mm, width 0.73 mm, and thickness 0.19 mm), especially in L5–S1. That is why during biportal endoscopic flavectomy, the surgeon must attempt a gentle detachment to avoid dural injuries.

At the thoracic level, meningovertebral ligaments have been found and also divided according to their morphology into four types: "Y"-shaped type, stripe type, slice type, and cord type [20]. In addition, the meningovertebral ligaments in the thoracic region are also related to fat and dorsal epidural venous plexuses (Fig. 7.10).

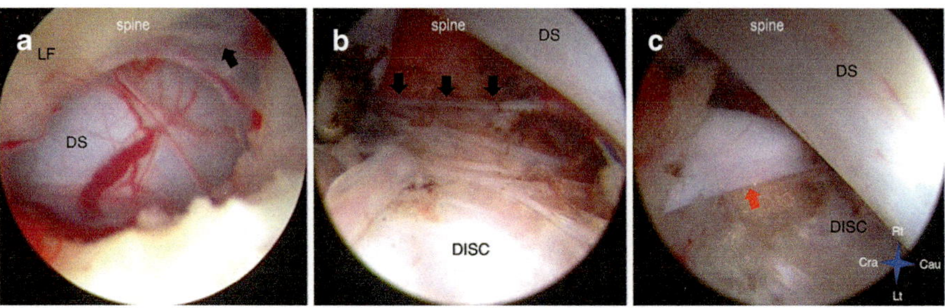

Fig. 7.9 Left L4–L5 lateral recess UBE decompression. (**a**) Part of ligamentum flavum removed, and dorsal epidural space exposed. The black arrow points to a dorsal meningovertebral ligament. (**b**) The black arrows in the ventral epidural space show the so-called Hofmann ligaments or ventral meningovertebral ligaments. (**c**) Considerable dimensions of an epidural ventrolateral venous vessel (red arrow). *Cra* cranial, *Cau* caudal, *Rt* right, *Lt* left, *DS* dural sac, *LF* ligamentum flavum, *UBE* unilateral biportal endoscopy

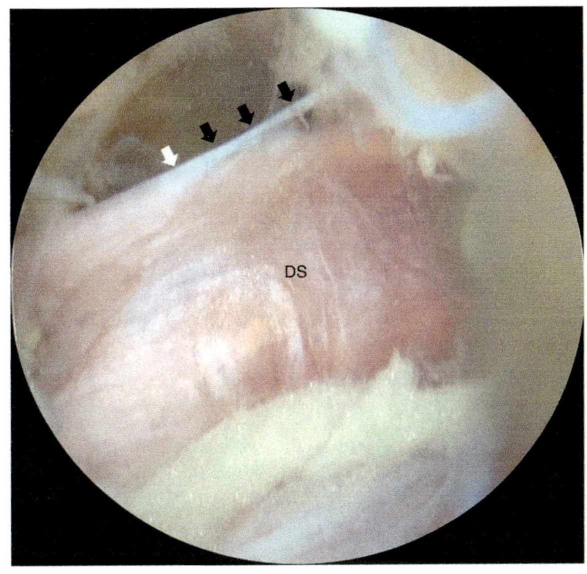

Fig. 7.10 T8–T9 UBE-ULBD. The white arrow points to the meningovertebral ligament's tight dural attachment. The black arrows show the ligament trajectory. *DS* dural sac, *UBE-ULBD* biportal endoscopic unilateral laminotomy bilateral decompression

Vascular Supply and Drainage of Epidural Space

The arterial supply of the dural sac and epidural space follows a bilateral pattern and depends on the ventral division of each dorsal spinal trunk bilaterally, which comes from the corresponding segmental or intercostal arteries (Fig. 7.11).

An arterial arch located below the PLL supplies the posterior surface of the vertebral body. Other arterial branches run into the posterior epidural space to supply the anterior aspect of the lamina and the spinous process. The dorsal division of the dorsal spinal trunk ultimately passes posteriorly and under the ipsilateral transverse process and alongside the outer surface of the lamina, forming an arterial plexus close to the spinous process that provides arterial supply to dorsal muscles (Fig. 7.12a). There are also direct lateral muscle branches from a segmental or intercostal artery [22].

Also, there are intraspinal and extraspinal anastomoses formed at each spinal level and derived from segmental arteries. Transverse anastomoses within the spinal canal are present in the ventral and dorsal epidural space, supplying arterial blood to the dural sac (Fig. 7.12b, c). These epidural branches in the anterior space are recognizable angiographically as a hexagonal arterial pattern or retrocorporeal collateral arch [22].

The cervical region's predominant extravertebral longitudinal anastomotic trunk will establish ascending, vertebral, and deep arterial vascularization [22]. The spinal venous drainage is divided into three compartments—an internal and external venous network and epidural venous plexuses (Fig. 7.11). The epidural veins usually consist of two or more longitudinally interconnected veins in the dorsal and ventral epidural space (Fig. 7.12d). These veins drain into an emissary foraminal vein [22].

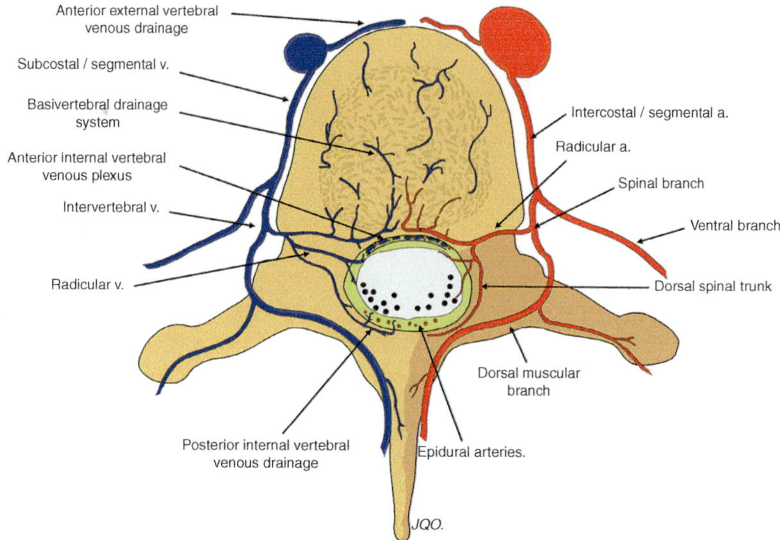

Fig. 7.11 Arterial supply and venous drainage of the spine

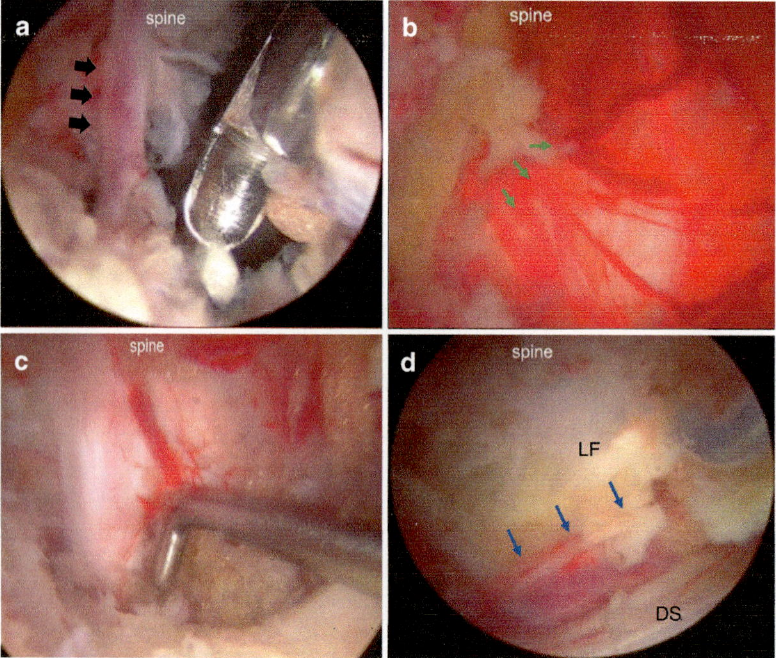

Fig. 7.12 (**a**) The black arrows point to a muscular arterial vessel that comes from the ipsilateral transverse process. (**b**) Endoscopic view of the arterial arch (green arrows) from the ventrolateral epidural space that runs to the dorsal epidural space. (**c**) The neural elements observed after coagulation of the arterial arch showed in (**b**). (**d**) The blue arrows point to a longitudinal, lateral epidural vein. *DS* dural sac, *LF* ligamentum flavum

UBE-Paramedian Lumbar Approach

This approach is of particular interest to the spine surgeon who intends to start the learning curve in biportal endoscopy. This approach was widely described by Eun et al. [23]. However, it has significant historical precedents reviewed in another chapter of this book. The paramedian approach aims to reach the interlaminar space and then address the biportal endoscopic procedure to different objectives depending on the surgical indication.

The procedures derived from the paramedian approach are the following:

1. Lumbar central decompression
2. Decompression of the lateral recess (ipsilateral)
3. Unilateral laminotomy and bilateral decompression
4. Subspinous and sublaminar contralateral decompression to reach the lateral recess, foraminal, and extraforaminal areas

All these procedures will be described in specific chapters of this book.

Overview

The surgical technique consists of placing the patient prone over the abdominal support frame, and the procedure can be done under general anesthesia, epidural or conscious sedation, depending on the surgeon's experience, planned operative time, and patient features. The C-arm is required during the surgery. Then, an orthogonal AP view to locate the interlaminar space of the index level is done.

It is advisable to place the incisions as follows: A medial interpedicular line of the index level is drawn in the skin. Then, the midline is also marked. The intervertebral space is projected in the skin and drawn. It will allow the surgeon guidance during the approach. The superior and inferior incisions are located slightly lateral to the medial interpedicular line, which generally occurs between 1 and 1.5 cm lateral to the midline and at the level of the superior and inferior pedicles, respectively. Thus, the distance between both incisions is usually around 2.5–3 cm (Fig. 7.13a). Subsequently, a 5–7 mm longitudinal or transverse incision in the skin and thoracolumbar fascia is sufficient in length for inferior and superior incisions. In this chapter, we focus on the general technical aspects of the paramedian approach.

The surgeon introduces a blunt-tip dilator of 6 mm outer diameter through the incision used as a working portal. In the left-side approach, the inferior incision is intended for this purpose. On the right side is the contrary. The dilator is addressed to the inferior third of upper lamina and the spinous process junction in a caudocranial and lateromedial trajectory. This trajectory enables the dilator to be inserted, and a working channel is created medially to the multifidus muscle. The surgeon can enlarge the space medial to the multifidus with soft lateral movements with the dilator tip. Finally, the position of the dilator is confirmed in an AP fluoroscopic projection, and the semi-tubular working sheath is advanced along the dilator (Fig. 7.13b).

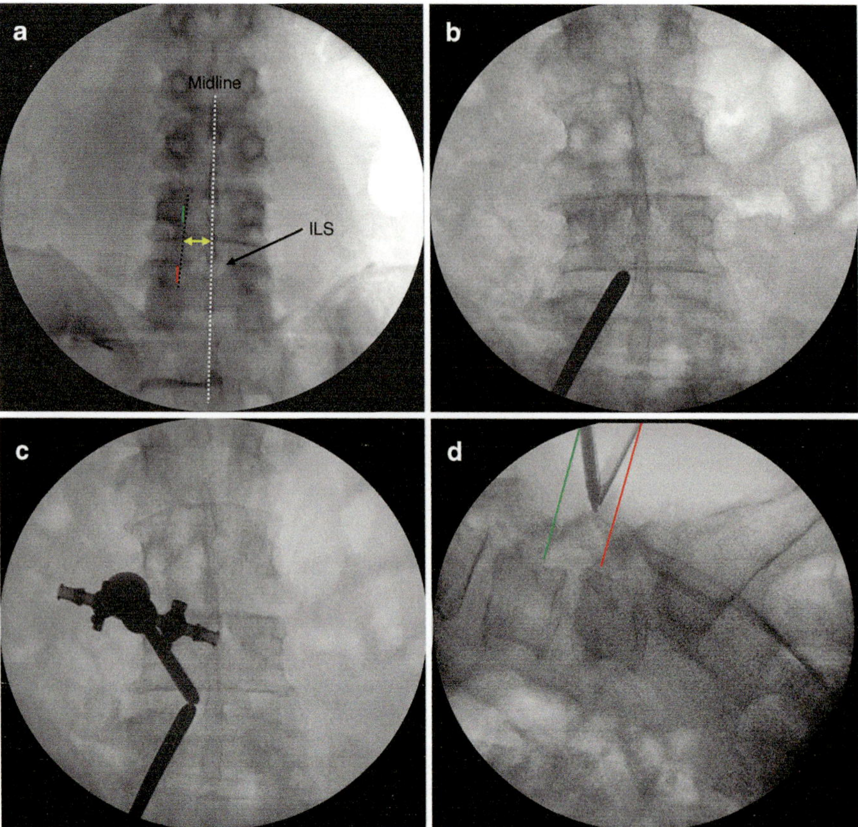

Fig. 7.13 Left paramedian biportal approach. (**a**) An orthogonal AP fluoroscopic view showing the lumbar spine. The cranial and caudal incisions were drawn in green and red lines, respectively. The bi-arrow yellow line represents the distance between the midline and the medial interpedicular line (black dotted line). (**b**) Dilator introduced through the caudal incision. (**c**) Endoscopic trocar introduced through the cranial incision. (**d**) Lateral view obtained from C-arm showing a paramedian lumbar biportal approach. Green and red lines show the cranial and caudal incision planned between both pedicles of the index level. *ILS* interlaminar space

When the thoracic spine is approached, the surgeon should palpate the lamina and feel it with the dilator, but keeping in mind that the thoracic lamina is the highest and thickest than the other areas of the spine, which means that the space between incisions could be a little bit larger than ordinary, especially in the more caudal thoracic levels, with T2 being the least and T11 the highest. Here, the attachments of the ligamentum flavum remain similar to those in the cervical spine. The ligamentum flavum attaches to the cranial lamina's ventral aspect and the caudal lamina's superior border in the thoracic region.

Xu et al. studied 851 vertebrae and reported results of the laminae anatomy from C2 to L5. Measurements were larger in male than female specimens. The highest lamina was T11 (25.1 ± 2.5 mm), and the lowest was C4. From T9 to L4, the height is between 20 and 25 mm. In L5, the height decreases to 16.6 mm [24].

The widest lamina was seen at L5 (15.7 ± 2.0 mm), and the smallest was at T4 (5.8 ± 0.8 mm). The width of the laminae decreases progressively from C3 to T4. From there, it progressively increases to L5. The slightest width angle of the lamina was seen at L3 (99.9 ± 6.3°), and from there, it increased to L5 (106 ± 10.2°) [24]. It is crucial since a more medial entry during UBE at L3 may be sufficient to cross to the contralateral side undercutting the spinous process. However, a more lateral approach may be necessary at L5 because its width angle is more significant. Based on the anatomy described, the ipsilateral lateral recess decompression through a UBE-paramedian approach will require more lateral bone remodeling in upper lumbar segments than in lower ones (Video 7.3).

Another study showed that the width of the interlaminar space increases in lower lumbar levels, and the height of the interlaminar space increases in upper lumbar segments [25]. In this situation, it is crucial to feel not only the inferior edge of the cranial lamina with the dilator but also its union with the spinous process, especially in upper segments where the interlaminar space is narrower; this will guide the surgeon and will be a point of confluence between the endoscope trocar and dilator.

The endoscope trocar will be inserted craniocaudally and lateromedially through the superior incision of the biportal approach. Next, the surgeon must palpate the upper lamina of the index level with the trocar's blunt tip and complete the instruments' triangulation with both hands, which will be confirmed by fluoroscopy using AP and lateral views. At this point, it is crucial that the surgeon feels the tips of both instruments touching and together palpating the spinolaminar junction. Finally, the surgeon can introduce the endoscope inside the trocar for starting the surgery (Fig. 7.13c, d).

Through the endoscope, the surgeon can identify connective tissue and fat. The radiofrequency probe can control any slight bleeding until the bone limits, and the interlaminar space can be observed (Video 7.4).

The authors recommend that the spinolaminar junction always be identified (Fig. 7.1c); this bone landmark will guide the surgeon and direct his or her approach towards any other bone structure of the posterior joint complex.

The ligamentum flavum in the lumbar spine is a structure that the surgeon performing the UBE-paramedian approach will deal with. One study concluded that the ligamentum flavum does not have a two-layer arrangement, but rather the so-called superficial layer is an extension of the interspinous ligament, which attaches laterally to the zygapophyseal joints [10].

When dissecting the ligamentum flavum in the lumbar region, the surgeon can observe through the biportal endoscopic approach that the interspinous portion (superficial layer) of the ligamentum flavum reaches the dorsal surfaces of cranial and caudal laminae. For this reason, it is necessary to detach it to visualize these bone elements during circumferential bone decompression, for example, in UBE-ULBD. The interlaminar portion or the so-called deep layer of the ligamentum flavum usually has a more extensive attachment on the ventral aspect of the cranial lamina, covering more of its surface than on the caudal lamina. The ligamentum flavum laterally extends until it meets the capsular ligament on the anteromedial surface of the SAP [10]. That is why when a lateral decompression is performed, it must be detached to observe the most medial part of the SAP.

Tips for a Left-Sided Paramedian Approach

1. Keep in mind that the biportal approach aims not to make a perfect triangle.
2. An essential feature about the triangle is where it is addressed, not the distance between the portals.
3. The most important step during triangulation is to place both portals independently but towards the same landmark. This ensures a perfect functional triangulation (Fig. 7.14).

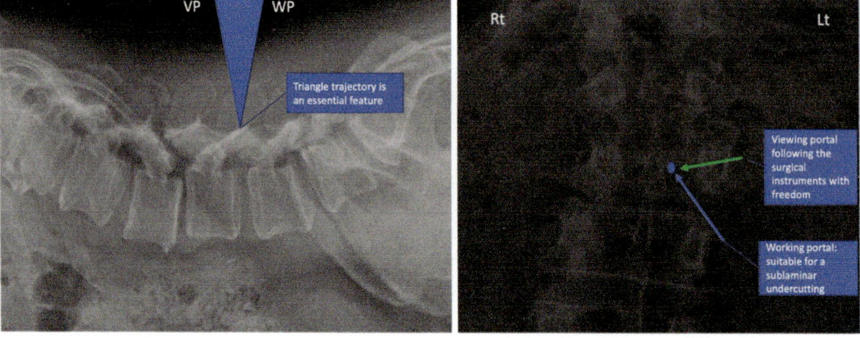

Fig. 7.14 Lateral and AP view of the lumbar X-rays showing a left biportal endoscopic paramedian approach addressed to the spinolaminar junction (blue circle). *VP* viewing portal, *WP* working portal, *Rt* right, *Lt* left

Tips for a Right-Sided Paramedian Approach

1. The surgeon must create the working portal regarding the surgical target in addition to considering radiological references such as the lateral edge of the pedicles.
2. Both ports are created slightly more caudal on the right side than on the left side.
3. The surgeon should consider the trajectory of the triangulation in the preoperative plan. The triangle trajectory depends on the working channel addressed.
4. The most important thing for the surgeon is to plan the working portal properly, and the viewing portal depends on the first (Fig. 7.15).

These recommendations can be effective in a right-handed surgeon determining how the biportal approach's triangulation is on each side (right or left) (Fig. 7.16).

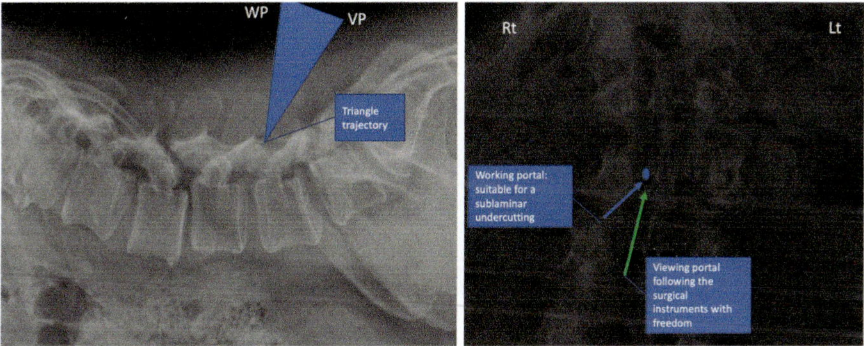

Fig. 7.15 Lateral and AP views of the lumbar X-rays showing a right biportal endoscopic paramedian approach addressed to the spinolaminar junction (blue circle). *WP* working portal, *VP* viewing portal, *Rt* right, *Lt* left

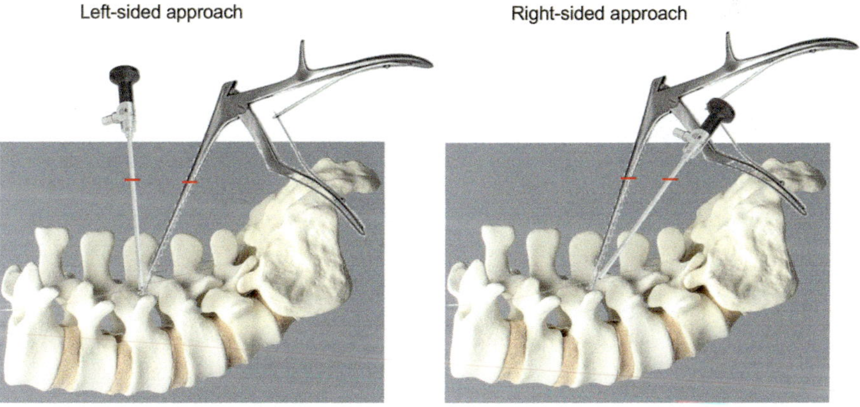

Fig. 7.16 Unilateral biportal endoscopic paramedian approach for both sides

UBE-Paraspinal Lumbar Approach

For the spine surgeon, the paraspinal approach is a familiar technique. Wiltse et al. described a direct route between the multifidus and longissimus muscle to reach the lamina's most lateral part, the laminofacetal junction, and the foraminal area through transforaminal procedures via posterior approach [26]. The procedure-related advantages seen in patients who underwent a paraspinal approach compared with midline spine procedure were a decreased risk of wound breakdown and infection, less blood loss, and fewer reoperations, and the risk of adjacent segment failure in short posterior constructs is lower in those who underwent spinal fusion through Wiltse approach [27]. The biportal endoscopic approach makes it possible to use the route described by Wiltse and more lateral modifications through the longissimus and iliocostalis muscle reported by other expert authors in UBE [28–30].

The indications of UBE through a paraspinal approach are the same as in conventional surgery:

1. Lumbar foraminal stenosis
2. Lumbar extraforaminal degenerative pathology (extraforaminal lumbar disc herniation)
3. Far-lateral degenerative pathologies (far-lateral lumbar disc herniation, far-out syndrome at L5–S1)
4. Biportal endoscopic transforaminal lumbar interbody fusion
5. Symptomatic lumbar facet joint syndrome (biportal endoscopic facet medial branch rhizotomy)
6. Revision surgery requiring a paraspinal entry (repositioning transpedicular screws under direct biportal endoscopic vision, foraminal restenosis in a fused segment, and foraminal stenosis due to adjacent segment disease)

Overview

Like other posterior thoracolumbar approaches, the patient is prone over the abdominal support frame, and the procedure can be done under general anesthesia, epidural or conscious sedation, depending on the surgeon's experience, planned operative time, and patient features. The C-arm is required throughout the surgery. Then, an orthogonal AP view is done to locate the intertransverse space and the well-defined ipsilateral pedicles' outline of the index level. Depending on surgical goals, the paraspinal biportal approach can be performed slightly lateral to the pedicle contour or 3 cm lateral, which means to perform a Wiltse-type or a lateral modified paraspinal approach, respectively (Fig. 7.17a).

Then, the caudal incision, used in the left-sided paraspinal approach as a working channel, will be located lateral to the pedicle silhouette over the inferior transverse process of the index level. A 5–7 mm longitudinal or transverse incision in the skin

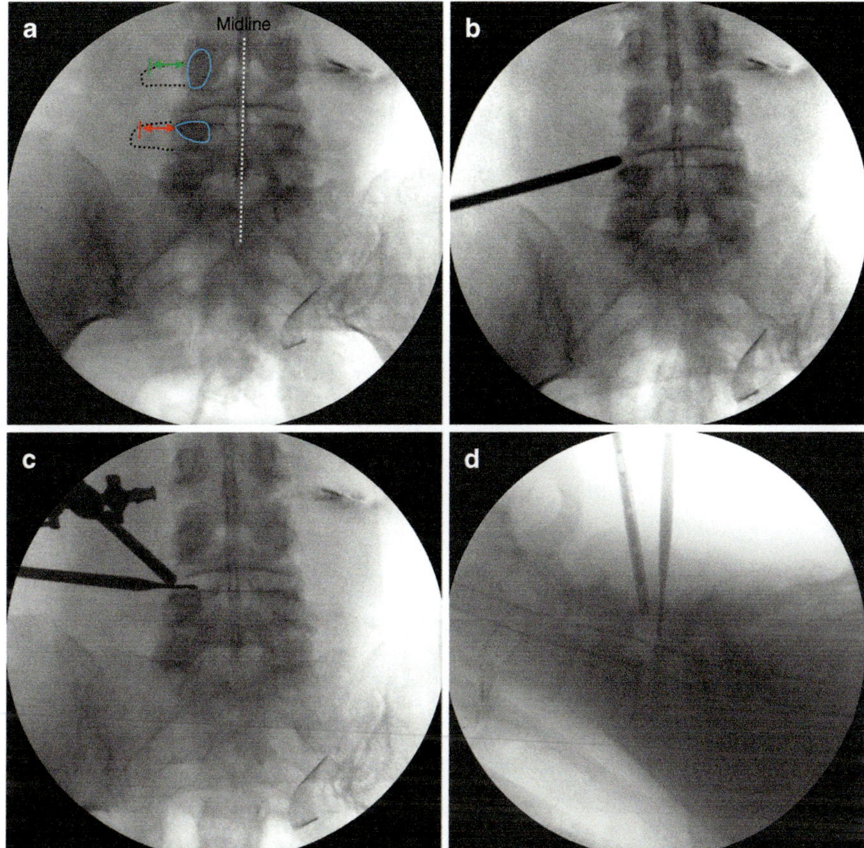

Fig. 7.17 The paraspinal biportal approach. (**a**) An orthogonal AP fluoroscopic view showing the lumbar spine. The cranial and caudal incisions were drawn in green and red lines, respectively. The bi-arrow green and red lines represent the distance between the lateral wall of the pedicle and the biportal entries. The pedicles are outlined in blue. The transverse processes are outlined with a black dotted line. (**b**) Dilator introduced through the caudal incision. (**c**) The endoscope passes through the cranial incision and (**d**) is confirmed with a lateral C-arm view

and fascia is done. The incision is slightly larger in unilateral biportal endoscopic transforaminal fusion cases to introduce the intervertebral cage and transpedicular screw.

The dilator will be inserted caudocranial and lateromedial through the caudal incision, and with it, the surgeon will palpate the junction of the inferior transverse process and the facet joint of the index level. However, if a foraminotomy was planned, the dilator could be addressed to the superior transverse process. More details about unilateral biportal endoscopic lumbar foraminotomy will be discussed in another chapter.

Careful dissection is recommended since a facet joint artery branch that comes directly from the segmental artery can be damaged, causing bleeding. The surgeon should not damage the intertransverse muscle membrane during dissection with the initial dilator since it is a safety margin towards the retroperitoneal space. The anatomical safety margins will always be bony structures. In this biportal paraspinal approach, the initial dilator could land at one of these three points: the proximal surface of the superior or inferior transverse process or the lateral and superior margin of the SAP of the index level (Fig. 7.17b), depending on surgical objectives.

The cranial incision is located lateral to the superior pedicle over the transverse process of the index level. A 5–7 mm transverse or longitudinal incision in the skin and fascia is sufficient to introduce the endoscopic system. In unilateral biportal endoscopic transforaminal fusion cases, the incision is slightly larger to introduce the transpedicular screw. The endoscope trocar will be inserted craniocaudally and lateromedially through the cranial incision. Next, the surgeon must feel the facet joint of the index level with the trocar and subsequently complete the triangulation of the instruments with both hands, confirmed by fluoroscopy using AP and lateral views (Fig. 7.17c, d).

The surgeon should identify anatomical landmarks usually seen in the biportal endoscopic paraspinal approach. For example, the ventrolateral surface of SAP and superior/inferior transverse processes can be observed depending on the craniocaudal approach trajectory and its purposes, and another important landmark is the foraminal ligamentum flavum since below this is the exiting nerve (Fig. 7.18).

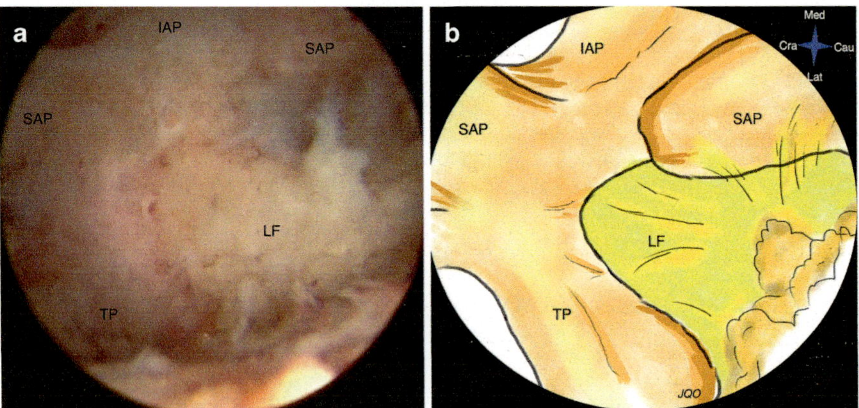

Fig. 7.18 Left L4–L5 UBE-paraspinal approach. (**a**) Endoscopic view of the paraspinal area. (**b**) Anatomic scheme of the paraspinal area showing the bone landmarks observed through the endoscope. *UBE* unilateral biportal endoscopy, *Cra* cranial, *Cau* caudal, *Med* medial, *Lat* lateral, *SAP* superior articular process, *IAP* inferior articular process, *TP* transverse process, *LF* ligamentum flavum

Conclusion

There are different approaches through the UBE technique to treat a broad spectrum of cervical, lumbar, and thoracic degenerative diseases. However, an essential advantage of UBE is the direct visualization of anatomy and pathology. For this reason, it should pay off in guidance for the surgeon and safety for the patient during any biportal endoscopic procedure.

References

1. Theodore N. Degenerative cervical spondylosis. N Engl J Med. 2020;383(2):159–68.
2. Smith AC, Albin SR, Abbott R, et al. Confirming the geography of fatty infiltration in the deep cervical extensor muscles in whiplash recovery. Sci Rep. 2020;10(1):11471.
3. Kim JY, Kim DH, Lee YJ, et al. Anatomical importance between neural structure and bony landmark: clinical importance for posterior endoscopic cervical foraminotomy. Neurospine. 2021;18(1):139–46.
4. Wu PF, Liu BH, Wang B, et al. Complications of full-endoscopic versus microendoscopic foraminotomy for cervical radiculopathy: a systematic review and meta-analysis. World Neurosurg. 2018;114:217–27.
5. Zdeblick TA, Zou D, Warden KE, McCabe R, Kunz D, Vanderby R. Cervical stability after foraminotomy. A biomechanical in vitro analysis. J Bone Joint Surg Am. 1992;74(1):22–7.
6. Chen BH, Natarajan RN, An HS, Andersson GB. Comparison of biomechanical response to surgical procedures used for cervical radiculopathy: posterior keyhole foraminotomy versus anterior foraminotomy and discectomy versus anterior discectomy with fusion. J Spinal Disord. 2001;14(1):17–20.
7. Hernandez RN, Wipplinger C, Navarro-Ramirez R, et al. Ten-step minimally invasive cervical decompression via unilateral tubular laminotomy: technical note and early clinical experience. Oper Neurosurg (Hagerstown). 2020;18(3):284–94.
8. Carr DA, Abecassis IJ, Hofstetter CP. Full endoscopic unilateral laminotomy for bilateral decompression of the cervical spine: surgical technique and early experience. J Spine Surg. 2020;6(2):447–56.
9. Lirk P, Kolbitsch C, Putz G, et al. Cervical and high thoracic ligamentum flavum frequently fails to fuse in the midline. Anesthesiology. 2003;99(6):1387–90.
10. Iwanaga J, Ishak B, Saga T, et al. The lumbar ligamentum flavum does not have two layers and is confluent with the interspinous ligament: anatomical study with application to surgical and interventional pain procedures. Clin Anat. 2020;33:34–40.
11. Rahmani MS, Terai H, Akhgar J, et al. Anatomical analysis of human ligamentum flavum in the cervical spine: special consideration to the attachments, coverage, and lateral extent. J Orthop Sci. 2017;22(6):994–1000.
12. Bosscher HA, Grozdanov PN, Warraich II, MacDonald CC, Day MR. The peridural membrane of the spine has characteristics of synovium. Anat Rec (Hoboken). 2021;304(3):631–46.
13. Wiltse LL. Anatomy of the extradural compartments of the lumbar spinal canal. Peridural membrane and circumneural sheath. Radiol Clin N Am. 2000;38(6):1177–206.
14. Miyauchi A, Sumida T, Manabe H, Mikami Y, Kaneko M, Sumen Y, Ochi M. Morphological features and clinical significance of epidural membrane in the cervical spine. Spine (Phila Pa 1976). 2012;37(19):E1182–8.
15. Luyendijk W. Canalography. Roentgenological examination of the peridural space in the lumbo-sacral part of the vertebral canal. J Belg Radiol. 1963;46:236–54.

16. Blomberg R. The dorsomedian connective tissue band in the lumbar epidural space of humans: an anatomical study using epiduroscopy in autopsy cases. Anesth Analg. 1986;65(7):747–52.
17. Hofmann M. Die befestigung der dural sacim wirbelcanal. Arch F Anat Physio (Anat ABT). 1898;18:403–12.
18. Shi B, Zheng X, Min S, Zhou Z, Ding Z, Jin A. The morphology and clinical significance of the dorsal meningovertebra ligaments in the cervical epidural space. Spine J. 2014;14(11):2733–9.
19. Shi B, Li X, Li H, Ding Z. The morphology and clinical significance of the dorsal meningovertebra ligaments in the lumbosacral epidural space. Spine (Phila Pa 1976). 2012;37(18):E1093–8.
20. Chen R, Shi B, Zheng X, et al. Anatomic study and clinical significance of the dorsal meningovertebral ligaments of the thoracic dura mater. Spine (Phila Pa 1976). 2015;40(10):692–8.
21. Scapinelli R. Anatomical and radiologic studies on the lumbosacral meningo-vertebral ligaments of humans. J Spinal Disord. 1990;3(1):6–15.
22. Becske T, Nelson PK. The vascular anatomy of the vertebro-spinal axis. Neurosurg Clin N Am. 2009;20(3):259–64.
23. Eun SS, Eum JH, Lee SH, Sabal LA. Biportal endoscopic lumbar decompression for lumbar disk herniation and spinal canal stenosis: a technical note. J Neurol Surg A Cent Eur Neurosurg. 2017;78(4):390–6.
24. Xu R, Burgar A, Ebraheim NA, Yeasting RA. The quantitative anatomy of the laminas of the spine. Spine (Phila Pa 1976). 1999;24(2):107–13.
25. Sakçı Z, Önen MR, Fidan E, Yaşar Y, Uluğ H, Naderi S. Radiologic anatomy of the lumbar interlaminar window and surgical considerations for lumbar interlaminar endoscopic and microsurgical disc surgery. World Neurosurg. 2018;115:e22–6.
26. Wiltse LL, Spencer CW. New uses and refinements of the paraspinal approach to the lumbar spine. Spine (Phila Pa 1976). 1988;13(6):696–706.
27. Street JT, Andrew Glennie R, Dea N, et al. A comparison of the Wiltse versus midline approaches in degenerative conditions of the lumbar spine. J Neurosurg Spine. 2016;25(3):332–8.
28. Heo DH, Eum JH, Jo JY, Chung H. Modified far lateral endoscopic transforaminal lumbar interbody fusion using a biportal endoscopic approach: technical report and preliminary results. Acta Neurochir. 2021;163(4):1205–9.
29. Ahn JS, Lee HJ, Choi DJ, Lee KY, Hwang SJ. Extraforaminal approach of biportal endoscopic spinal surgery: a new endoscopic technique for transforaminal decompression and discectomy. J Neurosurg Spine. 2018;28(5):492–8.
30. Quillo-Olvera J, Quillo-Reséndiz J, Quillo-Olvera D, Barrera-Arreola M, Kim JS. Ten-step biportal endoscopic transforaminal lumbar interbody fusion under computed tomography-based intraoperative navigation: technical report and preliminary outcomes in Mexico. Oper Neurosurg (Hagerstown). 2020;19(5):608–18.

Chapter 8
Basic Principles of Unilateral Biportal Endoscopic Surgery: Intraoperative Radiation Exposure During UBE Procedures

Xinchun Liu

Abbreviations

ALARA	As low as reasonably achievable
AP	Anteroposterior
CT	Computed tomography
DNA	Deoxyribonucleic acid
MIS	Minimally invasive spine
MRI	Magnetic resonance imaging
OEL	Occupational exposure limit
PESSTS	Percutaneous endoscopic spine surgery through saline
TLIF	Transforaminal lumbar interbody fusion
UBE	Unilateral biportal endoscopy

Introduction

Intraoperative radiation is inevitable nowadays in spine surgeries when the localization of the target segment, the position of the spinal instrumentation, the distribution of the bone cement, the introduction of minimally invasive surgical tools, or the spine alignment need to be confirmed in intraoperative fluoroscopic imaging studies. Radiation exposure is a significant concern for the patients, surgeons, and personnel in the operation room [1, 2]. During the exposure, radiation acts in a direct

X. Liu (✉)
Department of Orthopedics, The First Hospital of China Medical University, Shenyang, Liaoning Province, People's Republic of China
e-mail: xcliu@cmu.edu.cn

J. Quillo-Olvera et al. (eds.), *Unilateral Biportal Endoscopy of the Spine*,
https://doi.org/10.1007/978-3-031-14736-4_8

or scattered way. Ionizing radiation from intraoperative imaging leads to cellular damage through the induction of direct or indirect DNA lesions and the production of reactive oxygen species [3, 4]. The pathologic effects manifest as deterministic effects including hair loss, skin erythema, skin burns, and cataract formation or stochastic effects including carcinogenesis and teratogenesis [2].

Minimally invasive spine (MIS) surgery is becoming well accepted by the patients and the surgeons with smaller incisions, less blood loss, quicker return to daily activities, decreased postoperative pain medication requirements, and increased visualization [5]. Although the enthusiasm for minimally invasive approaches to the spine has grown substantially, the MIS technique usually relies heavily on intraoperative fluoroscopy navigation. MIS lumbar surgeries expose the surgeon to significantly more radiation than open surgery [6].

As one of the MIS techniques, percutaneous endoscopic spine surgery through saline media (PESSTS) can provide perfect solutions for disc herniation [7–10], stenosis [11–15], and instability of the spine [16–19]. Basically, PESSTS can be performed through posterolateral transforaminal approaches or posterior interlaminar approaches with a uniportal spinal endoscope or a biportal arthroscope. In transforaminal approaches, the radiation exposure is roughly thought to be similar to MIS pedicle screw insertion and MIS TLIF, whereas the radiation dose in PESSTS is somewhat less than that in percutaneous vertebroplasty or kyphoplasty [20]. At the same time, it seems that more radiation exposure exists in posterolateral transforaminal approaches than in posterior interlaminar approaches [21–22].

Unilateral biportal endoscopic spinal surgery (UBE) is performed using the posterior approach with an arthroscope [10, 14, 23]. The intraoperative radiation exposures during the UBE procedures happen mainly during the establishment of the surgical corridors. In other situations, confirmation of the decompression range or the position of the intervertebral surgical tools and implants usually needs fluoroscopic image guidance. The UBE procedures will be introduced in the following chapters including the lumbar spine, cervical spine, and thoracic spine. This chapter gives a general view of intraoperative radiation exposure during UBE procedures. Similarly, as one of the posterior approaches, the radiation exposure in the UBE procedures has been proven less than posterolateral transforaminal approaches [24]. It is estimated that the number of cases for UBE was 9519 for the whole body, 1208 for the hand, and 1125 for the eye according to the latest yearly occupational exposure limit (OEL) by the National Council on Radiation Protection and Measurements. However, according to the radiation exposure guidelines ALARA (as low as reasonably achievable), efforts should still be made to decrease the exposure as much as possible [25].

Strategies for Intraoperative Radiation Protection During UBE Procedures

There are three different types of ionizing radiation exposure in the operating room: the primary X-ray beam, scattered X-rays, and leakage X-rays. The primary X-ray beam usually affects the patient. Although exposure to the patient is inevitable, a specially designed lead radiation protector is used to reduce unintended radiation as much as possible [26]. The surgeons and other medical staff in the operating room are usually affected by the scattered X-rays and leakage X-rays with the lower dose. However, the cumulative effect should draw the greatest attention. A 29% incidence of cancer was reported among the orthopedic surgeons who were exposed to radiation compared to a 4% incidence of cancer among the workers who were not exposed to radiation [27]. The following contents focus on the reduction of medical staff radiation exposure.

Use Wearable Radiation Protective Equipment

Various types of protective devices have been developed to shield staff from radiation exposure, such as aprons, thyroid shields, gloves, and eyewear (Fig. 8.1a). Although many radiation protection tools come with drawbacks, such as heavy and uncomfortable, shields should be used whenever possible to keep personnel exposure as low as reasonably achievable without lengthening the procedure or compromising patient safety [28].

Use Non-wearable Shields

A mobile shield mounted on wheels can be used (Fig. 8.1a). The radiation is eliminated in the shadow of the shield. If possible, the surgeon and operating room personnel can step out of the operating room and the radiation-protective doors and walls of the room are used as shields. In this way, nearly complete protection from radiation can be acquired. But it is not fully protected if the surgeon stands in a substerile room with an unleaded door during imaging [6].

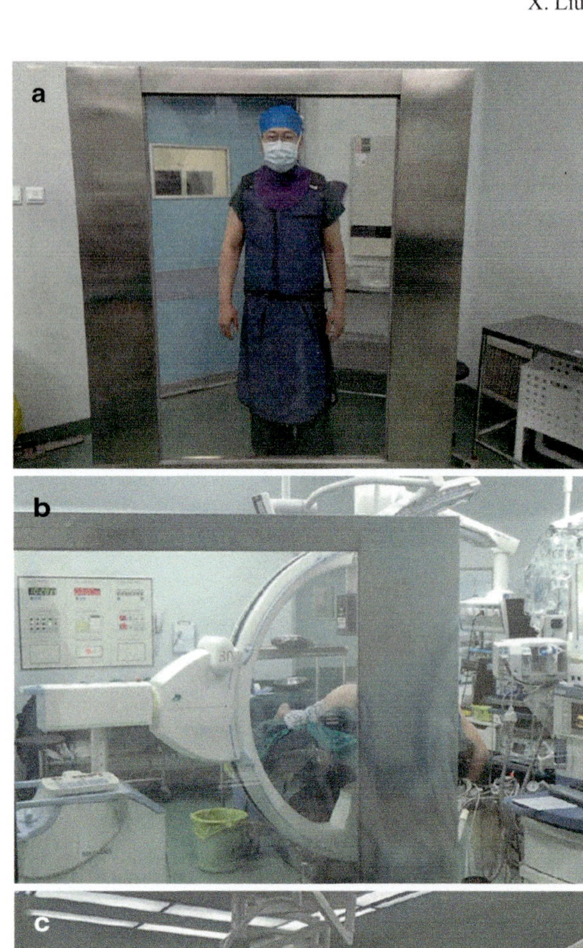

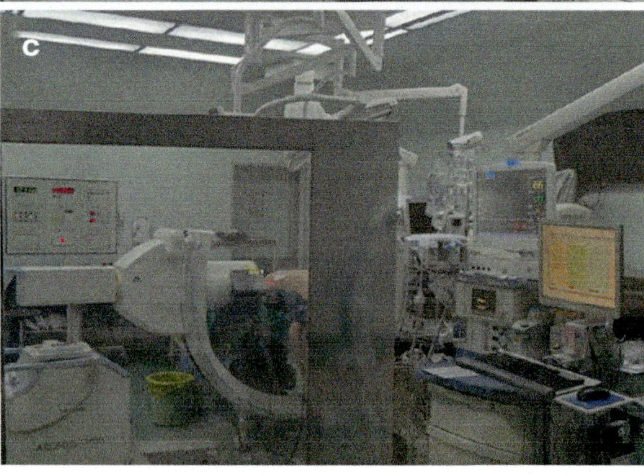

Fig. 8.1 The C-arm and shield are set up in the operating room. (**a**) Wearable and non-wearable shields. (**b**) AP views are obtained with the X-ray tube on the bottom. (**c**) Lateral views are obtained with the medical staff standing on the side of the transmitted beam behind a mobile shield during the X-ray exposure

Maximize the Distance

This principle derives from the fact that radiation intensity follows an inverse square law, decreasing substantially with increasing distance from the radiation or scatter source [29]. For scatter radiation, radiation doses decreased according to the distance from the central radiation beam [30]. The distance between the patient surface and the surgeon or the operative room personnel should be maximized.

Use the "Hands-Off" Technique

Hand exposure is significantly higher in minimally invasive spine surgeries compared to open surgeries [6]. Although sterile protective surgical gloves provide radiation attenuation levels in the range of 15–30%, studies have shown that they provide minimal protection when hands are placed in the primary X-ray beam. Forward and backscattered X-rays within the glove add to hand exposure [28]. Whenever possible, the surgeon should move their hands out of the primary X-ray beam.

Setup with the X-Ray Tube on the Bottom

With the X-ray tube on the bottom, most of the scattered radiation is towards the legs and feet of the surgeon [25]. In this way, the radiation to vital organs will be reduced (Fig. 8.1b).

Stand on the Side of the Transmitted Beam

Surgeons who stand on the same side of the table as the X-ray source were exposed to significantly more radiation than those who did not [6] (Fig. 8.1c).

Reduce Fluoroscopic Dose

Dose reduction techniques such as intermittent exposures, last image hold, dose spreading, beam filtration, pulsed fluoroscopy, and others should be used [31]. Although using pulsed and low-dose settings does pose a risk for producing lower image quality, pulsed and low-dose fluoroscopy modes reduce overall exposure times by 56.7% [32].

Wear Dosimeters

All surgeons and medical staff are exposed to cumulative doses of ionizing radiation. Dosimeters should be used to monitor their annual exposure. This monitoring enables medical professionals to take actions to keep their occupational radiation exposure as low as reasonably achievable, especially when increased doses are measured [33].

Tricks to Avoid Unintended Radiation Exposure

Make a Reasonable Preoperative Planning

Reasonable preoperative planning relies on careful reading and understanding of the preoperative imaging studies. The preoperative imaging studies (X-ray plain radiograph, CT, MRI) should be carefully read. The accurate position of the pathological target (usually the disc herniation or the stenosis) should be clearly identified. The approach-related anatomical features should be noticed such as the position and the size of the interlaminar window, the hypertrophy of the facet joints, the direction of the spinous processes, and the mutual spatial location relationships between the pathological target and palpable surface bony markers. A reasonable surgical plan will smooth the operation and reduce the incidence of unnecessary radiation exposure.

Obtain "Standard" AP and Lateral of Radiographic Views of the Target Segment

In order to increase the accuracy of fluoroscopic guided percutaneous procedures, the "standard" AP and lateral radiographic views of the target segment are important. Owing to the walls and ground of the operating room being used as references, the direction which is perpendicular or parallel to the ground is easy to be identified and controlled by the surgeon. During the surgery, the C-arm radiation beam is used perpendicular or parallel to the ground. Then the patient is coordinated with the C-arm by setting the axial plane of the target intervertebral disc space perpendicular to the ground and the coronal plane parallel to the ground. Thus, the "standard" fluoroscopic views are obtained. In the "standard" fluoroscopic images, the surface radiopaque markers will accurately reflect the inner spinal structures, which helps to reduce potential radiation exposure. In addition, the intervertebral cage can be inserted with less fluoroscopic guidance when the disc space is perpendicular to the ground than the other angles. To set the target segment accurately, the preoperative plane radiographs can provide references to adjust the operation table after the patient is positioned, which helps to reduce radiation exposure as much as possible (Fig. 8.2).

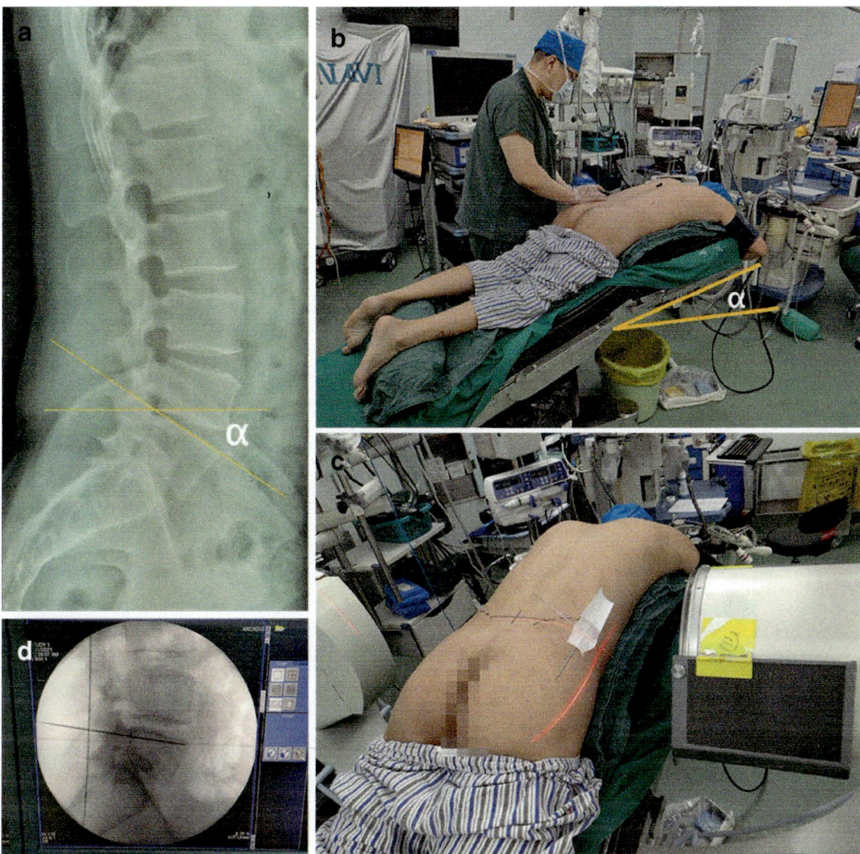

Fig. 8.2 Obtain the "standard" AP and lateral images of the target segment. (**a**) The L4/5 disk space has an angle α with the perpendicular line to the ground, as shown in the preoperative lateral view. (**b**) The cranial end is raised upwards to tilt the operating table from the ground at an angle of α. (**c**) A cross-mental radiopaque marker is placed on the lateral side of the patient to evaluate the orientation of the disc space. The marker wires are placed parallel and perpendicular to the ground. A lateral fluoroscopic view is then obtained. (**d**) The disc space is nearly perpendicular to the ground, as shown in the lateral view

Make a Careful Body Surface Marking

The visible or palpable body surface markers, such as the iliac crests, the spinous processes, and the ribs, should be carefully marked (Fig. 8.2b). The target segment is marked according to the surface marking and the preoperative imaging studies. Then the target segment is confirmed by using a C-arm after the radiopaque markers were placed onto the target segment. In this way, confirming the target segment under continuous fluoroscopic monitoring can be avoided (Fig. 8.3).

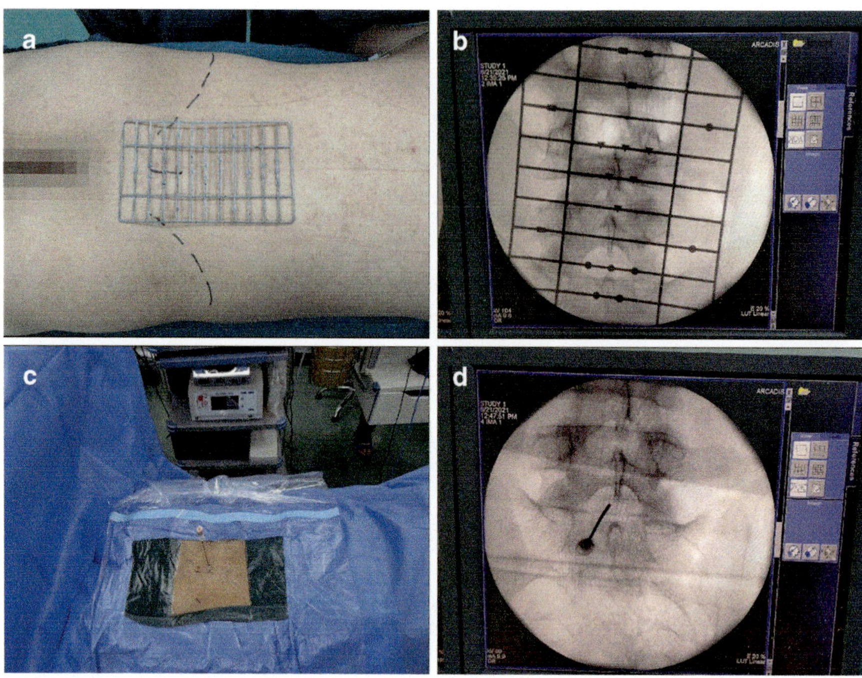

Fig. 8.3 Patient surface marking and radiopaque markers. (**a**) A metal mesh is used as a radiopaque marker. The dotted lines are body surface marking indexing the iliac crests and the spinal processes of the target segment. (**b**) The AP fluoroscopic view of the metal mesh. (**c**) A spine needle is used as a radiopaque marker. (**d**) The AP fluoroscopic view of the spinal needle

Make a Good Exposure of the Interlaminar Window

It is easy to get lost when the interlaminar window could not be identified under direct endoscopic view. Additional X-ray exposure will be required to confirm the right position. Thus, a good exposure of the interlaminar window is important to avoid unintended radiation exposure. A good tissue dissection will help to expose the interlaminar window clearly. For a narrow interlaminar window, placing the patient in a prone position on a curved chest frame with slight flexion of the hip joints is helpful to open the interlaminar space (Fig. 8.2b).

Future Directions for Intraoperative Radiation Reduction in UBE Procedures

Add Skin Markers to Preoperative Imaging Studies

Choi et al. [34] attached the skin markers to the patients before an MRI scan. After acquiring and analyzing the MRI images, the entry points of the posterolateral transforaminal approach were decided based on the MRI markers. As the study hints, adding skin markers when the patients accept preoperative imaging examination will probably decrease the radiation exposure during UBE procedures. Considering the relatively less requirement of fluoroscopic guidance in the UBE procedures, the intraoperative X-ray radiation will probably decrease to zero.

3D Computed Tomography Navigation or Robotic Guidance

It has been reported that 3D computed tomography navigation and robotic guidance can improve the overall accuracy of localization, temper learning curve, and reduce radiation exposure in posterolateral transforaminal approaches [35]. Theoretically, the intraoperative radiation to the staff will be decreased if the navigation or robotic system is used in the UBE procedures. However, extra radiation to patients needs to be considered [36].

Surgical Instruments

As stated above, more radiation exposure is required in a posterolateral transforaminal approach than in a posterior interlaminar approach. However, in fact, this situation is changing. The working style of the posterolateral approach is quite different nowadays. Fan et al. [37] reported that the radiation exposure to the surgeons was reduced by about 40% with the aid of specially designed instruments for posterolateral transforaminal puncture. Ouyang et al. [38] reported that full-endoscopic foraminoplasty using a visualized reamer is safe and effective and can decrease intraoperative fluoroscopy time in posterolateral transforaminal approaches. To decrease the requirement for fluoroscopic guidance, Liu et al. [39] used a foraminoplasty working tube to increase the accuracy for localization and reaming in single portal spinal endoscopic surgeries. As for the UBE procedures, instruments should be designed especially in case of getting lost during the establishment of the working space.

Ultrasound Guidance

Liu et al. [40] used volume navigation with the fusion of real-time ultrasound and CT images to guide posterolateral transforaminal puncture in percutaneous endoscopic lumbar discectomy. This helps to accurately guide percutaneous posterolateral transforaminal puncture while reducing puncture time and exposure to intraoperative radiation. However, the surgeons need to be trained in this technique. As for the UBE procedures, ultrasound guidance should be a good candidate to decrease intraoperative radiation exposure.

Conclusion

The future designs of intraoperative navigation and other devices for guiding biportal endoscopy are opportunities for technological innovation that will lead to safer and more accurate biportal endoscopic procedures with less radiation generation. However, at this time, the C-arm remains a valuable tool that should be used with caution to expose the patient and operating room staff to a lower dose of intraoperative radiation. It is also necessary to highlight that in biportal endoscopic surgery, lower intraoperative radiation exposure can be expected compared to uniportal endoscopic transforaminal approaches.

References

1. Kruger R, Faciszewski T. Radiation dose reduction to medical staff during vertebroplasty: a review of techniques and methods to mitigate occupational dose. Spine (Phila Pa 1976). 2003;28(14):1608–13.
2. Narain AS, Hijji FY, Yom KH, Kudaravalli KT, Haws BE, Singh K. Radiation exposure and reduction in the operating room: perspectives and future directions in spine surgery. World J Orthop. 2017;8(7):524–30.
3. Vozenin-Brotons MC. Tissue toxicity induced by ionizing radiation to the normal intestine: understanding the pathophysiological mechanisms to improve the medical management. World J Gastroenterol. 2007;13(22):3031–2.
4. Morgan WF, Day JP, Kaplan MI, McGhee EM, Limoli CL. Genomic instability induced by ionizing radiation. Radiat Res. 1996;146(3):247–58.
5. Momin AA, Steinmetz MP. Evolution of minimally invasive lumbar spine surgery. World Neurosurg. 2020;140:622–6.
6. Mariscalco MW, Yamashita T, Steinmetz MP, Krishnaney AA, Lieberman IH, Mroz TE. Radiation exposure to the surgeon during open lumbar microdiscectomy and minimally invasive microdiscectomy: a prospective, controlled trial. Spine (Phila Pa 1976). 2011;36(3):255–60.
7. Yeung AT, Tsou PM. Posterolateral endoscopic excision for lumbar disc herniation: Surgical technique, outcome, and complications in 307 consecutive cases. Spine (Phila Pa 1976). 2002;27(7):722–31.
8. Schubert M, Hoogland T. Endoscopic transforaminal nucleotomy with foraminoplasty for lumbar disk herniation. Oper Orthop Traumatol. 2005;17(6):641–61.
9. Ruetten S, Komp M, Merk H, Godolias G. A new full-endoscopic technique for cervical posterior foraminotomy in the treatment of lateral disc herniations using 6.9-mm endoscopes: prospective 2-year results of 87 patients. Minim Invasive Neurosurg. 2007;50(4):219–26.
10. Soliman HM. Irrigation endoscopic discectomy: a novel percutaneous approach for lumbar disc prolapse. Eur Spine J. 2013;22(5):1037–44.
11. Lee CK, Rauschning W, Glenn W. Lateral lumbar spinal canal stenosis: classification, pathologic anatomy and surgical decompression. Spine (Phila Pa 1976). 1988;13(3):313–20.
12. Ahn Y. Percutaneous endoscopic decompression for lumbar spinal stenosis. Expert Rev Med Devices. 2014;11(6):605–16.
13. Ruetten S, Komp M, Merk H, Godolias G. Surgical treatment for lumbar lateral recess stenosis with the full-endoscopic interlaminar approach versus conventional microsurgical technique: a prospective, randomized, controlled study. J Neurosurg Spine. 2009;10(5):476–85.

14. Soliman HM. Irrigation endoscopic decompressive laminotomy. A new endoscopic approach for spinal stenosis decompression. Spine J. 2015;15(10):2282–9.
15. Liu X, Zhu Y. Endoscopic bilateral decompression for cervical stenosis caused by calcification of ligamentum flavum through unilateral approach: technical note [published online ahead of print, 2020 Sept 22]. Clin Spine Surg. 2020; https://doi.org/10.1097/BSD.0000000000001071.
16. Osman SG. Endoscopic transforaminal decompression, interbody fusion, and percutaneous pedicle screw implantation of the lumbar spine: a case series report. Int J Spine Surg. 2012;6:157–66.
17. Wang MY, Grossman J. Endoscopic minimally invasive transforaminal interbody fusion without general anesthesia: initial clinical experience with 1-year follow-up. Neurosurg Focus. 2016;40(2):E13.
18. Ahn Y, Youn MS, Heo DH. Endoscopic transforaminal lumbar interbody fusion: a comprehensive review. Expert Rev Med Devices. 2019;16(5):373–80.
19. Heo DH, Son SK, Eum JH, Park CK. Fully endoscopic lumbar interbody fusion using a percutaneous unilateral biportal endoscopic technique: technical note and preliminary clinical results. Neurosurg Focus. 2017;43(2):E8.
20. Ahn Y, Kim CH, Lee JH, Lee SH, Kim JS. Radiation exposure to the surgeon during percutaneous endoscopic lumbar discectomy: a prospective study. Spine (Phila Pa 1976). 2013;38(7):617–25.
21. Nie H, Zeng J, Song Y, et al. Percutaneous endoscopic lumbar discectomy for L5-S1 disc herniation via an interlaminar approach versus a transforaminal approach: a prospective randomized controlled study with 2-year follow up. Spine (Phila Pa 1976). 2016;41(Suppl 19):B30–7.
22. Li Y, Wang B, Wang S, Li P, Jiang B. Full-endoscopic decompression for lumbar lateral recess stenosis via an interlaminar approach versus a transforaminal approach. World Neurosurg. 2019;128:e632–8.
23. Lin GX, Huang P, Kotheeranurak V, et al. A systematic review of unilateral biportal endoscopic spinal surgery: preliminary clinical results and complications. World Neurosurg. 2019;125:425–32.
24. Merter A, Karaeminogullari O, Shibayama M. Comparison of radiation exposure among 3 different endoscopic diskectomy techniques for lumbar disk herniation. World Neurosurg. 2020;139:e572–9.
25. Kaplan DJ, Patel JN, Liporace FA, Yoon RS. Intraoperative radiation safety in orthopaedics: a review of the ALARA (As low as reasonably achievable) principle. Patient Saf Surg. 2016;10:27.
26. Ishii K, Iwai H, Oka H, Otomo K, Inanami H. A protective method to reduce radiation exposure to the surgeon during endoscopic lumbar spine surgery. J Spine Surg. 2019;5(4):529–34.
27. Hayda RA, Hsu RY, DePasse JM, Gil JA. Radiation exposure and health risks for orthopaedic surgeons. J Am Acad Orthop Surg. 2018;26(8):268–77.
28. Schueler BA. Operator shielding: how and why. Tech Vasc Interv Radiol. 2010;13(3):167–71.
29. Singer G. Occupational radiation exposure to the surgeon. J Am Acad Orthop Surg. 2005;13(1):69–76.
30. Lee K, Lee KM, Park MS, Lee B, Kwon DG, Chung CY. Measurements of surgeons' exposure to ionizing radiation dose during intraoperative use of C-arm fluoroscopy. Spine (Phila Pa 1976). 2012;37(14):1240–4.
31. Mahesh M. Fluoroscopy: patient radiation exposure issues. Radiographics. 2001;21(4):1033–45.
32. Goodman BS, Carnel CT, Mallempati S, Agarwal P. Reduction in average fluoroscopic exposure times for interventional spinal procedures through the use of pulsed and low-dose image settings. Am J Phys Med Rehabil. 2011;90(11):908–12.
33. McCulloch MM, Fischer KW, Kearfott KJ. Medical professional radiation dosimeter usage: reasons for noncompliance. Health Phys. 2018;115(5):646–51.
34. Choi G, Modi HN, Prada N, et al. Clinical results of XMR-assisted percutaneous transforaminal endoscopic lumbar discectomy. J Orthop Surg Res. 2013;8:14.

35. Liounakos JI, Basil GW, Urakawa H, Wang MY. Intraoperative image guidance for endoscopic spine surgery. Ann Transl Med. 2021;9(1):92.
36. Jenkins NW, Parrish JM, Sheha ED, Singh K. Intraoperative risks of radiation exposure for the surgeon and patient. Ann Transl Med. 2021;9(1):84.
37. Fan G, Feng C, Yin B, et al. Concentric stereotactic technique of percutaneous endoscopic transforaminal discectomy and radiation exposure to surgeons. World Neurosurg. 2018;119:e1021–8.
38. Ouyang ZH, Tang M, Li HW, et al. Full-endoscopic foraminoplasty using a visualized bone reamer in the treatment of lumbar disc herniation: a retrospective study of 80 cases. World Neurosurg. 2021;149:e292–7.
39. Liu X, Peng Y. A novel foraminoplasty technique for posterolateral percutaneous transforaminal endoscopic lumbar surgery. Oper Neurosurg (Hagerstown). 2020;19(1):E11–8.
40. Liu YB, Wang Y, Chen ZQ, et al. Volume navigation with fusion of real-time ultrasound and CT images to guide posterolateral transforaminal puncture in percutaneous endoscopic lumbar discectomy. Pain Physician. 2018;21(3):E265–78.

Part III
The Learning Process

Chapter 9
The Learning Process of the Unilateral Biportal Endoscopic Spine Surgery: What Does the Surgeon Need to Perform the Technique?

Diego Quillo-Olvera, Javier Quillo-Reséndiz, Michelle Barrera-Arreola, and Javier Quillo-Olvera

Abbreviations

AKA	As known as
AP	Anteroposterior
BESS	Biportal endoscopic spinal surgery
Cau	Caudal
CPK	Creatine phosphokinase
Cra	Cranial
CRP	C-reactive protein
EBL	Estimated blood loss
Lat	Lateral
MD	Microdiscectomy
Med	Medial
MISS	Minimally invasive spine surgery
PEID	Percutaneous endoscopic interlaminar discectomy
PELD	Percutaneous endoscopic lumbar discectomy
RF	Radiofrequency
SAP	Superior articular process
UBE	Unilateral biportal endoscopy
ULBD	Unilateral laminotomy bilateral decompression

D. Quillo-Olvera (✉) · J. Quillo-Reséndiz · M. Barrera-Arreola · J. Quillo-Olvera
The Brain and Spine Care, Minimally Invasive Spine Surgery Group, Hospital H+ Querétaro, Spine Clinic, Querétaro, México
e-mail: drquilloolvera86@gmail.com; kitnoz@hotmail.com; michelle.barrera@anahuac.mx; neuroqomd@gmail.com

J. Quillo-Olvera et al. (eds.), *Unilateral Biportal Endoscopy of the Spine*,
https://doi.org/10.1007/978-3-031-14736-4_9

Introduction

Unilateral biportal endoscopy (UBE) is considered a minimally invasive spine procedure. This technique uses an arthroscope under continuous fluid irrigation to achieve a high-quality surgical field visualization, magnification, and illumination. However, this technique requires a triangular approach by two ports addressed to a particular target on the spine. Each port has a specific role; one is used for viewing and the other for working. The saline inflow is for the endoscopic portal, and the outflow is for the working channel.

The biportality of the technique allows the independent use of both ports. That enables the endoscope to follow the working instrument in the surgical field, which in turn will facilitate overcoming bone anatomical barriers to achieve successful decompression.

The other situation that should be highlighted in biportal endoscopic surgery is that standard surgical tools for the spine can be used most of the time in the procedures, although different brands have recently started to launch special equipment for UBE.

In general, UBE is performed through a posterior or posterolateral route. The two main approaches that the surgeon must know are the paramedian approach that allows treating spinal pathologies in the central canal and lateral recesses, and the paraspinal approach gives access to the foraminal and extraforaminal space (Fig. 9.1). However, the current UBE techniques have led to paramedian entry approaches for foraminal and extraforaminal pathologies in the lumbar spine, the same as paraspinal entry to cover foraminal and lateral recess injuries [1–17].

As we have mentioned, in the biportal technique, the surgeon holds the working tool with one hand, independent of the arthroscope, which allows moving both instruments more freely. That makes it easy to reach anatomical structures in a complex environment or perform maneuvers requiring different viewing angles. The contralateral sublaminar approach through a paramedian biportal endoscopy is a clear example of the latter [18] (Fig. 9.2).

There are different minimally invasive methods to deal with various spinal pathologies; therefore, there is a wide variety of techniques and technology to

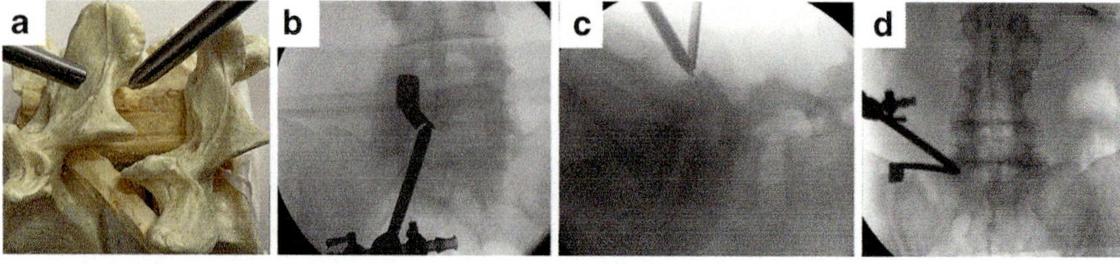

Fig. 9.1 Paramedian and paraspinal UBE lumbar approaches. (**a**) The viewing and working ports in a spine model. The triangle is addressed to the spinolaminar junction. (**b**) A paramedian triangulation was successfully confirmed in an AP view of the C-arm at L5–S1. (**c**) The same approach in a lateral view. (**d**) Paraspinal UBE lumbar approach at L5–S1

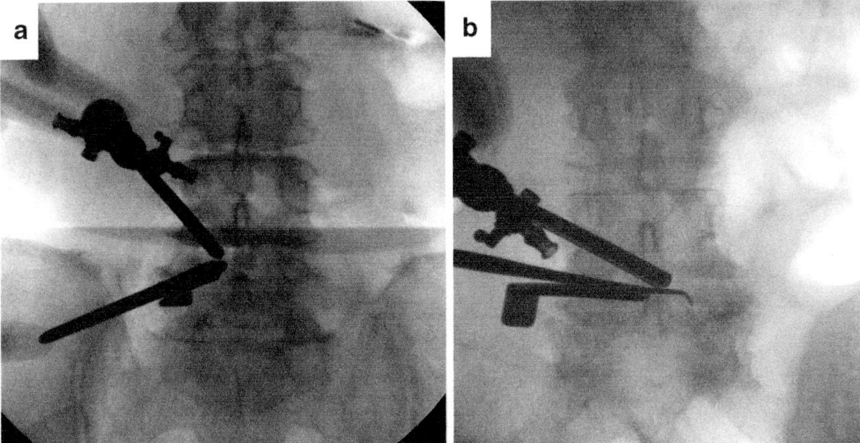

Fig. 9.2 Paramedian approach planned for central and contralateral decompression. (**a**) Paramedian approach addressed to spinolaminar junction and base of the spinous process. (**b**) Contralateral sublaminar approach

overcome challenging spinal pathologies [1, 5, 19]. In addition, biportal endoscopy has also expanded its indications.

Despite having this knowledge and the experiences of other opinion leaders, it is necessary to mention that the learning curve and the access and use of new technologies can be a limitation for implementing these minimally invasive techniques. That is why a deep knowledge of the disease and its anatomy is required first, and then a comprehensive understanding of the different surgical alternatives to solve it, including conventional and minimally invasive techniques.

A deep understanding of MISS then includes the rational use of technology to reduce spinal and paraspinal tissue destruction, reduce systemic damage associated with the procedure, and allow the patient to return to their daily activities more quickly [20].

Biportal endoscopy requires the following technology: displays connected to a high-definition camera coupled to an image-magnifying lens and a light source that allows maintaining a light intensity. In addition, the image and video recorders will enable the capture of the surgical events. The radiofrequency (RF) equipment will permit hemostasis. The high-speed drill system is used for bone removal, and standard surgical tools are used for spine surgery [2, 18] (Fig. 9.3).

UBE is similar to open surgery or microsurgery regarding a posterior route used in both. However, in UBE, two 6–8 mm skin and fascia incisions separated by 3 cm are made. Then, a muscular dilation addressed to the epiperiosteal space in paramedian approaches or intertransverse area in paraspinal approaches is done. Finally, both ports are created to insert the endoscope and the surgical instrument [2, 18] (Fig. 9.4).

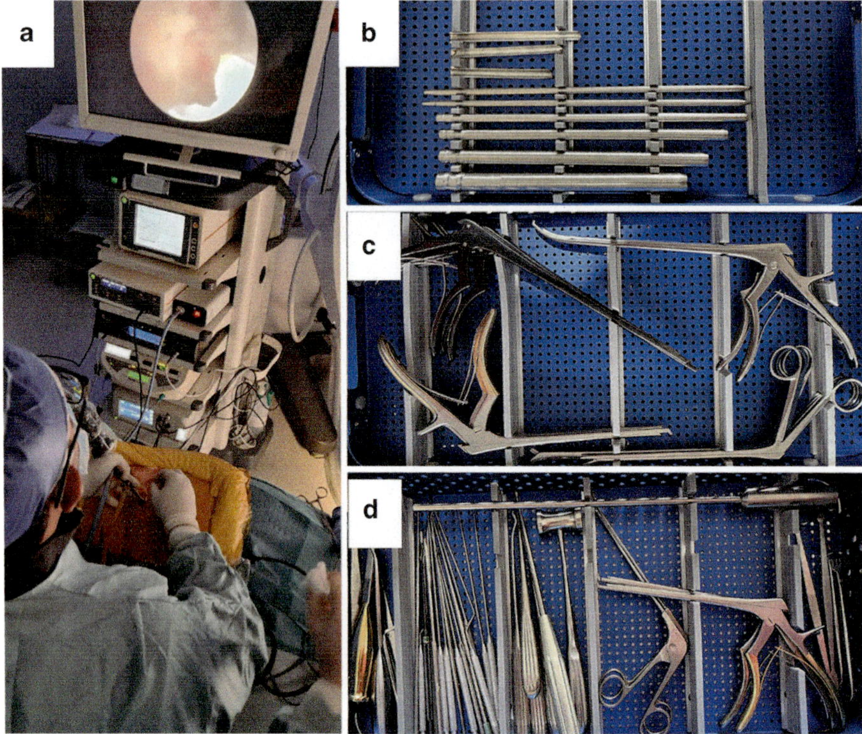

Fig. 9.3 Different devices and tools for UBE. (**a**) Endoscopic tower. (**b**) Dilators and working cannulas. (**c**) Kerrison punches and pituitary forceps. (**d**) Dissectors, curettes, and other surgical tools

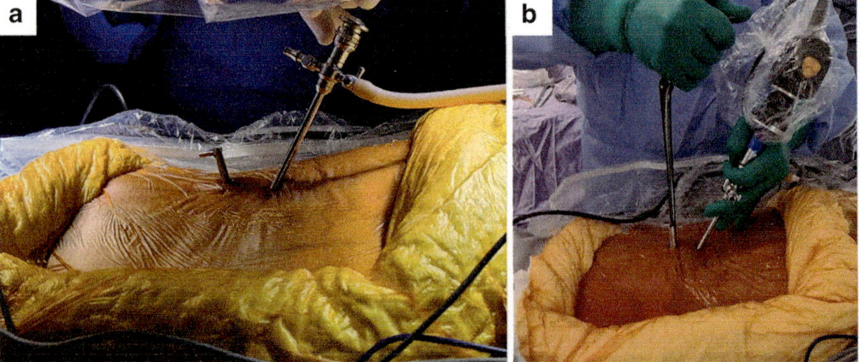

Fig. 9.4 Intraoperative picture of UBE approaches. (**a**) The working cannula was docked and the endoscopic trocar placed cranially. (**b**) Unrestricted motion with the endoscope and surgical tools thanks to independent portals

The surgeon must know the following before beginning his or her learning curve in biportal endoscopic surgery:

1. Anatomical knowledge of the spine
2. Radiological spinal anatomy understanding
3. Palpation of the surgical target
4. Endoscopic visualization of the target emphasizing the paramedian approach

Anatomical Knowledge of the Spine

Because UBE is a targeted endoscopic technique, the surgeon needs to plan the target before the procedure. For example, in cases where only decompression of the ipsilateral traversing nerve root is required, decompression of the lateral recess through a direct paramedian approach should be planned; in this case, identification through the endoscope of the spinolaminar and laminofacet junction is critical for starting with the bone removal.

Knowledge of the interlaminar space, dimensions, and features between the different lumbar levels will allow us to decide between an ULBD-type approach and a contralateral sublaminar or interlaminar approach. These examples are intended to tell the reader that the fact that there are two major approaches (paramedian and paraspinal) for biportal endoscopy does not mean that these should be inflexibly applied to all spinal pathologies. On the contrary, variations of classical routes allow us to be highly specific in reaching the planned target, but we must know the surgical anatomy that will be identified during the procedure to guide us or achieve the intended goals.

Another advice for the surgeon is to become familiar with the epiperiosteal space or the multifidus triangle (Fig. 9.5). This triangular area medial to the multifidus muscle is relevant for a successful paramedian biportal endoscopic approach. This area is bounded medially by the lateral surface of the spinous process and laterally by the multifidus muscle, and its base is the multifidus muscle of the inferior lumbar level.

This area filled with loose connective tissue and fat allows us to work precisely medial and below the deep stabilizing muscles of the lumbar spine. This transfers the characteristic of minimal invasion to the biportal paramedian endoscopic approach.

Also, performing only the dilation of the tissues adjacent to the spine to introduce the two ports causes minimal aggression. As a result, the muscles are not denervated or detached, and injury to the muscle-tendinous structures that stabilize the spine is avoided. It is similar to what is perceived in classic tubular approaches.

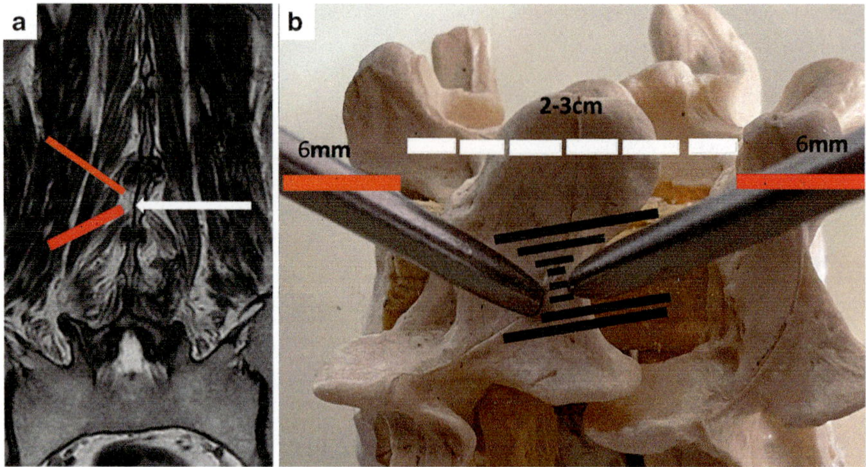

Fig. 9.5 Paramedian surgical window in UBE. (**a**) Coronal view of the lumbar MRI showing the window medial to the multifidus (white arrow) AKA "multifidus triangle." The orange line represents the working port, and the red represents the viewing port during a right paramedian UBE approach. The multifidus muscle is preserved thanks to this surgical window. (**b**) Spine model representing a paramedian biportal triangular approach. The black lines are the spinolaminar junction. Both dilators reached the spinolaminar junction passing through the multifidus triangle—the skin incision's length is 6 mm for each. *AKA* as known as

Radiological Spinal Anatomy Understanding

The C-arm views commonly used for UBE are anteroposterior (AP) and lateral (Lat). The AP view should have the following features:

- The endplates should be aligned.
- Equidistant and symmetric pedicles.
- The spinous process is central regarding the pedicles and representing the midline.
- The lateral view should show the pedicles' boundaries and the endplates aligned.

The lordosis and sacral inclination at L5–S1 play a crucial role in docking both ports. The surgeon should consider each patient's spinopelvic parameters undergoing the lumbosacral junction's UBE procedure and confirm any step with the C-arm.

For central and contralateral biportal endoscopic lumbar decompression, the landmark is the spinolaminar junction. The triangulation of this surgical reference with both dilators must be verified with AP and lateral C-arm projections before inserting the endoscope or any surgical instrument through the ports.

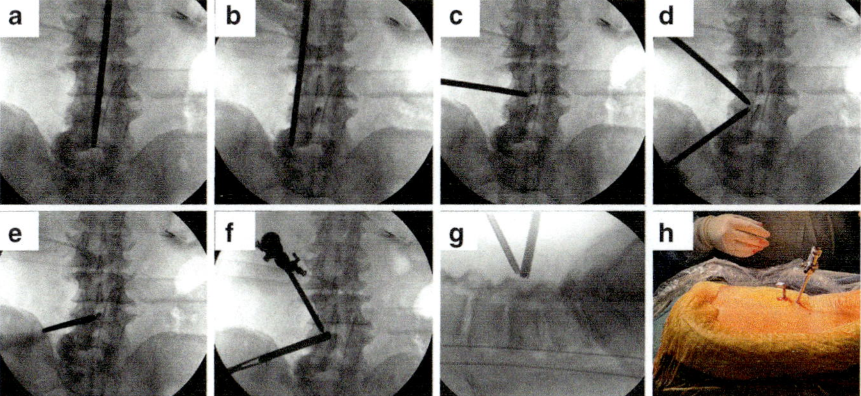

Fig. 9.6 Radiological steps for a left-sided paramedian L3–L4 UBE approach. (**a**) Midline. (**b**) Mid-pedicle line. (**c**) Disc space. (**d**) Triangular approach. (**e**) Working port. (**f**) Viewing and working ports docked in the interlaminar space. (**g**) The biportal approach was confirmed with lateral projection. (**h**) Intraoperative picture of the biportal approach in the surgical field

The reference lines to mark in the AP projections are:

- Midline through the spinous processes
- Mid-pedicle through the medial edge of the index level's pedicles
- The disc space

Lateral projection:

The lateral view will confirm the trajectory of the approach (Fig. 9.6).

Palpation of the Surgical Target

For this purpose, it is crucial to make proper skin and fascia incisions to introduce the dilators. Then, sequential dilators will be introduced through both incisions. The authors usually dilate the paraspinal tissues from 6 mm to 8 mm. That is sufficient for placing the endoscopic trocar and the semi-tubular customized working cannula. However, to create enough working space is the objective of the proper palpation-dissection with the dilators.

1. Each dilator will be introduced independently and addressed to the target for a paramedian approach to the spinolaminar junction.
2. The surgeon should palpate the lamina, the inferior border of the superior lamina, the base, and the lateral surface of the spinous process and dissect them with each dilator.

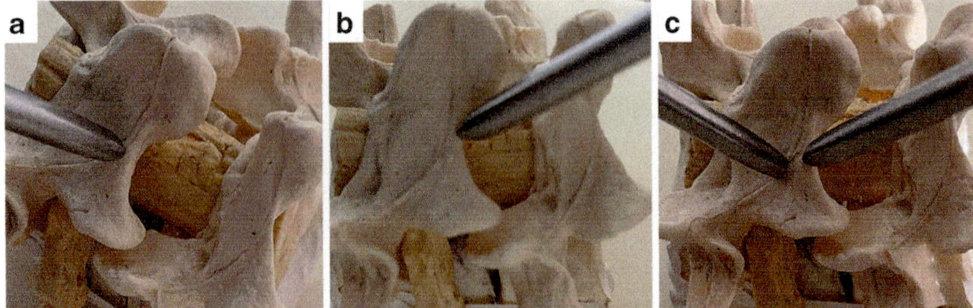

Fig. 9.7 Palpation sequence of spinolaminar junction through a paramedian approach. (**a**) Palpation of the inferior border of the lamina with the cranial dilator. (**b**) Palpation of the same reference with the caudal dilator. (**c**) Both dilators joined in the bone reference after enlarging the working space

3. Soft lateral movements with each dilator will enlarge the multifidus triangle.
4. After both dilators are placed, the surgeon will palpate the bone references mentioned above with both and will also be able to feel the touch of one with the other.

These maneuvers will ensure orientation in the procedure because the bone landmarks are being identified by palpation, and with dissection of the working space, the surgeon will co-locate the instruments with the endoscope in the surgical field easier and allow for the procedure a correct flow of the irrigated fluid. As already mentioned, these maneuvers should be verified with fluoroscopy in AP and lateral projections (Fig. 9.7).

Endoscopic Visualization of the Target Emphasizes the Paramedian Approach

After successfully performing the triangular approach and confirming it with the C-arm, the surgeon can introduce the endoscope through the viewing portal and the radiofrequency probe through the working channel. Then, the first thing the surgeon needs to do is confirm that the irrigated fluid is coming out through the working channel. After that, the surgeon must locate his or her working instrument with the endoscope (Fig. 9.8). The following steps to identify the landmarks and drive the endoscopic approach are cited in order:

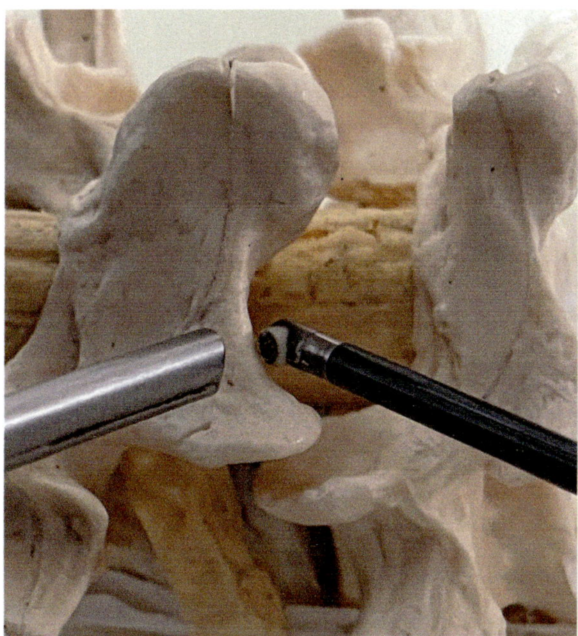

Fig. 9.8 The endoscope has located the radiofrequency in the surgical field. That is what we call co-location of surgical instruments

1. The working (epiperiosteal) space filled with connective loose tissue and fat is cleaned using pituitary forceps and radiofrequency probe (Fig. 9.9a).
2. The spinolaminar junction (3), interlaminar space (2), and ipsilateral lamina are observed (1) (Fig. 9.9b).
3. Ipsilateral laminotomy using different surgical tools (Fig. 9.9c) and contralateral undercutting of the lamina are performed (Fig. 9.9d).
4. The ipsilateral and contralateral SAPs are removed (Fig. 9.9e).
5. The bone references mentioned were removed in an over-the-top fashion. Ligamentum flavum preservation is critical to care for the neural elements during bone removal, and the ligamentum flavum acts as a protecting barrier against the neural elements.
6. The flavectomy is performed under direct visualization (Fig. 9.9f).
7. Finally, after bone removal and flavectomy, the dural sac, traversing nerves, or exiting nerves, depending on the surgical goals of decompression, can be identified (Fig. 9.9g).

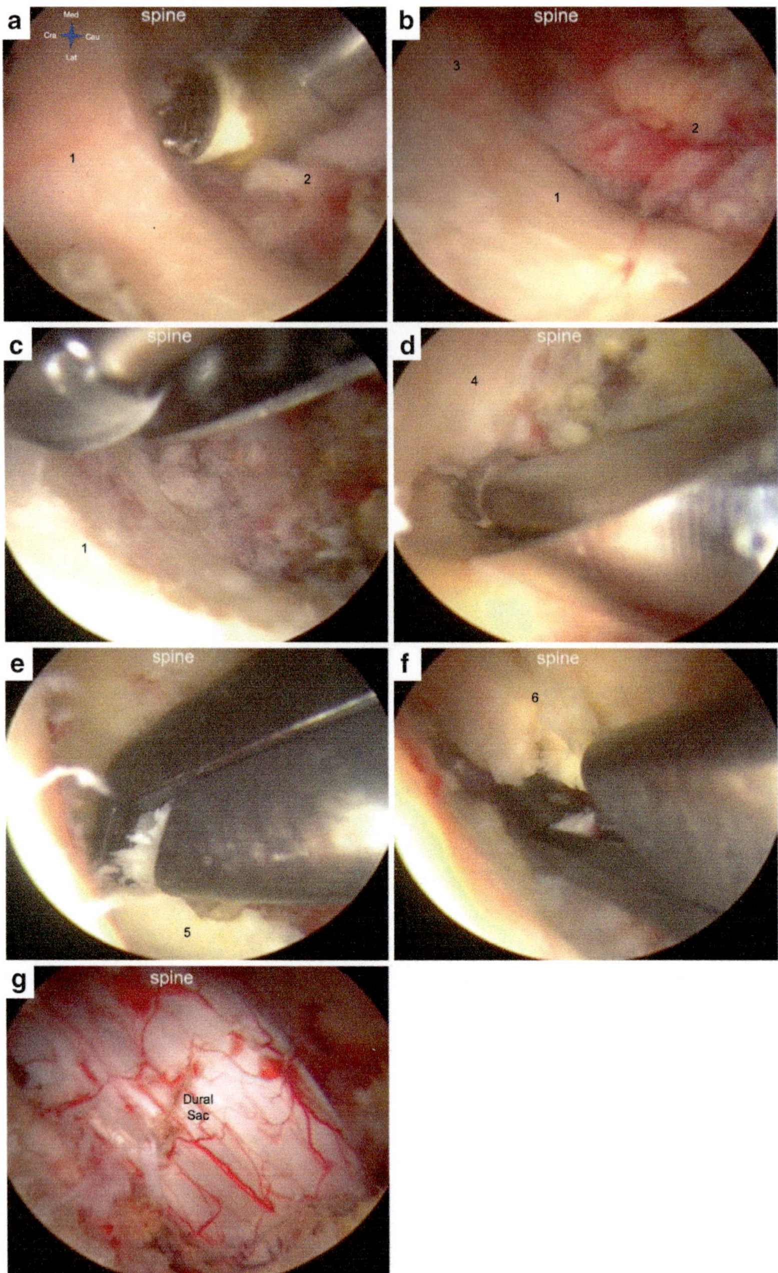

Fig. 9.9 Anatomical landmarks that should be identified in a paraspinal UBE lumbar approach. (**a**) The lamina (1) and interlaminar space (2) are cleaned with the RF probe. (**b**) Panoramic view of 1, 2, and 3. (**c**) Ipsilateral laminotomy. (**d**) Contralateral sublaminar undercut. (**e**) Ipsilateral SAP (5) removal. (**f**) Flavectomy. (**g**) Dural sac decompressed. *Cra* cranial, *Cau* caudal, *Lat* lateral, *Med* medial, *RF* radiofrequency, 1: lamina, 2: interlaminar space, 3: spinolaminar junction, 4: contralateral lamina, 5: superior articular process (SAP), 6: ligamentum flavum

Tips and Tricks

- A slight flexion in the operating table allows the opening of the interlaminar space.
- We recommend palpate-confirm-dissect the bone references. So, this process includes the surgeon's hands, the C-arm, and the feeling-deep structures to get oriented before starting with the endoscopic procedure, ensuring the proper approach of the target.
- We recommend always confirming with an AP and lateral views your surgical approach as routine.
- Do not continue with the next step if proper hemostasis is not achieved.
- The pump-water pressure should be set at 25–30 mmHg. It will allow tissue dissection underwater and maintain enlarged working space, high-quality visualization, illumination, and magnification, and a protective effect against infection has been observed due to continuous washing of the surgical field.
- Be careful with the outflow of saline. Muscle edema and other paraspinal tissues could result if continuous irrigation is stagnant.

The above recommendations could shorten your learning curve and make your UBE procedure safer, quicker, and efficient.

Discussion

Biportal endoscopic spinal surgery (BESS) has proven to be an effective MISS technique like tubular microsurgery and uniportal endoscopic surgery [1]. BESS tries to combine the usefulness of conventional spinal surgical procedures with the benefits of spinal endoscopy [2–4].

Choi et al. [1] reported the inflammatory biological profile of different surgical techniques for discectomy measuring the C-reactive protein (CRP) and creatine phosphokinase (CPK). Percutaneous endoscopic lumbar discectomy (PELD) was the less disruptive technique for discectomy. However, UBE discectomy was less aggressive in biological terms than microdiscectomy (MD).

Heo et al. [5], in 2019, compared three techniques for central decompression in lumbar stenosis (MD, PEID, and UBE). The authors concluded that lesser violation of the facet joint was found in UBE compared to the other techniques. Moreover, an acceptable clinical and radiological outcome has been reported by other authors using the UBE technique for neural decompression [6–8].

The rate of complications reported in UBE is around 6.7%: dural tear, persistent back pain, paresthesia, postoperative headache, numbness, incomplete decompression, and epidural hematoma are the most frequently reported [9].

However, UBE has proven to be an effective technique for treating various spinal pathologies with some advantages such as minor trauma to the paraspinal tissues, less estimated blood loss (EBL), faster recovery, less postoperative pain, and an acceptable rate of postoperative satisfaction using the Macnab criteria reported by the patient with a shorter hospital stay [9, 10].

The advantages observed in UBE over other MISS techniques are the independent use of the surgical tool under direct endoscopic visualization. It allows independent and unrestricted motion with the endoscope and the instrument and the feasibility for reaching complex and challenging anatomy of the spine [11–15]. But the main advantage is still the excellent visualization, illumination, and magnification through a truly water-based endoscopic procedure [16].

Finally, the surgeon must know that complications can occur even with an experienced surgeon's hands performing the UBE procedure. A study reported that the learning curve of UBE is achieved in the 30th case. This learning curve is shorter than the uniportal endoscopic technique, with approximately 100 patients. However, this curve could be reduced if the surgeon has experience with conventional spinal surgery, microsurgery, or uniportal endoscopy [3, 21].

Conclusion

Throughout this chapter, relevant aspects regarding the biportal technique were discussed, including the anatomical landmarks that the surgeon must identify in intraoperative radiology and the bone references that must be palpated and observed during the biportal endoscopic procedure. In addition, recommendations were given to drive a biportal endoscopic procedure safely and efficiently. Despite this, it is essential to mention that, like any technique, biportal endoscopic surgery requires a learning process, during which the surgeries could take more time than expected or seem complex, but later the learning curve is overcome.

References

1. Choi KC, Shim HK, Hwang JS, et al. Comparison of surgical invasiveness between microdiscectomy and 3 different endoscopic discectomy techniques for lumbar disc herniation. World Neurosurg. 2018;116:e750–8.
2. Choi CM, Chung JT, Lee SJ, Choi DJ. How I do it? Biportal endoscopic spinal surgery (BESS) for treatment of lumbar spinal stenosis. Acta Neurochir. 2016;158(3):459–63.
3. Choi DJ, Choi CM, Jung JT, Lee SJ, Kim YS. Learning curve associated with complications in biportal endoscopic spinal surgery: challenges and strategies. Asian Spine J. 2016;10(4):624–9.
4. Hwa Eum J, Hwa Heo D, Son SK, Park CK. Percutaneous biportal endoscopic decompression for lumbar spinal stenosis: a technical note and preliminary clinical results. J Neurosurg Spine. 2016;24(4):602–7.
5. Heo DH, Lee DC, Park CK. Comparative analysis of three types of minimally invasive decompressive surgery for lumbar central stenosis: biportal endoscopy, uniportal endoscopy, and microsurgery. Neurosurg Focus. 2019;46(5):E9.
6. Ahn Y. Percutaneous endoscopic decompression for lumbar spinal stenosis. Expert Rev Med Devices. 2014;11(6):605–16.
7. Kim HS, Paudel B, Jang JS, et al. Percutaneous full endoscopic bilateral lumbar decompression of spinal stenosis through uniportal-contralateral approach: techniques and preliminary results. World Neurosurg. 2017;103:201–9.

8. Komp M, Hahn P, Oezdemir S, et al. Bilateral spinal decompression of lumbar central stenosis with the full-endoscopic interlaminar versus microsurgical laminotomy technique: a prospective, randomized, controlled study. Pain Physician. 2015;18(1):61–70.
9. Lin GX, Huang P, Kotheeranurak V, et al. A systematic review of unilateral biportal endoscopic spinal surgery: preliminary clinical results and complications. World Neurosurg. 2019;125:425–32.
10. Fishchenko I, Balan S, Blonskyi R, Borzykh N, Kravchuk L. Georgian Med News. 2020;301:21–7.
11. Torudom Y, Dilokhuttakarn T. Two portal percutaneous endoscopic decompression for lumbar spinal stenosis: preliminary study. Asian Spine J. 2016;10(2):335–42.
12. Ahn JS, Lee HJ, Choi DJ, Lee KY, Hwang SJ. Extraforaminal approach of biportal endoscopic spinal surgery: a new endoscopic technique for transforaminal decompression and discectomy. J Neurosurg Spine. 2018;28(5):492–8.
13. Choi G, Prada N, Modi HN, Vasavada NB, Kim JS, Lee SH. Percutaneous endoscopic lumbar herniectomy for high-grade down-migrated L4-L5 disc through an L5-S1 interlaminar approach: a technical note. Minim Invasive Neurosurg. 2010;53(3):147–52.
14. Soliman HM. Irrigation endoscopic decompressive laminotomy. A new endoscopic approach for spinal stenosis decompression. Spine J. 2015;15(10):2282–9.
15. Soliman HM. Irrigation endoscopic discectomy: a novel percutaneous approach for lumbar disc prolapse. Eur Spine J. 2013;22(5):1037–44.
16. Kim JE, Choi DJ, Park EJJ, et al. Biportal endoscopic spinal surgery for lumbar spinal stenosis. Asian Spine J. 2019;13(2):334–42.
17. Park SM, Kim GU, Kim HJ, et al. Is the use of a unilateral biportal endoscopic approach associated with rapid recovery after lumbar decompressive laminectomy? A preliminary analysis of a prospective randomized controlled trial. World Neurosurg. 2019;128:e709–18.
18. Eun SS, Eum JH, Lee SH, Sabal LA. Biportal endoscopic lumbar decompression for lumbar disk herniation and spinal canal stenosis: a technical note. J Neurol Surg A Cent Eur Neurosurg. 2017;78(4):390–6.
19. Kim W, Kim SK, Kang SS, Park HJ, Han S, Lee SC. Pooled analysis of unsuccessful percutaneous biportal endoscopic surgery outcomes from a multi-institutional retrospective cohort of 797 cases. Acta Neurochir. 2020;162(2):279–87.
20. Schmidt FA, Wong T, Kirnaz S, et al. Development of a curriculum for minimally invasive spine surgery (MISS). Global Spine J. 2020;10(2 Suppl):122S–5S.
21. Pao JL, Lin SM, Chen WC, Chang CH. Unilateral biportal endoscopic decompression for degenerative lumbar canal stenosis. J Spine Surg. 2020;6(2):438–46.

Chapter 10
How to Go Further with My Clinical Practice on Unilateral Biportal Endoscopy

Ghazwan Abdulla Hasan

Abbreviations

DDD	Degenerative disc disease
EBM	Evidence-based medicine
MIS	Minimally invasive surgery
MISST	Minimally invasive spinal surgery techniques
OR	Operating room
PELD	Percutaneous endoscopic lumbar decompression
PLIF	Posterior lumbar interbody fusion
SMART	Specific, Measurable, Attainable, Reliable, Time-bound
UBE	Unilateral biportal endoscopy
ULBD	Unilateral laminotomy for bilateral decompression

Introduction

Each year, more than 1.62 million instrumented spine surgeries are performed in the United States, according to the iData Report. This number is increasing each year due to improving life expectancy of the people; with this increasing number of surgeries each year, the number of complications is also increasing that include perioperative and postoperative complications; some of these complications are approach related that have wound complications, delay rehabilitation, blood loss, and more.

G. A. Hasan (✉)
Royal Private Hospital, Orthopedic Spine Surgery Center, Baghdad, Iraq
e mail: dr.bayaty@gmail.com

J. Quillo-Olvera et al. (eds.), *Unilateral Biportal Endoscopy of the Spine*,
https://doi.org/10.1007/978-3-031-14736-4_10

The history of spine surgery goes back to at least 5000 years; at the beginning of early civilization (Egyptian and Mesopotamian), the first evidence of spine surgery was found in Egyptian mummies from 3000 BC, which was elucidated 15 centuries later in the Edwin Smith Papyrus in 1550 BC [1], while the first documented operative treatment of the spine belonged to Paulus of Aegina in the seventh century [2].

The early spine surgeries carried many complications and poor outcomes until 1829 when Alban G. Smith was the first who performed a laminectomy in the United States with partial improvement in his neurology postoperatively [3]. After that, many surgical techniques were developed to improve the surgical outcome and treat many spine pathologies, including infection, trauma, deformities, trauma, and tumors.

With the growth of technologies and applications in surgeries, a vast improvement and variety in spine surgery happened in the twentieth and twenty-first centuries, including spine instrumentation, drills, microscope, radiology, and others.

The development and progress in spine surgery are continuous and never stop. For example, the introduction of the microscopic interlaminar approach by G. Yasargil and W. Casper in 1977 and the tubular system by Hijikata in 1975 opened the door to minimally invasive spine surgery to decrease the approach-related complication with open surgeries [4].

In 1986, Parviz Kambin described the Kambin triangle for percutaneous endoscopic discectomy, while A. Yeung, in 1990, first applied the transforaminal approach under continuous irrigation, followed by Sabastian Rutten in 2000, who described the endoscopic interlaminar approach [5].

De Antoni and Soliman first described the unilateral biportal endoscopy (UBE) [6], followed by Eum et al. who expanded the indication to involve spine decompression in spinal stenosis [7], Kim et al. known for cervical spine [8], and Heo et al. known for interbody fusion [9]; now, UBE technique has become more popularized and is done by many surgeons worldwide with wide varieties of indication including most of the spine regions and pathologies.

Do We Need to Upgrade to Endoscopic Spine?

The AOSpine four principles for proper spinal patient management, including stability, alignment, biology, and function, should be considered in every patient to be treated with spine pathologies.

These principles are applied to all spine pathologies that include degenerative, trauma, infection, tumor, and deformities. In contrast, each spine surgery aims to resolve the patient's clinical problem by treating the underlying pathology, we can consider these pathologies as a target, and each spine surgery aims to treat the target pathology whether this surgery is carried out by conventional, MIS, or endoscopy; to get the target pathology we have to access it. The access differs by the technique to be used (traditional, MIS, or endoscope).

In conventional spine surgeries, which were started decades before, the degree of muscle, soft tissue, and adjacent bony structure damage is high that threatens the stability and biology. Moreover, it might impact the postoperative outcome (function) in many cases and postoperative complications related to access approach that include blood loss, extended hospital stays, infection, and iatrogenic instability.

Applying the AOSpine principles, avoiding postoperative complications, decreasing soft-tissue damage, and giving attention to spine unit stabilities all should alert us to think about upgrading the techniques to be used in treating different spine pathologies; that is why minimally invasive spine surgery and endoscopic spine surgery should be applied in our practice.

Unilateral biportal endoscope (UBE) has been one of the rapidly growing techniques in the last decade that had emerged in spine surgery and become popularized among many surgeons all over the world, not only in the country where it delivered (South Korea); nowadays, we have many expert surgeons treating their patients who are presenting with different spine pathologies using UBE techniques.

So currently, as we live in an innovation era, with enormous upgrades in the surrounding that involve technologies, artificial intelligence, and automotive, we must continue our practice to outdo the surgical outcome, decrease the postoperative complications, improve our carrier, and satisfy our esteem.

What Is the EBM That Supported UBE and Its Clinical Applications?

When we talk about endoscopic spine surgeries, the first things that appear in our mind are the limitation of evidence-based support and the learning curve; in this section, we will deal with the evidence base that supports the UBE technique and how this technique extends the indication of treating spine pathologies with minimal learning curve effort compared with other methods.

Many kinds of literature have been published comparing UBE techniques with other surgical techniques that include:

- UBE vs. tubular microendoscopy [10]
- UBE vs. open microdiscectomy [11]
- UBE vs. PELD [12]
- UBE interbody fusion vs. conventional PLIF [13]
- UBE vs. uniportal endoscope vs. microdiscectomy [14]
- UBE vs. microscopic decompression for spinal stenosis [15]
- The clinical and radiologic outcome between UBE and ULBD [16, 17]
- Radiation exposure among three endoscopic techniques [18]
- Cost-effectiveness of microdiscectomy versus endoscopic discectomy for lumbar disc herniation [19]
- UBE lumbar interbody fusion vs. MIS fusion [20]

The pathologies treated by UBE techniques as reviewed in the literature are as follows:

- Primary lumbar disc herniation [6, 21]
- Recurrent lumbar disc herniation [22]
- Cervical disc herniation [8, 23]
- Degenerative lumbar spine decompression [24, 25]
- Dorsal spine decompression
- Cervical spine decompression [26]
- Lumbar interbody fusion [9, 27–30]
- Facet cyst excision [31, 32]
- Foraminal stenosis [33–36]
- Spinal epidural lipomatosis [37]

Systematic review, outcome, and clinical trial:

- Clinical results and complications [38]
- UBE approach related to rapid recovery [39]
- Clinical and radiological outcome of UBE [40]

Complications:

- Dural injury [41]
- Hidden blood loss [42]
- Postoperative epidural hematoma [43]

How to Overcome the Obstacles?

After reviewing the scope of application of UBE techniques in the treatment of different spine pathologies, we start to realize how this technique is an effect in the treatment of a wide range of pathologies and can be applied and how it substitutes the conventional spine surgeries, but what about the other obstacles that include the learning curve, operating room setting, and dealing with the complications?

Endoscopic spine surgeries got attraction from most spine surgeons all over the world, and most spine surgeons embraced MISST as mainstream and considered it as an integral part of their clinical practice [44], so being an endoscopic spine surgeon is the aim of most surgeons all over the world including the author.

In our experience in the last 5 years, we showed how the endoscopic spine surgery topic had got an interest among spine surgeons in international, regional, and local events, so the motivation to learn this technique is high and many learning activities are available that include mentorships, fellowships, cadaver courses, workshops, and simulation training that open the scope to extend this technique globally and get more surgeons to involve.

As per Lewandrowski et al., in the global survey about surgeon training and clinical implementation of spinal endoscopy in routine practice, few minimally invasive spinal surgery techniques (MISST) surgeons are fellowship trained. Still, they attend workshops and various meetings, suggesting that many are self-taught. Orthopedic surgeons were more likely to implement endoscopic spinal surgery into routine clinical practice. As endoscopic spine surgery gains more traction and patient demand, minimal adequate training will be part of the ongoing debate field [44].

Most surgeons are motivated to learn endoscopic spine surgeries and apply them in their practice. Still, there are some obstacles in their way that include learning curve, instrument cost, evidence-based references, and dealing with complications.

A review about the motivation and obstacles concludes that the number of spine surgeries was high but was impeded by the high cost of equipment and disposables. The primary motivators for spine surgeons' desire to implement were personal interest and patients' demands [45].

So, one of the obstacles to being involved in endoscopic spine surgery is the cost of the instruments. Still, when we talk about and compare the price of UBE instruments (which is like most of the conventional spine instruments) to uniportal endoscopic spine instruments, we see that UBE instruments are much cheaper and do not require new purchasing of most devices as they are using some tools for conventional surgeries like the Kerrisons.

Another point to be considered is the learning curve; some reviews conclude that UBE techniques have a shorter learning curve compared to uniportal spine endoscope, and this concept is logical as most of the spine surgeons are familiar with the interlaminar approach compared to the transforaminal and the field is much like microscopic tubular one [46–48].

Many learning activities are available that start from references (articles and books), online events, international conferences, fellowships, and industry-sponsored cadaver workshops; each mentioned reference is critical in some point of training journey, but Kim et al., in their review, conclude that industry-sponsored weekend cadaver workshops have remained the mainstay of training-aspiring endoscopic spinal surgeons in North America and Europe leaving many of them to become autodidacts [49].

Starting a new technique will not be easy, but UBE techniques are familiar with joint arthroscopy. The concept of triangulation will give us a leap forward. It is essential to start with easily selected cases at last in the beginning. Wu et al. describe the endoscopic ladder of competence progression model by reviewing the challenges and defining each step starting from easy to complex [50].

Our 12 Steps to Start UBE

1. *Define your why*

   This is the first step in the journey for any new technique you want to learn, and invest your time and carrier in it. Only then can you understand the reason why (the purpose) you will be more capable of pursuing the things that give you fulfillment.

As we are surgeons and working in the field dealing with patients' pathologies, we have to have a clear why or purpose in our work, so in UBE, which is our example here, each one has to define why they want to start the UBE technique as to improve the patients' outcome and his or her carrier, because finding the purpose makes us to put a plan to our next step after the Why, which are the How and What.

2. *Set a goal*

The next step in the journey is setting a specific goal to achieve it, and the simple framework is using the SMART (Specific, Measurable, Attainable, Reliable, Time-bound) mnemonics (Fig. 10.1); in UBE, we follow the SMART goal formula (Fig. 10.1) by planning our goal as follows:

S: I want to start UBE surgery for DDD as a first step.
M: When I start my first case, I can measure my progression.
A: I must know my limit and capability, so I have enough experience in conventional and MIS so the UBE step will be attenable; Learning is a step ladder and in the case of Endoscopic spine surgeries, conventional and Microscopic spine surgeries are essential to the initial steps to learning endoscopic spine surgeries.
R: UBE surgery should be relevant to your work, and it will impact your carrier positively; as you are a spine surgeon, investing your time, effort, and money in the UBE technique will be relevant and affordable, so you have to have a good number of spine cases per year so when you learn this technique, you can apply it in your daily practice.
T: Put a timetable in each step in your goal setting till you achieve the entire goal by starting UBE surgery, so in your list, you will measure your progression.

Specific
Measurable
Attainable
Relevant
Time-bound
S
M
A
R
T
G
O
A
L
S
What *exactly* are you trying to achieve?
How will you know when you've achieved it?
Is it genuinely possible to achieve it?
Does it contribute to your agency's revenue growth?
When do you want to achieve this by?

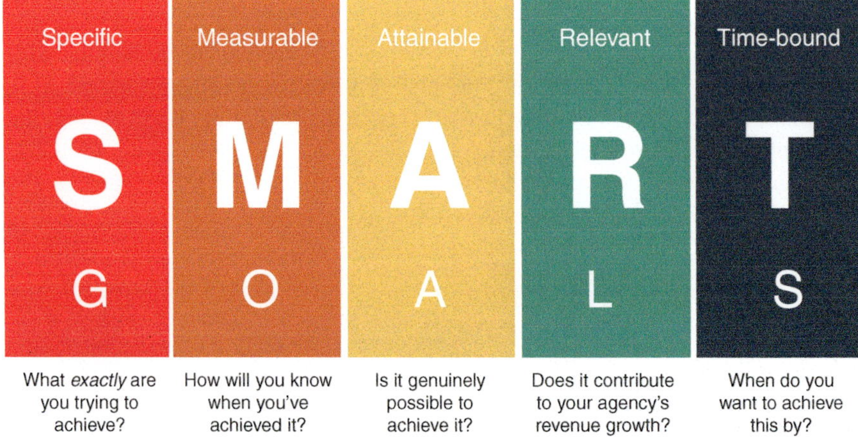

Fig. 10.1 SMART goal formula, https://doi.org/10.21182/jmisst.2020.00024, Figure 6 in the article

3. *References*

   After setting a SMART goal, the next step is to find a reference to learn the UBE technique; you will collect the references from published articles, books, videos, recorded presentations, and other resources and start to dig into the knowledge of the UBE technique so that you will build a base from which you can begin your next step. For references, many resources are available right now. You can find them.
4. *Mentoring*

   Finding a mentor is crucial in learning in our field (UBE surgery) and our lives. Your mentor will help, direct, motivate, and guide you in each step till you reach your goal. UBE surgery mentorship is critical as your mentor will teach you the basics of UBE surgery and show you how to start and deal with the initial obstacle. The author has mentors who help him create and overcome the initial obstacles in UBE surgeries, and fortunately, all the masters of UBE surgery are welcome to support any surgeon. Therefore, the author recommends that anyone who start their journey in the UBE technique contact masters and ask for help.
5. *Overcome the struggles*

   In each new technique to apply in our practice, we will face many struggles that prevent us from starting. Some of these struggles are related to setting the OR, local healthcare system, financial support, or others. The author recommends dealing with these struggles and trying to overcome them, especially initially to start by asking help from the companies and hospitals or using the available resources to apply it in UBE surgery. As we mentioned before, most UBE surgery instruments should be available in hospitals, not like other techniques.
6. *Easy start*

   The learning curves are stepping ladder process, so in UBE surgery, it is essential to start with the easy, straightforward case as a start, review all the preoperative data and radiology, and discuss with your mentor about the tips and tricks to be applied, how to avoid the struggles, the level to be operated (L5–S1 is preferable), the pathology (posterolateral disc prolapse is preferable), the age of the patient (young is preferable), and any associated pathologies (like deformity, revision, or stenosis).
7. *Backup surgeon*

   Starting UBE surgery will be the first practical step in the journey. To start with UBE surgeries the author recommends being done in the presence of an expert surgeon as a backup, that will be available if any struggles you face or any complications that can be dealt with, the author start initial cases in the presence of one of the expert UBE surgeons during his visit to one of the conferences. So, you can start with confidence.

8. *Plan B*

   When you start UBE surgery, you should have a plan B, or what is called conversion surgery, as you might find difficulties that prevent you from finishing the surgery like bleeding, or approach disorientation, or you face intraoperative complications that you cannot deal with UBE technique like a dural tear, especially when you do not have a backup surgeon. The author uses tubular microscopic system as a backup option and discusses the possibility of conversion with the patient, so knowing other techniques will help you deal with initial obstacles. Conversion from UBE to tubular will be easier than conversion from UBE to open from the patient perspective.
9. *Feedback loops*

   After each surgery, you have to collect all the data about the surgery, including the preoperative planning, intraoperative events, video recording, and difficulties that you faced, and review it with your mentor to learn and improve your skills; this is called feedback loops, and it is one of the fundamental steps of deliberate practice concept in learning.
10. *Ask the expert*

    Your mentor will be your expert; as we mentioned before, they will help you overcome the initial struggles and teach you to master UBE surgery. Initially, you can discuss with your mentor each step. Then, they will provide you with an expert opinion about your questions and provide you with the needed resources.
11. *Measure the progression*

    After doing initial cases in UBE, you will start to measure the progression of your learning curve (this is one of the steps in the SMART goal formula setting as mentioned before), so the time of the surgery, the difficulties of the pathologies, and dealing with complications and any other factors that determine your progression are essential to know the level you reached.
12. *Mastering*

    Mastering UBE surgeries is the last step in our approach in which UBE surgeon are able to perform and deals with different pathologies, complications, have a fair number of cases operated per year, start to publish your work, invent a new way to expand the indications, and improve the outcome and be a mentor to teach the others.

Conclusion

UBE surgery is one of the endoscopic techniques applied for different spine pathologies, and it is a safe and innovative technique to match patients' outcomes. Setting a roadmap of steps to learn and master UBE surgeries will improve our knowledge and decrease the risk of surgical complications. Every initial step in new technologies will not be easy, but following our 12-steps recommendations will help surgeons start UBE techniques and join the experts.

References

1. Lang JK, Kolenda H. First appearance and sense of the term "spinal column" in ancient Egypt. Historical vignette. J Neurosurg. 2002;97(1 Suppl):152–5.
2. Knoeller SM, Seifried C. Historical perspective: history of spinal surgery. Spine (Phila Pa 1976). 2000;25(21):2838–43.
3. Patwardhan RV, Hadley MN. History of surgery for ruptured disk. Neurosurg Clin N Am. 2001;12(1):173–9, x.
4. Castro I, Santos DP, Christoph Dde H, Landeiro JA. The history of spinal surgery for disc disease: an illustrated timeline. Arq Neuropsiquiatr. 2005;63(3A):701–6.
5. Mayer HM. A history of endoscopic lumbar spine surgery: what have we learnt? Biomed Res Int. 2019;2019:4583943.
6. Soliman HM. Irrigation endoscopic discectomy: a novel percutaneous approach for lumbar disc prolapse. Eur Spine J. 2013;22(5):1037–44.
7. Hwa Eum J, Hwa Heo D, Son SK, Park CK. Percutaneous biportal endoscopic decompression for lumbar spinal stenosis: a technical note and preliminary clinical results. J Neurosurg Spine. 2016;24(4):602–7.
8. Wang MC, Yu KY, Zhang JG, Wang YP. Zhonghua Wai Ke Za Zhi. 2020;58(11):892–6.
9. Heo DH, Son SK, Eum JH, Park CK. Fully endoscopic lumbar interbody fusion using a percutaneous unilateral biportal endoscopic technique: technical note and preliminary clinical results. Neurosurg Focus. 2017;43(2):E8.
10. Aygun H, Abdulshafi K. Unilateral biportal endoscopy versus tubular microendoscopy in management of single level degenerative lumbar canal stenosis: a prospective study. Clin Spine Surg. 2021;34(6):E323–8.
11. Kim SK, Kang SS, Hong YH, Park SW, Lee SC. Clinical comparison of unilateral biportal endoscopic technique versus open microdiscectomy for single-level lumbar discectomy: a multicenter, retrospective analysis. J Orthop Surg Res. 2018;13(1):22.
12. Hao J, Cheng J, Xue H, Zhang F. Clinical comparison of unilateral biportal endoscopic discectomy with percutaneous endoscopic lumbar discectomy for single L4/5-level lumbar disk herniation. Pain Pract. 2021; https://doi.org/10.1111/papr.13078.
13. Park MK, Park SA, Son SK, Park WW, Choi SH. Clinical and radiological outcomes of unilateral biportal endoscopic lumbar interbody fusion (ULIF) compared with conventional posterior lumbar interbody fusion (PLIF): 1-year follow-up. Neurosurg Rev. 2019;42(3):753–61.
14. Heo DH, Lee DC, Park CK. Comparative analysis of three types of minimally invasive decompressive surgery for lumbar central stenosis: biportal endoscopy, uniportal endoscopy, and microsurgery. Neurosurg Focus. 2019;46(5):E9.
15. Pranata R, Lim MA, Vania R, July J. Biportal endoscopic spinal surgery versus microscopic decompression for lumbar spinal stenosis: a systematic review and meta-analysis. World Neurosurg. 2020;138:e450–8.
16. Min WK, Kim JE, Choi DJ, Park EJ, Heo J. Clinical and radiological outcomes between biportal endoscopic decompression and microscopic decompression in lumbar spinal stenosis. J Orthop Sci. 2020;25(3):371–8.
17. Kim HS, Choi SH, Shim DM, Lee IS, Oh YK, Woo YH. Advantages of new endoscopic unilateral laminectomy for bilateral decompression (ULBD) over conventional microscopic ULBD. Clin Orthop Surg. 2020;12(3):330–6.
18. Merter A, Karaeminogullari O, Shibayama M. Comparison of radiation exposure among 3 different endoscopic diskectomy techniques for lumbar disk herniation. World Neurosurg. 2020;139:e572–9.
19. Choi KC, Shim HK, Kim JS, Cha KH, Lee DC, Kim ER, et al. Cost-effectiveness of microdiscectomy versus endoscopic discectomy for lumbar disc herniation. Spine J. 2019;19(7):1162–9.
20. Gatam AR, Gatam L, Mahadhipta H, Ajiantoro A, Luthfi O, Aprilya D. Unilateral biportal endoscopic lumbar interbody fusion: a technical note and an outcome comparison with the conventional minimally invasive fusion. Orthop Res Rev. 2021;13:229–39.

21. Heo DH, Sharma S, Park CK. Endoscopic treatment of extraforaminal entrapment of L5 nerve root (far out syndrome) by unilateral biportal endoscopic approach: technical report and preliminary clinical results. Neurospine. 2019;16(1):130–7.
22. Lee DY, Shim CS, Ahn Y, Choi YG, Kim HJ, Lee SH. Comparison of percutaneous endoscopic lumbar discectomy and open lumbar microdiscectomy for recurrent disc herniation. J Korean Neurosurg Soc. 2009;46(6):515–21.
23. Park JH, Jun SG, Jung JT, Lee SJ. Posterior percutaneous endoscopic cervical foraminotomy and diskectomy with unilateral biportal endoscopy. Orthopedics. 2017;40(5):e779–83.
24. Pao JL, Lin SM, Chen WC, Chang CH. Unilateral biportal endoscopic decompression for degenerative lumbar canal stenosis. J Spine Surg. 2020;6(2):438–46.
25. Kim JE, Choi DJ, Park EJJ, Lee HJ, Hwang JH, Kim MC, et al. Biportal endoscopic spinal surgery for lumbar spinal stenosis. Asian Spine J. 2019;13(2):334–42.
26. Kim J, Heo DH, Lee DC, Chung HT. Biportal endoscopic unilateral laminotomy with bilateral decompression for the treatment of cervical spondylotic myelopathy. Acta Neurochir (Wien). 2021;163(9):2537–43.
27. Kim JE, Choi DJ. Biportal endoscopic transforaminal lumbar interbody fusion with arthroscopy. Clin Orthop Surg. 2018;10(2):248–52.
28. Quillo-Olvera J, Quillo-Resendiz J, Quillo-Olvera D, Barrera-Arreola M, Kim JS. Ten-step biportal endoscopic transforaminal lumbar interbody fusion under computed tomography-based intraoperative navigation: technical report and preliminary outcomes in Mexico. Oper Neurosurg (Hagerstown). 2020;19(5):608–18.
29. Kang MS, Chung HJ, Jung HJ, Park HJ. How I do it? Extraforaminal lumbar interbody fusion assisted with biportal endoscopic technique. Acta Neurochir. 2021;163(1):295–9.
30. Eun SS, Eum JH, Lee SH, Sabal LA. Biportal endoscopic lumbar decompression for lumbar disk herniation and spinal canal stenosis: a technical note. J Neurol Surg A Cent Eur Neurosurg. 2017;78(4):390–6.
31. Sharma SB, Lin GX, Jabri H, Siddappa ND, Kim JS. Biportal endoscopic excision of facetal cyst in the far lateral region of L5S1: 2-dimensional operative video. Oper Neurosurg (Hagerstown). 2020;18(6):E233.
32. Akbary K, Kim JS, Park CW, Jun SG, Hwang IC. The feasibility and perioperative results of bi-portal endoscopic resection of a facet cyst along with minimizing facet joint resection in the degenerative lumbar spine. Oper Neurosurg (Hagerstown). 2020;18(6):621–8.
33. Choi DJ, Kim JE, Jung JT, Kim YS, Jang HJ, Yoo B, et al. Biportal endoscopic spine surgery for various foraminal lesions at the lumbosacral lesion. Asian Spine J. 2018;12(3):569–73.
34. Kim JS, Park CW, Yeung YK, Suen TK, Jun SG, Park JH. Unilateral bi-portal endoscopic decompression via the contralateral approach in asymmetric spinal stenosis: a technical note. Asian Spine J. 2021;15(5):688–700.
35. Park JH, Jung JT, Lee SJ. How I do it: L5/S1 foraminal stenosis and far-lateral lumbar disc herniation with unilateral bi-portal endoscopy. Acta Neurochir. 2018;160(10):1899–903.
36. Akbary K, Kim JS, Park CW, Jun SG, Hwang JH. Biportal endoscopic decompression of exiting and traversing nerve roots through a single interlaminar window using a contralateral approach: technical feasibilities and morphometric changes of the lumbar canal and foramen. World Neurosurg. 2018;117:153–61.
37. Kang SS, Lee SC, Kim SK. A novel percutaneous biportal endoscopic technique for symptomatic spinal epidural lipomatosis: technical note and case presentations. World Neurosurg. 2019;129:49–54.
38. Lin GX, Huang P, Kotheeranurak V, Park CW, Heo DH, Park CK, et al. A systematic review of unilateral biportal endoscopic spinal surgery: preliminary clinical results and complications. World Neurosurg. 2019;125:425–32.
39. Park SM, Kim GU, Kim HJ, Choi JH, Chang BS, Lee CK, et al. Is the use of a unilateral biportal endoscopic approach associated with rapid recovery after lumbar decompressive laminectomy? A preliminary analysis of a prospective randomized controlled trial. World Neurosurg. 2019;128:e709–18.

40. Kim JE, Choi DJ. Clinical and radiological outcomes of unilateral biportal endoscopic decompression by 30 degrees arthroscopy in lumbar spinal stenosis: minimum 2-year follow-up. Clin Orthop Surg. 2018;10(3):328–36.
41. Lee HG, Kang MS, Kim SY, Cho KC, Na YC, Cho JM, et al. Dural injury in unilateral biportal endoscopic spinal surgery. Global Spine J. 2021;11(6):845–51.
42. Wang H, Wang K, Lv B, Li W, Fan T, Zhao J, et al. Analysis of risk factors for perioperative hidden blood loss in unilateral biportal endoscopic spine surgery: a retrospective multicenter study. J Orthop Surg Res. 2021;16(1):559.
43. Ahn DK, Lee JS, Shin WS, Kim S, Jung J. Postoperative spinal epidural hematoma in a biportal endoscopic spine surgery. Medicine (Baltimore). 2021;100(6):e24685.
44. Lewandrowski KU, Soriano-Sanchez JA, Zhang X, Ramirez Leon JF, Soriano Solis S, Rugeles Ortiz JG, et al. Surgeon training and clinical implementation of spinal endoscopy in routine practice: results of a global survey. J Spine Surg. 2020;6(Suppl 1):S237–48.
45. Lewandrowski KU, Soriano-Sanchez JA, Zhang X, Ramirez Leon JF, Soriano Solis S, Rugeles Ortiz JG, et al. Surgeon motivation, and obstacles to the implementation of minimally invasive spinal surgery techniques. J Spine Surg. 2020;6(Suppl 1):S249–59.
46. Kang T, Park SY, Kang CH, Lee SH, Park JH, Suh SW. Is biportal technique/endoscopic spinal surgery satisfactory for lumbar spinal stenosis patients? A prospective randomized comparative study. Medicine (Baltimore). 2019;98(18):e15451.
47. Kim JE, Yoo HS, Choi DJ, Hwang JH, Park EJ, Chung S. Learning curve and clinical outcome of biportal endoscopic-assisted lumbar interbody fusion. Biomed Res Int. 2020;2020:8815432.
48. Choi DJ, Choi CM, Jung JT, Lee SJ, Kim YS. Learning curve associated with complications in biportal endoscopic spinal surgery: challenges and strategies. Asian Spine J. 2016;10(4):624–9.
49. Kim JS, Yeung A, Lokanath YK, Lewandrowski KU. Is Asia truly a hotspot of contemporary minimally invasive and endoscopic spinal surgery? J Spine Surg. 2020;6(Suppl 1):S224–36.
50. Wu PH, Kim HS, Choi DJ, Gamaliel Y-HT. Overview of tips in overcoming learning curve in uniportal and biportal endoscopic spine surgery. J Minim Invasive Spine Surg Tech. 2021;6(Suppl 1):S84–96.

Chapter 11
From Conventional to Biportal Endoscopic Surgery: The Transition Observed by an Expert Surgeon

Yanting Liu, Claudia-Angélica Covarrubias-Rosas, and Jin-Sung Kim

Abbreviations

BESS	Biportal endoscopic spinal surgery
CPK	Creatine phosphokinase
CRP	C-reactive protein
LBP	Lower back pain
MISS	Minimally invasive spine surgery
ODI	Oswestry Disability Index
RCT	Randomized controlled trial
TLIF	Transforaminal lumbar interbody fusion
UBE	Unilateral biportal endoscopy
ULBD	Unilateral laminotomy bilateral decompression
VAS	Visual analog scale

Y. Liu (✉) · J.-S. Kim
Neurosurgery and Minimally Invasive Spine Surgery, Department of Neurosurgery, Seoul St. Mary's Hospital, College of Medicine, The Catholic University of Korea, Seoul, South Korea
e-mail: yantingliu02@gmail.com; mddavidk@gmail.com

C.-A. Covarrubias-Rosas
Department of Experimental Surgery, McGill University, Montreal, QC, Canada
e-mail: claudia.covarrubias@mcgill.ca

J. Quillo-Olvera et al. (eds.), *Unilateral Biportal Endoscopy of the Spine*,
https://doi.org/10.1007/978-3-031-14736-4_11

Introduction

Globally, low back pain is the leading cause of years lost to disability [1]. In the United States alone, it is estimated that approximately 1 million spine procedures are performed annually, with current trends indicating increased demand [2]. In addition, spinal surgery procedures have rapidly evolved during the past few decades through breakthrough technological development in image-based intraoperative navigation systems and disruptive technologies. As a result, there has been a shift towards minimally invasive spine surgery (MISS) techniques.

Furthermore, when compared to conventional open spine surgery, MISS techniques have proven to be less damaging to adjacent spinal tissues, offering safer and less aggressive procedures through reduced hospital stay, blood loss, infection rate, and perioperative pain, thus allowing for faster return to functional life for the patient [3].

With a steep learning curve, endoscopic spinal surgery is one of the techniques among the MISS approaches that offer precision from guided intraoperative navigation, which has undergone generational evolution since it was first introduced in the 1990s [4, 5].

Indications for endoscopic spinal surgery are categorized in terms of generations, most often employed for degenerative disc diseases such as total intervertebral disc removal or as an adjuvant to lumbar fusion. They are described to offer more advantages proportional to the complexity of the disease present [4, 6].

Unilateral biportal endoscopy (UBE), conducted through unilateral access with two ports, is one of the variants of endoscopic procedures frequently utilized for decompression and fusion of the spine. This chapter describes the evolution and transition of conventional spine procedures to biportal endoscopic spinal surgery (BESS) as observed by an expert spinal surgeon (JSK).

Considerations of Endoscopic Technique

Technical Characteristic of Open Techniques

Decades ago, surgery was mainly performed with open surgical techniques as the gold standard for the treatment of lumbar spinal disease; however, it requires excessive dissection of the paraspinal structures, leading to postoperative muscle apoptosis and denervation [7]. Meanwhile, traditional discectomy and facetectomy exacerbate postoperative instability by excessive lamina and facet joint disruption with additional fusion surgery [8–10].

All of the above factors represent an elevated hidden risk of postoperative infection and long recovery times. With the promotion of microsurgery, spine surgical techniques have undergone a paradigm shift, regarding the microscopic tubular approach on the spine; however, these existing clinical performances are far from sufficient for meeting the needs of patients.

First, it is challenging to manipulate instruments through a narrow working tube under unclear visualization to access the contralateral surgical field, even when the microscope is tilted to the contralateral side, especially in obese patients. Second, surgical visualization and instrumental range of motion are restricted due to crowding within the surgical field, which can potentially result in inadequate decompression, leading to the presence of remnant lesions and revision surgery.

Technical Characteristic of Endoscopic Techniques

Based on the primary principle of surgical treatment to amend symptomatic relief and functional improvement with minor invasion, various MISS techniques have emerged as alternatives to conventional surgery and thus have become the current prevailing procedures in East Asian countries, reaching the consensus of the development of endoscopic techniques.

Such transmutation appreciates the introduction of the safe triangular zone discovered by Kambin and Hijikata and the technological progress of surgical instruments in high-resolution cameras, high-speed burr, and high-performance light source systems [11, 12].

Compared with microscopic surgery, the advantage of endoscopic surgery has minimal damage to the paraspinal muscles and better preservation of posterior structures and direct neural decompression without violation of the central nucleus [13–19]. Additionally, the endoscope allows the surgeon's eye to extend to the area adjacent to the lesion and dural sac. It can help explore the corner of the lateral recess and assess neural decompression by inspecting the dural sac pulsation.

Meanwhile, continuous saline irrigation gentles the plane dissection of the epidural space intraoperatively, providing more spacious intervening space between the ligament and neural structure, thus significantly reducing the risk of nerve injury and epidural bleeding.

In general, saline pressure is recommended to maintain an optimal pressure of 30 mmHg, preventing cerebrospinal fluid hypertension and tissue edema. Moreover, it can also prevent the accumulation of thermal energy, which predisposes to severe tissue-related thermal necrosis during high-speed drill and electrocautery operations.

In the present moment, the percutaneous uniportal and biportal endoscopic techniques are the two most common and widely used techniques in endoscopic spinal surgery. However, compared to the uniportal endoscopic technique, biportal endoscopic surgery has different technical characteristics (Fig. 11.1).

Biportal endoscopic technique utilizes two independent and transmuscular portals that are installed on the unilateral side, one being the endoscopic portal, which allows for continuous saline irrigation and provides real-time magnification view, and the other serving as a working portal that allows flexible manipulation of various instruments for bleeding control or bone work. Therefore, biportal endoscopic surgery yields independent movement and familiar anatomic orientations similar to open surgery, which is impossible using uniportal endoscopy as it restricts one-directional view and motion.

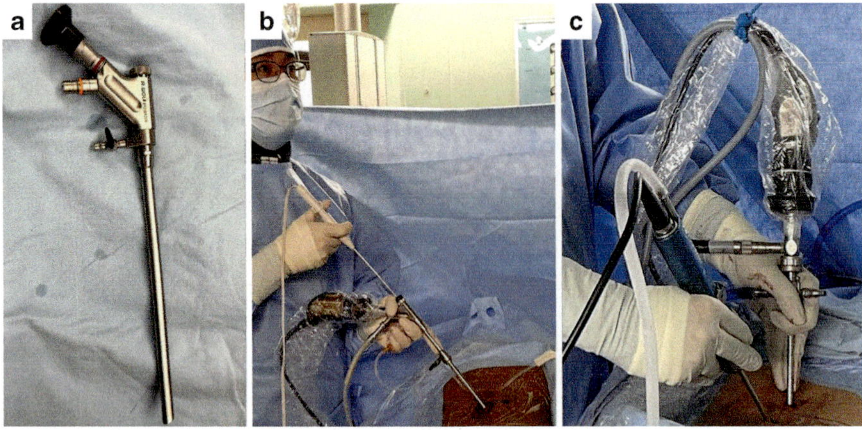

Fig. 11.1 (**a**) Transforaminal endoscopic lens, (**b**) uniportal endoscopic surgery (transforaminal full-endoscopic discectomy), (**c**) biportal endoscopic surgery

Two independent portals provide a broader surgical view of the intracanalicular area, especially in decompression around the corner of lateral recess or broadened spinal stenosis. It also achieves a superior range of motion of instruments with familiar manipulation feeling similar to open or arthroscopic surgery. It is worthy to note that the biportal endoscopic working cannula does not require specialized endoscopic tools, as an open surgery or arthroscopic instruments can also be adapted for its use.

Therefore, biportal endoscopy could be used as a transition tool for learning uniportal endoscopy on adapting to the magnified field of endoscopic view. And also, because of the relatively low-cost technology, the biportal endoscopy offers benefit and is used widespread in underdeveloped countries. However, even though the biportal system is similar to conventional or arthroscopic surgery, it still requires basic techniques with a steep learning curve, being more complicated than the microscope technique by one-handed manipulation.

Park et al. [20] reported a learning curve cumulative summation test to evaluate the learning curve of biportal endoscopy in novice surgeons with no previous endoscopic experience, reporting sufficient competency to perform decompression surgery at the 58th operation.

Broadening of the Indications of Endoscopic Techniques

It has been emphasized that the goal of a novel technique is to fulfill clinical results commensurate with current methods, being less invasive and avoiding adverse long-term outcomes.

There was a concern that endoscopic surgery could potentially be labeled as "incomplete decompression" or "few indications." However, with the development of the endoscopic equipment and accumulation of experience in surgeons, the indication of endoscopic surgery has broadened after the technique has seen improvement on laminectomy, foraminotomy, and transforaminal lumbar interbody fusion (TLIF) surgery.

Up until this moment, uniportal and biportal endoscopic techniques are the indicated treatment options for single lumbar disc herniation and juxtafacet cysts that can be treated via foraminal technique or the high-"keyhole" technique; unilateral asymmetrical spinal stenosis can be treated with unilateral laminectomy for bilateral decompression (ULBD); and spinal instability or significant intervertebral disc collapse can be treated with TLIF [11, 12].

The therapeutic effect of two endoscopic techniques compared with the microscopic technique has been previously reported as "noninferiority" in the literature [21]. A previous meta-analysis found no significant difference in visual analog scale (VAS) score for low back and lower extremity pain and Oswestry Disability Index (ODI) at 2–3 months and the final follow-up [22–24]. Interestingly, the VAS score for low back pain was higher in the microscopic technique than in two endoscopic procedures in other prospective and retrospective studies [14, 24, 25]. This may be related to the inflammatory response generated by surgical injury, described later in the chapter.

Furthermore, one intention-to-treat and per-protocol analysis confirmed similar clinical results with no differences in length of hospital stays or complications between the microscopic and biportal endoscopic surgery [24, 26]. Despite a series of researches that included RCTs for meta-analysis, the efficacy of UBE remains unclear, such as there is no consensus on the operative time in UBE and microsurgery [16, 22, 23, 27].

Recently, a large multicenter, prospective randomized controlled trial (RCT), an assessor-blind trial, is expected to solve the puzzle and provide high-level clinical evidence for developing clinical guidance of biportal endoscopic technique in spine surgery [28].

From the authors' point of view, uniportal endoscopic surgery is usually much faster than microsurgery in simple spinal diseases, and it depends on the complexity of lesions and the proficiency of endoscopic surgeons. In addition, based on the authors' personal experience, the following patient selection could achieve a satisfactory treatment with endoscopic technique:

1. Radiating pain on lower extremities, low back pain, or intermittent claudication related to index-level lesion.
2. Radiological evidence correlated to the symptoms such as persistent intermittent claudication or neurological symptoms.
3. Mono-segmental pathology.
4. Patients with grade I or II degenerative spondylolisthesis or isthmic spondylolisthesis.
5. Concomitant foraminal stenosis with intermediate-degree spinal stenosis. Additional criteria would be the persistence in the patient's symptoms with no response to appropriate conservative treatment over three months.

In contrast, the contraindication of endoscopic spine surgery is as follows:

1. Severe ligamentum flavum ossification
2. Complex trauma, oncology, or inflammatory spondylolisthesis with musculoskeletal disorders
3. Multi-segmental spinal instability
4. High-grade degenerative or isthmic spondylolisthesis
5. Severe adhesion in revision surgery
6. Advanced adult spinal deformity (Cobb angle >20°)

Lumbar Spinal Stenosis

Lumbar spinal stenosis is a significant cause of lower back pain (LBP), neurogenic claudication, and decreased walking ability, and is a common and disabling condition mainly affecting daily function and overall quality of life [29, 30].

The pathological characteristic of degenerative spinal stenosis is defined by the facet joint arthropathy, ligament flavum hypertrophy or ossification, and degenerative intervertebral disc that narrows the spaces for the dural sac and nerve root [31].

In general, conventional treatments such as physiotherapy or steroid injection have been clinically recommended for patients with mild-to-moderate symptoms [16]. The clinical outcomes of non-surgery are unsatisfactory, failing to meet patients' expectations compared with decompressive surgery in treating a patient with lumbar spinal stenosis [32]. For less pain and effective treatment, percutaneous endoscopic surgery is often the first choice for surgeons.

However, most consider the unsatisfactory outcomes with revision surgery caused by incomplete decompression with the endoscopic technique. If surgeons were to embrace the standard principle of the surgical procedure, the unfavorable outcome would often be correlated with a patient preoperative clinical condition, such as long-term claudication or severe stenosis, and not with the technique.

In the case of unbroadened asymmetric spinal stenosis, manipulating biportal endoscopy from the non-diseased side could grant an easier decompression. First, approaching the contralateral side achieves more expansive bony undercutting space in the cross-sectional area through the center of the vertebral body and spinolaminar junction [33]. Meanwhile, more strength and meticulous motion can be applied to the tip of the instruments through more extended arm movement achieved with the principle of leverage. At the same time, the less pathologically constraint space on the normal side could effectively prevent accidental intraoperative injuries on the way to the intended target point. Secondly, the whole process of instrument manipulation follows the principle of leverage, and the ipsilateral facet joint can be used as a fulcrum bearing to change the force orientation of the high-speed drill or Kerrison rongeurs away from the neural structures.

The deep-layer ligament flavum can be used as a protective barrier recommended for resection after laminectomy. Great attention should be given to the "in-out" bony work undercutting the ventral side of the contralateral lamina, as it can cause fracture of the lamina if proper attention to the interface between the cancellous and cortical bone is not given, especially in cases with accompanying osteoporosis.

Additionally, most of the anatomical planes between healthy and pathological tissue can be identified with 0° endoscopy overhead the dural from the contralateral side. However, under endoscopic manipulation, further decompression of the lateral recess or foraminal area is challenging. Prospective studies in the literature have also reported that uniportal endoscopy has limited visualization of the lateral recess and foraminal area [34].

However, we found that changing to 30°, a 4 mm endoscope is an excellent strategy to access foraminal regions and lateral recess [35]. Therefore, uniportal endoscopy proficiently can achieve the same surgical effects as biportal endoscopy treatment while achieving less surgical injury to the musculoligamentous structures. To note, the monetary cost of the uniportal endoscopic system is undeniably higher.

Lumbar Interbody Fusion

First introduced by Harms and Jeszenszky, TLIF has become a popular and well-established technique to restore the height of the interbody without nerve structure retraction [36].

Conventional interbody fusion has a higher risk of incomplete decompression of neural element, inadequate endplate preparation, and iatrogenic ischemia in deep layers of muscle tissue due to the narrow and deep working space consisting of the tubular retractor. Presently, the emergence of endoscopic surgery has made up for that disadvantage by introducing the working cannula.

It could provide the magnified real-time intraoperative visual inspection at the location of the interbody, improving the efficiency of removal of the disc and cartilaginous material. Also, it could further reduce the surgical trauma of paraspinal muscle retraction, eliminating the patient's need to take opioids and only necessitating simple oral analgesics like acetaminophen [37–39].

In degenerative scoliosis cases, a tridimensional deformity consisting of rotation and lateral deviation of the spine is the most common presentation. The surgical corridor starting from the concave side will produce a long vertical distance from the skin surface to the bone with complex foraminal pathology. Therefore, we recommend operating on the contralateral side, providing a safe surgical corridor to place the cage and acquire decompression. Meanwhile, the contralateral approach allows surgeons to keep an ergonomic position with an upright posture instead of leaning forward intraoperatively. On the other hand, surgeons have some concerns regarding the negative impact of graft material loss and decreasing fusion rate because of continuous fluid irrigation. Nevertheless, some previous reports pointed out that irrigation does not affect the postoperative spinal fusion [37, 40].

Discussion

The surgical injury will cause paravertebral muscle denervation and necrosis, resulting in postoperative spinal instability, which is common and unavoidable in spine surgery, even in uniportal endoscopic surgery. Because the dorsal ramus's medial branch innervates the paraspinal multifidus muscles, the surgical approach plays a crucial role in protecting this paraspinal structure [41, 42]. Therefore, lateral recess decompression via the ipsilateral approach has a higher risk of dorsal rami injury.

The endoscopic technique provides an obvious advantage of tissue-sparing preserving facet joint and ligament complex structures. In the contralateral approach, oblique blunt dissection from lateral transverse incision to the spinolaminar junction through the potential space between the multifidus fascicles medially creates a unique corridor that does not communicate between muscle layers under the natural anatomical position, improving the tightness of the postoperative incision. Meanwhile, a more lateral superficial incision is recommended for a larger movement angle of instruments without excessive skin tension and less excursion force in the multifidus structures during leverage.

Although the surgical related paraspinal muscle injury is related to the time and extent of muscle retraction, the multifidus change shows a tendency to reverse back to normal condition without causing long-term postoperative pain and disability in endoscopic surgery. Choi et al. [13] reported that the level of creatine phosphokinase (CPK) and C-reactive protein (CRP) in the uniportal endoscopic technique was lower than that in the biportal endoscopy and microscopy for discectomy, especially on the postoperative days 1 and 3.

A similar previous laboratory also explained the postoperative surgical related muscle pain that lowers the elevation of biomarkers of serum CRP and CPK level in endoscopic surgery than microscopic surgery in the early postoperative period, with no difference in serum CPK level between the microscopic and endoscopic techniques at the 3-, 6-, or 12-month follow-up [26, 37, 43].

On the other hand, the preservation of facet joint plays a critical role in preventing postoperative spinal instability. In general, interbody fusion is necessary for additional surgery to avoid potential spinal column instability after spinal decompression in conventional surgery. However, radiography evidence found that the resection area is only 15.8% of the total articular process in lateral recess stenosis with the foraminal area using the UBE technique [44]. Further, the mean angle of the resection area of facetectomy is significantly lower than microscopic surgery [14, 25]. Therefore, the above evidence shows that endoscopic techniques are a good substitute for decreasing the fusion rate with faster pain relief than microscopic techniques.

Future Perspective

Nowadays, prospective studies, RCT studies, and cost-benefit analyses are rare and require a longer follow-up time and larger sample sizes from different regions to continue to explore the benefits of endoscopy. Until now, endoscopic surgery has achieved satisfactory data in East Asia, which has laid a strengthened foundation for the third-generation surgical revolution of spinal surgery. It can be believed that shortly, the technological convergence in navigation and augmented reality technology will provide more advanced intraoperative navigation.

In the future, artificial intelligence deep learning projects would become the robot's brain to analyze real-time intraoperative images and identify critical anatomical structures. Likewise, the endoscopic skills of surgeons would become the learning objects of the robot to access the lesion automatically. Future advances can also facilitate long-distance real-time sharing under low-latency communication technology, achieving globalization of knowledge and technology.

Conclusion

Endoscopic spine surgery is not a "panacea"; the first surgical principle is thorough the removal of pathology rather than blindly pursuing less invasiveness. Meanwhile, the degree of preservation of paraspinal structures and nerve decompression in endoscopic surgery often depends on the proficiency of surgeons, according to our perspective. Uniportal endoscopic techniques benefit simple disc herniation and unilateral foraminal and lateral recess lesions, and for central stenosis or other complex conditions, the biportal endoscopic approach looks better.

Despite the restricted manipulation in uniportal endoscopy, it could achieve the same satisfactory clinical results as microscopy or biportal endoscopy with better protection of the paraspinal structure. However, complication rates may be higher in the learning stage of endoscopic surgery, and the operation is recommended to be performed under the senior endoscopic surgeon after strictly selecting proper patient candidates.

References

1. Grotle M, Småstuen MC, Fjeld O, et al. Lumbar spine surgery across 15 years: trends, complications and reoperations in a longitudinal observational study from Norway. BMJ Open. 2019;9(8):e028743.
2. McDermott KW, Freeman WJ, Elixhauser A. Overview of operating room procedures during inpatient stays in U.S. hospitals, 2014: statistical brief #233. Healthcare Cost and Utilization Project (HCUP) statistical briefs. Washington, DC: Agency for Healthcare Research and Quality (US); 2006.
3. Nerland US, Jakola AS, Solheim O, et al. Minimally invasive decompression versus open laminectomy for central stenosis of the lumbar spine: pragmatic comparative effectiveness study. BMJ. 2015;350:h1603.
4. Kim M, Kim HS, Oh SW, et al. Evolution of spinal endoscopic surgery. Neurospine. 2019;16(1):6–14.
5. Akbary K, Kim JS. Recent technical advancements of endoscopic spine surgery with disparate or disruptive technologies and patents. World Neurosurg. 2021;145:693–701.
6. Ahn Y, Youn MS, Heo DH. Endoscopic transforaminal lumbar interbody fusion: a comprehensive review. Expert Rev Med Devices. 2019;16(5):373–80.

7. Sihvonen T, Herno A, Paljärvi L, Airaksinen O, Partanen J, Tapaninaho A. Local denervation atrophy of paraspinal muscles in postoperative failed back syndrome. Spine (Phila Pa 1976). 1993;18(5):575–81.
8. Mobbs RJ, Li J, Sivabalan P, Raley D, Rao PJ. Outcomes after decompressive laminectomy for lumbar spinal stenosis: comparison between minimally invasive unilateral laminectomy for bilateral decompression and open laminectomy: clinical article. J Neurosurg Spine. 2014;21(2):179–86.
9. Eum JH, Heo DH, Son SK, Park CK. Percutaneous biportal endoscopic decompression for lumbar spinal stenosis: a technical note and preliminary clinical results. J Neurosurg Spine. 2016;24(4):602–7.
10. James A, Laufer I, Parikh K, Nagineni VV, Saleh TO, Härtl R. Lumbar juxtafacet cyst resection: the facet sparing contralateral minimally invasive surgical approach. J Spinal Disord Tech. 2012;25(2):E13–7.
11. Kambin P. Arthroscopic microdiscectomy. Arthroscopy. 1992;8(3):287–95.
12. Hijikata S. Percutaneous nucleotomy. A new concept technique and 12 years' experience. Clin Orthop Relat Res. 1989;238:9–23.
13. Choi KC, Shim HK, Hwang JS, et al. Comparison of surgical invasiveness between microdiscectomy and 3 different endoscopic discectomy techniques for lumbar disc herniation. World Neurosurg. 2018;116:e750–8.
14. Heo DH, Lee DC, Park CK. Comparative analysis of three types of minimally invasive decompressive surgery for lumbar central stenosis: biportal endoscopy, uniportal endoscopy, and microsurgery. Neurosurg Focus. 2019;46(5):E9.
15. Lin GX, Huang P, Kotheeranurak V, et al. A systematic review of unilateral biportal endoscopic spinal surgery: preliminary clinical results and complications. World Neurosurg. 2019;125:425–32.
16. Chen T, Zhou G, Chen Z, Yao X, Liu D. Biportal endoscopic decompression vs. microscopic decompression for lumbar canal stenosis: a systematic review and meta-analysis. Exp Ther Med. 2020;20(3):2743–51.
17. Khandge AV, Sharma SB, Kim JS. The evolution of transforaminal endoscopic spine surgery. World Neurosurg. 2021;145:643–56.
18. Liu Y, Kim J-S, Chen C-M, et al. A review of full-endoscopic interlaminar discectomy for lumbar disc disease: a historical and technical overview. J Minim Invasive Spine Surg Tech. 2021;6(Suppl 1):S109–16.
19. Chen KT, Jabri H, Lokanath YK, Song MS, Kim JS. The evolution of interlaminar endoscopic spine surgery. J Spine Surg. 2020;6(2):502–12.
20. Park SM, Kim HJ, Kim GU, et al. Learning curve for lumbar decompressive laminectomy in biportal endoscopic spinal surgery using the cumulative summation test for learning curve. World Neurosurg. 2019;122:e1007–13.
21. Kim SK, Kang SS, Hong YH, Park SW, Lee SC. Clinical comparison of unilateral biportal endoscopic technique versus open microdiscectomy for single-level lumbar discectomy: a multicenter, retrospective analysis. J Orthop Surg Res. 2018;13(1):22.
22. Pranata R, Lim MA, Vania R, July J. Biportal endoscopic spinal surgery versus microscopic decompression for lumbar spinal stenosis: a systematic review and meta-analysis. World Neurosurg. 2020;138:e450–8.
23. Kang T, Park SY, Kang CH, Lee SH, Park JH, Suh SW. Is biportal technique/endoscopic spinal surgery satisfactory for lumbar spinal stenosis patients? A prospective randomized comparative study. Medicine (Baltimore). 2019;98(18):e15451.
24. Heo DH, Quillo-Olvera J, Park CK. Can percutaneous biportal endoscopic surgery achieve enough canal decompression for degenerative lumbar stenosis? Prospective case-control study. World Neurosurg. 2018;120:e684–9.
25. Min WK, Kim JE, Choi DJ, Park EJ, Heo J. Clinical and radiological outcomes between biportal endoscopic decompression and microscopic decompression in lumbar spinal stenosis. J Orthop Sci. 2020;25(3):371–8.

26. Park SM, Park J, Jang HS, et al. Biportal endoscopic versus microscopic lumbar decompressive laminectomy in patients with spinal stenosis: a randomized controlled trial. Spine J. 2020;20(2):156–65.
27. Kaito T. In lumbar spinal stenosis, biportal endoscopic decompressive laminectomy did not differ from microscopic lumbar decompressive laminectomy for low back-associated disability and QoL at 1 year. J Bone Joint Surg Am. 2020;102(16):1467.
28. Park HJ, Park SM, Song KS, et al. Evaluation of the efficacy and safety of conventional and biportal endoscopic decompressive laminectomy in patients with lumbar spinal stenosis (ENDO-B trial): a protocol for a prospective, randomized, assessor-blind, multicenter trial. BMC Musculoskelet Disord. 2021;22(1):1056.
29. Hall S, Bartleson JD, Onofrio BM, Baker HL Jr, Okazaki H, O'Duffy JD. Lumbar spinal stenosis. Clinical features, diagnostic procedures, and results of surgical treatment in 68 patients. Ann Intern Med. 1985;103(2):271–5.
30. Whitman JM, Flynn TW, Childs JD, et al. A comparison between two physical therapy treatment programs for patients with lumbar spinal stenosis: a randomized clinical trial. Spine (Phila Pa 1976). 2006;31(22):2541–9.
31. Choi CM, Chung JT, Lee SJ, Choi DJ. How I do it? Biportal endoscopic spinal surgery (BESS) for treatment of lumbar spinal stenosis. Acta Neurochir (Wien). 2016;158(3):459–63.
32. Malmivaara A, Slätis P, Heliövaara M, et al. Surgical or nonoperative treatment for lumbar spinal stenosis? A randomized controlled trial. Spine (Phila Pa 1976). 2007;32(1):1–8.
33. Van Schaik JP, Verbiest H, Van Schaik FD. Isolated spinous process deviation. A pitfall in the interpretation of AP radiographs of the lumbar spine. Spine (Phila Pa 1976). 1989;14(9):970–6.
34. Komp M, Hahn P, Ozdemir S, et al. Operation of lumbar zygoapophyseal joint cysts using a full-endoscopic interlaminar and transforaminal approach: prospective 2-year results of 74 patients. Surg Innov. 2014;21(6):605–14.
35. Akbary K, Kim JS, Park CW, Jun SG, Hwang IC. The feasibility and perioperative results of bi-portal endoscopic resection of a facet cyst along with minimizing facet joint resection in the degenerative lumbar spine. Oper Neurosurg (Hagerstown). 2020;18(6):621–8.
36. Harms JG, Jeszenszky D. Die posteriore, lumbale, interkorporelle Fusion in unilateraler transforaminaler Technik. Oper Orthop Traumatol. 1998;10(2):90–102.
37. Kang MS, You KH, Choi JY, Heo DH, Chung HJ, Park HJ. Minimally invasive transforaminal lumbar interbody fusion using the biportal endoscopic techniques versus microscopic tubular technique. Spine J. 2021;21(12):2066–77.
38. Quillo-Olvera J, Quillo-Reséndiz J, Quillo-Olvera D, Barrera-Arreola M, Kim JS. Ten-step biportal endoscopic transforaminal lumbar interbody fusion under computed tomography-based intraoperative navigation: technical report and preliminary outcomes in Mexico. Oper Neurosurg (Hagerstown). 2020;19(5):608–18.
39. Park SM, Kim GU, Kim HJ, et al. Is the use of a unilateral biportal endoscopic approach associated with rapid recovery after lumbar decompressive laminectomy? A preliminary analysis of a prospective randomized controlled trial. World Neurosurg. 2019;128:e709–18.
40. Kim JE, Yoo HS, Choi DJ, Park EJ, Jee SM. Comparison of minimal invasive versus biportal endoscopic transforaminal lumbar interbody fusion for single-level lumbar disease. Clin Spine Surg. 2021;34(2):E64–71.
41. Binder DS, Nampiaparampil DE. The provocative lumbar facet joint. Curr Rev Musculoskelet Med. 2009;2(1):15–24.
42. Shuang F, Hou SX, Zhu JL, et al. Clinical anatomy and measurement of the medial branch of the spinal dorsal ramus. Medicine (Baltimore). 2015;94(52):e2367.
43. Choi DJ, Kim JE. Efficacy of biportal endoscopic spine surgery for lumbar spinal stenosis. Clin Orthop Surg. 2019;11(1):82–8.
44. Akbary K, Kim JS, Park CW, Jun SG, Hwang JH. Biportal endoscopic decompression of exiting and traversing nerve roots through a single interlaminar window using a contralateral approach: technical feasibilities and morphometric changes of the lumbar canal and foramen. World Neurosurg. 2018;117:153–61.

Chapter 12
Put It into Practice: The Unilateral Biportal Endoscopic Surgery

Henry-David Nava-Dimaano

Abbreviations

e.g.	exempli gratia (For example)
i.e.	id est
OR	Operating room
RF	Radiofrequency
UBE	Unilateral biportal endoscopy

Introduction

Since Mixter and Barr first described their fully open laminectomy technique for decompression of the lumbar spine in 1934, surgeons have continually sought to improve on this original technique, making the surgical exposure smaller, less disruptive, and less destabilizing as possible while still being able to achieve adequate decompression of impinged neurologic structures inside the bony spine [1]. The next paradigm shift in this pursuit would come in 1977 in the form of Caspar and Yasargil's open microdiscectomy technique, which enabled surgeons to adequately decompress the lumbar spine while using a smaller exposure, with visualization that is aided by operative microscopy, thus requiring less muscle injury and less bony removal [1].

However, the minimally invasive nature of microscope-assisted lumbar spine surgery would be further improved by introducing the tubular dilator system

H.-D. Nava-Dimaano (✉)
Department of Orthopedic Surgery, Fe del Mundo Medical Center (Mount Grace Hospitals Inc.), Quezon City, Metro Manila, Philippines
e-mail: drhenrydimaano@gmail.com

J. Quillo-Olvera et al. (eds.), *Unilateral Biportal Endoscopy of the Spine*,
https://doi.org/10.1007/978-3-031-14736-4_12

independently devised by Destandau and Foley in 1990 [2, 3]. This technique allowed for the smallest possible opening that would be compatible with an "air-medium" visualization device (i.e., either operative microscope or magnifying loupes).

The limitations of visualization of the surgical site through an air medium would be both focal length (i.e., the surgeon's eyes are still outside of the patient's body, viewing the spine structures through a progressively narrow tunnel) and bleeding at the surgical site (which would necessitate the use of a suction tube, Cottonoid pads, coagulation packing, and vigorous hemostasis with bipolar electrocautery). And while image magnification can be increased to compensate, this would, in turn, decrease both field of view and flexibility of a line of sight.

Innovation of Lumbar Endoscopic Access

The workaround for limitations of a microscope-based technique for spine surgery would come in the form of the percutaneously inserted endoscope (Fig. 12.1). By 1988, Kambin demonstrated that the nucleus pulposus of a lumbar disc could be safely accessed with an arthroscope by passing through a triangular zone on the posterolateral corner of the intervertebral disc bordered by the exiting nerve root, the traversing nerve root, and the superior endplate margin of the lower vertebra

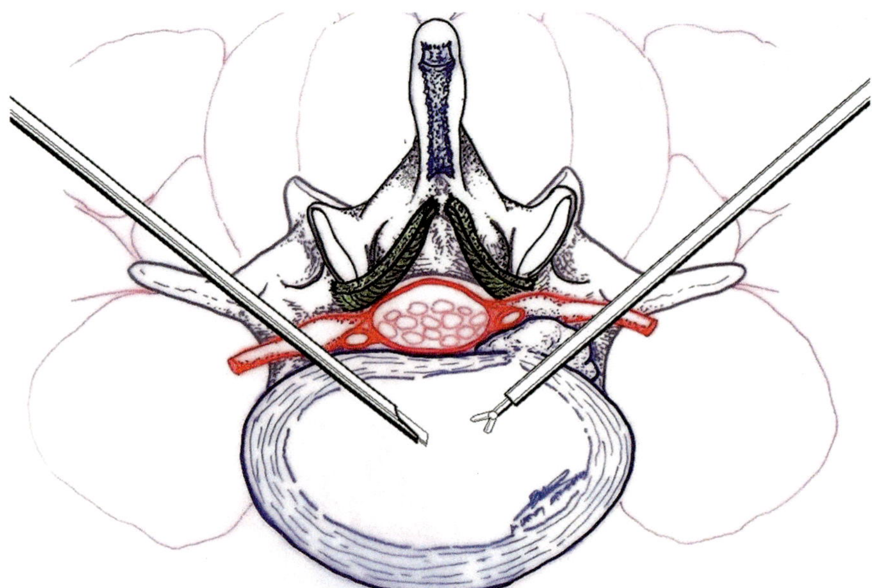

Fig. 12.1 Diagram of bilateral biportal approach for discectomy used by Kambin

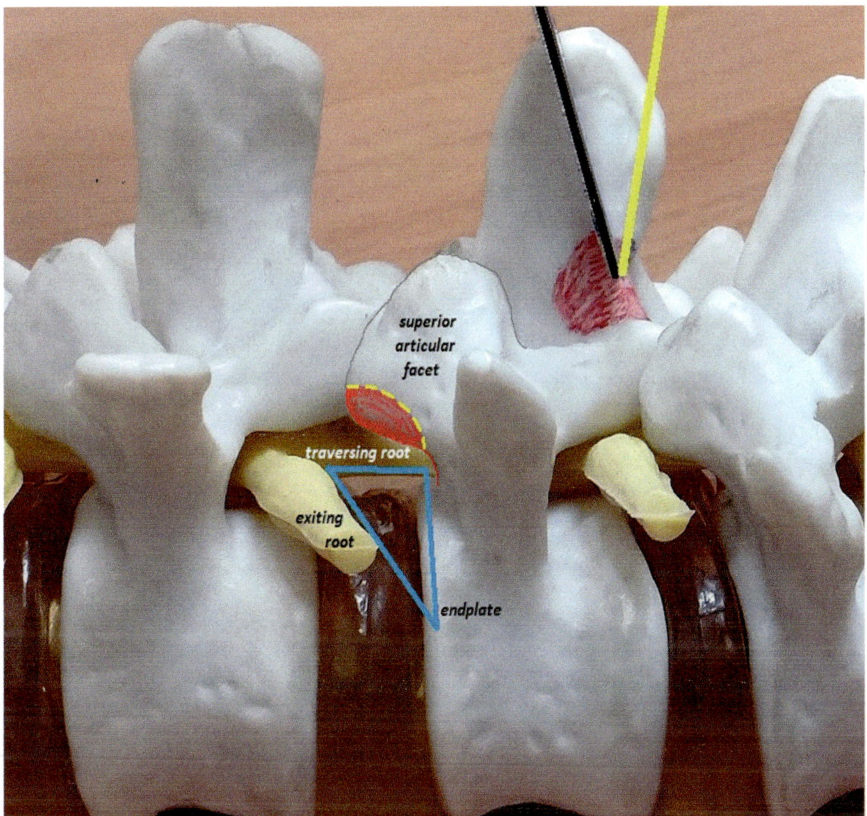

Fig. 12.2 The Kambin's triangle is represented in blue

(Fig. 12.2). The Kambin's triangle is the anatomic foundation of uniportal endoscopic lumbar spine surgery [1, 2, 4, 5].

With the rapid development of multichannel endoscopes and percutaneous drills and burrs, as well as innovations in operative techniques—e.g., those by Yeung and Tsou (1997), by Schubert and Hoogland (2005), or by Choi (2008)—uniportal transforaminal decompression evolved into a subspecialty of minimally invasive spine surgery (Fig. 12.3) [1, 2, 5].

Coinciding with the rapid development of uniportal transforaminal endoscopic spine surgery techniques during the turn of the millennium, there was a growing interest in repurposing the arthroscope used for orthopedic knee and shoulder surgery (Fig. 12.4), with a purpose of creating a comparable minimally invasive lumbar technique based on the more familiar interlaminar approach.

Note that by this time, the current standard of minimally invasive spine surgery, which used an interlaminar approach, was the technique based on serially enlarging tubular muscle retractors popularized by Destandau and Foley in the 1990s, basically a uniportal system [2, 3].

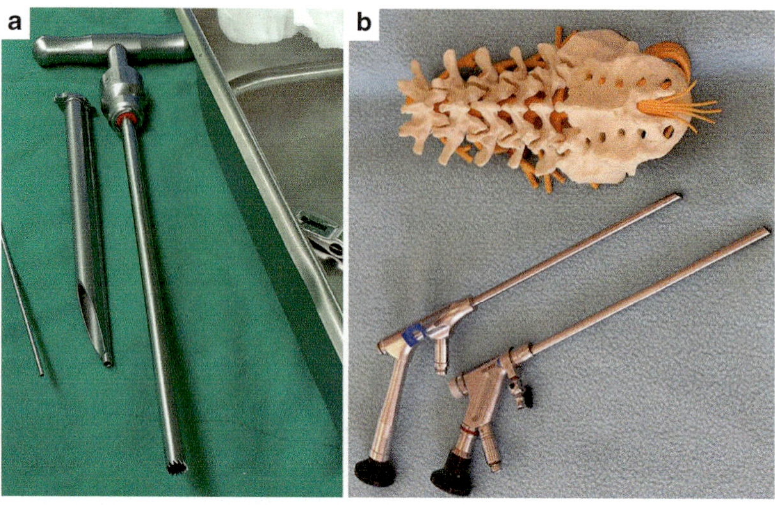

Fig. 12.3 Specialized devices for uniportal endoscopy. (**a**) Percutaneous cannulated trephine system for transforaminal resection of the underside of superior articular process. (**b**) Percutaneous multichannel endoscopes for transforaminal discectomy

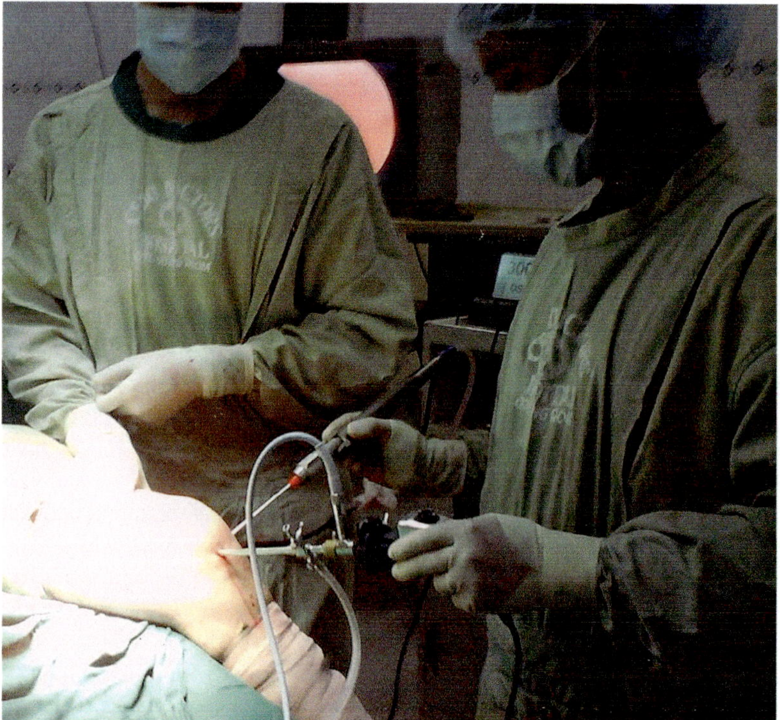

Fig. 12.4 Knee arthroscopy uses a biportal endoscopic approach to visualize and manipulate cartilaginous and bony intra-articular structures without needing a direct line of sight

As a biportal modification of the tubular retractor technique, De Antoni demonstrated his translaminar lumbar epidural endoscopy technique in 1996 [6]. And half a decade later, a similar biportal visualization technique for arthroscopic discectomy was introduced by Abdul Gaffar Shaikh Ahmed in Bahrain Defense Force Hospital.

Transition to Biportal Endoscopic Access

From these initial attempts at using the arthroscope as a makeshift endoscope (with the working channel now separate from the viewing channel), it slowly became apparent that both the mini-open microscope-assisted interlaminar lumbar decompression technique and uniportal endoscopic transforaminal decompression technique were destined to produce a hybridized approach to minimally invasive spine surgery: one that would bring the surgeon's eyes inside the patient's body and maximize the preservation of spinal muscle and bone as uniportal spine endoscopy does while allowing the surgeon to use both hands familiarly (akin to the haptics of minimally invasive "air-medium" lumbar surgery) (Fig. 12.5).

True enough, as early as 2001, South Korean spine surgeons led by Jin Hwa Eum and Sang Kyu Son began pioneering what would eventually be known today as "UBE" or "unilateral biportal endoscopy" [7].

The UBE technique would initially find use in lumbar disc herniations treated with an ipsilateral interlaminar approach (Fig. 12.6). Still, not surprisingly, this approach would later evolve to techniques that include contralateral lumbar decompression for degenerative central and lateral stenosis and superiorly migrated disc herniations, as well as transforaminal approaches for far-lateral disc herniations and degenerative foraminal canal stenosis. In addition, UBE techniques would later find use in patients with thoracic or cervical (Fig. 12.7) compressive pathologies and low-grade lumbar instabilities that can be treated with endoscopic interbody fusion.

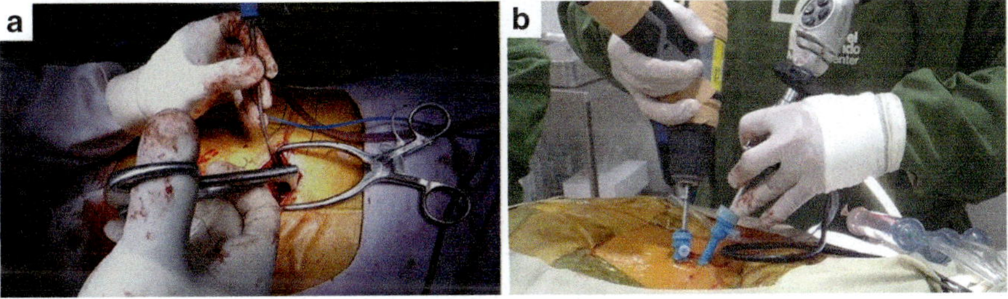

Fig. 12.5 From open to biportal endoscopic surgery. (**a**) Open lumbar discectomy. (**b**) Unilateral biportal endoscopic discectomy

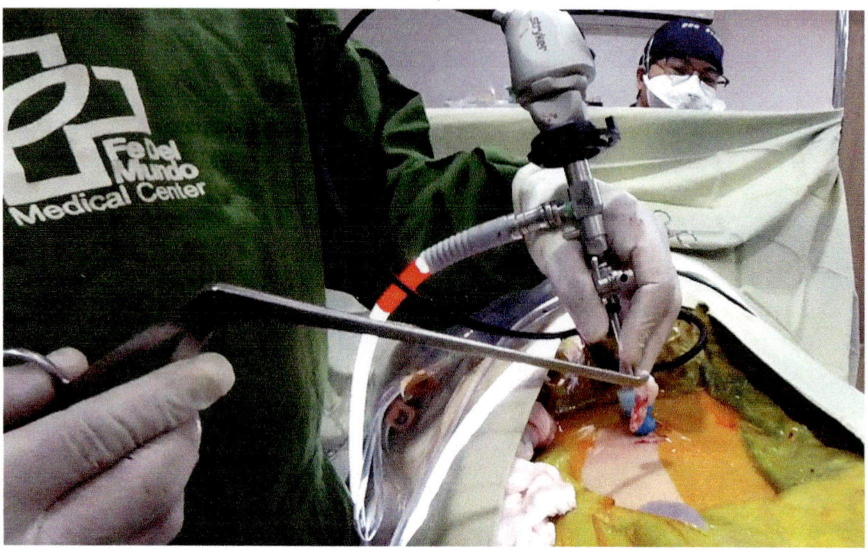

Fig. 12.6 Lumbar disc herniation removed via UBE discectomy technique

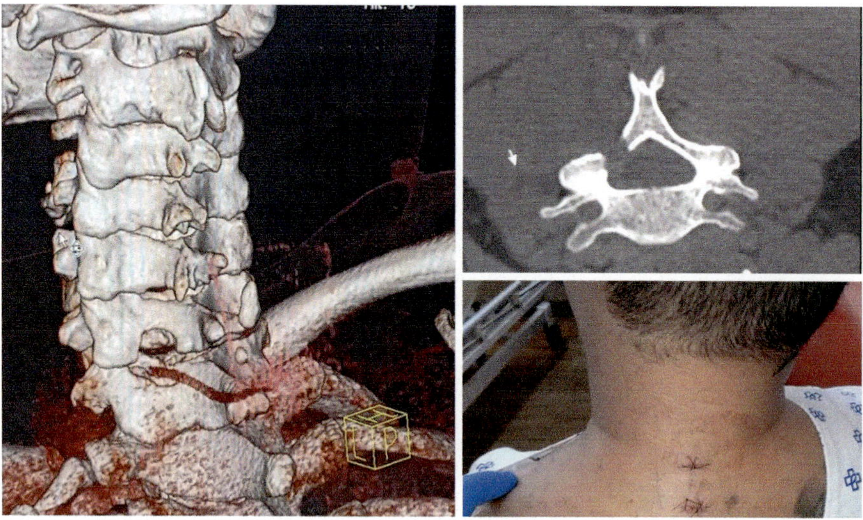

Fig. 12.7 UBE posterior cervical discectomy

Preoperative Preparation

Surgical Indications and Endpoints

The most basic UBE procedure is that of lumbar ipsilateral laminotomy combined with discectomy (or simply sequestrectomy or hernioplasty, as some instances may require) [8, 9]. This basic technique is indicated for clinically significant central and posterolateral lumbar disc herniations, which occur at L4–L5 and L5–S1 levels. The surgical endpoints of this technique are quite straightforward:

- Create the least possible damage to intrinsic spinal muscles.
- Preserve the posterior central ligamentous tension band.
- Remove the least possible amount of bony vertebra.
- Create adequate visualization of neural structures.
- Preserve as much of the facet joint as possible—so as not to create iatrogenic instability that would necessitate fusion (using pedicle screws and rods and interbody cages).
- Adequately decompress the neurologic structures while avoiding mechanical and hydrostatic injury.

Paracentral and lateral disc herniations are the most common indications for UBE lumbar surgery. In addition, far-lateral herniations can also be treated with UBE techniques—e.g., via paramedian contralateral sublaminar route or paraspinal transforaminal approach (Fig. 12.8). However, these approaches are technically in the realm of "advanced techniques" [10, 11], in which case, we shall exclude these techniques from this discussion of basic UBE and instead focus on pathologies illustrated in Fig. 12.9.

Surgical Preoperative Planning

The side from which the surgeon approaches is of major consideration in the planning of the actual procedure. It is easier for most right-handed surgeons to use their dominant right hand to handle the cutting and grasping instruments while using the nondominant left hand for holding the endoscope. Add to this the anterosuperior-to-posteroinferior slope of the laminae, thus making it more optimal for the opening of the working port to be placed about 1–1.5 cm inferior to the level of the disc [12, 13].

With this positioning, a right-handed surgeon would find it easier standing on the left side of the prone patient (Fig. 12.10). With the slope of the laminae making the inferior approach of the working instruments more optimal, the endoscope would now naturally have to originate from a port opening at about 1–1.5 cm superior to the level of the disc. This usually places the endoscopic trajectory nearly perpendicular to the lamina and practically in line with the anteroposterior orientation of the disc (Fig. 12.11).

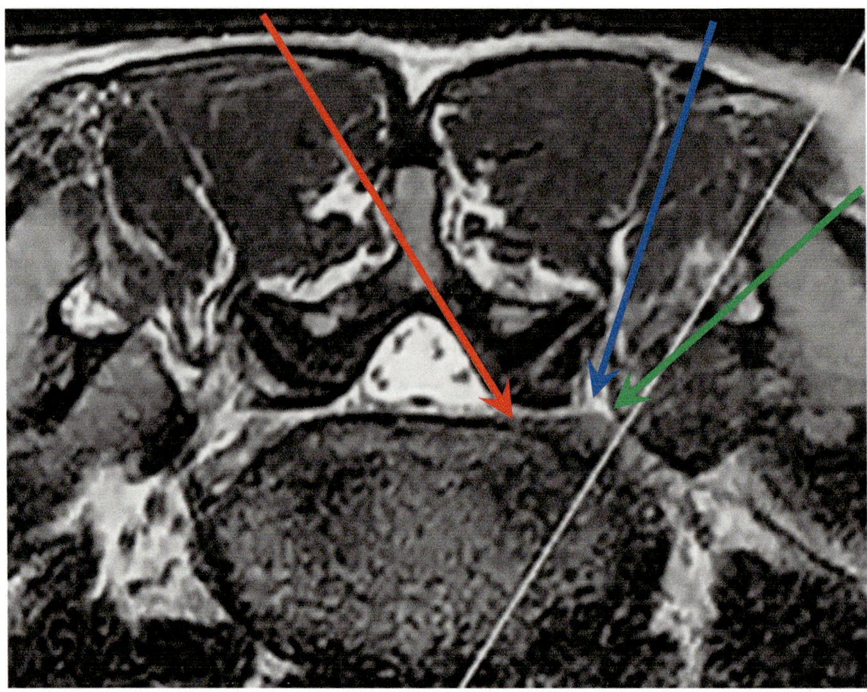

Fig. 12.8 Approaches for far-lateral disc herniations: contralateral UBE approach (red arrow), transforaminal UBE approach (blue arrow), uniportal transforaminal approach (green arrow)

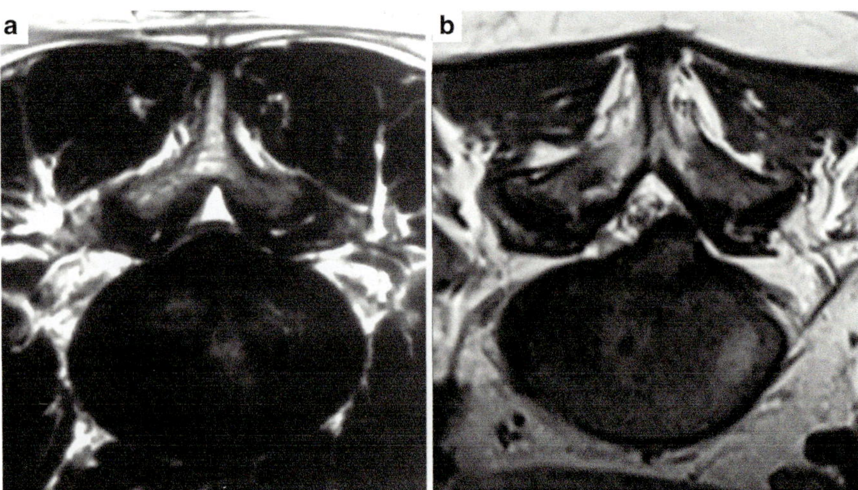

Fig. 12.9 Indications for UBE discectomy. (**a**) Central broad-based lumbar disc herniation. (**b**) Lateral lumbar disc herniation

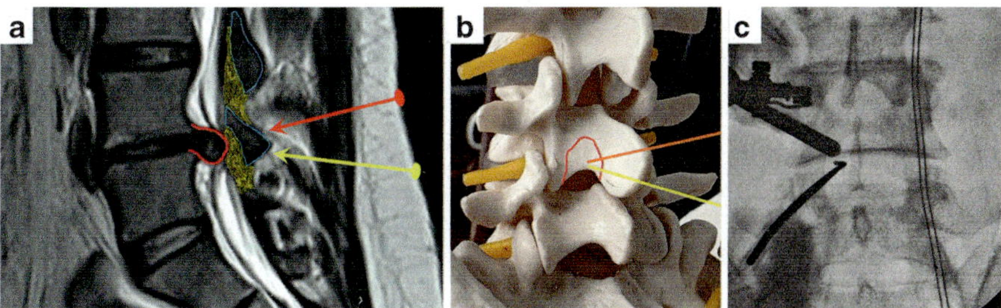

Fig. 12.10 Paramedian approach for UBE discectomy. (**a**) Scope port trajectory (red arrow) and working port trajectory (yellow arrow) on the lateral view of lumbar MRI. (**b**) Left oblique view showing port trajectories (orange and yellow lines). (**c**) AP fluoroscopic view showing scope and probe

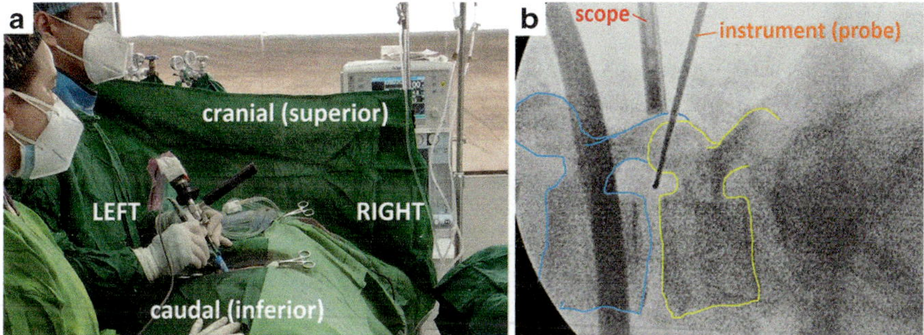

Fig. 12.11 Biportal approach confirmed with the C-arm. (**a**) Surgeon and assistant standing on the patient's left side. (**b**) Lateral fluoroscopic view showing scope and probe

As part of preoperative planning, it is typically prudent to digitally pre-measure the distances and angles of the viewing and working ports on the MRI (Fig. 12.12) to understand how deep and steep your instruments will be positioned during the surgery. While seasoned surgeons may already have a "second-nature" feel for estimating distances and angles, nothing is lost with observing due diligence in preparing for every patient's unique anatomy.

As pointed in Fig. 12.13, it is also prudent to note that the interlaminar windows of every motion segment (yellow lines) have varying-level relationships to their respective discs (red lines)—i.e., the interlaminar L5–S1 window is most in line along the horizontal plane of its corresponding disc, in contrast with those of L4–L5, L3–L4, L2–L3, and L1–L2. That means a more superiorly positioned disc will likely require a relatively taller laminotomy to provide adequate exposure of the posterior aspect of the annulus.

In contrast, an L5–S1 discectomy may not require the surgeon to do a laminotomy and instead merely necessitates a partial ipsilateral flavectomy—i.e., by adequately flexing the patient in the prone position, the interlaminar window might open up enough, such that both the scope and working instrument can easily move down into the central canal after removal of the ligamentum flavum.

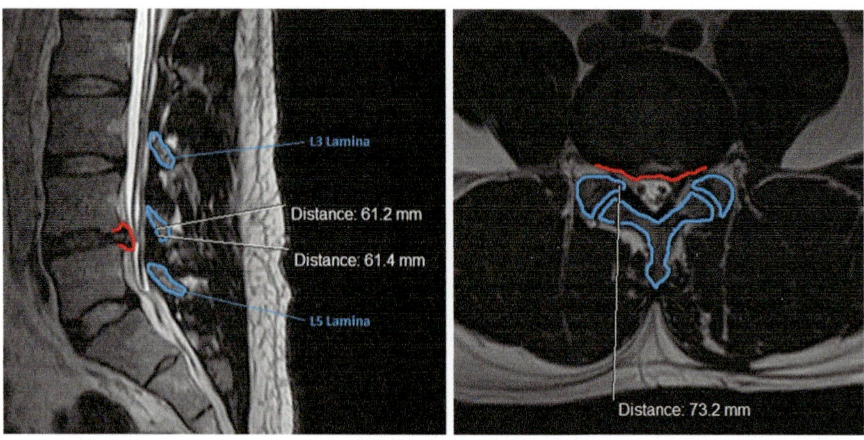

Fig. 12.12 Measurements from the skin to lamina and facet using the digital caliper function of the MRI software. The measurements are likely to be underestimated since the patient is in a supine position upon MRI scanning, thus compressing the soft tissues of the back and shortening the distance from skin to bony spine

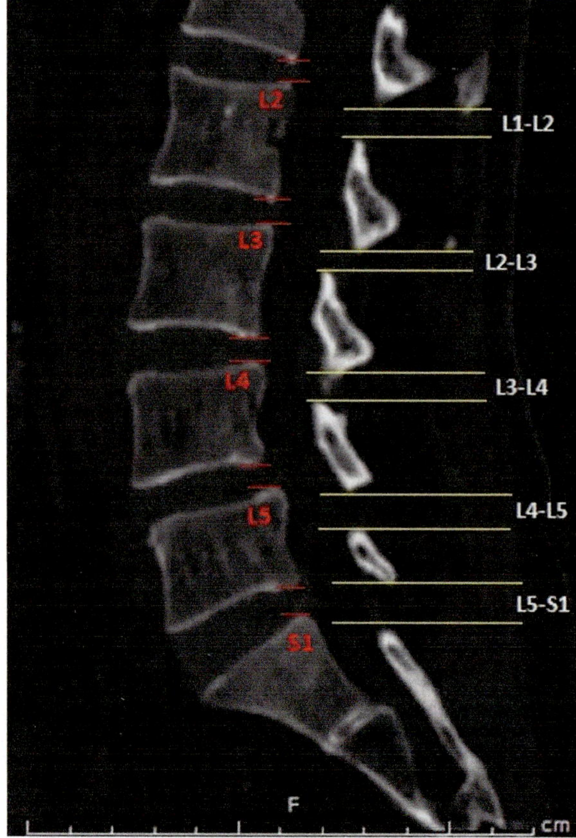

Fig. 12.13 Lateral CT scan bone window along the sagittal plane of the laminae

Operating Room Setup

Placing the patient in a prone position with partial trunk flexion on an appropriately cushioned operating table serves as the optimal setup. Figure 12.14 shows a typical operating room (OR) configuration for a UBE procedure. In addition, it is recommended that the lumbar spine and sacrum be placed a bit lower than the head (Fig. 12.15) to minimize the risk of gravity-driven increased intracranial pressure from saline infusion into the epidural space [12].

Depending on the requirements of the procedure, the patient may be asleep (intubated and under general anesthesia) or awake to a certain degree (under lumbar epidural anesthesia, with or without an epidural catheter) while lying prone.

Saline infusion pressure may be preset via gravity (Fig. 12.16a) or with the help of an automated infusion pump (Fig. 12.16b). The recommended infusion pressure is 30–50 mmHg (saline bottles raised to a height of 1.5–1.7 m)—strong enough to stop capillary bleeding but mild sufficient to reveal arterial bleeding that requires coagulation. Also, by maintaining saline pressure within this range, increased intracranial pressure risk is significantly lessened, thus avoiding postoperative headache and delayed recovery [13].

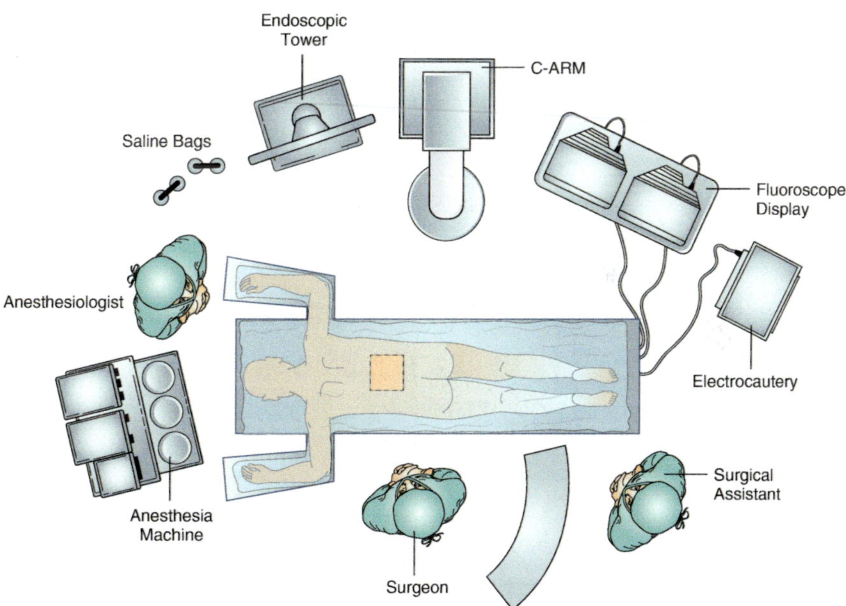

Fig. 12.14 OR setup

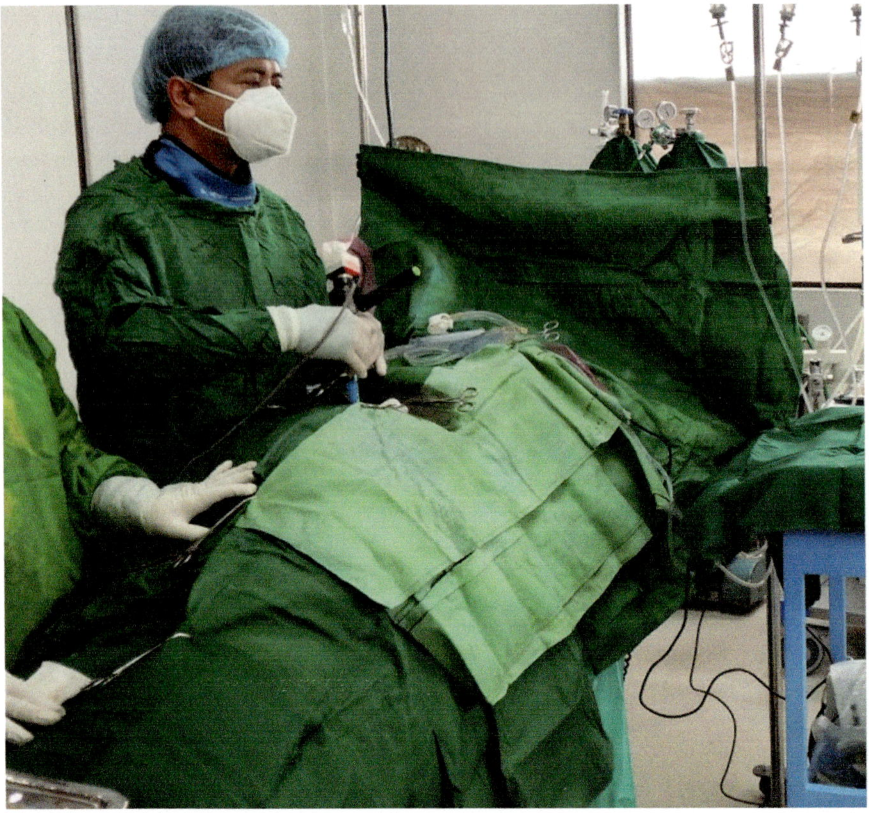

Fig. 12.15 OR table in slight Fowler's (head up) position

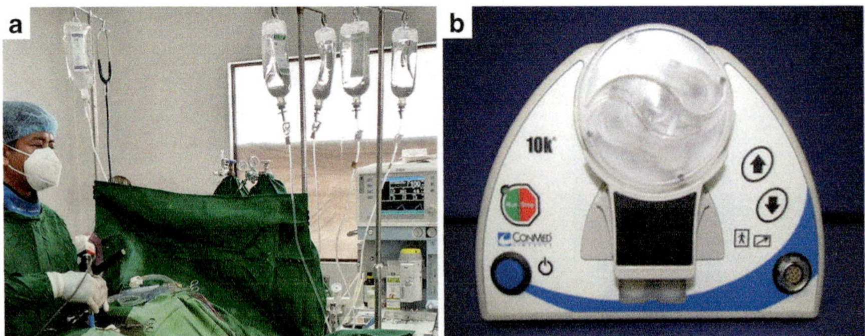

Fig. 12.16 Saline infusion during UBE. (a) Gravity infusion. (b) Water pump

Surgical Instruments

One of the biggest advantages of the UBE technique is its compatibility with standard open spine surgery instruments—i.e., classic Kerrison rongeurs, classic hook probes and micro-forceps, small curettes, narrow osteotomes, and even modified bipolar electrocautery probes—as well as standard arthroscopy equipment—e.g., the arthroscopic shaver which also doubles as a bone drill and burr, radiofrequency (RF) coagulator wands for both hemostasis and soft-tissue debridement, and of course the standard arthroscope (Fig. 12.17). The advantage of this equipment is that it is less expensive to procure and more familiar to use than the uniportal endoscopic instrument system.

A standard 0° "front-facing" scope (with a diameter of 4 mm and a length of 175 mm) that inserts into a 6-mm-wide saline infusion endoscope sleeve is usually sufficient for basic UBE work. However, depending on the demands of the surgery, a 30° "glancing" endoscope (typically used by arthroscopists/well-trained general orthopedic surgeons) can also be used to provide the surgeon a wider field of rotational view. As an added feature, the scope's sleeve can be designed with a "tongue" at its tip, making it similar in function to the uniportal endoscope's sleeve—i.e., for use as a nerve root retractor (Fig. 12.18).

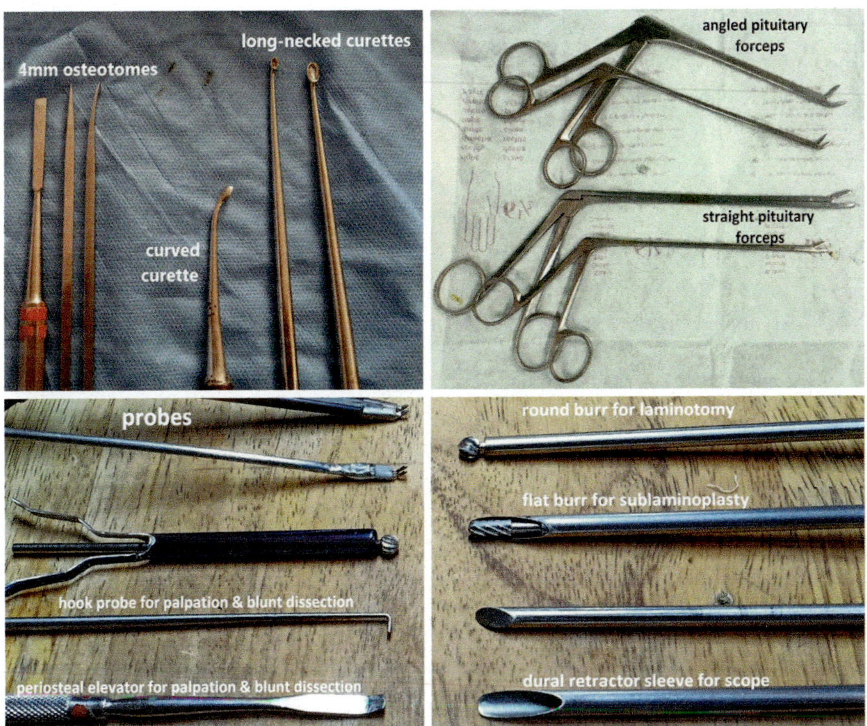

Fig. 12.17 Spine instruments used for classic open surgery can be used for UBE

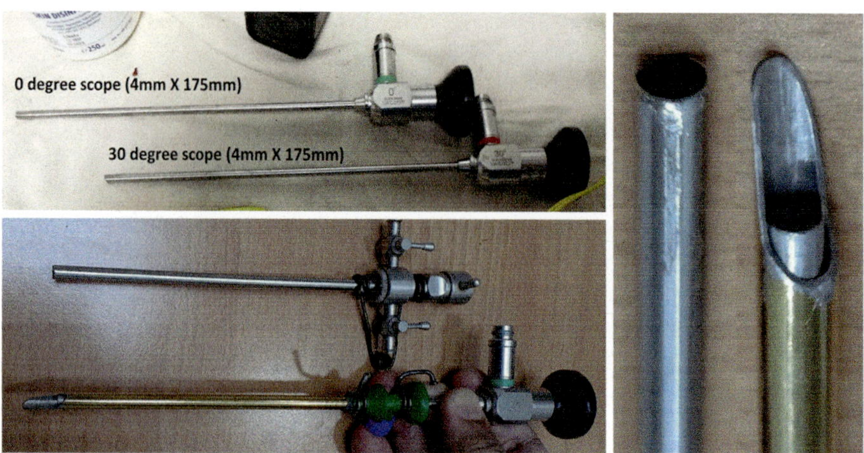

Fig. 12.18 Standard arthroscopes for UBE and modified "tongue" tip of scope sleeve for retraction

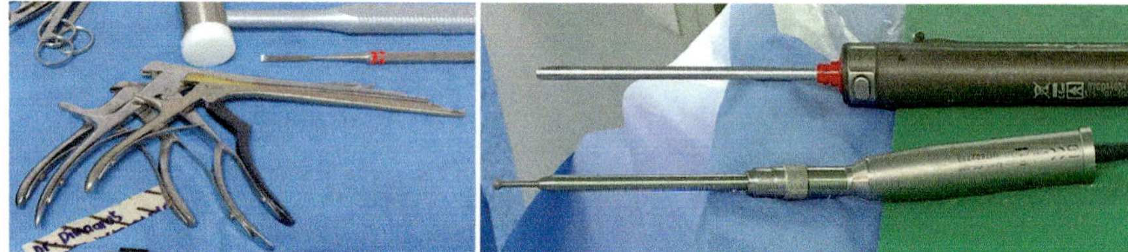

Fig. 12.19 Kerrison punches, arthroscopic shaver, and high-speed drill

A power drill of sufficient length (e.g., an arthroscopic burr or neurosurgical burr) combined with various Kerrison bone rongeurs is typical of all the bone-cutting laminotomy equipment that a UBE surgeon will need (Fig. 12.19). The drill is used to thin out the lamina from the dorsal (posterior) cortex to the cancellous bone; then, the Kerrison punches are used for removing the remaining ventral (anterior) laminar cortex. An osteotome may be used in place of the burr; however, osteotomy requires that an assistant will have to pound the osteotome with a mallet—unlike a burr which does not need a "third hand" to work.

Achieving hemostasis is essential to UBE surgery, given that any bleeding in the endoscopic working space can make the saline turbid and cause a "red out" of the endoscope's view. In addition, fluent saline flow helps wash out capillary extravasation, and judicious use of saline pressure helps in tamponading low-pressure bleeders. However, for persistent bleeding, electrocoagulation or electrocautery is necessary. The preferred system for hemostasis would be the RF ablator (or "RF probe/wand"). This coagulator probe quickly burns and contracts soft tissues and efficiently stops bone bleeding. However, RF probes rapidly generate a lot of heat that can cause thermal damage to neural structures—so cautiously use it with only short, targeted bursts. (As a personal preference, I use bipolar electrocautery probes normally used in open spine surgery—these generate less heat but work slower at stopping bleeds and contracting soft tissue) (Fig. 12.20).

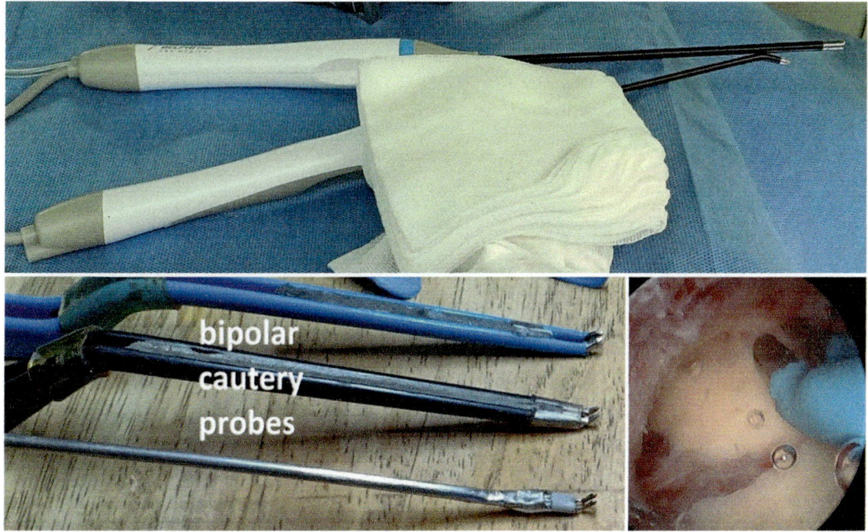

Fig. 12.20 Top: RF wands—large flat tip and small round curved tip. Bottom: Bipolar cautery probes for open surgery repurposed for UBE

Surgical Technique

Fluoroscopic Landmarks

After patient positioning, instrument and equipment preparation, and operating room setup, fluoroscopic localization of the surgical level and targeting of the starting point of the endoscopic working space can be done (Fig. 12.21). Two small-bore spinal needles (G22, 10 cm length) can be used as directional guides for creating the scope and working ports. For single disc-level procedures, skin openings are made 2–3 cm apart and centered on the disc's X-ray projection on the skin. Both ports are placed about 1.5 cm left of midline (Fig. 12.22). Keep the X-ray beam axis straight down and adequately centered on your target disc.

Two points of convergence need to be considered when reviewing the MRI and when starting the fluoroscopic triangulation:

1. The spinolaminar junction, where muscle clearance and bone exposure for the creation of the working space are most accessible (Fig. 12.23)
2. The posterior annulus of the disc itself, where the surgeon can safely retract the nerve roots and access the herniation (Fig. 12.24)

As the working space is enlarged by laminotomy and flavectomy, expect the tip of the inverted triangle to go deeper—and the instrument angle to get steeper. This is why it is recommended that the port skin openings be at least 1–1.5 cm equidistant from the level of the disc—to avoid crowding of the surgeon's hands when the scope and instrument tips dive deeper.

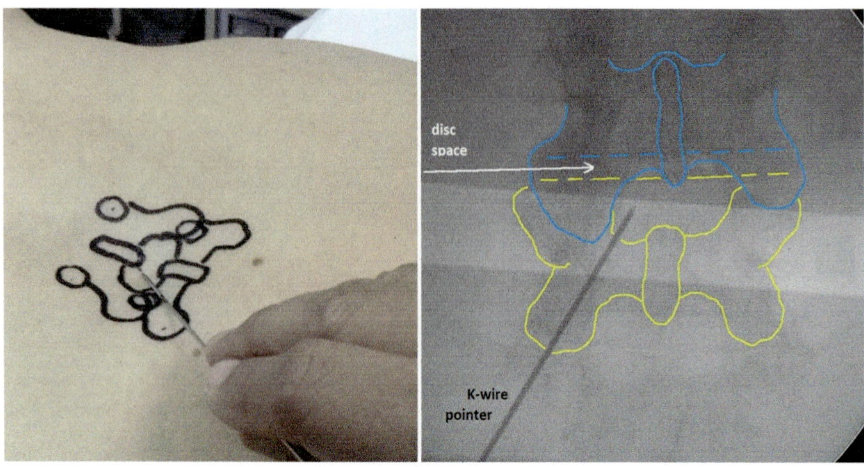

Fig. 12.21 Fluoroscopic outline of interlaminar space using a K-wire as a pointer. Disc space location is also mapped here

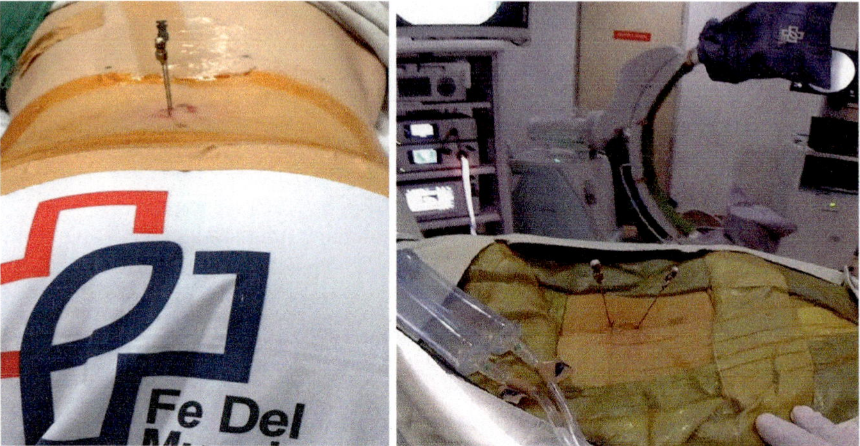

Fig. 12.22 Fluoroscopic insertion of triangulation needles can then be done to facilitate dissection of the working space

Creating the Working Space

Once the creation of the ports and targeting of the inferior spinolaminar junction are done, the multifidus and rotatores muscle fascicles are stripped off their bony attachments. This is easiest if the dissection begins inside the multifidus triangle, where the intermuscular gap provides a low-resistance starting point for soft-tissue dissection and bony exposure [12]. As muscles are lifted off the lamina, the entering saline solution acts as a hydro-dissector and enlarges the working space, allowing for an

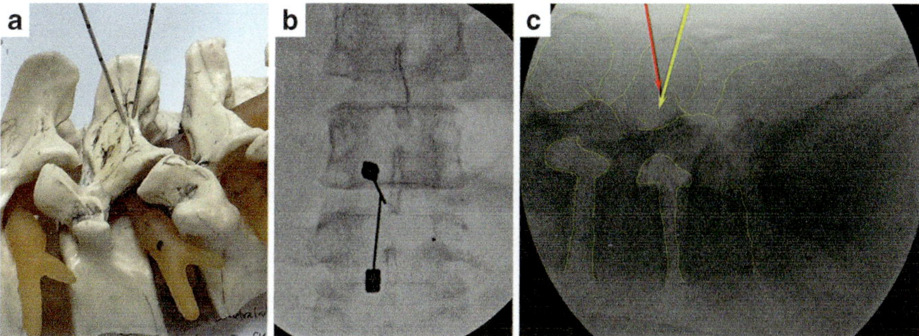

Fig. 12.23 Paramedian UBE approach addressed to the spinolaminar junction. (**a**) Simulation with needles in an anatomical model. (**b**) Triangular approach on the AP view of the C-arm. (**c**) Triangular approach on the lateral view of the C-arm. The bony structures are highlighted in yellow

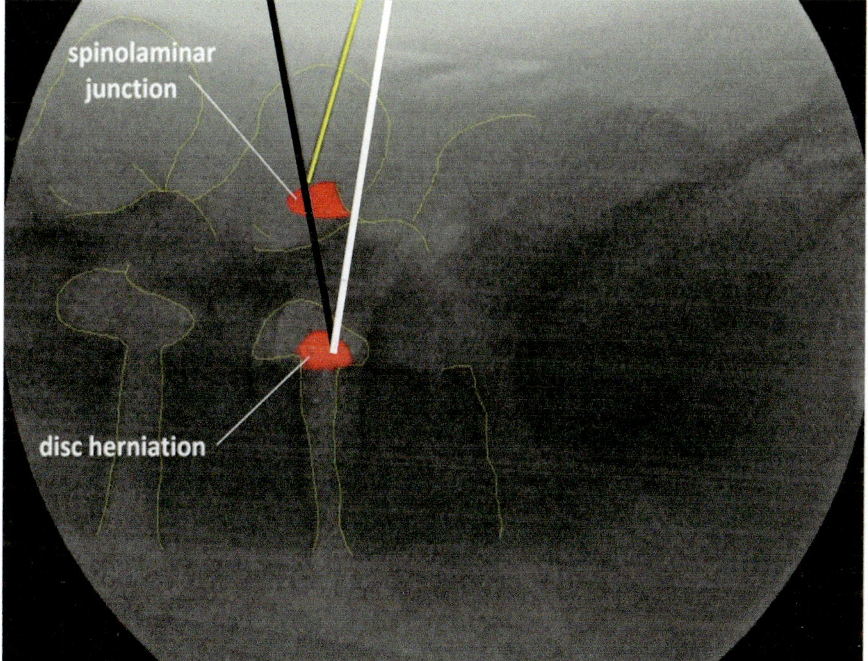

Fig. 12.24 Planning on C-arm's lateral projection, the trajectory of both ports according to the disc pathology. First, the approach was addressed to the spinolaminar junction (black and yellow lines), and then it is advanced to the disc (black and white lines)

even wider view of the inferior half of the lamina and base spinous process (Fig. 12.25). In addition, RF coagulation on muscles and tendons controls bleeding, thus keeping the saline environment blood-free while also detaching the soft tissue off the bone.

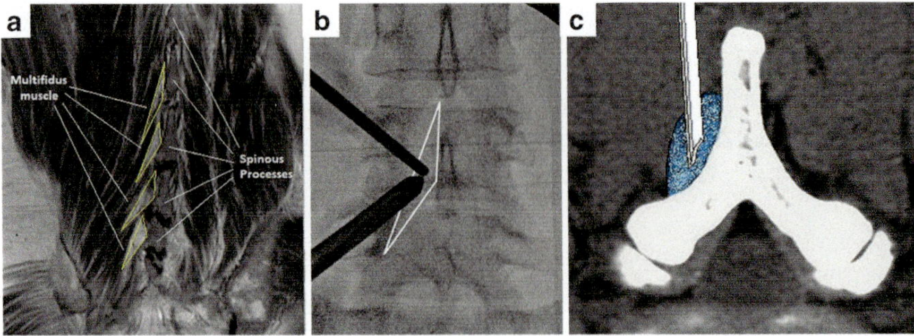

Fig. 12.25 Epiperiosteal space or the so-called multifidus triangle. (**a**) Coronal view of the lumbar MRI showing the multifidus triangle (yellow triangles) at different levels. (**b**) Paramedian UBE approach through the multifidus triangle (white triangle). (**c**) Working space enlarged by the continuous irrigated fluid

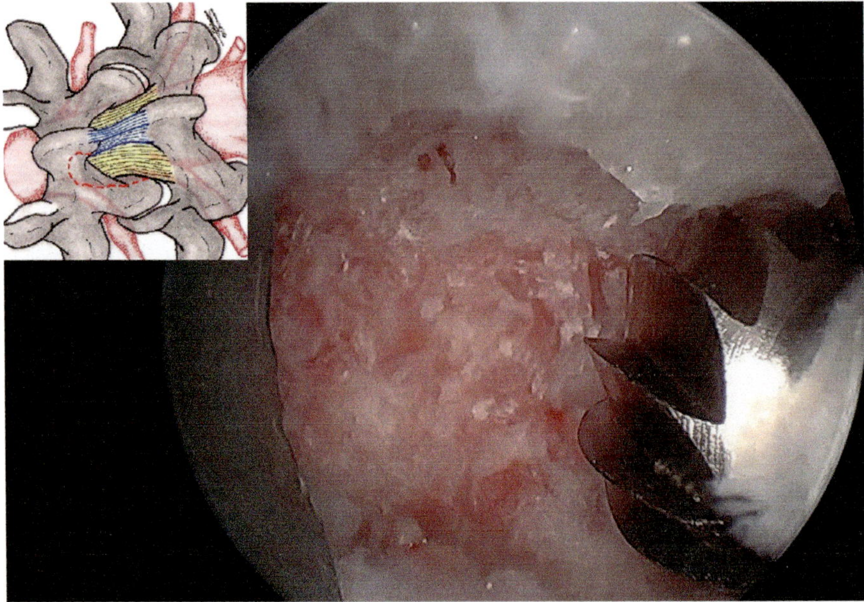

Fig. 12.26 Intraoperative endoscopic view of the drilled lamina

After initially docking into the multifidus triangle, the surgeon further enlarges the working space by burring the lamina high enough to allow access to the disc (Fig. 12.26). To avoid inadvertent laceration of the underlying flavum (and possibly tearing the dural sac), the laminar bone is burred down to its anterior or ventral cortex. To facilitate removal of the anterior cortex, the underlying flavum is stripped off using a curved curette, which is insinuated in between cortex and flavum (Fig. 12.27). This creates room for the Kerrison's footplate to insert before cutting the cortex.

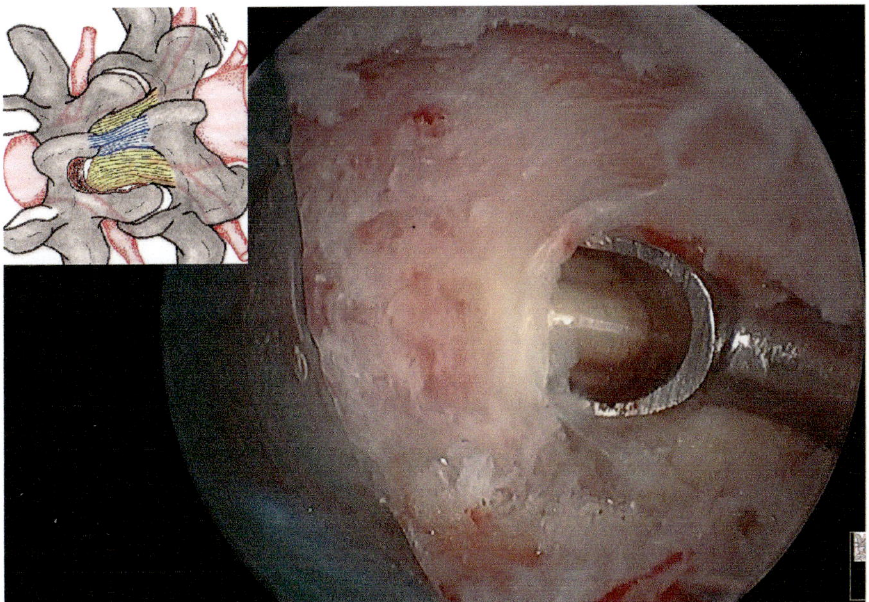

Fig. 12.27 A curette is used to detach the ligamentum flavum from the ventral aspect of the lamina

Gaining Access to the Spinal Canal

Once thinned, the anterior laminar cortex can be safely removed in a piecemeal manner to expose the underlying ligamentum flavum using Kerrison punches typically of the size 3 and 4 mm (Fig. 12.28). One useful endoscopic landmark for easier removal of the ligamentum flavum is its median raphe (Fig. 12.29), located at midline, between left and right halves of the flavum [10]. Exposure of this median cleft is achieved by doing a sufficiently sized laminotomy beginning at the spinolaminar junction (Fig. 12.30). The superomedial edge of the ipsilateral flavum can be easily and safely grasped and lifted away from the dural sac due to the presence of ample epidural fat interpositioned between dura and flavum at the midline. Lifting the flavum also allows the saline to dissect the epidural space and push down the dura (away from the flavum being lifted).

Detaching the ipsilateral flavum from its lateral moorings can be aided by performing a small medial facetectomy (using the burr), followed by elevation of the lateral flavum off the underside of the lamina and medial facet (using a curved curette). This further mobilizes the flavum, making it easier to peel it off in a superior to an inferior direction (Fig. 12.31).

To avoid the bothersome situation of difficult-to-control arterial bleeding, it is advisable to prevent lacerating the interarticular artery and the superior/inferior articular arteries (Fig. 12.32) during muscle stripping and laminar burring. Avoiding periarticular arterial injury is one other reason why beginning the creation of your

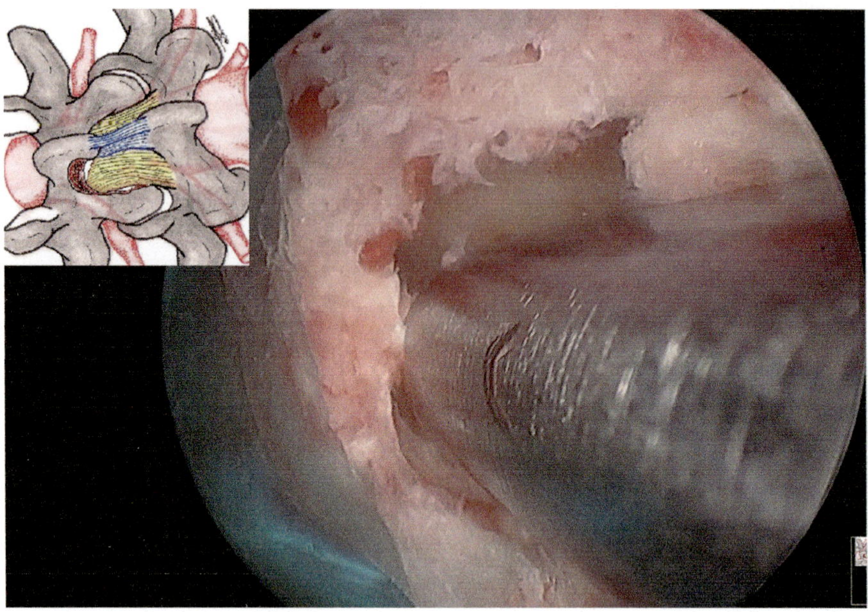

Fig. 12.28 The lamina is removed using Kerrison punches

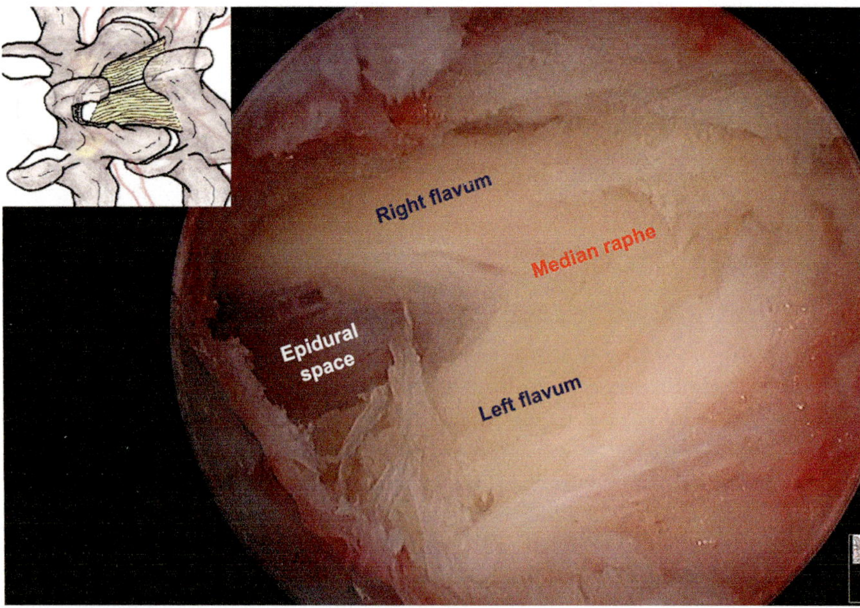

Fig. 12.29 The ligamentum flavum has been exposed after partial laminotomy

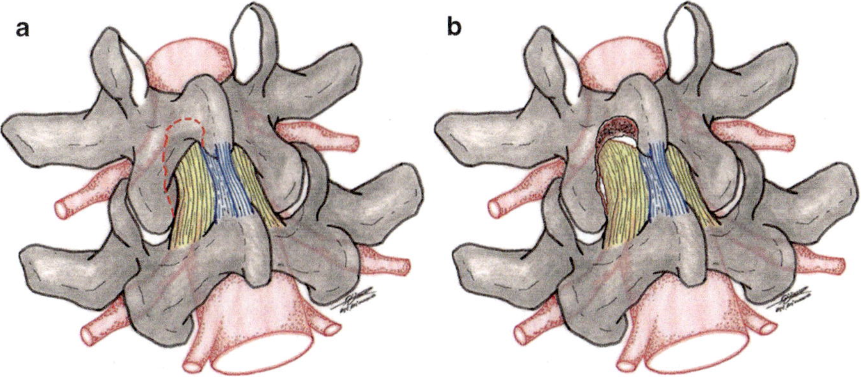

Fig. 12.30 The drawings show an ipsilateral partial laminotomy highlighted in red (**a**) and drilling out of the base of the spinous process (**b**). Then, the cranial attachment of the ligamentum flavum can be identified

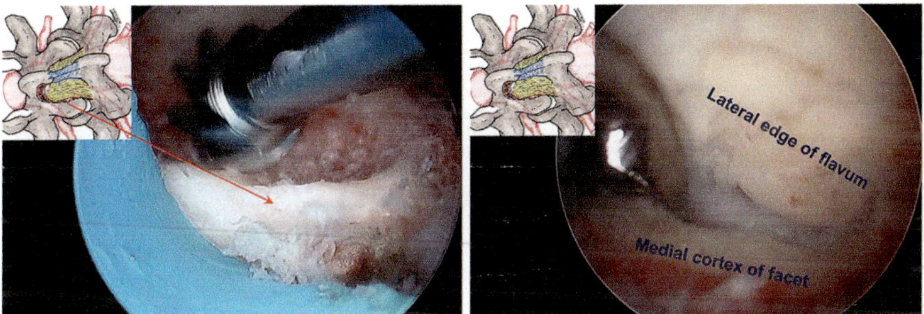

Fig. 12.31 The medial aspect of the facet joint is drilled out (left) to reach the lateral attachment (right) of the ligamentum flavum

working space from within the multifidus triangle and at the inferior spinolaminar junction is desirable—because this starting point allows for keeping distance from these arteries for as long as possible. After completing the flavectomy, the endoscope can now be inserted deeper into the epidural space to focus on the lateral edge of the dural sac (which contains the traversing nerve root) (Fig. 12.33). With careful but adequate dural sac retraction, unmigrated disc herniations can be easily accessed and removed from this location.

Discectomy/Sequestrectomy

The standard arthroscope normally has a sleeve or cannula with a flat end that is flush with the terminus of the scope. As such, the tip of the standard scope sleeve cannot be used to retract the nerve roots, and an endoscopic nerve root retractor

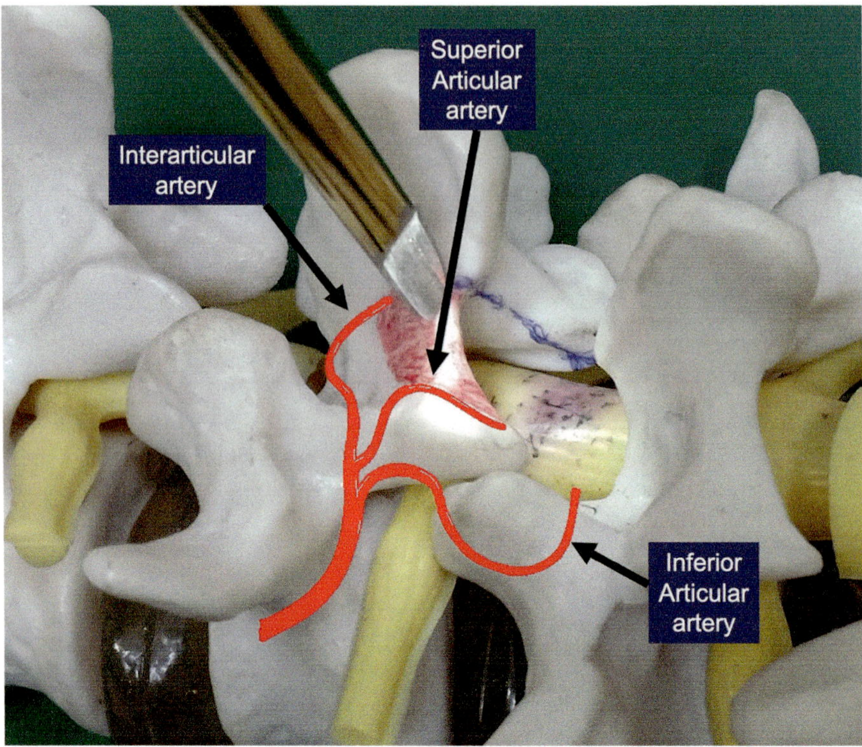

Fig. 12.32 Arterial supply of the lumbar facet joints

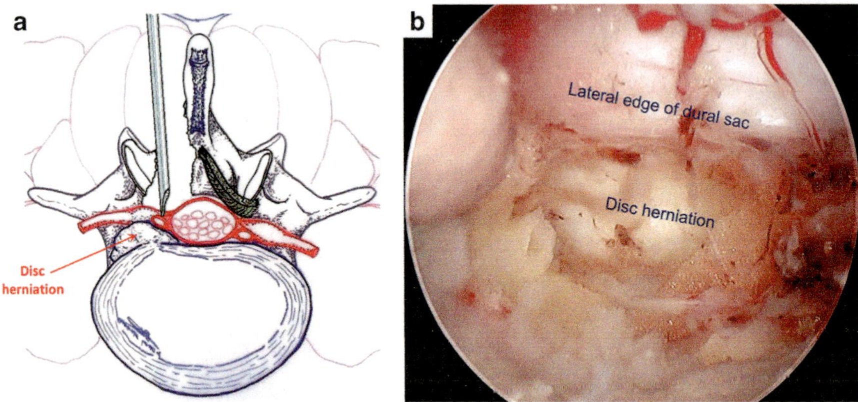

Fig. 12.33 Exploration of epidural space. (**a**) Drawing showing the endoscope within the spinal canal. (**b**) Endoscopic view of the lateral edge of the dural sac and the disc herniation

(which needs to be held by the surgeon's assistant) will have to be inserted (usually through the working port) to protect the nerve root or dural sac while the herniated disc is being exposed [13]. Hence, I recommend using a tongue-tipped scope sleeve (Fig. 12.34), which functions much like the cannula tip of a uniportal endoscopy. The tongue tip doubles as a retractor but does not require an assistant for its positioning. This helps avoid pauses in the performance of surgery, thus affording a more efficient workflow.

It was standard to do complete discectomy with open surgical approaches to achieve decompression—i.e., the entire nucleus pulposus is removed. But with UBE, adequate nerve root decompression is achievable by removing only the herniated or sequestered disc—i.e., only the unstable nuclear material or that readily extrudes is removed [8, 9].

After dural retraction and annulotomy, the herniated nucleus is pulled out with a hook probe or micro-forceps; meanwhile, the nucleus pulposus, which remains contained in the disc, is left intact. This is done to prolong the use of the intact nucleus and delay the collapse of the disc space. The exiting and traversing nerve roots are inspected for adequacy of decompression after the unstable nuclear material has been extracted. Return of blood perfusion to the nerve root sheath should be noticeable after adequate decompression. In addition, the presence of free space and absence of adhesions around the nerve root are also noted (i.e., tested with a hook probe). Once the surgeon is satisfied with the adequacy of decompression, the

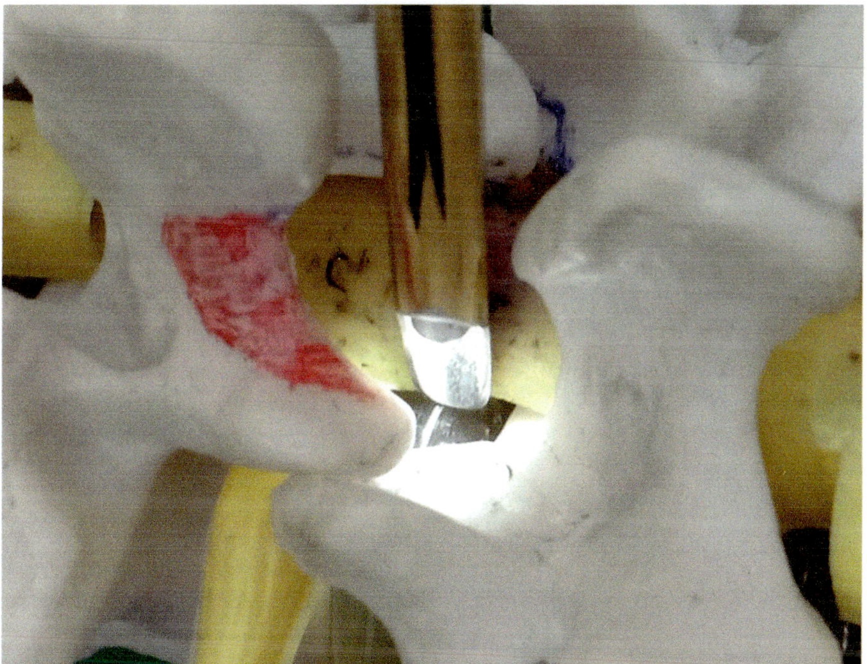

Fig. 12.34 Self-retraction of the dural sac by using a customized bevel-ending endoscope sleeve

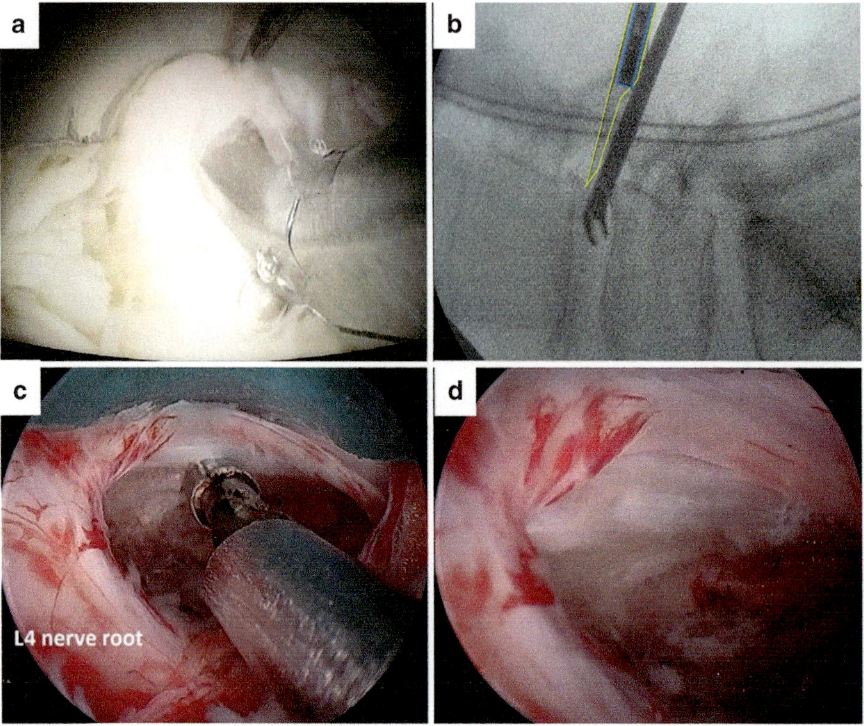

Fig. 12.35 L4–L5 UBE sequestrectomy. (**a**) The pituitary forceps are located in the subannular area, and the sleeve bevel is retracting the thecal sac. (**b**) The latter is confirmed with a lateral projection of the C-arm. (**c**) After disc particle removal, RF annuloplasty is performed in the annular tear. (**d**) Inspection of the epidural space is done to ensure complete decompression of the neural elements

annular opening is located and heat-sealed with electrocautery, and then reinspected (Fig. 12.35).

After a final review of hemostasis, a silicone suction drain tube is inserted into the epidural space via the working port (Fig. 12.36), and skin port openings are closed with Nylon or Vicryl sutures. Drain position and absence of any hematoma are verified on the postoperative imaging scan, and drain output is monitored for the next 24 h.

Postoperative Management

A postoperative MRI or CT scan is taken to review the decompression site and the surrounding soft tissues.

Scan images are correlated with recorded intraoperative endoscope videos and are presented to the patient the next day. If clinically improved, the patient is

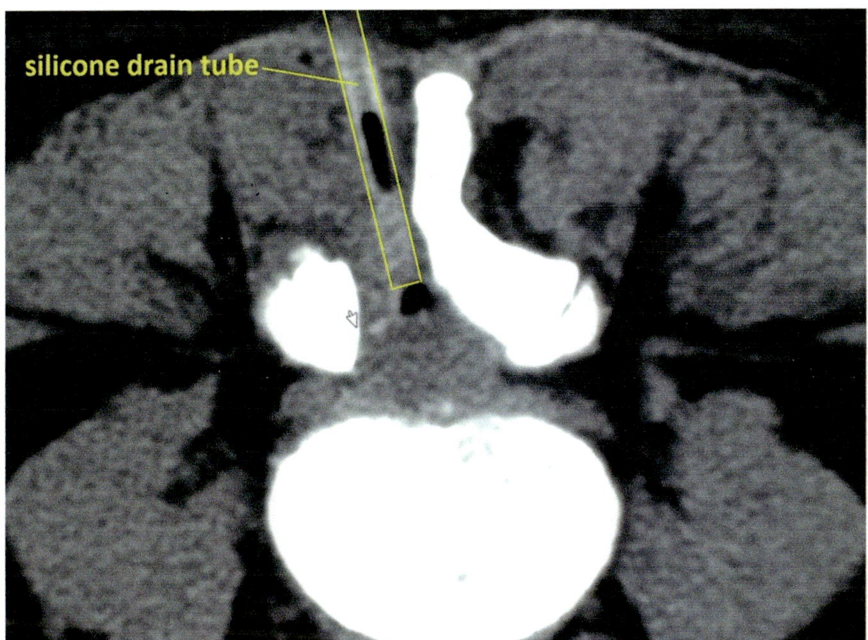

Fig. 12.36 Drain inserted after UBE

clinically re-evaluated for symptom resolution and is discharged as early as 24–36 h postoperatively. Intravenous analgesics are commonly given within the immediate 24-h postoperative period and then shifted to oral analgesics in preparation for discharge. A single dose of intravenous antibiotic is given upon anesthesia induction but may or may not be repeatedly given after the procedure (depending on whether the operating time exceeded the antibiotic's half-life or not).

Antibiotic coverage is typically not required after the immediate 24-h postoperative period. The drain tube is removed within 24 h if no arterial blood is present or if the total output of diluted venous blood is under 60 mL. If the patient has been fitted with an epidural catheter for surgical anesthesia or postoperative analgesia, this is also pulled out before discharge.

Evaluating Symptom Resolution

Among the clinical endpoints that significantly impact the patient's postoperative satisfaction is pain, specifically radicular pain that substantially hinders the patient's posture and mobility. As such, it is a good idea to compare and document the patient's preoperative and postoperative leg pain and back pain levels using clinically useful scoring tools (e.g., Visual Analog Scale, Numeric Rating Scale) as well as to compare preoperative and postoperative motor strength and gait (since sciatic or neuropathic pain can significantly hinder lumbopelvic or hip joint range of motion and balance).

Protective lumbar and pelvic reflexive muscle spasms may cause a patient to walk with a list or tilt, and traction on the sciatic nerve upon forwarding foot swing, heel strike, and full weight bearing on the affected side may all provoke shooting pain from lumbar spine to leg and foot, causing the patient to limp and avoid walking on the affected side. Therefore, the success of the surgical technique should be measured by how much these primary symptoms have resolved following the UBE decompression.

Discussion

Why Do UBE Lumbar Surgery Instead of Open Lumbar Surgery?

The benefits of adding the UBE lumbar surgery technique to one's skill set can be summed up as belonging to "benefits gained by the patient" and "benefits gained by the surgeon and surgical team." Comparing UBE technique with open surgery (even tubular microdiscectomy) for herniated lumbar discs, the advantages of going minimally invasive are quite clear-cut [3, 14–21] (Tables 12.1 and 12.2).

On the other side of the coin, the UBE technique is not without its own set of risks and disadvantages. In that case, here are recognized issues with the lumbar UBE discectomy procedure [3, 10–13, 15, 16, 22].

Risks and Disadvantages for the Patient

1. Increased intracranial pressure due to the epidural saline infusion is a known risk (albeit easily mitigated with better technique).
2. Paraspinal hematoma has been reported in literature once (due to arterial bleeding).

Table 12.1 Benefits gained by the patient

1. Less intraoperative EBL
2. Less dissection and destruction of muscle tissue
3. Less removal of bone (including facet joints)
4. Less postoperative surgical site pain
5. Less risk of surgical site infection
6. Less risk of developing iatrogenic instability
7. Less need for fusion
8. Less chance of needing general anesthesia
9. Less overall expense for treatment [4]

Table 12.2 Benefits gained by surgeon

1. 30-fold magnification due to scope
2. Wider field of view (especially with 30° endoscope)
3. The familiar feel of open "two-handed" surgery
4. OR setup is similar to knee/shoulder arthroscopy
5. Portable "on-the-go" endoscope systems are now available (i.e., no strict need for endoscope tower)
6. Instruments for open surgery can be used in UBE
7. Localization of vertebral level/landmarks can be done with ultrasonography (if intraoperative imaging intensifier is unavailable)
8. Having fallback of open surgery if UBE fails
9. Targeted technique

3. Inadvertent dural tears due to difficulty in scope and instrument triangulation have been reported by surgeons who are new to the UBE technique.
4. Possible thermal injury with indiscriminate RF coagulator wands is a theoretical risk.
5. A recurrent herniation is a risk in lumbar discectomies, open or endoscopic—but literature shows comparable rates of re-herniation for both.

Disadvantages for the Surgeon

1. Requires familiarization with equipment and OR setup (if the surgeon or surgical team does not regularly do arthroscopic procedures already)
2. Requires good ambidexterity and triangulation skills on the part of the surgeon

It can be argued that endoscopic spine surgery, whether uniportal or biportal, would provide similar benefits and incur similar risks as far as the patient is concerned. The surgeon's decision to adopt UBE techniques is thus mainly influenced by personal capability and institutional resource availability. Here are some points to consider with regard to either endoscopic approach.

Uniportal Endoscopy

- *Approaches*: transforaminal and interlaminar
- *Anesthesia*: local (Kambin's triangle) for transforaminal approach; epidural or general for interlaminar approach
- *Dexterity requirement*: the ambidextrous or unidextrous surgeon can easily handle both scope and instruments (i.e., practically no triangulation needed)
- *Equipment*: transforaminal and interlaminar specialized spinal endoscopes, instruments compatible with either endoscope
- *Intraoperative imaging*: highly dependent on fluoroscopy (especially for transforaminal surgery)

Biportal Endoscopy

- *Approaches*: paramedian and paraspinal
- *Anesthesia*: general or epidural, depending on the length of the procedure and patient requirements, comorbidities, and expected comfort level

- *Dexterity requirement*: endoscope in the nondominant hand, instruments in the dominant hand (i.e., requires some degree of ambidexterity for triangulation)
- *Equipment*: 4 mm × 175 mm scope, standard instruments used in open spine surgery
- *Intraoperative imaging*: fluoroscopy or still-shot X-ray for verifying the level

Comparison of UBE and Full Endoscopy of the Spine

A noteworthy feature of UBE, compared to its uniportal predecessor, is the versatility of the endoscopic hardware. UBE surgery requires only one size of lens—the 4 mm × 175 mm rigid arthroscope—for various approaches and procedures. In addition, having the soft-tissue working port separated from the endoscope sleeve means that instruments are not constrained by the diameter of the endoscopic self-integrated working channel nor by the movement of the endoscope itself.

Pearls and Pitfalls of UBE

- A discussion on the UBE technique would not be complete without mentioning a few hacks and bodges unique to this relatively new field of specialty. Let us start with pitfalls, beginning with the most basic—difficulty of triangulation.
- Making two instruments held in each hand meet at a given point in space is easy if the operator can directly see the instruments. This condition, however, is not possible in UBE surgery. While fluoroscopic guidance can get the surgeon started, the bulk of the procedure is done mainly by feel. The experience is quite similar to playing a computer video game, with the player looking at the action on the screen while their hands moving the game controller's joysticks and buttons without needing to look at the controller itself.
- The only solution to this pitfall of difficulty in triangulation is to develop a familiarity with the feel of "playing the game" by constant practice. (Incidentally, practicing on video/computer games that require independent hand control has proven to benefit the development of endoscopic skills in other surgical specialties and most likely can also provide training value to the field of UBE surgery) [23–27].
- One recommendation to surgical colleagues on how to develop the feel of doing biportal endoscopic work would be to find opportunities that allow for hands-on practice—e.g., anything from cadaver workshops to actual knee arthroscopy procedures, to fluoroscopic percutaneous orthopedic procedures, and even ultrasound-guided percutaneous procedures such as nerve blocks and plane blocks. These learning experiences, while using different visualization instruments, all train a surgeon's muscle memory and hand coordination for the task of bi-dextrously manipulating instruments while looking at a screen instead of at the actual surgical site.
- Cadaver workshops and conventions are understandably difficult to come by in this age of COVID-19. And not many surgery departments have access to simu-

lation training labs in their respective institutions. However, for those who want to train without having to be dependent on institutions continually, there is the option of constructing your training station—by using anatomy lab human bone models or orthopedic sawbones, or even animal cadaver spines as raw material, and using a portable endoscopy station for practicing triangulation. All that is needed are (Fig. 12.37):

- Your laptop computer
- A high-definition USB endoscope camera head
- All of the other instruments for endoscopic spine work

Underwater visualization and manipulation can be done using plastic containers with covers of varying opacity.

- Another common pitfall is running into a bloody field when clearing muscle and tendinous soft tissue. Muscle easily bleeds when agitated, thus easily obscuring the operative field with blood-tinged saline. The primary countermove for this is a combination of fluent saline flow and judicious electrocoagulation. Make your working port opening large enough to allow continuous fluid outflow; both the skin and the thoracolumbar fascia should have stab wounds that will enable your saline to drain out. Expect chunks of subcutaneous fat sometimes to block your outflow and remove them as they pop into your working channel.
- Use electrocoagulation in a precise manner to avoid overheating your entire workspace. Move the scope tip closer to the RF probe tip so that you can see what you are burning and burn only that which is bleeding. Then wait for the saline to clear the field slowly and continue hunting for bleeders until the field stops being bloody.
- Bleeding from the cancellous bone of the lamina can be another challenging issue. Bone continuously bleeds once you burr away the posterior cortex. The

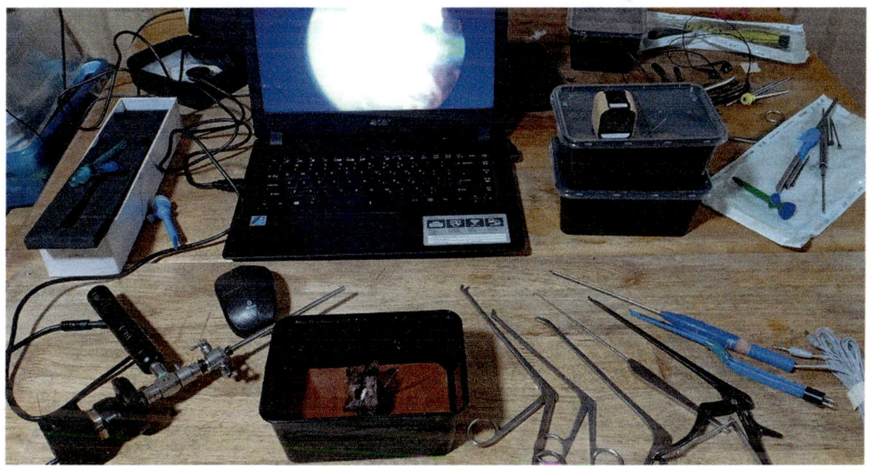

Fig. 12.37 Customized UBE simulator for training

easiest way to stop bone bleeds in UBE is by using your RF wand on the bleeding trabecular openings. However, this is not the only way to prevent bone bleeding.

- A classic way of stopping bone bleeding is by spreading bone wax into open trabecular bone. However, it is more easily done in open surgery and can be frustrating to do in a UBE setting (as the bone wax may keep falling from your applicator tip before you even manage to push the wax onto the bone). A more mechanical way to address the problem of bone bleed is to "crimp" the trabecula by pushing the bleeding point with your Kerrison or curette tip, thus collapsing the marrow and closing the bleeders. Or, if you are using a burr, simply burr the bone down to the anterior cortex, reverse the burr rotation, and impact the marrow (similar to crimping with a Kerrison) to close bleeding trabeculae.
- Speaking of bone work, it is of benefit to use preoperative MRI or CT scans in planning your laminotomy and flavectomy. Be mindful of the shape of the flavum (especially the deep layer adjacent to the epidural space) and the laminotomy size and shape necessary for allowing you biportal endoscopic access to the disc. Remember that the laminotomy has to allow two different instruments to enter the spinal canal from two different angles. Otherwise, the instrument tips end up competing for space on their way to the disc.
- During the surgery, complete your bone work before removing the ligamentum flavum. The flavum acts as a protective barrier, so only remove it when you have done all the burring and cutting that is required. That helps you avoid injuring the dura and epidural vessels.
- A quick note on fluoroscopy and triangulation: keep your X-ray beam centered as much as possible on the target anatomic structure to avoid landmark shifting on-screen. Your ports are based on your target disc level. Taking an off-centered fluoroscopic projection will shift skin markings by a small but spatially significant amount, thus shifting your port placement off your target.
- Last but certainly not least, a word on doing UBE surgery on a right-sided lesion. The right-handed UBE surgeon has three options for attacking this problem:
  - Open from the patient's left side as usual, but use a contralateral approach (i.e., go over the top of the dural sac to reach the right side of the spinal canal).
  - Open from the right side, but hold your endoscope and instruments in standard fashion (i.e., scope port becomes the caudal port, still held by the left hand).
  - Open from the right side, but switch hands, thus creating a mirror image of your left-sided approach (i.e., viewing port is the cranial port, but the surgeon's left hand will have to do the bulk of the work).
- The first option is probably the least difficult to adapt to since it does not involve flipping the operating room setup and the endoscopic projection into a mirror image. However, a contralateral decompression does require more bone removal and epidural dissection, so extra planning is to be expected with a contralateral "over-the-top" approach [10, 11].

- The second option (maintaining a right-handed port orientation while opening from the patient's right side) is expected to create some instrument-to-lamina mismatch. The surgeon would need to rotate the Kerrison punch by 180° to effect laminotomy from inferior lamina to mid-lamina. (Even with a rotatable Kerrison punch, this position would be cumbersome.) The surgeon also loses the utility of the widely spacious interlaminar gap (allowing for more freedom of movement of instruments approaching the spinal canal from the caudal port). Thus, working tools entering from the cranial port would have to settle for whatever space the laminotomy will allow.
- The third option (switching to a "southpaw" grip of the endoscope and instruments) is probably the most challenging option for the right-handed surgeon needing to operate on a right-sided disc herniation. Not as tricky for a left-handed surgeon to switch hands and operate from the left side, though, since all southpaws have to learn to adjust to a predominantly orthodox world anyway. In this scenario, everything is flipped to mirror image—and this takes a lot more adjustment on the surgeon's part.
- Learning a southpaw technique is really learning a new technique altogether. Of course, it requires a lot more practice from the right-handed surgeon, but having the ability to do a southpaw-style UBE approach will practically extend the surgeon's range of skills to double that of his/her original.
- Consider a different scenario wherein a patient has a far-lateral lumbar disc herniation on the left side, which can be more conveniently approached by doing an interlaminar contralateral UBE approach from the patient's right—imagine doing this surgery in both orthodox grip and southpaw grip. In which situation would your working instruments have more room to maneuver?
- That said, whichever side a UBE surgeon learns to approach from, there will undoubtedly be more approach options and techniques that open up as he/she becomes more proficient and comfortable with fully utilizing two hands holding two instruments that are passed into two ports.
- However, the approaches are mixed and matched, and the goals remain the same: perform the least invasive indicated procedure possible while providing the most effective treatment of the pathology.

Conclusion

In summary, UBE has, in less than two decades of evolution, extended the range of minimal invasiveness and maximal efficacy of endoscopic spine surgery. As the technology gets better and the boundaries of what this technique can achieve are pushed further into the realm of lumbar fusion, thoracic decompression, and cervical anterior-posterior surgery, we shall expect endoscopic spine surgery to eventually become the new standard of care for degenerative spine pathology.

As for UBE discectomy, in particular, the most significant advantages of this technique are its minimal invasiveness, its versatility in instrument usage, its ability to adequately decompress the spinal canal while preserving the still-functional part of the disc, its nature of maintaining segment stability by avoiding the disruption of crucial bony and soft-tissue structures (thus avoiding the necessity of doing instrumented fusion), and its economy in terms of resource utilization and overall cost of care.

Contrary to what some may believe, the level of evolution of endoscopic spine technique and technology in general—and UBE spine surgery in particular—is not the biggest obstacle to its development and use. (We have had the adequate technology and technique available to us for nearly three decades now.)

Conceptually speaking, the biggest obstacles to this technique are a lack of an open mind, an unfounded fear of change, and a self-doubting attitude towards global inclusivity and knowledge sharing. But, unfortunately, the harsh reality in today's world is that we must find and use better ways of achieving worthwhile goals—especially in an era where pandemics and increasing limitations of global resources continue to threaten the sustainability and adequate delivery of specialized health care to those who direly need it.

In closing, regardless of whether a surgeon comes from the classic school of open spine surgery, or from the school of microdiscectomy and mini-open surgery, or even from the uniportal school of endoscopic surgery—and regardless of whether a surgeon comes from the neurosurgical specialty or the orthopedic specialty—UBE spine surgery proves to be an all-inclusive field of specialization for any surgical practitioner in search of a better means of providing affordable quality healthcare to spine patients the world over. And it is with this outlook, we hope that the greater medical community will eventually see and appreciate the UBE movement and the professionals behind its continued evolution and success.

References

1. Telfeian AE, Veeravagu A, Oyelese AA, Gokaslan ZL. A brief history of endoscopic spine surgery. Neurosurg Focus. 2016;40(2):E2.
2. Choi G, Pophale CS, Patel B, Uniyal P. Endoscopic spine surgery [published correction appears in J Korean Neurosurg Soc. 2019 May;62(3):366]. J Korean Neurosurg Soc. 2017;60(5):485–97.
3. Kang T, Park SY, Kang CH, Lee SH, Park JH, Suh SW. Is biportal technique/endoscopic spinal surgery satisfactory for lumbar spinal stenosis patients? A prospective randomized comparative study. Medicine (Baltimore). 2019;98(18):e15451.
4. Wu PH, Kim HS, Jang IT. A narrative review of development of full-endoscopic lumbar spine surgery. Neurospine. 2020;17(Suppl 1):S20–33.
5. Kim M, Kim HS, Oh SW, et al. Evolution of spinal endoscopic surgery. Neurospine. 2019;16(1):6–14.
6. De Antoni DJ, Claro ML, Poehling GG, Hughes SS. Translaminar lumbar epidural endoscopy: anatomy, technique, and indications. Arthroscopy. 1996;12(3):330–4.

7. Eun SS, Eum JH, Lee SH, Sabal LA. Biportal endoscopic lumbar decompression for lumbar disk herniation and spinal canal stenosis: a technical note. J Neurol Surg A Cent Eur Neurosurg. 2017;78(4):390–6.
8. Ran J, Hu Y, Zheng Z, et al. Comparison of discectomy versus sequestrectomy in lumbar disc herniation: a meta-analysis of comparative studies. PLoS One. 2015;10(3):e0121816.
9. Fakouri B, Shetty NR, White TC. Is sequestrectomy a viable alternative to microdiscectomy? A systematic review of the literature. Clin Orthop Relat Res. 2015;473(6):1957–62.
10. Park JH, Jang JW, Park WM, Park CW. Contralateral keyhole biportal endoscopic surgery for ruptured lumbar herniated disc: a technical feasibility and early clinical outcomes. Neurospine. 2020;17(Suppl 1):S110–9.
11. Heo DH, Kim JS, Park CW, Quillo-Olvera J, Park CK. Contralateral sublaminar endoscopic approach for removal of lumbar juxtafacet cysts using percutaneous biportal endoscopic surgery: technical report and preliminary results. World Neurosurg. 2019;122:474–9.
12. Choi CM, Chung JT, Lee SJ, Choi DJ. How I do it? Biportal endoscopic spinal surgery (BESS) for treatment of lumbar spinal stenosis. Acta Neurochir. 2016;158(3):459–63.
13. Kim JE, Choi DJ, Park EJJ, et al. Biportal endoscopic spinal surgery for lumbar spinal stenosis. Asian Spine J. 2019;13(2):334–42.
14. Aygun H, Abdulshafi K. Unilateral biportal endoscopy versus tubular microendoscopy in management of single level degenerative lumbar canal stenosis: a prospective study. Clin Spine Surg. 2021;34(6):E323–8.
15. Kim JE, Yoo HS, Choi DJ, Park EJ, Jee SM. Comparison of minimal invasive versus biportal endoscopic transforaminal lumbar interbody fusion for single-level lumbar disease. Clin Spine Surg. 2021;34(2):E64–71.
16. Choi DJ, Kim JE. Efficacy of biportal endoscopic spine surgery for lumbar spinal stenosis. Clin Orthop Surg. 2019;11(1):82–8.
17. Gadjradj PS, Harhangi BS, Amelink J, et al. Percutaneous transforaminal endoscopic discectomy versus open microdiscectomy for lumbar disc herniation: a systematic review and meta-analysis. Spine (Phila Pa 1976). 2021;46(8):538–49.
18. Feng F, Xu Q, Yan F, et al. Comparison of 7 surgical interventions for lumbar disc herniation: a network meta-analysis. Pain Physician. 2017;20(6):E863–71.
19. Kim HS, Paudel B, Jang JS, et al. Percutaneous full endoscopic bilateral lumbar decompression of spinal stenosis through uniportal-contralateral approach: techniques and preliminary results. World Neurosurg. 2017;103:201–9.
20. Lee CW, Yoon KJ, Ha SS. Comparative analysis between three different lumbar decompression techniques (microscopic, tubular, and endoscopic) in lumbar canal and lateral recess stenosis: preliminary report. Biomed Res Int. 2019;2019:6078469.
21. Wong AP, Smith ZA, Lall RR, Bresnahan LE, Fessler RG. The microendoscopic decompression of lumbar stenosis: a review of the current literature and clinical results. Minim Invasive Surg. 2012;2012:325095.
22. Kim W, Kim SK, Kang SS, Park HJ, Han S, Lee SC. Pooled analysis of unsuccessful percutaneous biportal endoscopic surgery outcomes from a multi-institutional retrospective cohort of 797 cases. Acta Neurochir. 2020;162(2):279–87.
23. Datta R, Chon SH, Dratsch T, et al. Are gamers better laparoscopic surgeons? Impact of gaming skills on laparoscopic performance in "Generation Y" students. PLoS One. 2020;15(8):e0232341.
24. Sammut M, Sammut M, Andrejevic P. The benefits of being a video gamer in laparoscopic surgery. Int J Surg. 2017;45:42–6.
25. Rosser JC Jr, Lynch PJ, Cuddihy L, Gentile DA, Klonsky J, Merrell R. The impact of video games on training surgeons in the 21st century. Arch Surg. 2007;142(2):181–6.
26. Griffith JL, Voloschin P, Gibb GD, Bailey JR. Differences in eye-hand motor coordination of video-game users and non-users. Percept Mot Skills. 1983;57(1):155–8.
27. Sedlack RE, Kolars JC. Computer simulator training enhances the competency of gastroenterology fellows at colonoscopy: results of a pilot study. Am J Gastroenterol. 2004;99(1):33–7.

Part IV
Lumbar

Chapter 13
Unilateral Biportal Endoscopy for Non-migrated Lumbar Disc Herniation

Cigdem Mumcu

Abbreviations

AP	Anteroposterior
LDH	Lumbar disc herniation
LM	Lumbar microdiscectomy
MISS	Minimally invasive spine surgery
MRI	Magnetic resonance imaging
PELD	Percutaneous endoscopic lumbar discectomy
RF	Radiofrequency
UBE	Unilateral biportal endoscopy

Introduction

Lumbar disc herniation (LDH) is a common degenerative spinal disease. The current standard surgery for LDH is lumbar microdiscectomy (LM). However, muscle and ligament injury from surgery can lead to postoperative back pain and muscle atrophy [1–3]. Therefore, more time may be required for functional recovery and pain control after LM.

Supplementary Information The online version contains supplementary material available at [https://doi.org/10.1007/978-3-031-14736-4_13].

C. Mumcu (✉)
Sultanbeyli State Hospital, Spine Surgery Clinic, Istanbul, Turkey
e-mail: drmumcu@gmail.com

J. Quillo-Olvera et al. (eds.), *Unilateral Biportal Endoscopy of the Spine*,
https://doi.org/10.1007/978-3-031-14736-4_13

Thus, in recent years, minimally invasive spine surgery (MISS) techniques have been developed to reduce the damage to surrounding tissues [4–7]. Percutaneous endoscopic lumbar discectomy (PELD) is one of the MISS techniques and has been performed using only one portal [8–11]. This conventional endoscopic surgery which is called uniportal transforaminal and interlaminar PELD is an appropriate surgical method. It can protect the posterior musculoligamentous structures better than LM. Although these procedures can remove soft disc herniation and ruptured LDH without foraminal obstruction by well-designed surgical tools, they have limited indications due to the restricted movements of the endoscope and instruments and obstructed intervertebral foramen following degenerative changes [1, 12].

Unilateral biportal endoscopy (UBE) is a new endoscopic technique that combines the advantages of interlaminar endoscopy and microscopic surgery [13–17]. In this method, two portals are used. One is for viewing with the endoscope, and the other is for using instruments, and these two portals move independently. This is enormous progress compared to the uniportal method; its property allows the surgeon to overcome the limitation of surgical indication of uniportal endoscopy [18]. Moreover, the endoscopic trajectory has the same steps as conventional microsurgery with a clear view; thus, it may help the learning curve earlier [19, 20]. UBE has many advantages such as protection of the musculoligamentous complex, a smaller incision, less postoperative back pain, and a short hospitalization period. Another advantage is that UBE causes less postoperative morbidity by reducing the incidence of epidural fibrosis and by raising the preservation of the epidural venous system [21]. Furthermore, complicated cases such as highly migrated disc herniation and herniated disc with concomitant spinal stenosis can be treated with UBE.

Such benefits of UBE surgery including simple discrimination of anatomic structures, tender manipulation of pathology with a magnified endoscopic view, and detailed operative information might contribute to getting successful results in the lumbar disc herniations.

Indications

UBE has a wider range of spectrum for indications that are similar to those for conventional LM [22].

All herniated discs such as central, lateral, foraminal, and extraforaminal; upward migrated or downward migrated; moderate to large; and recurrent lumbar disc herniations can be treated under UBE.

Limitations

1. Decompression of the exiting nerve is difficult in the foraminal stenosis with the narrow disc space and bony spur through a paraspinal approach.

2. Advanced spinal deformity and unstable stenotic spine: Instrumentation for distraction and stabilization is required in these cases.

Equipment

Endoscope: 0° or 30°, 4 mm diameter (Conmed Linvatec, Utica, NY) (Fig. 13.1)
Radiofrequency probe (ArthroCare Sports Medicine Quantum-II, USA)

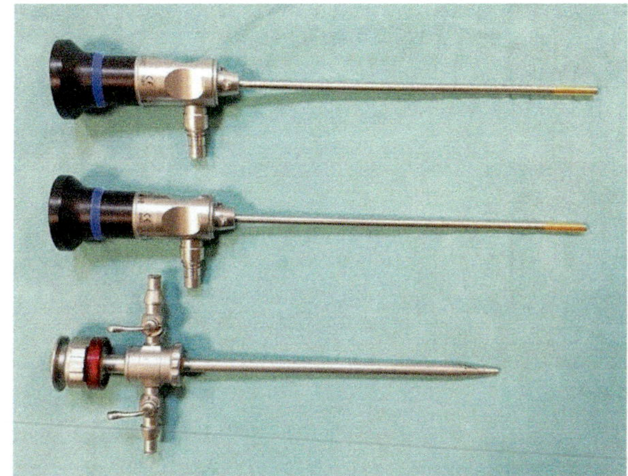

Fig. 13.1 0° and 30° endoscope and trocar

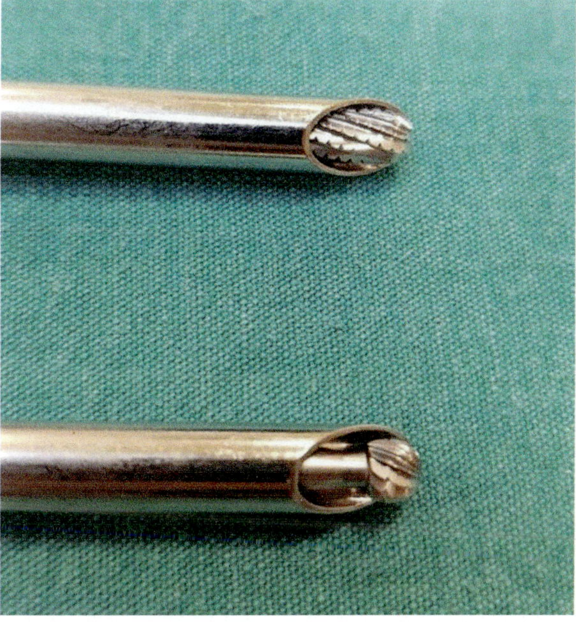

Fig. 13.2 One-side protected drill, oval and spherical

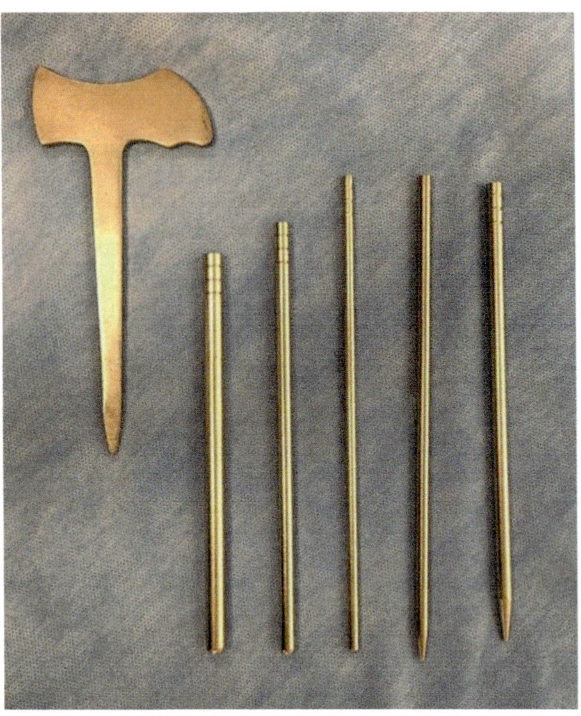

Fig. 13.3 Blunt muscle detacher and serial dilators

One-sided protected drill burr, spherical or oval (Conmed Linvatec, Utica, NY) (Fig. 13.2)
Pressure pump irrigation system (Conmed Linvatec, Utica, NY)
Standard laminectomy instruments
Blunt muscle detacher and serial dilators (Fig. 13.3)

Surgical Procedure

There are two basic approaches which are paramedian and paraspinal (Fig. 13.4). However, modified and targeted approaches can also be adopted depending on the pathology and location [23].

Paramedian Approach

The paramedian approach is applied for pathologies of central and lateral recess on the spine.

1. Position and anesthesia

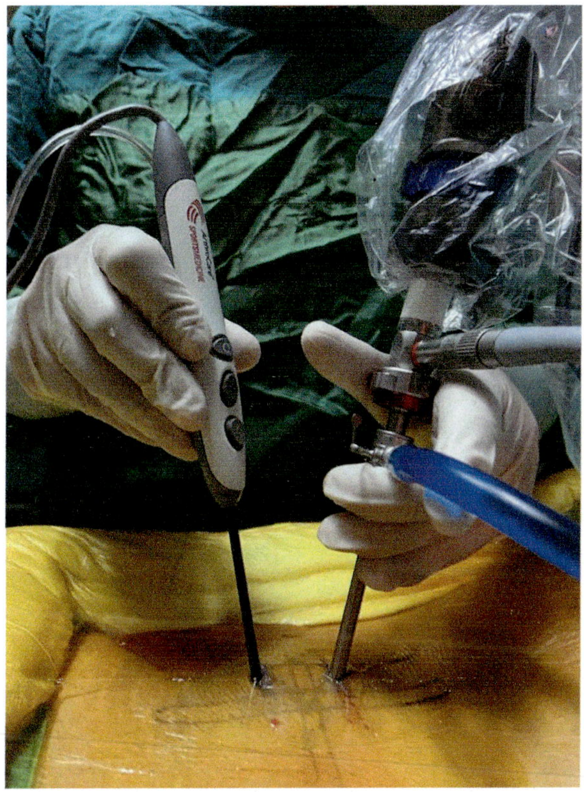

Fig. 13.4 Intraoperative image of UBE

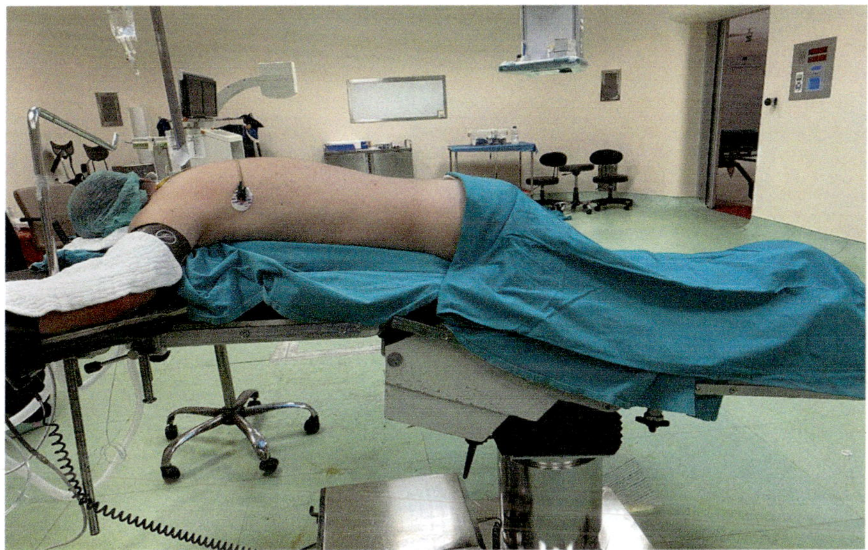

Fig. 13.5 Patient position

The UBE is performed with the patient under general anesthesia on a radiolucent operating table. The patient is placed in the prone position over the rolling pad in a flexed position (Fig. 13.5). A waterproof surgical drape is applied after sterile preparation.

2. Target point

The spinous process is identified on the anteroposterior (AP) position, and the midline is created on that spinous process under C-arm fluoroscopic guidance. Then, the interpedicular line is determined on the medial side of the pedicle. After that, the target level is identified. Two entry points for endoscopic and working portals are made about 1 cm above and 1 cm below the ruptured disc level at the ipsilateral interpedicular line for the paramedian approach (Fig. 13.6).

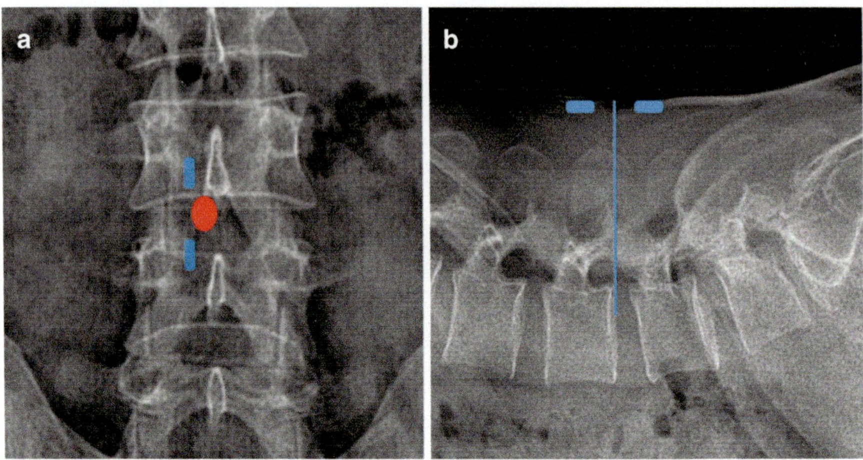

Fig. 13.6 Skin points of the two portals for paramedian approach in the lumbar spine. (**a**) AP view. (**b**) Lateral view

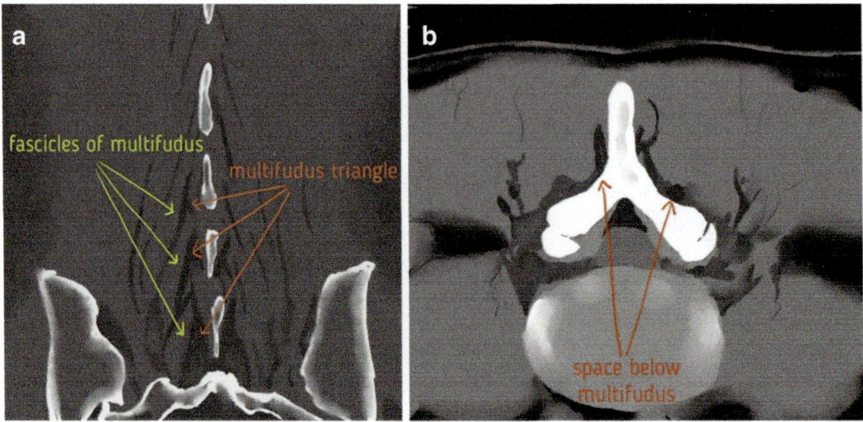

Fig. 13.7 Here are the potential spaces between fascicles of the multifidus muscle, which is also defined as the multifidus triangle for the paramedian approach. Two portals are made in the multifidus triangle. (**a**) Coronal view. (**b**) Axial view

3. Working portal

   The first skin incision for the working (caudal) portal is opened around 1 cm horizontally above the target point. Then, serial dilators are inserted into the potential space located between fascicles of the multifidus muscles, which is also defined as the multifidus triangular space in the lamina (Fig. 13.7). Interlaminar soft tissue is dissected from the distal margin of the spinolaminar junction to the medial side of the facet joint to prepare enough visual space for allowing to work in earnest with blunt muscle detacher.

4. Endoscopic portal

   The second skin incision for the endoscope (cranial) portal is opened 7 mm horizontally about 2–3 cm away from the first incision (Video 13.1). Either a 0° or 30° endoscope is inserted through the cranial portal after insertion of the trocar.

   For continuous saline irrigation, a pressure pump irrigation system is connected to the endoscope and is set to a pressure of 30–50 mmHg during the procedure. Simple water pressure control using the height of the saline bag on the fluid stand is also possible. For this, hanging the saline bag 170 cm high from the ground or holding it 100 cm high from the patient would be enough to achieve the safe pressure practically. A controlled continuous fluid flow is essential to prevent the extreme rise of the epidural pressure. Furthermore, the continuous flow of saline irrigation clears the endoscopic surgical view and prevents bleeding in the operative field. The irrigation saline flows from the cranial portal to the caudal portal.

5. Triangulation

   Surgical instruments are inserted through the working portal (Fig. 13.8). Then, these two portals make a triangular shape on the interlaminar space (Figs. 13.9 and 13.10). After triangulation, the soft tissue overlying the lamina and ligamentum flavum is cleaned with the radiofrequency probe. Following this

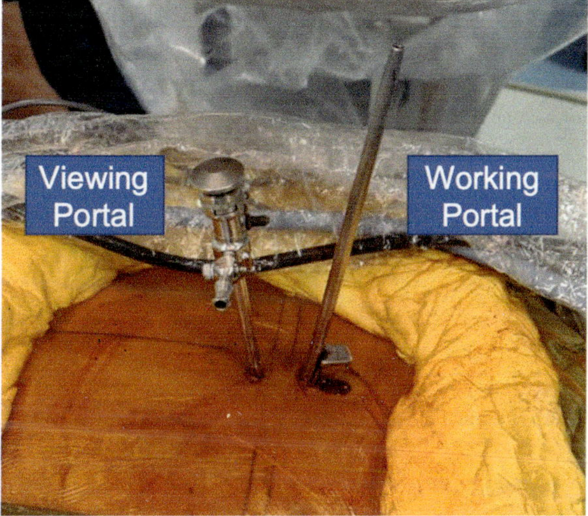

Fig. 13.8 Both portals are created in a triangular shape. (*Image courtesy of Javier Quillo-Olvera M.D.*)

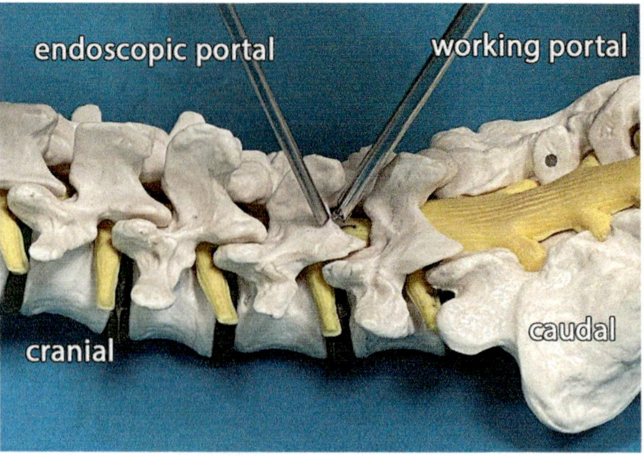

Fig. 13.9 Example with an anatomical model of how triangulation should be performed with both ports addressed to the target

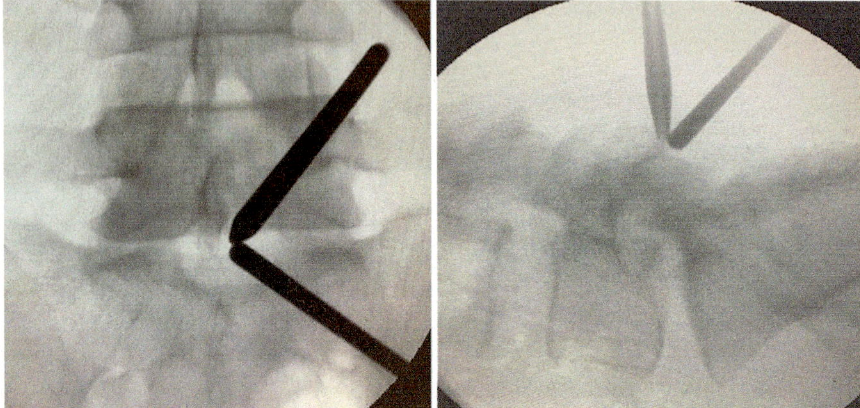

Fig. 13.10 Triangular approach was verified with the C-arm. Left: AP view. Right: Lateral view

completed exposure, the surgical endoscopic view is clearer due to the expansion of the interlaminar space with irrigation saline.

6. Laminotomy and discectomy

   The upper border of the lower lamina and medial border of the facet are removed ipsilaterally as needed with a one-side protected drill and Kerrison punches (Fig. 13.11). The ligamentum flavum is dissected and removed until full identification of the lateral border of the nerve root (Fig. 13.12). However, the ligamentum flavum should be left intact as much as possible to act as a protective shield for neural structures.

   The nerve root is gently retracted (Fig. 13.13). Annular incision, disc fragment dissection, and ruptured fragment removal are performed carefully. After

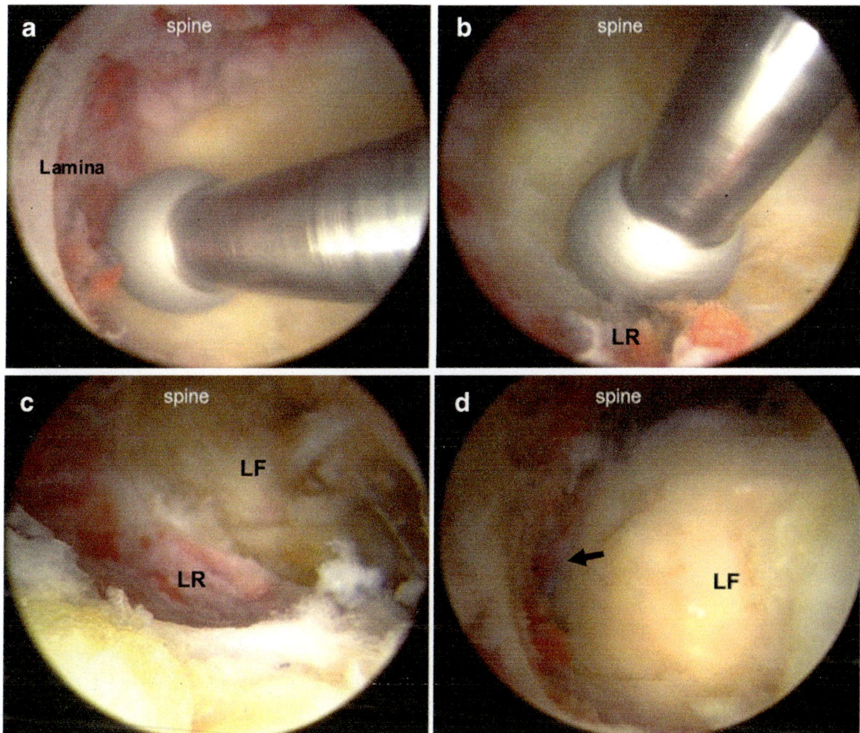

Fig. 13.11 Limited laminotomy is performed until identifying the ligamentum flavum attachments. (**a**) Circumferential bone removal starting with superior lamina. (**b**) The lateral recess (LR) is undercutting ipsilaterally. (**c**) The ligamentum flavum (LF) is identified. (**d**) Bone removal stops until the LF attachments (black arrow) are observed. (*Images courtesy of Javier Quillo-Olvera M.D.*)

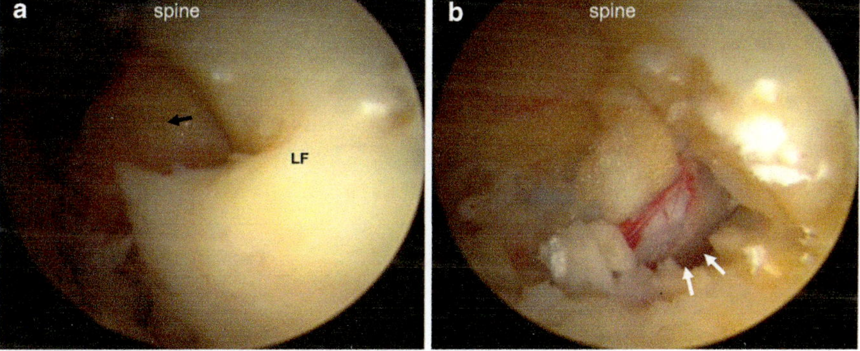

Fig. 13.12 Ligamentum flavum (LF) is dissected from the lamina and removed until identifying the lateral border of the dural sac and the traversing nerve. (**a**) The epidural space (black arrow) is exposed after partial flavectomy. (**b**) The lateral border of the dural sac (white arrows) is apparent after lateral flavectomy. (*Images courtesy of Javier Quillo-Olvera M.D.*)

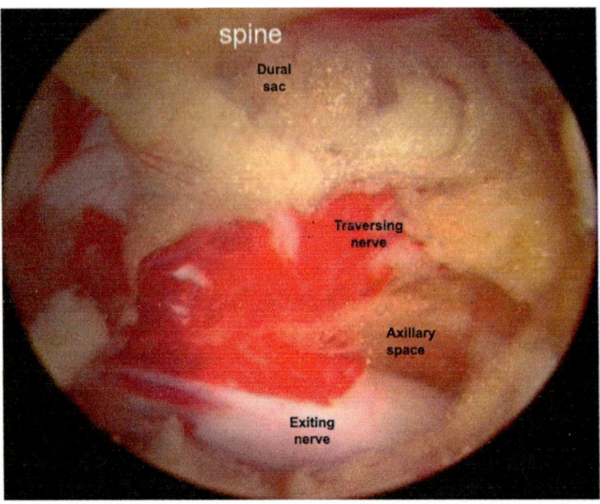

Fig. 13.13 The neural elements were confirmed with the endoscope. (*Image courtesy of Javier Quillo-Olvera M.D.*)

checking the nerve root is free and disc space is decompressed using a 90° hook dissector, a minivac drain is placed temporarily and the skin is sutured with a 3:0 absorbable suture.

Illustrated Cases

Case 1

A 66-year-old male presented severe pain in both legs, with being more severe on the left side. Preoperative lumbar MRI showed a central ruptured disc of L4–L5 level (Fig. 13.14). We performed UBE discectomy successfully (Fig. 13.15). After surgery, the ruptured disc was thoroughly removed. Postoperative MRI showed complete removal of the disc particles (Fig. 13.16 and Video 13.2).

Case 2

A 49-year-old female patient had severe radicular pain in the left leg. Preoperative lumbar MRI showed extruded disc herniation in the L5–S1 level (Fig. 13.17). We performed a paramedian UBE approach (Fig. 13.18). After UBE discectomy, post-operative MRI showed that extruded disc was completely removed and S1 root was well decompressed (Fig. 13.19 and Video 13.3).

Paraspinal Approach

In central, paracentral, and foraminal disc herniations, the paramedian approach is adequate. In disc herniations of far lateral and intraforaminal, basically, the pathologies which are on lateral of pedicle midline, the paraspinal (paravertebral) approach is applicable [23] (Fig. 13.20).

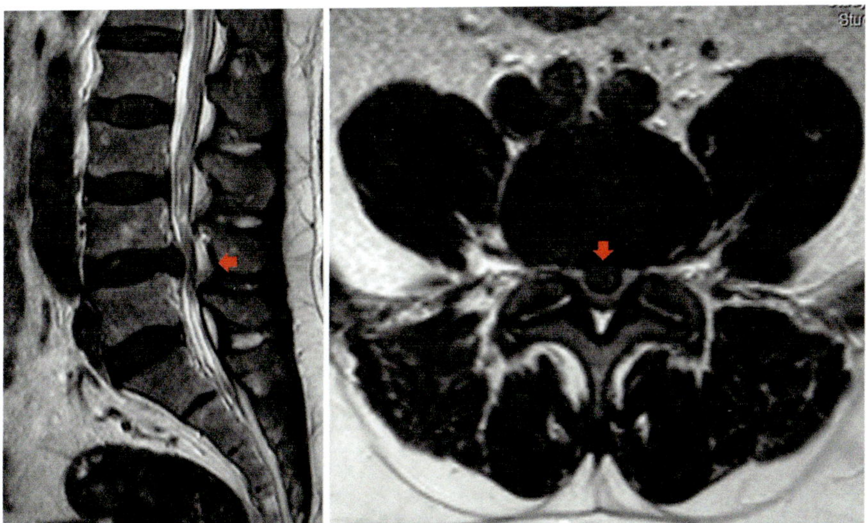

Fig. 13.14 Case 1: Preoperative lumbar MRI showing a central LDH at L4–L5 (red arrows) causing severe central spinal stenosis

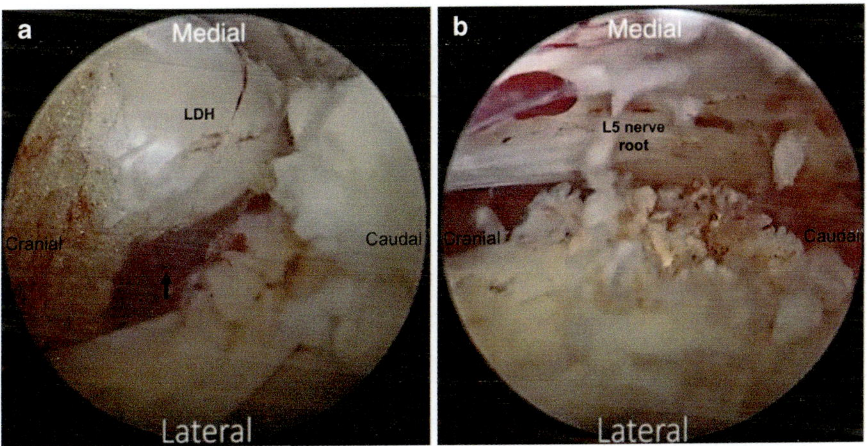

Fig. 13.15 Intraoperative endoscopic view during Case 1 surgery. (**a**) Identification of the lumbar disc herniation (LDH) in the ventral epidural space (black arrow). (**b**) The left-sided L5 nerve root was decompressed

Skin points in lateral position for the paraspinal approach are nearly the same as the paramedian approach. In this approach, the difference is about the AP position. Two portals are opened in the paraspinal area. These entry points are formed along the imaginary line connecting the tips of the transverse processes, which are 1 or 1.5 cm far from the vertebral body of the foraminal disc level for the paraspinal approach (Fig. 13.21). Initially, the working portal is formed at the junction of a point 1 cm lateral to the lateral border of the pedicle and the lower endplate.

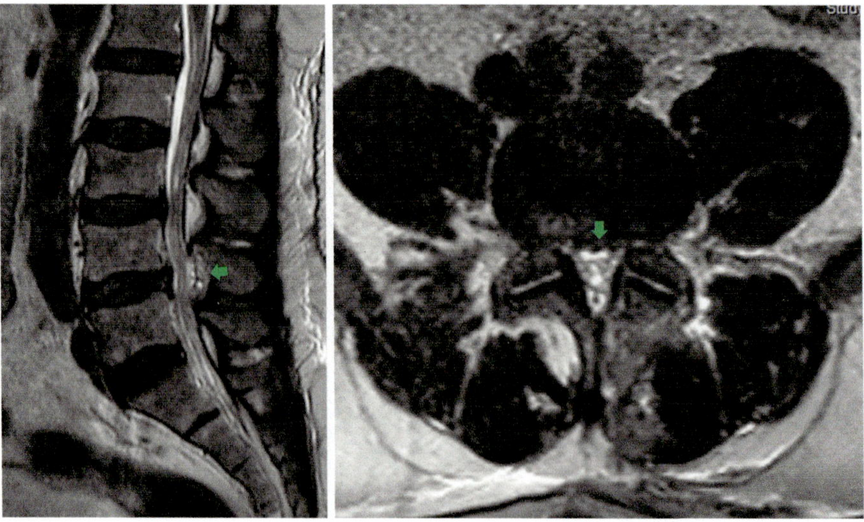

Fig. 13.16 Case 1: Postoperative lumbar MRI. Acceptable decompression was achieved at L4–L5 with the UBE technique

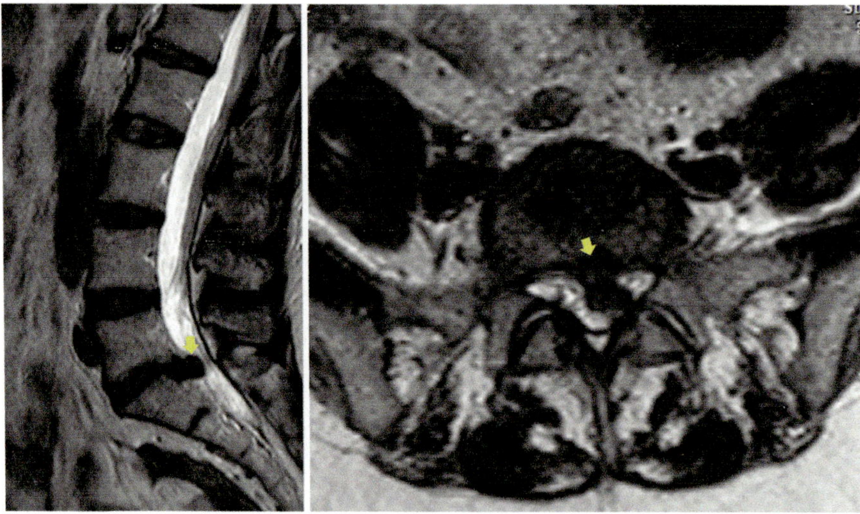

Fig. 13.17 Case 2: Preoperative lumbar MRI shows an extruded LDH (yellow arrows) on the left side at L5–S1

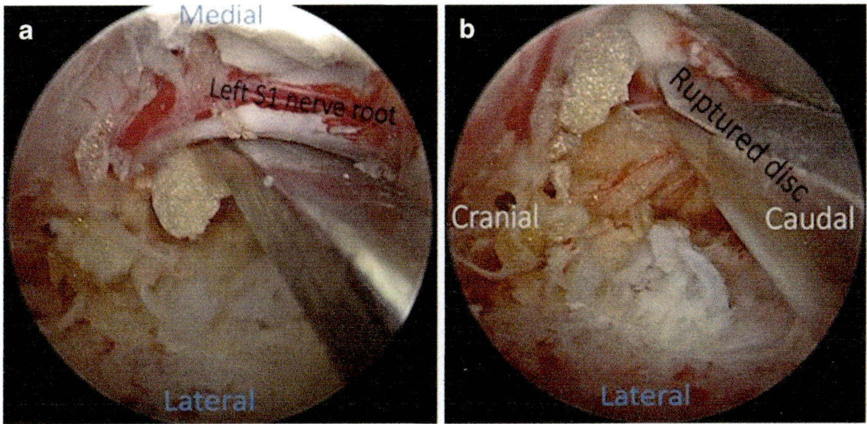

Fig. 13.18 Intraoperative images with the endoscope from Case 2. (**a**) After bone removal, the left S1 nerve root has been exposed. (**b**) The disc herniation is identified below the left S1 nerve

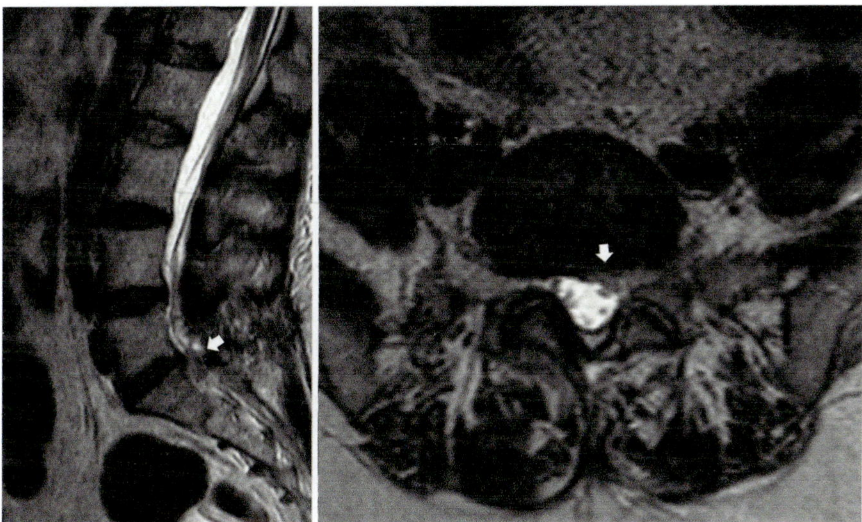

Fig. 13.19 Case 2: Postoperative lumbar MRI. The white arrows point to L5–S1 after discectomy

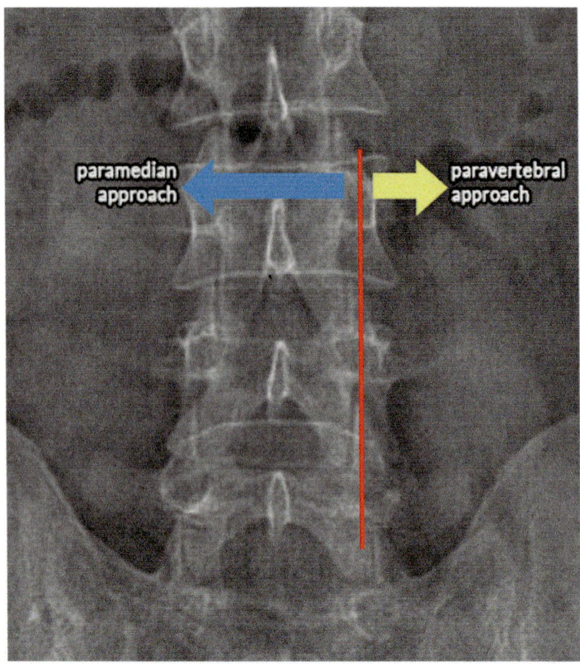

Fig. 13.20 The two basic approaches in UBE depend on the pathology and location

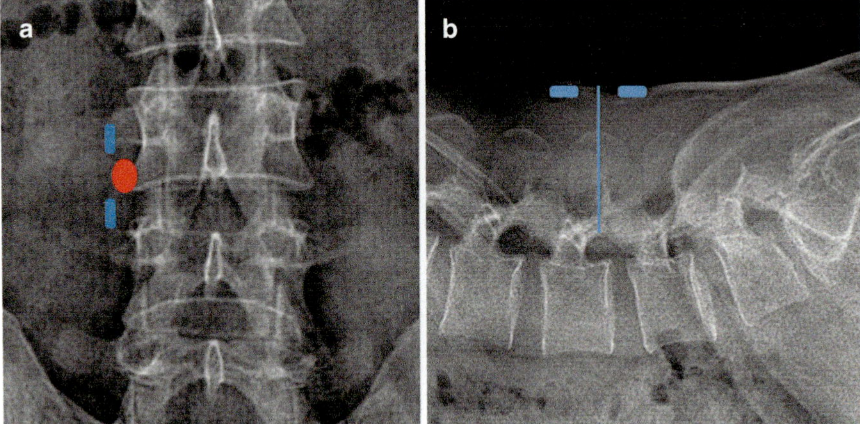

Fig. 13.21 Portal entrances for paramedian approach. (**a**) AP view. (**b**) Lateral view

Secondly, the endoscopic portal is formed on the lower margin of the transverse process of the upper vertebrae under the C-arm. The target points are the isthmus in the AP view, and the middle of the foramen in the lateral X-ray view.

Paravertebral UBE approach principles are the same as the paramedian UBE approach. This approach is no different from the endoscopic version of the "Wiltse" approach that is known in microsurgery.

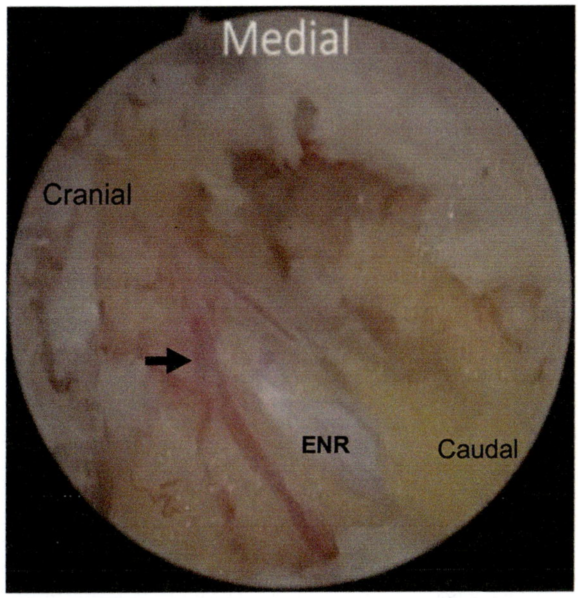

Fig. 13.22 Endoscopic view through a paraspinal (paravertebral) lumbar approach with UBE. (**a**) Dorsal branch of the segmental artery. (**b**) Exiting nerve root

Serial dilators are inserted through the skin incision in the direction of the isthmus. Following removal of the dilators, the blunt muscle detacher is moved into the transverse process, and soft tissue on the isthmus and the lateral border of the facet joint is dissected. Then, an endoscope is inserted into the trocar from its sheath, and an RF probe is inserted in the working portal. After triangulation, an RF probe is used to clean the soft tissue on the upper transverse process, isthmus, and superior facet joint. Firstly, the isthmus is found; in doubting situations after isthmus is viewed, a control check must be done with fluoroscopy. After that, lateral facetectomy is applied partially with an arthroscopic burr, and then it is enlarged with Kerrison punches. Here, the movement should be towards the distal pedicle, disc space should be reached, and bone resection should be applied cranially to find nerve root (Fig. 13.22). After the intertransverse ligament is carefully removed, then the exiting root is explored. Here, the dorsal branch of the segmental artery should be seen (Fig. 13.22). Then, this artery must be coagulated with an RF probe; otherwise, bleeding might be too much for surgery to continue with ease. Nerve root ganglion should not be manipulated at the best, and no irritation should be done with the help of a retractor [23]. The ruptured disc is removed, and discectomy is done under endoscopic view.

Illustrated Case

Case 3

A 54-year-old female complained of radicular pain in her left leg. The preoperative lumbar MRI showed disc herniation at the left extraforaminal area at L4–L5

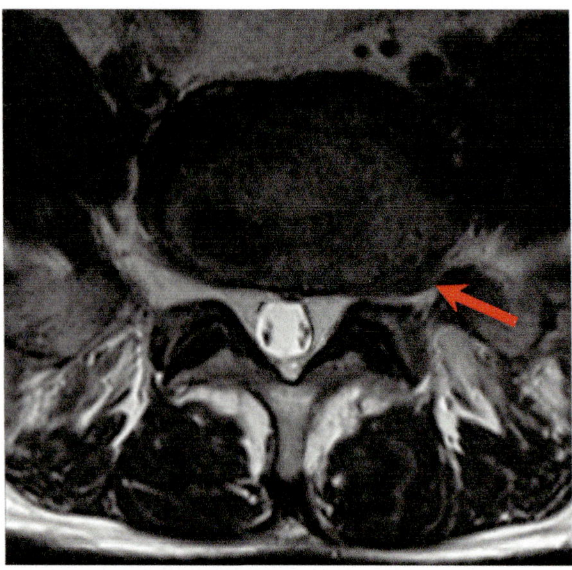

Fig. 13.23 Axial view at L4–L5 on the lumbar MRI from Case 3. The red arrow points to an extraforaminal LDH on the left side

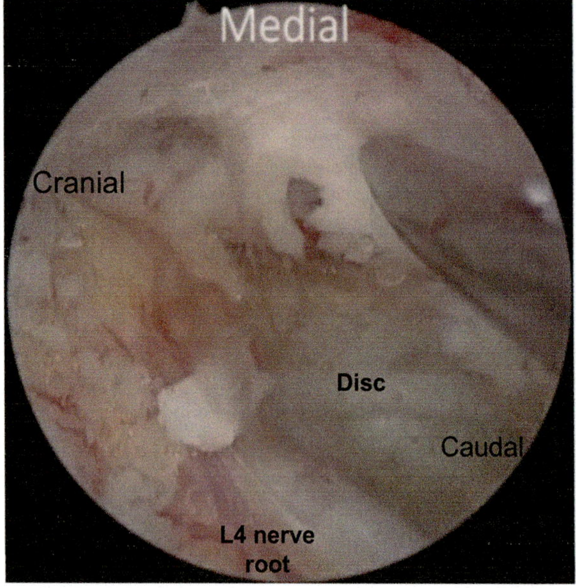

Fig. 13.24 Intraoperative endoscopic view of the L4 nerve root after discectomy through a UBE paraspinal approach. The extraforaminal disc space is observed

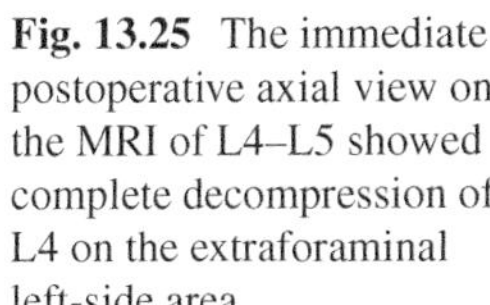

Fig. 13.25 The immediate postoperative axial view on the MRI of L4–L5 showed complete decompression of L4 on the extraforaminal left-side area

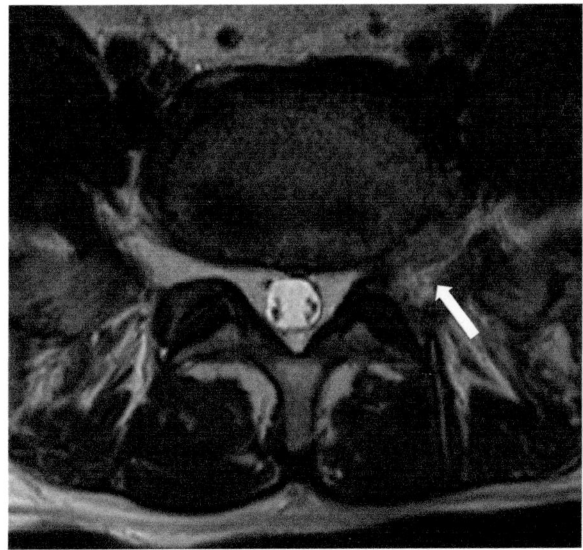

(Fig. 13.23). A paraspinal (paravertebral) approach for L4–L5 on the left side was planned with UBE. During the surgery, the LDH was ablating with the RF probe, and the exiting L4 nerve root was decompressed (Fig. 13.24). Postoperative lumbar MRI showed sufficient decompression at the extraforaminal area at L4–L5 on the left side (Fig. 13.25 and Video 13.4).

Advantages

For surgeons:

- Easy handling
- Familiar surgical anatomy and approach
- Minimal muscle injury
- Use of the standard surgical instruments as in microscopic discectomy
- Easy pressure control of continuous fluid irrigation thanks to biportal system
- Better and wider visualization
- Reduced bleeding: Continuous irrigation of saline allows better bleeding control
- A migrated ruptured disc can be handled

For patients:

- Minimal muscle and bone damage
- Less pain
- Early rehabilitation
- Reduced hospital stay
- Early return to work [24–26]

Complications and Avoidance

Possible complications of the UBE technique are classified into early and late.

1. Early complications

    - Dural tears: Incidental durotomy is a rare complication during the procedure. Using collagen fibrin patches such as TachoSil can be directly repaired for small dura tears with no neural incarceration under endoscopic view [27].
    - Increased cerebrospinal pressure and neurological dysfunction: Constant inflow of irrigation without proper outflow may cause fluid to collect in the limited area of the spinal canal, which may increase cerebrospinal fluid pressure; then, it can lead to neurological dysfunction such as headache, neck pain, seizure, or cerebral edema [28–30]. The surgeon should always attempt to ensure a good inflow and outflow system while maintaining irrigation pressure at an average of 30–50 mmHg [31].
    - Epidural hematoma: Careful hemostasis before the closure is a key to preventing hematoma formation. The surgeon should consider keeping a soft suction drainage tube to drain irrigation fluids and blood for the first postoperative day [32].

2. Late complications

    - Infection: The infection rate after UBE surgery is very low. However, excessive usage of RF may cause fat and tissue necrosis leading to a high risk of infection [23].
    - Recurrence: UBE allows a targeted approach to the annular rupture site without violation of the normal annulus. Annuloplasty can be done in all disc herniations, reducing the risk of recurrence.

Conclusion

UBE can be an effective treatment modality for LDH. The anatomic trajectory and endoscopic view are similar to that of conventional LM. It provides an exceptional and extraordinary navigation experience to the spinal canal, which makes the procedure safer by enhancing the view of neural and vascular structures. UBE discectomy has quite sufficient and direct fragmentectomy, and discectomy to that in LM resulted in the same clinical outcomes while preserving the spinal tissues. Considering adequate indications, UBE is a highly feasible alternative endoscopic technique to microsurgery.

References

1. Seung-Kook K, Sang-Soo K, Young-Ho H, Seung-Woo P, Su-Chan L. Clinical comparison of unilateral biportal endoscopic technique versus open microdiscectomy for single-level lumbar discectomy: a multicenter, retrospective analysis: research article. J Orthop Surg Res. 2018;13:22.
2. Wu CY, Jou IM, Yang WS, Yang CC, Chao LY, Huang YH. Significance of the mass-compression effect of postlaminectomy/laminotomy fibrosis on histological changes on the dura mater and nerve root of the cauda equina: an experimental study in rats. J Orthop Sci. 2014;19:798–808.
3. He J, Xiao S, Wu Z, Yuan Z. Microendoscopic discectomy versus open discectomy for lumbar disc herniation: a meta-analysis. Eur Spine J. 2016;25:1373–81.
4. Podichetty VK, Spears J, Isaacs RE, Booher J, Biscup RS. Complications associated with minimally invasive decompression for lumbar spinal stenosis. J Spinal Disord Tech. 2006;19(3):161–6.
5. Adams MA, Hutton WC. The mechanical function of the lumbar apophyseal joints. Spine. 1983;8(3):327–30.
6. Adams MA, Hutton WC, Stott JR. The resistance to flexion of the lumbar intervertebral joint. Spine. 1980;5(3):245–53.
7. Cusick JF, Yoganandan N, Pintar FA, Reinartz JM. Biomechanics of sequential posterior lumbar surgical alterations. J Neurosurg. 1992;76(5):805–11.
8. Yeung AT. The evolution and advancement of endoscopic foraminal surgery: one surgeon's experience incorporating adjunctive technologies. SAS J. 2007;1(3):108–17.
9. Ahn Y. Percutaneous endoscopic decompression for lumbar spinal stenosis. Expert Rev Med Devices. 2014;11(6):605–16.
10. Lee S, Kim SK, Lee SH, et al. Percutaneous endoscopic lumbar discectomy for migrated disc herniation: classification of disc migration and surgical approaches. Eur Spine J. 2007;16(3):431–7.
11. Lee SH, Kang BU, Ahn Y, et al. Operative failure of percutaneous endoscopic lumbar discectomy: a radiologic analysis of 55 cases. Spine. 2006;31(10):E285–90.
12. Jin Hwa E, Sang Kyu S, Ketan D, Alfonso G. Unilateral biportal endoscopic decompression for lumbar spinal stenosis. In: Kim DH, Choi G, Lee S-H, Fessler RG, editors. Endoscopic spine surgery. 2nd ed. Thieme Medical Publishers: New York; 2018. p. 75–80.
13. Komp M, Hahn P, Oezdemir S, et al. Bilateral spinal decompression of lumbar central stenosis with the full-endoscopic interlaminar versus microsurgical laminotomy technique: a prospective, randomized, controlled study. Pain Physician. 2015;18(1):61–70.
14. Hwa EJ, Hwa HD, Son SK, Park CK. Percutaneous biportal endoscopic decompression for lumbar spinal stenosis: a technical note and preliminary clinical results. J Neurosurg Spine. 2016;24(4):602–7.
15. De Antoni DJ, Claro ML, Poehling GG, Hughes SS. Translaminar lumbar epidural endoscopy: anatomy, technique, and indications. Arthroscopy. 1996;12(3):330–4.

16. Costa F, Sassi M, Cardia A, et al. Degenerative lumbar spinal stenosis: analysis of results in a series of 374 patients treated with unilateral laminotomy for bilateral microdecompression. J Neurosurg Spine. 2007;7(6):579–86.
17. Minamide A, Yoshida M, Yamada H, et al. Endoscope-assisted spinal decompression surgery for lumbar spinal stenosis. J Neurosurg Spine. 2013;19(6):664–71.
18. Dae-Jung C, Chang-Myong C, Je-Tea J, Sang-Jin L, Yong-Sang K. Clinical study learning curve associated with complications in biportal endoscopic spinal surgery: challenges and strategies. Asian Spine J. 2016;10(4):624–9.
19. Choi CM, Chung JT, Lee SJ, Choi DJ. How I do it? Biportal endoscopic spinal surgery (BESS) for treatment of lumbar spinal stenosis. Acta Neurochir. 2016;158:459–63.
20. Dong Hwa H, Jin Hwa E, Sang KS. Percutaneous unilateral biportal endoscopic diskectomy and decompression for lumbar degenerative disease. In: Daniel HK, Gun C, Sang-Ho L, Richard GF, editors. Endoscopic spine surgery. 2nd ed. New York: Thieme Medical Publishers; 2018. p. 81–7.
21. Garg B, Nagraja UB, Jayaswal A. Microendoscopic versus open discectomy for lumbar disc herniation: a prospective randomised study. J Orthop Surg. 2011;19(1):30–4.
22. Chang-Myong C. Biportal endoscopic spine surgery (BESS): considering merits and pitfalls review of techniques on full-endoscopic spine surgery. J Spine Surg. 2020;6(2):457–65.
23. Hayati A. Bölüm 47: Unilateral biportal endoskopik lomber disk ve spinal stenoz cerrahisi. In: Hüseyin Yener E, Onur Y, Ertuğrul Ş, editors. Omurga Cerrahisinde Yeni Yaklaşımlar ve Minimal İnvaziv Omurga Cerrahisi. Ankara: Akademisyen Kitabevi; 2021. p. 379–93.
24. Gibson JN, Cowie JG, Iprenburg M. Transforaminal endoscopic spinal surgery: the future 'gold standard' for discectomy? A review. Surgeon. 2012;10:290–6.
25. Lee DY, Shim CS, Ahn Y, et al. Comparison of percutaneous endoscopic lumbar discectomy and open lumbar microdiscectomy for recurrent disc herniation. J Korean Neurosurg Soc. 2009;46:515–21.
26. Ruetten S, Komp M, Merk H, et al. Recurrent lumbar disc herniation after conventional discectomy: a prospective, randomized study comparing full-endoscopic interlaminar and transforaminal versus microsurgical revision. J Spinal Disord Tech. 2009;22:122–9.
27. Kim HS, Raorane HD, Wu PH, et al. Incidental durotomy during endoscopic stenosis lumbar decompression: incidence, classification, and proposed management strategies. World Neurosurg. 2020. pii: S1878-8750(20)30260-6.
28. Choi G, Kang HY, Modi HN, et al. Risk of developing seizure after percutaneous endoscopic lumbar discectomy. J Spinal Disord Tech. 2011;24(2):83–92.
29. Joh JY, Choi G, Kong BJ, Park HS, Lee SH, Chang SH. Comparative study of neck pain in relation to increase of cervical epidural pressure during percutaneous endoscopic lumbar discectomy. Spine. 2009;34(19):2033–8.
30. Parpaley Y, Urbach H, Kovacs A, et al. Pseudohypoxic brain swelling (postoperative intracranial hypotension-associated venous congestion) after spinal surgery: report of 2 cases. Neurosurgery. 2011;68:E277–83.
31. Kim HS, Sharma SB, Wu PH, et al. Complications and limitations of endoscopic spine surgery and percutaneous instrumentation. Indian Spine J. 2020;3:78–85.
32. Pang HW, Hyeun-Sung K, Il-Tae J. A narrative review of development of full-endoscopic lumbar spine surgery, review article. Neurospine. 2020;17(Suppl 1):S20–33.

Chapter 14
Unilateral Biportal Endoscopy for Complex Lumbar Disc Herniations

Ariel Kaen, Takaki Yoshimizu, and Fernando Durand Neyra

Abbreviations

CLA	Contralateral approach
Cs	Central space
E-Fo	Extraforaminal
FLA	Far-lateral approach
Fo	Foraminal
IPA	Ipsilateral posterolateral approach
LBP	Lower back pain
LDH	Lumbar disc herniation
LR	Lateral recess
MRI	Magnetic resonance imaging
MSU	Michigan State University
NR	Nerve root
PC	Paracentral
PELD	Percutaneous endoscopic lumbar discectomy
RF	Radiofrequency
SAP	Superior articular process
UBE	Unilateral biportal endoscopy

Supplementary Information The online version contains supplementary material available at [https://doi.org/10.1007/978-3-031-14736-4_14].

A. Kaen (✉) · F. Durand Neyra
Department of Neurosurgery, Virgen del Rocio University Hospital, Sevilla, Spain
e-mail: kaenariel@hotmail.com; fdurandn@hotmail.com

T. Yoshimizu
Department of Orthopedic Surgery, Seirei Hamamatsu General Hospital, Shizuoka, Japan
e-mail: yossy8772@gmail.com

J. Quillo-Olvera et al. (eds.), *Unilateral Biportal Endoscopy of the Spine*, https://doi.org/10.1007/978-3-031-14736-4_14

Introduction

Herniation of the nucleus pulposus into or through the annulus fibrosus is a well-recognized cause of lower back pain (LBP) and sciatica. The surgery goal is to identify the lumbar disc fragment and remove it with as minor damage to surrounding structures as possible. The spectrum of endoscopic discectomy is expanding gradually, with some past contraindications now becoming indications [1, 2].

Before starting with the development of the chapter, the reader should know what we consider to be "complex" lumbar disc herniation. It means that there are "simple" herniated discs, which is a big mistake. Lumbar disc herniation can be the most straightforward spinal surgery or the most complex one, even worse than a fusion. Locating the lumbar disc herniation (LDH) position is critical to selecting the appropriate surgical technique. Numerous classifications have been proposed to estimate the difficulty in axial and sagittal planes. For all these reasons, we will define the main factors contributing to LDH surgery's complexity and how to solve it through biportal endoscopic surgery.

Preoperative Planning

When we are planning the surgical procedure in our patients with LDH, we must take into account four critical factors:

Sagittal Migration

The most widely used classification in a sagittal plane is the Lee modified [3]. This one includes seven zones (Fig. 14.1 and Table 14.1):

- "Zero" zone represents "non-migrated" LHD.
- "Low-grade" migrated LDH refers to disc migration limited to the line 3 mm below the inferior margin of the upper pedicle (rostral) or the line of the middle of the lower pedicle (caudal) from the disc margin.
- "High-grade" migrated LDH refers to disc migration beyond the reference line in either the rostral or the caudal direction.
- "Very-high-grade" migrated LDH refers to disc migration that extends beyond the inferior margin of the pedicle in either the rostral or the caudal direction.

UBE could be used to remove all types of migrated intervertebral disc herniation [4, 5].

In 2018, Kim et al. tried to determine the degree of difficulty in treating a lumbar disc herniation from the point of view of full-endoscopic surgery. Unfortunately, this level of complexity was aimed at the full-endoscopic approach. It cannot be

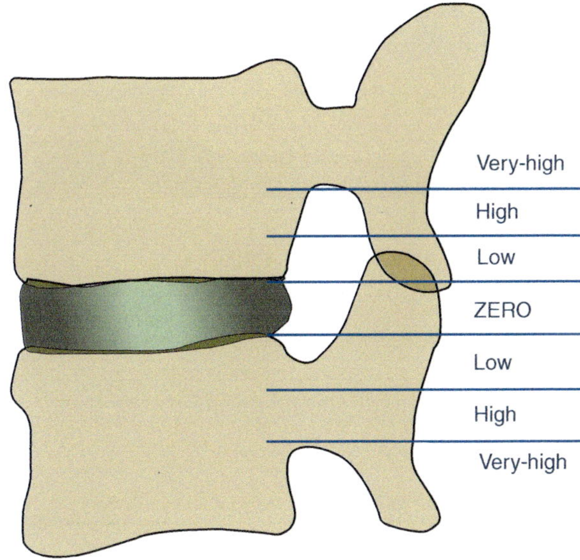

Fig. 14.1 Schematic representation of disc herniation. The direction and degree of migration of herniated discs are divided into seven zones

Table 14.1 Classification of the LDH in the sagittal plane

Degree/direction	Range of migration distance
Very high/upward	From the inferior margin of the upper pedicle
High/upward	From the inferior margin of the upper pedicle to 3 mm below the inferior margin of the upper pedicle
Low/upward	From 3 mm below the inferior margin of the upper pedicle to the superior disc margin
Non-migrated	From the superior disc margin to the inferior disc margin
Low/downward	From the inferior disc margin to the middle of the lower pedicle
High/downward	From the middle of the lower pedicle to the inferior margin of the lower pedicle
Very high/ downward	Beyond the inferior margin of the lower pedicle

extrapolated to biportal surgery since, for example, the "low-grade" downward migration is considered in this study to be of moderate difficulty for PELD, whereas with the biportal technique, the complexity is less [6]. We can assume that any herniated disc presenting as high or very high grade is "complex" LDH for UBE.

Axial Location

Based on the axial MRI, Michigan State University (MSU) classification can be used to precisely position the LDH in the axial plane (Fig. 14.2). To classify the location of the herniated disc, this group places three points along the intrafacet line,

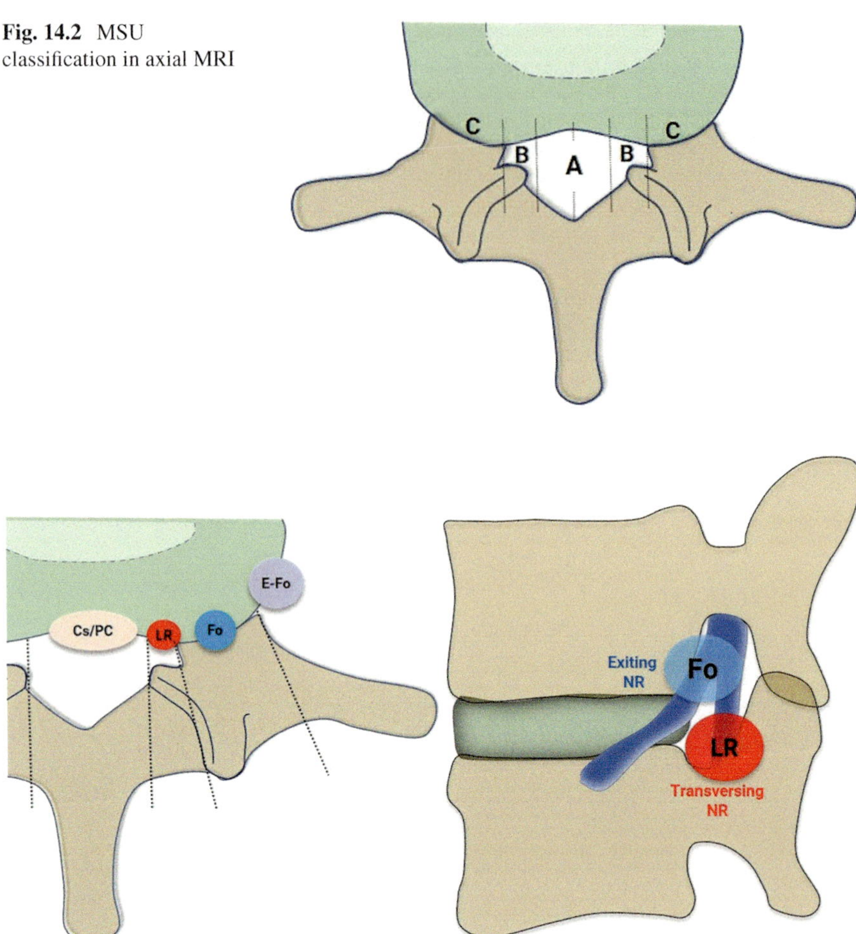

Fig. 14.2 MSU classification in axial MRI

Fig. 14.3 Classical classification of the LHD (left) and the difference between lateral recess and foraminal disc herniation (right). *Cs* central space, *PC* paracentral, *LR* lateral recess, *Fo* foraminal, *E-Fo* extraforaminal, *NR* nerve root

dividing it into four equal quarters [7, 8]. The left and right center quadrants represent zone A (central). The right and left lateral quadrants are zone B (lateral). A third zone C is represented at the level of the foramen by the area that extends beyond the medial margin of any facet joint, beyond the limit of the lateral quadrants. It is there, where the hernia extends into the intraforaminal space and beyond to the right and left sides, that the injury is traditionally known as the far lateral.

Unfortunately, most spine surgeons have not adopted this radiological classification. Instead, they prefer the classical nomenclature where herniated discs can be classified as central/paracentral, lateral recess, foraminal, and extraforaminal (Fig. 14.3) [9], where the main difficulty is in differentiating hernias located in the lateral recess (traversing NR clinic) from those found in the foramen (exiting NR clinic).

As will be discussed in the next section, these four areas in the axial plane allow us to plan the surgery with more precision; that is, if it is central/paracentral hernia or lateral recess (LR), an ipsilateral posterolateral approach (IPA) is indicated. While if the disc fragment is in the foramen, a good option is to perform a contralateral approach (CLA), especially if it is associated with central canal stenosis. Finally, the best suggestion is the far-lateral approach (FLA) if the herniated disc is extraforaminal.

Size and Consistency

The size and location of disc herniation are measured at the level of maximal extrusion in reference to a single intrafacet line drawn transversely across the lumbar canal, to and from the medial edges of the right and left facet joint articulations (Fig. 14.4). To represent the size of the herniated disc, the lesion is described as 1, 2, or 3. The intrafacet line determines whether the herniated disc extends to or less than 50% of the distance from the posterior aspect non-herniated from the disc to the intrafacet line (size 1), or more than 50% of that distance (size 2). If the hernia extends completely beyond the intrafacet line, it is called a size 3 disc [7]. It is important to note that the size of the LDH is not always associated with consistency. It has smooth LDHs that are technically easy to remove even when they are large (size 3), while smaller and generally long-term ones can be difficult to operate. Calcified lumbar disc herniation is a subtype of herniation, probably secondary to a longer course of the disease, changes in the development of the nucleus pulposus, and unknown triggers such as infections and microtrauma. Adhesion between calcification and nerve root or dura increases the surgical difficulty and can cause iatrogenic injuries, such as nerve root injury, dural tear, or both.

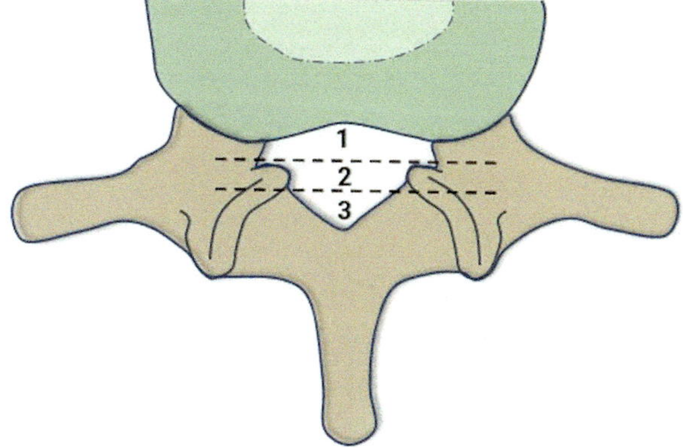

Fig. 14.4 Grading the disc herniation for size

Level

Most LDHs occur in the lower lumbar spine at the L4–L5 and L5–S1 (90–97%). The term upper LDH is not as uniformly defined. Some authors consider the term to include LDH at L1–L2, L2–L3, and L3–L4. However, others consider the term to refer to LDH occurring only at L1–L2 and L2–L3. We know that the postoperative outcomes for LDH at L3–L4 are significantly better than those occurring at L1–L2 and L2–L3 [10]. Furthermore, the anatomic characteristics of LDH at L3–L4 are more similar to those of the lower lumbar spine.

Compared with the lower lumbar spine facets, the upper facets are significantly more parallel to the midsagittal plane. This poses several surgical challenges in performing an ipsilateral endoscopic lumbar discectomy for paracentral and central LDH effectively and safely while preserving the integrity of the pars interarticularis and facet joints. This disparity is likely due to reduced motion and stress at the upper lumbar spine than the lower lumbar spine.

In addition, the upper spine has special anatomical features, including a narrow spinal canal, short nerve roots, and less distance between the dura and nerve roots (Fig. 14.5). Furthermore, the conventional posterior approach for a lumbar

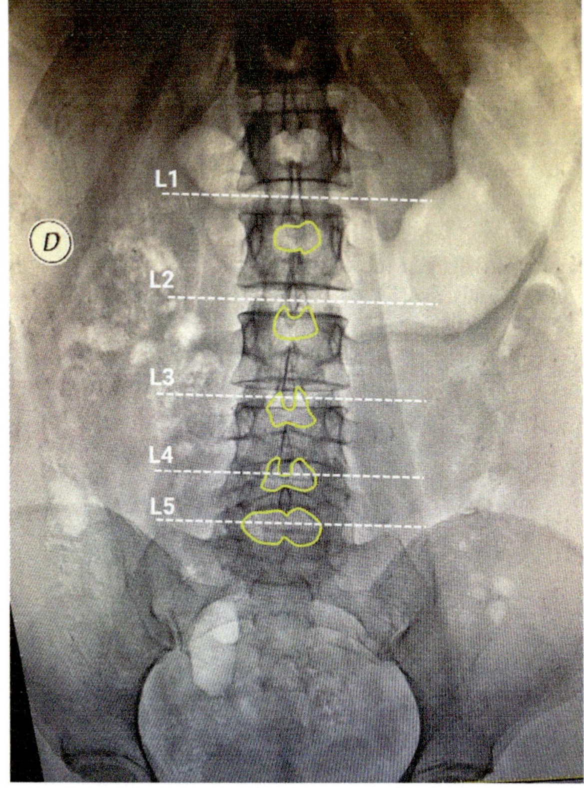

Fig. 14.5 Lumbar AP view. Note the location of the lumbar disc regarding the interlaminar space. In the upper lumbar disc, the window is smaller and the disc is higher regarding the spinolaminar junction

discectomy provides only limited surgical exposure in the upper lumbar spine. Performing a discectomy in such a narrow surgical field can result in over-retraction on the thecal sac and places the neural elements at an increased risk of injury. Alternatively, a near-complete facetectomy and possible pars interarticularis resection are required to obtain adequate bony exposure to safely perform an upper lumbar discectomy with a conventional posterior approach. There are no long-term studies on spinal fusion rates required following conventional ipsilateral open or endoscopic lumbar discectomy. However, as shown in reports performing a complete facetectomy or possible pars resection, or both, an upper lumbar discectomy theoretically accelerates spinal instability and likely requires a lumbar fusion surgery.

Surgical Technique

Anesthesia and Position

The physician can select local, spinal, and general anesthesia. For many years, the benefits of using local/epidural anesthesia to maintain patient collaboration have been published; however, in our experience, the complications associated with general anesthesia every day are less even in elderly patients. Remember that lumbar disc herniation will be one of your first procedures to perform UBE, and since the learning curve is not short, we strongly recommend using general anesthesia; if your patient is calm, you will be relaxed.

The prone position on a radiolucent table and Wilson frame is the gold standard position. C-arm fluoroscopy and a monitor for endoscopy were located at the contralateral side of the surgeon (remember that you will need an AP projection more frequently than in open surgery). A Wilson frame is recommendable because it induces distraction of the interlaminar space and makes a better view. To reduce brain complications associated with continuous saline irrigation, we recommend keeping the patient's head slightly above the lumbar spine (Fig. 14.6).

Surgical Steps

Unilateral biportal spine surgery can be performed using three different approaches:

1. The ipsilateral posterior approach (IPA) or paramedian is a good and formal way to perform an ipsilateral discectomy with or without bilateral decompression of the lateral recess stenosis (Fig. 14.7).

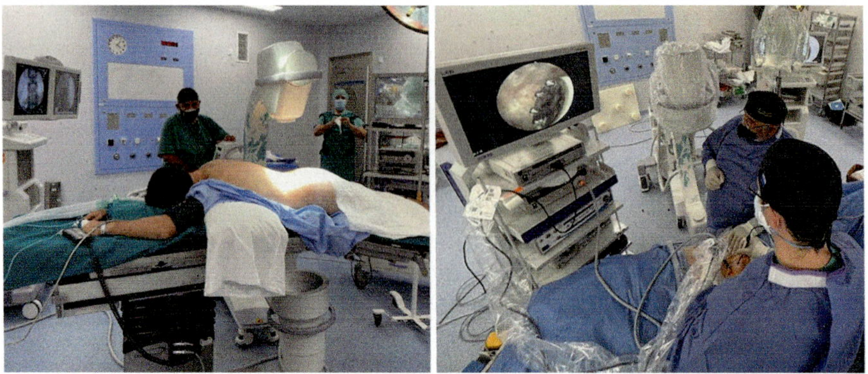

Fig. 14.6 OR setting. The C-arm and endoscopic tower are in front of the surgeon

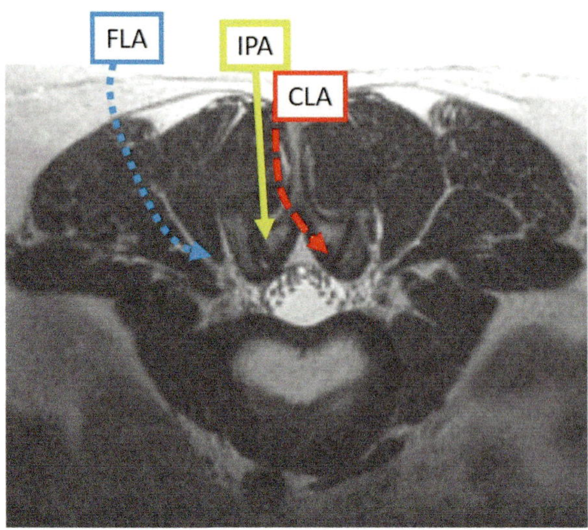

Fig. 14.7 Different biportal approaches to LDH. *CLA* contralateral approach, *FLA* far-lateral approach, *IPA* ipsilateral posterolateral approach

2. The contralateral approach (CLA) is an excellent option to decompress a foraminal disc herniation, especially in the upper lumbar space, to reduce the risk of postoperative instability.
3. The far-lateral approach (FLA) or paraspinal is the treatment of choice for foraminal LDH, especially those located in the extraforaminal area.

Skin Marking

Under fluoroscopic imaging, getting the "true" AP image of the target level (your C-arm not tilted) is very important (Fig. 14.8). Check the locations of two portals using the lateral C-arm fluoroscopic view. In the AP view, draw two lines, one in the midline coinciding with the spinous processes and the second as the

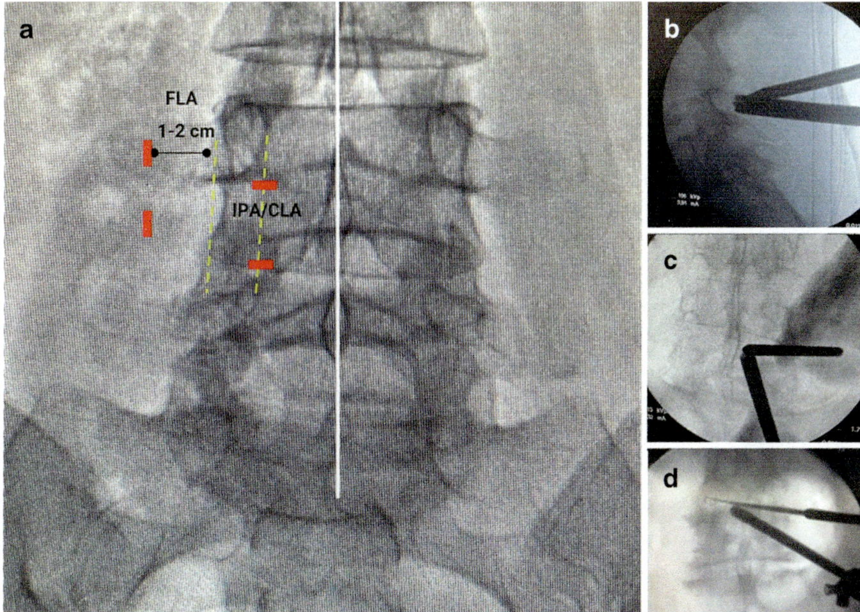

Fig. 14.8 The skin incision should be planned with the AP view of your C-arm (**a**), verify its correct trajectory in the lateral view (**b**, **c**), and carry out controls throughout the surgery, especially when performing a contralateral approach (**d**)

mid-interpedicular line. The third line is perpendicular to the previous ones at the disk level.

A viewing portal is made at 1 cm cranially, and the working portal can be set at 1 cm caudally from mid-intervertebral disc space. You can make vertical or horizontal incisions. In your first cases, the vertical incisions allow you to join both incisions if you need to transform the surgery into an open procedure. When planning an IPA or CLA technique, the two portals are located close to the midline to reach the ipsilateral or the contralateral spinal canal without or with a bit of bone resection as possible. For an FLA, the incision should be made 2 cm lateral to the outer margin of the pedicle to reduce the risk of damage to the lateral wall of the facet (Fig. 14.8). Incision of the portals is performed through penetration of skin and fascia. The fascia incision should be in the form of a cross for easy flow out of irrigation fluid and convenient use of instruments.

Making Working Space and Triangulation

First, we recommend introducing the dilators through the working portal for a craniocaudal disinsertion movement of the multifidus muscle until the spinolaminar angle is located. Next, make the viewing channel and begin irrigation; remember that to have a good vision, the inlet pressure of the irrigation is not so important (we usually use gravity) but a correct outflow through the work port; this allows a constant flow of saline solution and maintains the surgical view clear. To do the initial successful workspace, two distal portals at the endpoints must be found only in the laminar. This concept of "triangulation" has been conditioned by the distance between the incisions (Fig. 14.9). If you make incisions too far apart, it is very likely that you will not see your instruments, while if you make incisions too close together, your instruments get blocked (fighting for space), having to remove the scope to be able to insert the dissector.

Hemilaminectomy is performed using high-speed burr, Kerrison punch, or osteotome. The bone removal begins from the spinolaminar junction and the lower portion of the lamina of the superior vertebra until detaching the superior margin of the flavum ligament. The flavum ligament consists of a superficial layer and a deep layer. The lower portion of the deep layer attaches to the anterosuperior surface of

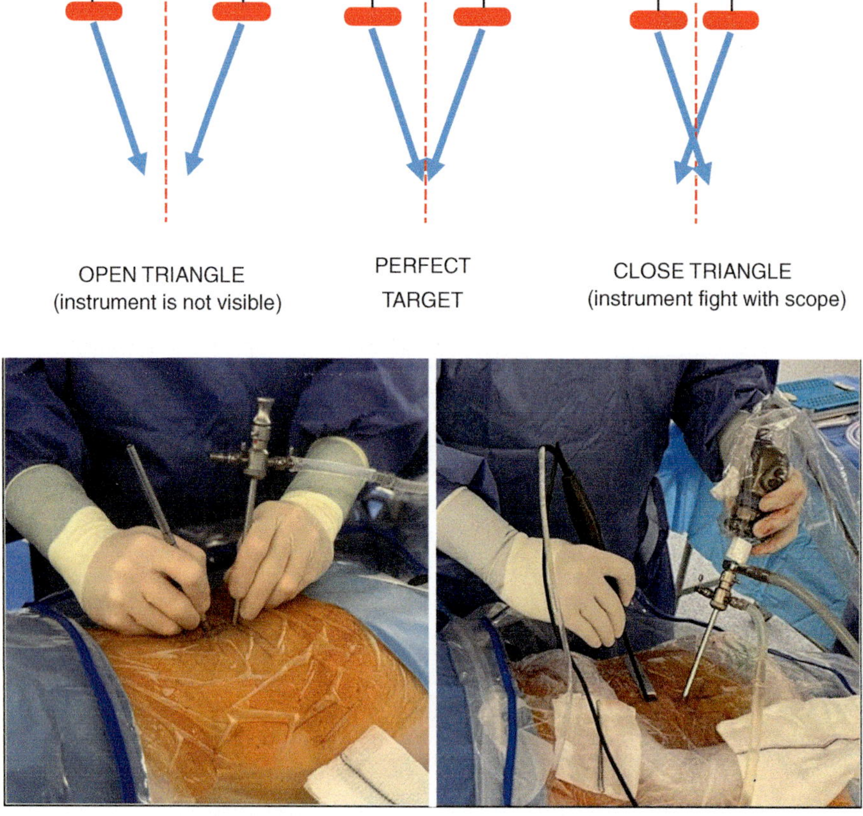

Fig. 14.9 Schematic illustration of the most common failures during instrument triangulation. Before introducing the endoscopy, you should check that the tips of your instruments are at the level of the desired surgical field

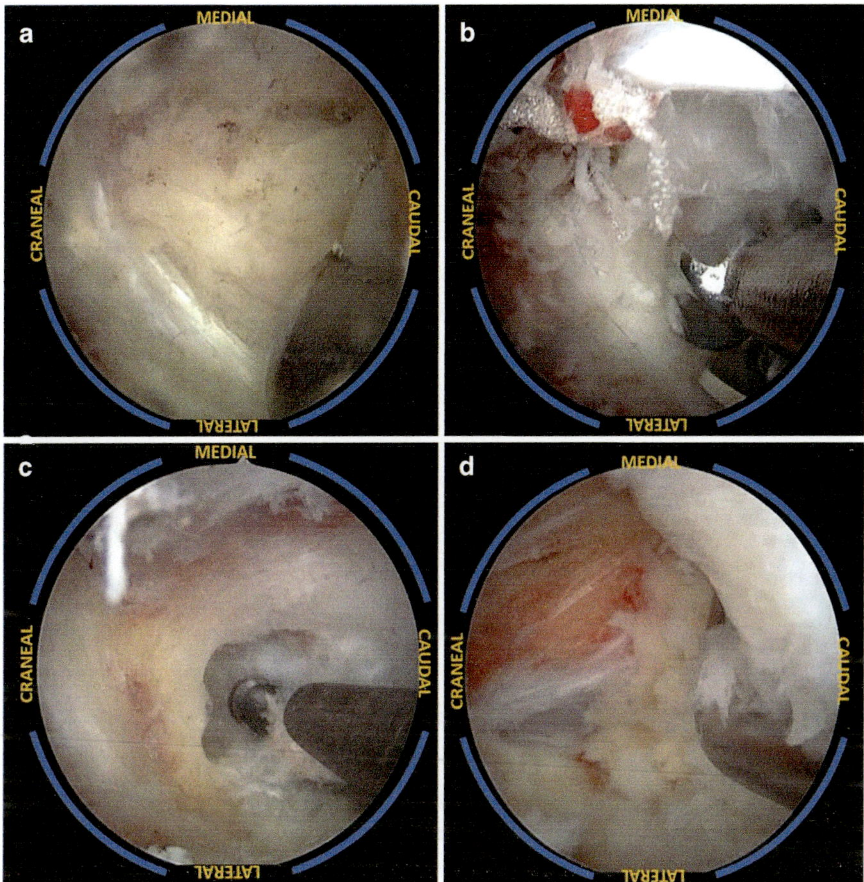

Fig. 14.10 Intraoperative endoscopic images. The initial target must be in a spinolaminar junction (**a**), and then you can drill (**b**) or bite with K-punch the upper lamina (**c**) until the flavum ligament is detached (**d**)

the caudal lamina (Fig. 14.10). The flavectomy is undergone from cranial to caudal and medial to lateral. The flavum ligament was carefully dissected and completely resected.

Discectomy

Once a bloodless field of operation is achieved (sometimes part of the epidural fatty tissue has to be removed), consider the LDH location if it is in the axilla or the shoulder of the nerve root. After gently retracting the nerve root medially, the extruded or sequestrated disc fragments are identified, and 2 mm pituitary forceps help you remove easily (Fig. 14.11). The physician should inspect the operating field entirely. Any remnant disc fragment or residual debris should be removed absolutely from the intracanal space.

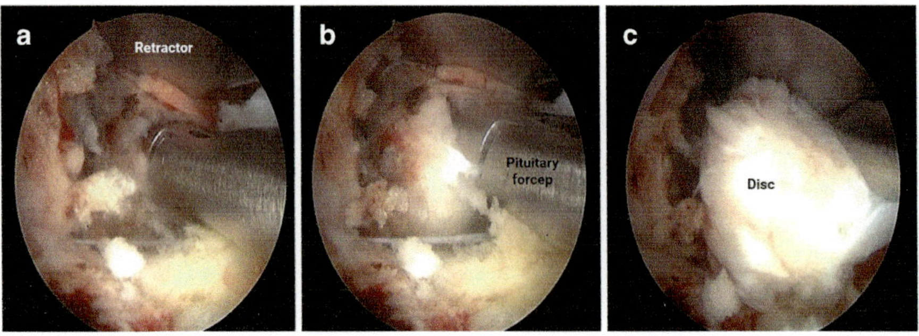

Fig. 14.11 Sequential endoscopic imaging during disc fragment removal (**a**–**c**)

Close and End the Procedure

Usually, before the surgery ends, we close the irrigation to detect bleeding that has gone unnoticed previously. Bleeding control is achieved using the RF and bone wax. If the surgical field is clear, we usually do not leave lumbar drainage unless a major laminectomy has been performed. Finally, we suture with stitches in a single plane. Patients are monitored 24 h after surgery for any complications.

Illustrated Cases

Case 1: L3–L4 High-Grade Migrated Hernia with Multilevel Canal Stenosis
A 67-year-old man has complained of severe back pain and bilateral sciatic pain 10 years prior. The last month presents a progressive worsening. MRI revealed multilevel canal stenosis (L2–L3, L3–L4, L4–L5) and a left high-grade upward migrated herniation on the L3–L4 level. We performed biportal endoscopic "over-the-top" decompression on L3–L4, and the disc fragment was removed ipsilaterally. Finally, we completed the decompression with a UBE on L2–L3 and L4–L5 levels. MRI showed multilevel well decompression and hernia resection (Fig. 14.12 and Video 14.1).

Case 2: L4–L5 Very-High-Grade Migrated Hernia with L4–L5 Disc Collapse
A 61-year-old man presented with progressively worsening back and right leg pain from 5 months before visiting. MRI revealed the very-high-grade downward migrated herniation at the L4–L5 level. The L4–L5 disc showed severe degenerative change with collapse of the disc space. We performed biportal endoscopic discectomy by IPA approach and completed the procedure with OLIF fusion (oblique lateral lumbar interbody fusion) (Fig. 14.13 and Video 14.2).

Case 3: Extraforaminal L2–L3 Disc Herniation
A 55-year-old man presented lower back pain (LBP) and 2 months of right radicular leg pain in the L2 dermatome. Preoperative MRI demonstrated an intra- and extraforaminal herniation at the right L2–L3 level. Therefore, we performed discectomy using the FLA approach associated with foraminoplasty, which means resecting the

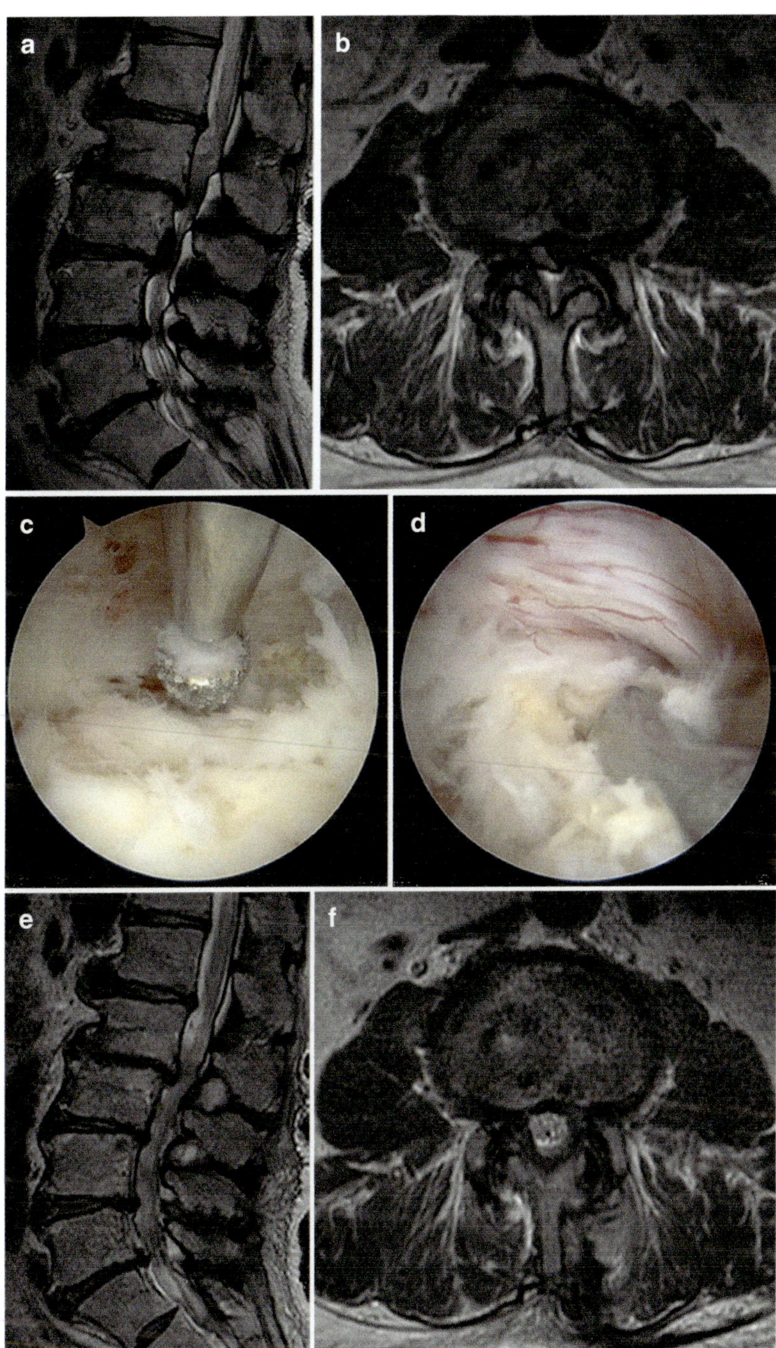

Fig. 14.12 Case 1. Preoperative T2-weighted images show multilevel lumbar spinal stenosis (**a**) and left high-grade upward-migrated L3–L4 herniation (**b**). Intraoperative endoscopic images show the contralateral decompression (**c**) and ipsilateral discectomy (**d**). Postoperative MRI demonstrated complete decompression and hernia fragment resection at L3–L4 on sagittal (**e**) and axial (**f**) views

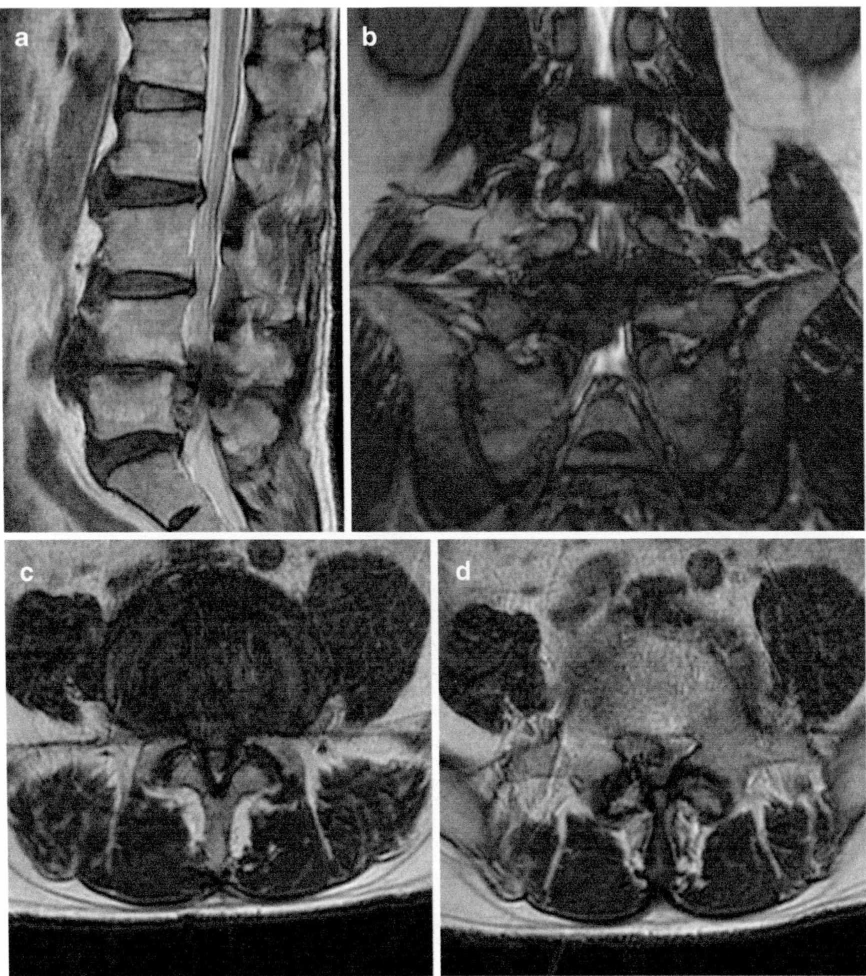

Fig. 14.13 Case 2. Preoperative T2-weighted images show a very-high-grade downward-migrated large herniation at the L4–L5 level on the sagittal (**a**) and coronal (**b**) views. The axial views of MRI show a disc herniation migrated from the L4–L5 (**c**) disc level to the parapedicular space at L5 (**d**). An intraoperative endoscopic image shows disc fragments in the shoulder (**e**) and axilla (**f**) of the L5 nerve root. Decompression was completed with an oblique lateral lumbar interbody fusion for stabilizing the segment (**g**, **h**)

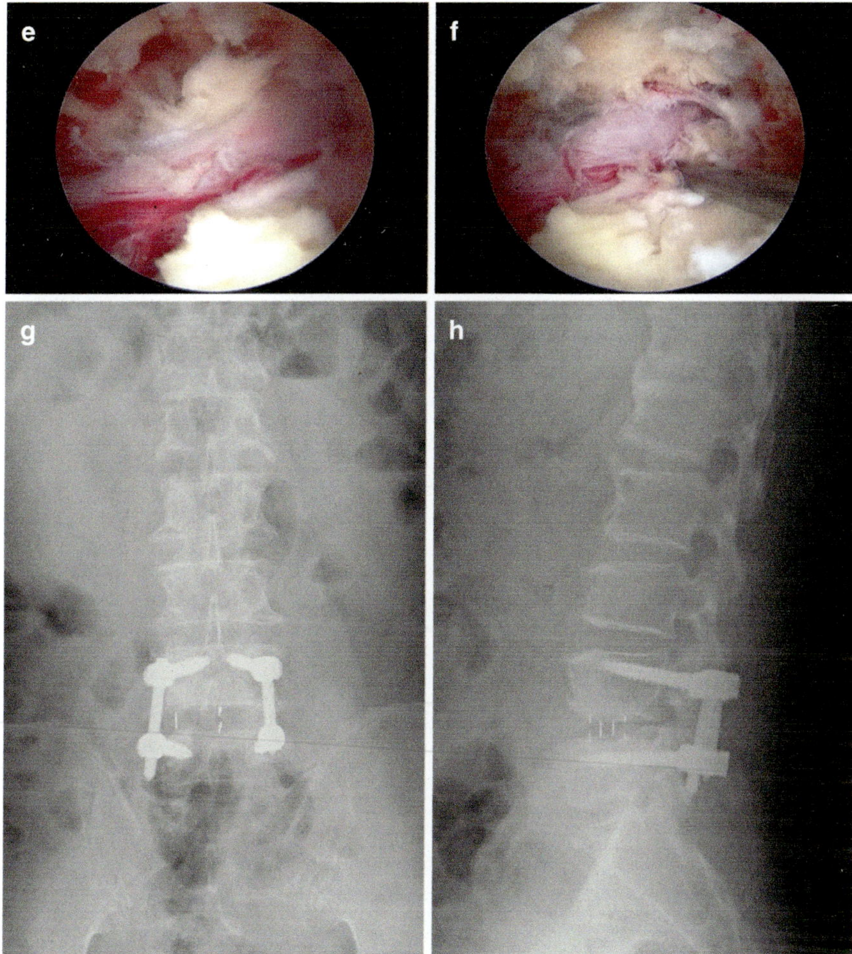

Fig. 14.13 (continued)

ventral part of SAP (superior articular process). Postoperative MRI revealed total removal of herniation (Fig. 14.14 and Video 14.3).

Case 4: Multiple Lumbar Discs: Right L2–L3 and Left L3–L4

A 70-year-old man presented LBP with left anterior thigh pain. The patient's symptom was mild, and he hoped for conservative treatment. However, a month after starting symptomatic therapy, he complained of another pain on the opposite thigh. MRI demonstrated a right low-grade upward migrated herniation at the L2–L3 level, and a left-side very-high-grade upward migrated herniation at the L3–L4 level. Therefore, we performed the endoscopic herniotomy by IPA for both levels. After surgery, the patient recovered from both legs' pain. Postoperative MRI revealed complete removal of HLD at L2–L3 and L3–L4 (Fig. 14.15 and Video 14.4).

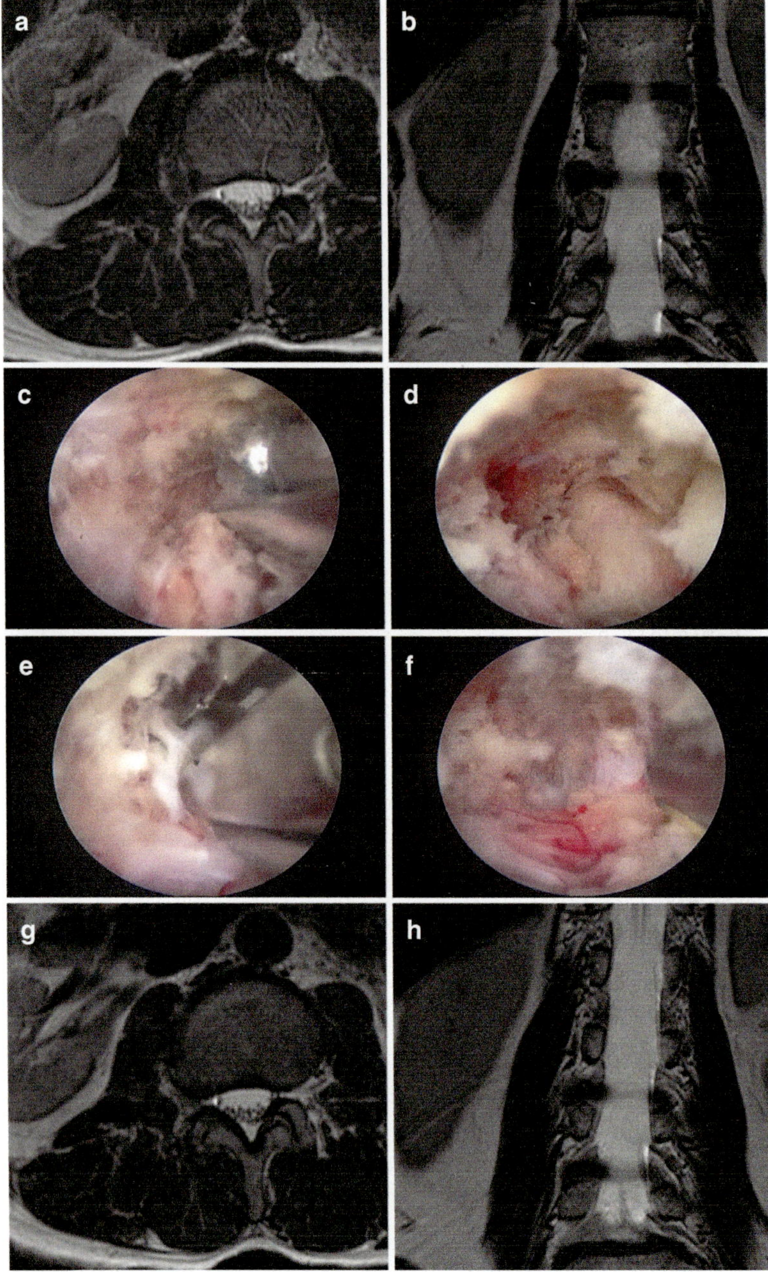

Fig. 14.14 Case 3. Preoperative axial (**a**) and coronal (**b**) T2-weighted images showing an extra- and intraforaminal herniation at L2–L3. Intraoperative endoscopic images show the foraminoplasty to reach the disc (**c**). A bulging disc can be observed (**d**). Disc removal (**e**). Foraminal decompression achieved (**f**). Postoperative MRI in axial (**g**) and coronal (**h**) T2-weighted views showing complete removal of the disc herniation

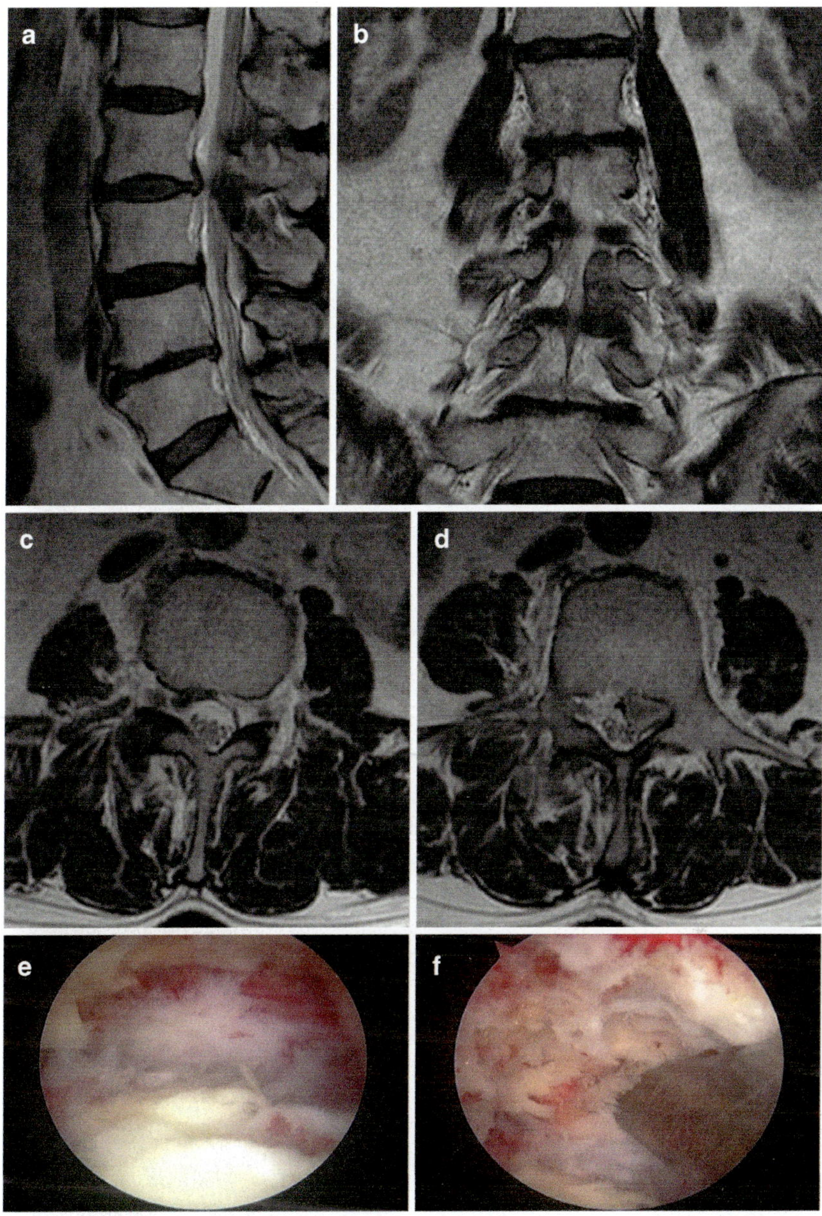

Fig. 14.15 Case 4. Preoperative T2-weighted images show low-grade upward-migrated L2–L3 herniation at the right side and high-grade upward-migrated herniation at the opposite side of one level below (**a**–**d**). Intraoperative photographs demonstrate L2–L3 herniotomy. The first intraoperative view uses 0° endoscopy, and the herniation is hidden behind the lamina and yellow ligament (**e**). In the second view, the hernia is revealed by using a 30° angled endoscope (**f**). The postoperative axial T2-weighted image shows complete removal of the herniations (**g**, **h**). Postoperative computed tomography image shows adequate laminectomy to get enough space for herniotomy while preserving the facet (**i**)

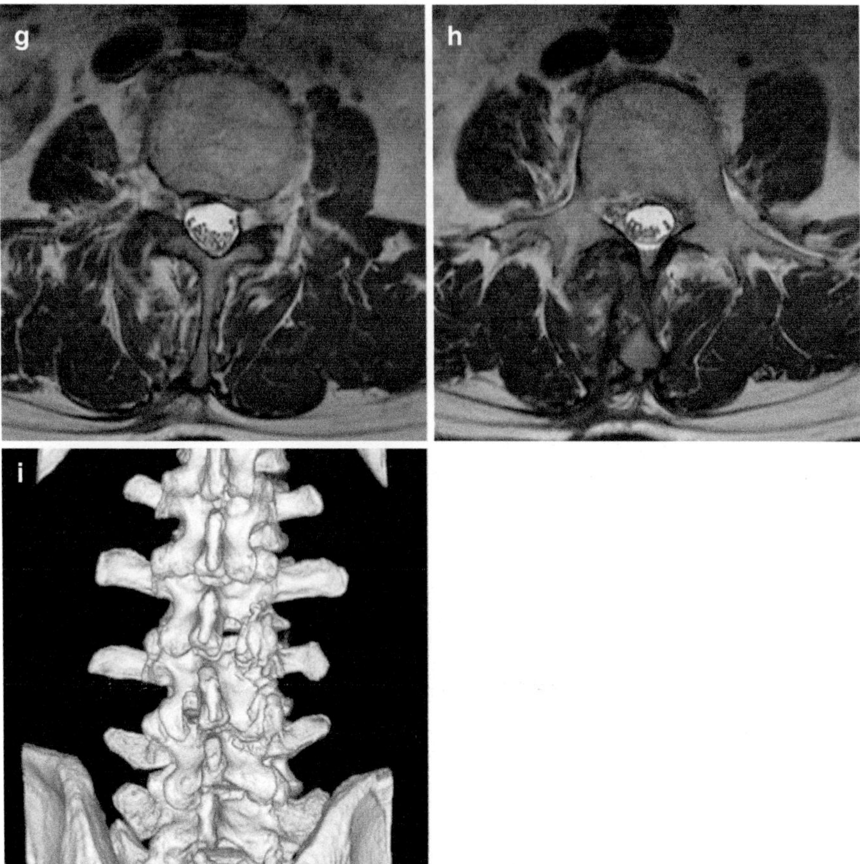

Fig. 14.15 (continued)

Discussion

Biportal endoscopic discectomy showed satisfactory clinical outcomes in all types of LDH and specialty in high-grade migrated disc herniations without increasing operation time [1, 2]. By using two portals, free movement, handling, and angulation of the surgical instruments and the arthroscope are allowed independently without crowding of instruments. In addition, this technique provides technical flexibility with sufficient bony and soft-tissue work, comparable to conventional surgery. Continuous saline perfusion can control bleeding and reduce the risk of infection and dural tear by a slight compression of the dura mater by continuous saline perfusion.

How to Avoid Complications

The complications of biportal endoscopic discectomy are similar to those of microdiscectomy. Especially, dura injury, intraoperative bleeding, epidural hematoma, and residual disc fragment are serious perioperative complications.

Dural Tear

Like conventional spinal operation, incidental durotomy or dural injury may occur during endoscopic procedures. The dural tear usually occurs during the flavectomy. Meticulous dissection of the dura and ligament flavum is encouraged before a complete flavectomy. Direct dural repair may be challenging through an endoscopic procedure. Dura-sealing materials like TachoSil (Takeda Pharma) can treat small dural tears. In a water environment, the adherent property of TachoSil is maintained. Therefore, some pieces of TachoSil (Takeda Pharma) can be applied to the dural defect. Even with the fibrin sealant patch, 5–7 days of absolute bed rest is recommended. Significant dural defects should be treated by direct repair, including suture and sealing materials. The authors suggest that endoscopic surgery should convert to microsurgery.

Bleeding and Epidural Hematoma

Bleeding obstructs the intraoperative view and should be staunched as quickly as possible. In most cases, this can be adequately achieved by a radiofrequency (RF) probe. The bleeding sources during the procedure included articular arteries, cancellous bone, and epidural veins.

Arterial bleeding that comes from branches of the segmental artery can be observed during much of the approach. They are known as articular arteries. In most patients, three arteries can be seen:

1. The superior articular artery at 9 o'clock
2. The interarticular artery at 7 o'clock
3. The inferior articular artery at 5 o'clock (UBE from the left side)

Bleeding coming from cancellous bone can be blocked with bone wax. But saline with a lower temperature could be difficult if spreading into tiny bleeding foci. Sometimes with the RF device, it is enough to stop bone bleeding. In addition, the diamond tip of the endoscopic burr can be beneficial to stop bone bleeding due to the thermal effect while drilling.

Bleeding from small epidural vessels is more complicated. Sometimes, the vessels are too close to the dural surface to be separated, and we have to perform procedures with the blurred visual field. If possible, you would better control even small bleeding in every possible way. If the bleeding foci are discriminated against, they can be controlled by an RF-tiny probe set at the lowest generation level (level 1 coagulation). But it comes from the underside of the proximal lamina just after proximal flavectomy, the foci are covered, and it cannot be coagulated easily. Besides increasing the pressure of continuous saline irrigation and hemostatic agents such as Gelfoam® sponge or Floseal®, hemostatic matrix might also help protect visualization and hemostasis.

After removing the herniated disc, epidural bleeding should also be meticulously coagulated with a bipolar RF probe to avoid epidural hematoma. Although a postoperative epidural hematoma can occur like conventional spine surgery, the incidence of "symptomatic" epidural hematoma may be very low. Keeping of drainage catheter may be effective for the prevention of epidural hematoma.

Residual Fragment

Residual disc fragments were observed in 2.8–15% of patients in several studies in which immediate postoperative MRI was performed after discectomy [11]. Although many factors were proposed for these complications, migration grade and surgical experience were the most frequent risk factors. Although the presence of a residual disc fragment with persistent compression is one cause of redo surgery, not all residual disc fragments observed on immediate postoperative MRI are symptomatic. Residual disc fragments are not always associated with poor longitudinal clinical outcomes. When the sequestrated disc is a large and fragile fragment, the total removal of the disc may be difficult through the small surgical corridor. The main take-away message is that "wait and see" is a good strategy for asymptomatic patients, even with persistent compression by a mixed tissue with a residual disc, retained fluid, and edematous tissue. The authors strongly recommend immediate postoperative MRI in patients with partial or complete radicular pain after surgery.

Conclusions

Biportal endoscopic discectomy has satisfactory results in complex herniated discs. Therefore, biportal endoscopic spine surgery can effectively treat all types of lumbar disc herniation. However, carefully evaluating preoperative radiographic images is essential for patient selection, planning the correct approach, and preventing complications.

References

1. Choi DJ, Jung JT, Lee SJ, Kim YS, Jang HJ, Yoo B. Biportal endoscopic spinal surgery for recurrent lumbar disc herniations. Clin Orthop Surg. 2016;8(3):325–9.
2. Kang MS, Hwang JH, Choi DJ, et al. Clinical outcome of biportal endoscopic revisional lumbar discectomy for recurrent lumbar disc herniation. J Orthop Surg Res. 2020;15(1):557.
3. Ahn Y, Jeong TS, Lim T, Jeon JY. Grading system for migrated lumbar disc herniation on sagittal magnetic resonance imaging: an agreement study. Neuroradiology. 2018;60(1):101–7.
4. Lee S, Kim SK, Lee SH, et al. Percutaneous endoscopic lumbar discectomy for migrated disc herniation: classification of disc migration and surgical approaches. Eur Spine J. 2007;16(3):431–7.
5. Zhao Y, Fan Y, Yang L, et al. Percutaneous endoscopic lumbar discectomy (PELD) via a transforaminal and interlaminar combined approach for very highly migrated lumbar disc herniation (LDH) between L4/5 and L5/S1 level. Med Sci Monit. 2020;26:e922777.
6. Kim HS, Paudel B, Jang JS, Lee K, Oh SH, Jang IT. Percutaneous endoscopic lumbar discectomy for all types of lumbar disc herniations (LDH) including severely difficult and extremely difficult LDH cases. Pain Physician. 2018;21(4):E401–8.
7. d'Ercole M, Innocenzi G, Ricciardi F, Bistazzoni S. Prognostic value of michigan state university (MSU) classification for lumbar disc herniation: Is It suitable for surgical selection? Int J Spine Surg. 2021;15(3):466–70.
8. Mysliwiec LW, Cholewicki J, Winkelpleck MD, Eis GP. MSU classification for herniated lumbar discs on MRI: toward developing objective criteria for surgical selection. Eur Spine J. 2010;19(7):1087–93.
9. Dowling Á, Lewandrowski KU, da Silva FHP, Parra JAA, Portillo DM, Giménez YCP. Patient selection protocols for endoscopic transforaminal, interlaminar, and translaminar decompression of lumbar spinal stenosis. J Spine Surg. 2020;6(Suppl 1):S120–32.
10. Jing Z, Li L, Song J. Percutaneous transforaminal endoscopic discectomy versus microendoscopic discectomy for upper lumbar disc herniation: a retrospective comparative study. Am J Transl Res. 2021;13(4):3111–9.
11. Baek J, Yang SH, Kim CH, Chung CK, Choi Y, Heo JH, et al. Postoperative longitudinal outcomes in patients with residual disc fragments after percutaneous endoscopic lumbar discectomy. Pain Physician. 2018;21(4):E457–66.

Chapter 15
Unilateral Biportal Endoscopy for Rostrally and Caudally Migrated Lumbar Disc Herniations

Javier Quillo-Olvera, Diego Quillo-Olvera, Javier Quillo-Reséndiz, and Michelle Barrera-Arreola

Abbreviations

CT	Computed tomography
EBL	Estimated blood loss
HLD	Herniated lumbar disc
IAP	Inferior articular process
IELD	Interlaminar endoscopic lumbar discectomy
MD	Microdiscectomy
MRI	Magnetic resonance imaging
PLL	Posterior longitudinal ligament
RF	Radiofrequency
SAP	Superior articular process
TELD	Transforaminal endoscopic lumbar discectomy
UBE	Unilateral biportal endoscopy
ULBD	Unilateral laminotomy for bilateral decompression

Supplementary Information The online version contains supplementary material available at [https://doi.org/10.1007/978-3-031-14736-4_15].

J. Quillo-Olvera (✉) · D. Quillo-Olvera · J. Quillo-Reséndiz · M. Barrera-Arreola
The Brain and Spine Care, Minimally Invasive Spine Surgery Group, Hospital H+ Querétaro, Spine Clinic, Querétaro, México
e-mail: neuroqomd@gmail.com; drquilloolvera86@gmail.com; kitnoz@hotmail.com; michelle.barrera@anahuac.mx

J. Quillo-Olvera et al. (eds.), *Unilateral Biportal Endoscopy of the Spine*, https://doi.org/10.1007/978-3-031-14736-4_15

Introduction

Migration of a disc fragment is not uncommon; 35–70% of herniated lumbar discs (HLDs) can migrate away from disc [1, 2]. This event represents a challenge in surgical planning since any procedure must achieve the decompression of the neural elements and at the same time avoid the damage of the paraspinal tissues. Therefore, lumbar discectomy has been a constantly evolving procedure.

In 1909, Krause and Oppenheim described the first lumbar discectomy [3]. And only 2 years later, Goldthwaite and Middleton associated a lumbar disc herniation with radicular symptoms and lower back pain [4, 5]. However, it was not until 1934 that Mixter and Barr published the first case series on herniated discs treated with a total laminectomy [6].

History showed that despite resolving the compressive nerve symptoms in the patients, the procedure-related collateral effect was considerable. The concept of microsurgery for herniated discs intended to reduce this collateral damage was incorporated worldwide by pioneers such as Yasargil [7] and Caspar [8] in 1977, Williams [9] in 1978, and McCulloch [10] during the 1990s. Hijikata, in 1973, introduced the concept of percutaneous discectomy, which he called "percutaneous nucleotomy" [11]. Kambin, in the 1980s, in addition to developing this technique, described a safe surgical corridor to approach the intervertebral disc, the "Kambin's triangle" [12]. The percutaneous nucleotomy procedure then evolved to the concept of percutaneous discoscopy by Schreiber et al., who introduced an endoscope to have optical control of the anatomy [13].

But not only reaching the surgical goal but also doing the minor damage in reaching it is even more relevant. Thanks to the evolution of minimally invasive techniques, the technology implemented, and the surgeon's needs, successful outcomes regarding water-based endoscopic procedures such as uniportal and biportal have been reported [14, 15].

However, migrated lumbar disc herniations' treatment can be challenging due to its intricate anatomy, leading to three serious situations:

1. The need for a broad bone resection, including laminectomy, medial facetectomy, and completely removing the ligamentum flavum, causing a biomechanical risk situation at the spine.
2. This pathology is technically demanding.
3. Finally, the risk of insufficient decompression due to the difficulty in removing the migrated fragment and sequestration in the epidural space.

Water-based endoscopic options for this condition can be uniportal or biportal [2, 16]. This chapter discusses the unilateral biportal endoscopic (UBE) technique for migrated lumbar disc herniation.

Generalities

A migrated herniated disc should be classified based on its direction and extent [2, 17] (Fig. 15.1).

1. High-grade up occurs when migration is located above the middle of the infrapedicular level.
2. Low-grade up occurs when migration is located between the upper margin of the intervertebral disc and the middle of the infrapedicular level.
3. High-grade down occurs when migration is located below the suprapedicular level.
4. Low-grade down occurs when migration is located between the lower margin of the intervertebral disc and the suprapedicular level.
5. Sequestration is a distal fragment without continuity to the original disc.

Biportal endoscopy has proven to have advantages that make it a very particular and accessible option for various diseases of the spine, including migrated HLD, due to the following:

1. Clear visualization of anatomical structures thanks to continuous saline irrigation allows underwater dissection. It helps to reduce the risk of postoperative hematomas since the source of bleeding in the surgical field can be found with relative ease. Another advantage to consider related to the excellent visualization obtained with the endoscope is that the surgeon can identify bone anatomical structures, allowing orientation during surgery preventing excessive bone removal.
2. During biportal endoscopic surgery, the surgical instrument is independent of the endoscope, and it can be used more freely than in uniportal endoscopic tech-

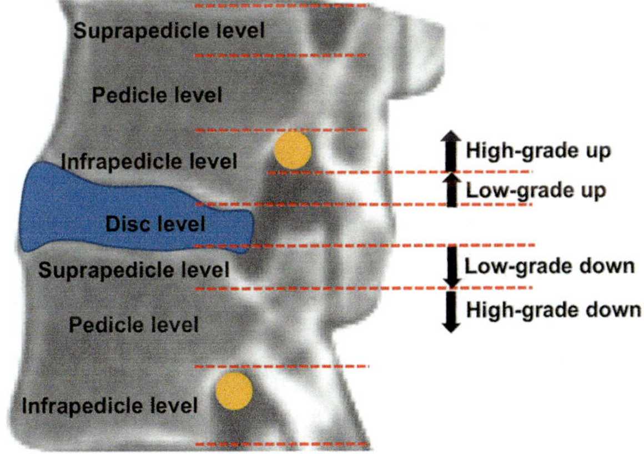

Fig. 15.1 Disc migration classification

niques. This feature is particularly advantageous since it is necessary to deal with complex anatomical barriers in some instances of migration or sequestration of lumbar discs. Therefore, the surgeon will need a reduced limitation using the instruments in these cases.

3. During biportal endoscopic procedures, a standard set of instruments for lumbar spinal surgery can be used.

Unilateral Biportal Endoscopic Approaches for Migrated Lumbar Disc Herniations

There are several biportal endoscopic approaches to remove migrated HLD. One of them is the lumbar sublaminar contralateral approach (Fig. 15.2). This approach is helpful for multiple indications such as proximal foraminal stenosis and foraminal disc herniation or synovial cysts.

The sublaminar contralateral approach lets crossing to the opposite side through a spinous process's base removal. This maneuver is familiar for surgeons who have experience with minimally invasive techniques with tubular accesses or uniportal endoscopy, mainly for bilateral decompression of the lumbar spinal canal through a unilateral laminotomy (ULBD).

When the surgeon is on the contralateral side, he or she can identify the contralateral structures such as the superior or inferior articular process (SAP, IAP), disc

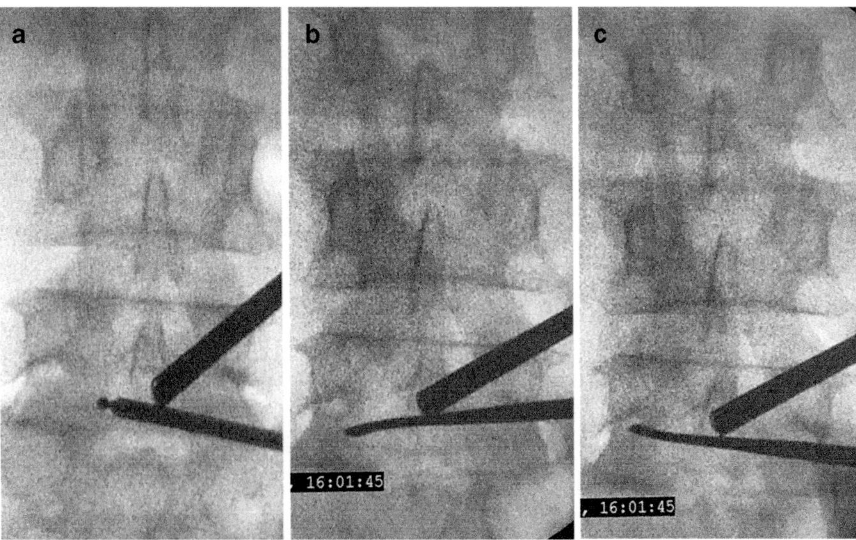

Fig. 15.2 Sequence of a biportal endoscopic contralateral sublaminar approach. (**a**) The base of the spinous process has been drilled out, and the tip of the drill is in the medial aspect of the facet joint. (**b**) The endoscope and the instrument are addressed to the contralateral lateral recess. (**c**) The instrument is in the foramen

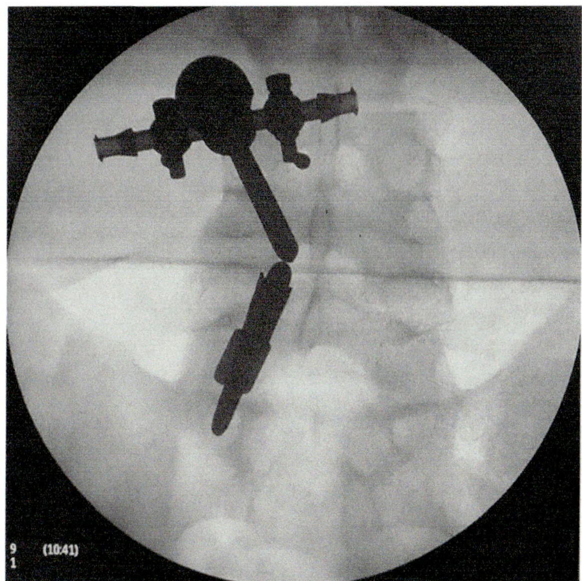

Fig. 15.3 Unilateral biportal endoscopic (UBE) paramedian approach

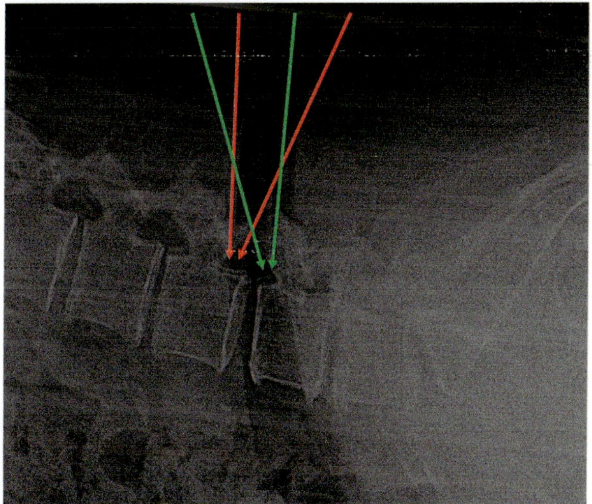

Fig. 15.4 The triangular approach should be addressed to the pathology. The red and green arrows show cranial and caudal trajectories, respectively

space, and neural elements such as the traversing nerves. Because of this, exploration of the contralateral epidural space is feasible [18–20].

The ipsilateral paramedian approach with biportal endoscopy is also often used, especially in patients who require decompression of the ipsilateral recess and subsequent removal of the migrated disc herniation [16] (Fig. 15.3).

It is advisable to consider the following anatomical aspects to decide on this approach:

1. The location and extent of migration to plan the trajectory of the triangular approach (Fig. 15.4).

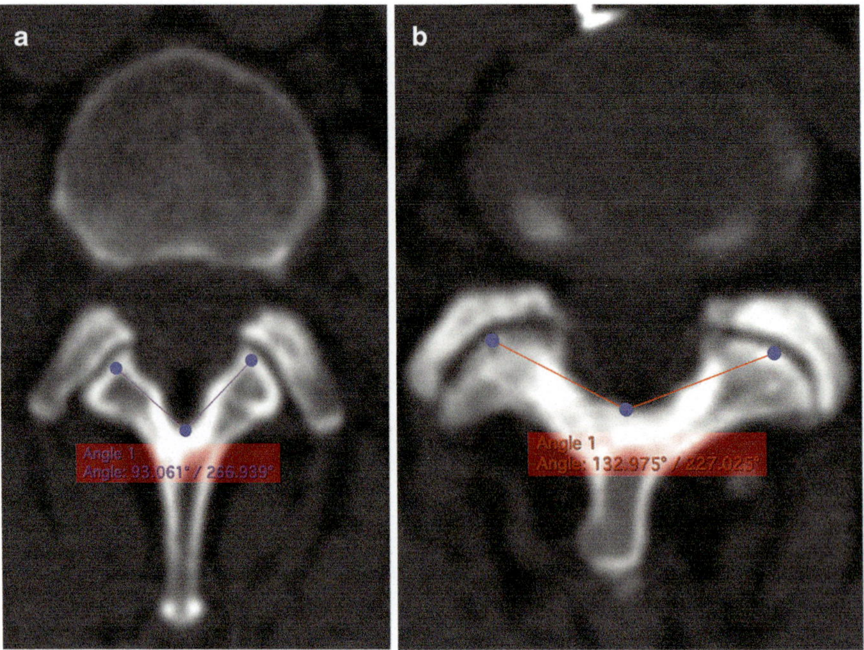

Fig. 15.5 Different laminar angles. (**a**) L2 laminar angle. (**b**) L5 laminar angle

2. The laminar angle is relevant. For example, in the lumbar cranial levels, it is lesser than that in caudal, and the risk of excessively removing the IAP with an ipsilateral paramedian approach may be greater than with a sublaminar contralateral approach. On the other hand, an ipsilateral approach may be a reasonable option at caudal levels with a greater laminar angle (Fig. 15.5).

Lastly, in cases of wide laminar angles in young patients, without considerable hypertrophy of the ligamentum flavum, or central spinal stenosis, especially at the L5–S1 level where we can find a wide interlaminar space, the authors have seen it feasible to perform an inclinatory approach.

The lumbar inclinatory approach would avoid removing the base of the spinous process and the dissection of a long sublaminar pathway preventing manipulation of the dural sac. As a result, the lateral attachment of the ligamentum flavum can be found easily, and access to the lateral and ventral epidural space is faster, identifying the S1 nerve root quickly. In addition, the inclination or oblique trajectory of the approach allows the medial facet to be undercut, avoiding excessive removal (Fig. 15.6).

The anesthesia generally used for this type of pathology will depend on variables such as the surgeon's experience, the features of the patient, and the complexity of the case. Therefore, general anesthesia, epidural anesthesia, or sedation can be used.

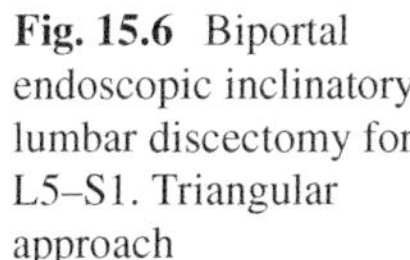

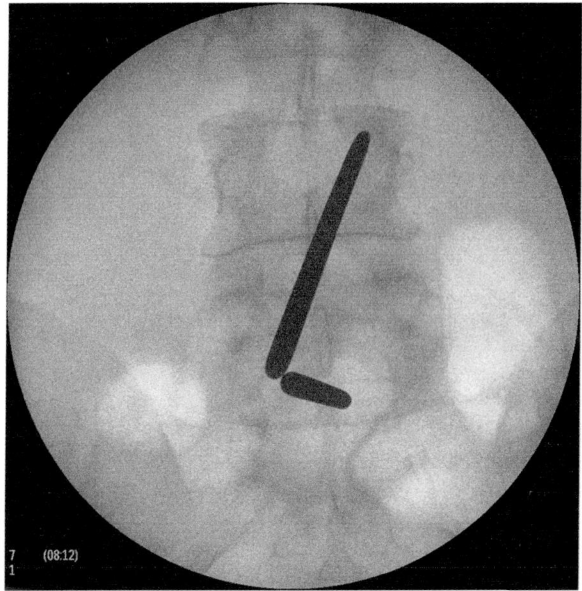

Fig. 15.6 Biportal endoscopic inclinatory lumbar discectomy for L5–S1. Triangular approach

The position to perform these procedures will be prone on an abdominal support frame to reduce intra-abdominal pressure and indirectly decrease excessive bleeding from the epidural venous plexuses during the surgery.

After the adequate positioning of the patient, the lumbar region is cleaned and draped in a sterile technique to begin the surgery. The location of the skin entries will depend on the approach used. In the paramedian method, the incisions can be planned ipsilateral to the pathology. On the right side, the cranial incision will be used for the working port and the caudal incision for the endoscope. On the left side, it will be the opposite.

Assistance with the fluoroscope is mandatory. After having triangulated both ports successfully, the endoscopic approach will begin. Continuous irrigation will be adjusted to 30 mmHg to prevent a drastic increase in epidural pressure with an undesirable impact on the nervous system. When starting the endoscopic procedure, the surgeon must confirm the adequate inflow and outflow of the solution to prevent edema or stagnation in the paraspinal soft tissues.

Indications

1. Patients with neurological symptoms such as radicular pain, sensory disorders, and muscle weakness caused by a localized migrated lumbar disc herniation on imaging studies such as MRI or myelotomography.
2. HLD with cranial or caudal migration in the spinal canal.
3. Failure of conservative treatment for 4–6 weeks.

4. Patients with previous spinal surgery, redo, or narrowing of the lumbar canal may require different endoscopic maneuvers.
5. Patients with HLD and significant instability with back pain as the predominant symptom should be studied and treated with other spinal surgical procedures.
6. Patients with extraforaminal HLD may be treated with other biportal endoscopic approaches.

Illustrated Cases

Case 1

A 53-year-old woman with a history of mild chronic back pain VAS 2/10 for 4 years presented progressive pain in her right leg that runs along the posterior surface until it reaches the lateral aspect of her right foot. Her symptoms have been present for 8 weeks, and recently they have become severe VAS 9/10 and resistant to analgesics of all kinds. Neurologic examination showed decreased strength in the right-ankle plantar flexion 4−/5.

The lumbar MRI demonstrated a broad-based chronic HLD at L5–S1 that did not compromise the dural sac. However, the lateral sagittal views on the right side showed a high-grade downward-migrated HLD at L5–S1, compressing the S1 nerve root on the right side as the cause of its chief complaint (Fig. 15.7).

A UBE approach was planned to address the S1 lamina on the right side and, after a small laminotomy, control the S1 axillary space (Fig. 15.8).

During surgery, the right S1 nerve root was identified, and a large number of enlarged epidural vessels were also seen over the S1 traversing nerve and the disc, confirming a considerable inflammation due to the HLD (Fig. 15.9). A subligamentous disc herniation was identified after opening the axillary space (Fig. 15.10). The disc was removed piecemeal until the S1 nerve root was confirmed free. Finally, an epidural drain was left to prevent the formation of an epidural hematoma (Video 15.1).

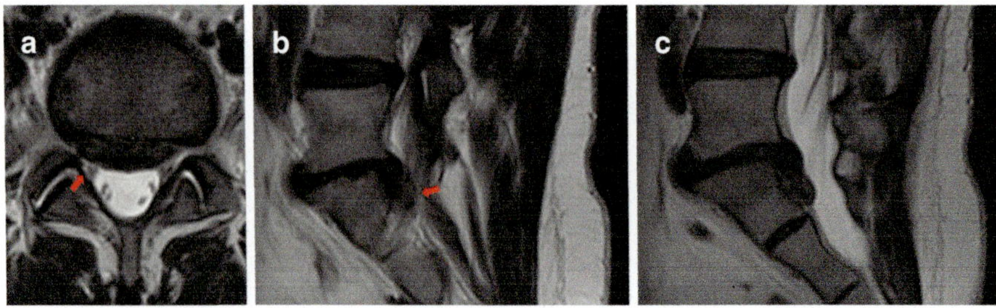

Fig. 15.7 Case 1: preoperative lumbar MRI. (**a**) Axial view showing a broad-based chronic HDL. However, the S1 nerve root compression is evident on the right side. (**b**, **c**) The sagittal views demonstrated a high-grade downward-migrated HDL touching the S1 nerve root (red arrow)

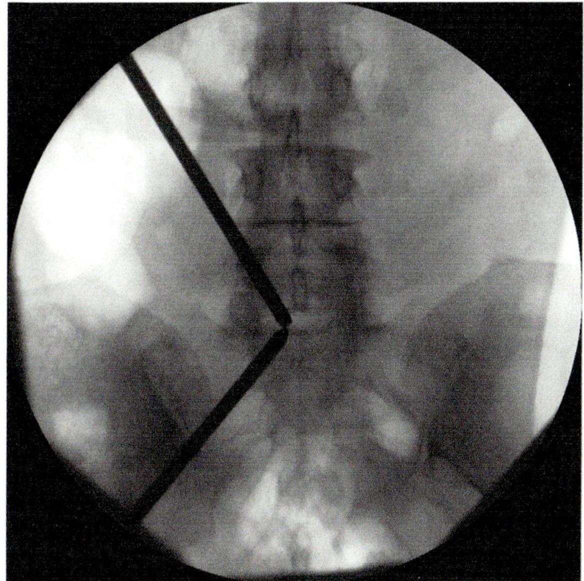

Fig. 15.8 The right-sided paramedian UBE approach was addressed to the S1 lamina

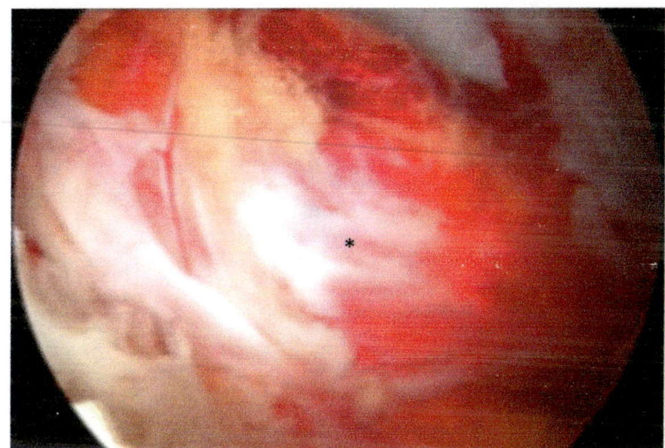

Fig. 15.9 Epidural vessels over the right S1(*) nerve root

The patient was discharged the following day. The postoperative clinical outcomes were encouraging, decreasing her leg pain to VAS 0/10 and back pain to VAS 1/10. In addition, at the 1-month postoperative follow-up, the plantar flexion strength of the right foot improved to 5/5.

Postoperative MRI demonstrated decompression of the S1 nerve root on the right side, the flavum ligament was respected, and the broad-based HLD was not removed because it was a radiological finding and not the cause of the patient's symptoms (Fig. 15.11).

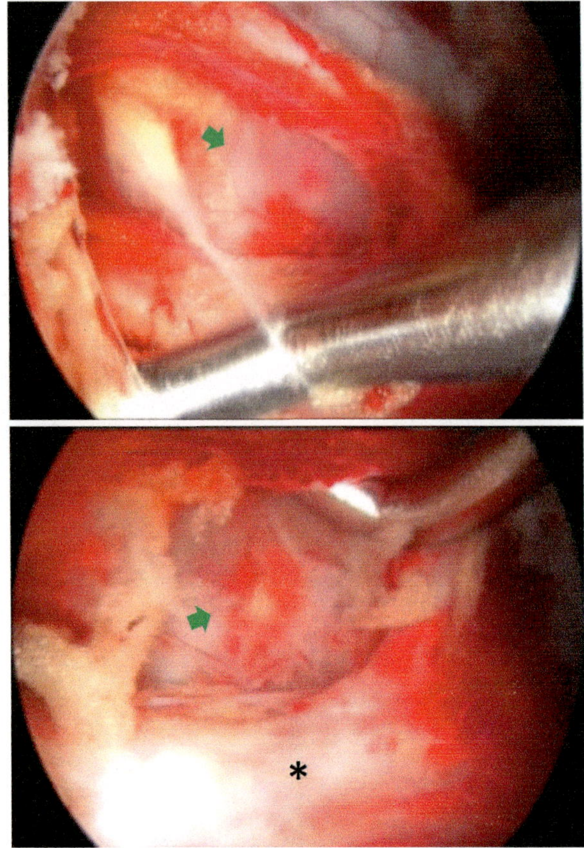

Fig. 15.10 Intraoperative images under endoscopic visualization from Case 1. The green arrows point to the migrated HLD in the axillary space. (*) S1 nerve root

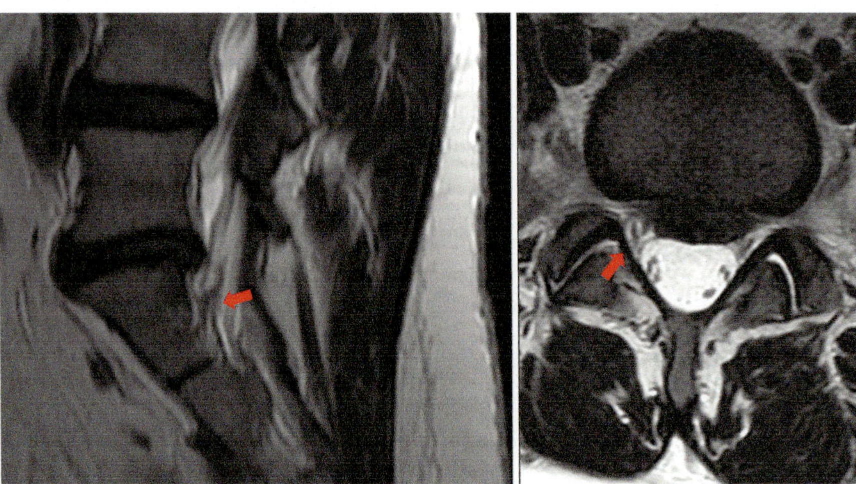

Fig. 15.11 Case 1: postoperative lumbar MRI. The red arrows point to an S1 nerve root of the right decompressed. The ligamentum flavum was preserved, and the broad-based HLD was left

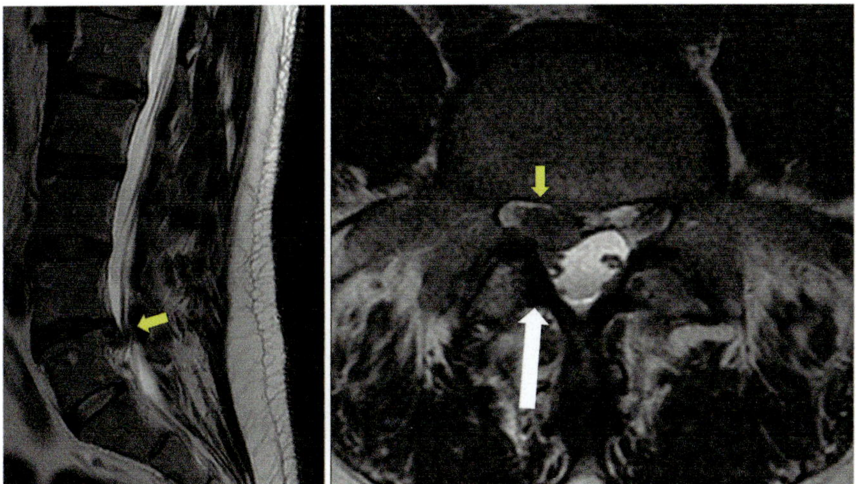

Fig. 15.12 Case 2: preoperative lumbar MRI. A low-grade downward-migrated HLD was identified at L4–L5 on the right side in the subarticular zone (yellow arrows). The white arrow points to the trajectory of the approach through an interlaminar trans-flavum route

Case 2
A 46-year-old man complained of pain in the right buttock that radiates to the leg reaching the calf. The severity of pain was VAS 8/10, associated with leg numbness and claudication when walking. A low-grade downward-migrated HLD at L4–L5 on the right side was identified in preoperative lumbar MRI, compressing the L5 nerve root in the subarticular area (Fig. 15.12).

The triangular approach was addressed to the upper edge of the L5 lamina on the right side (Fig. 15.13). The interlaminar space was enlarged only on the right side by minimum drilling of the laminae and the medial surface of the facet joint.

Later, the ligamentum flavum was detached and removed, only on the right side. The L5 nerve root was then identified and freed from ventral epidural adhesions with the nerve hook. This maneuver made it possible to remove the caudally migrated herniated disc. Then, hemostasis was performed in the ventral epidural space where the herniated disc was located, and the annular defect was coagulated with the radiofrequency (RF) probe. Finally, a remaining disc fragment was removed, and the right L5 nerve root decompression was confirmed (Fig. 15.14 and Video 15.2). Immediate postoperative MRI demonstrated a successful L4–L5 discectomy (Fig. 15.15). The patient was discharged a day after surgery with no pain in his leg, and no complications were reported during the procedure. In addition, claudication improved immediately after the surgery.

Case 3
A 36-year-old man complained of severe pain (VAS 8/10) in his right leg. The pain was associated with significant paresthesia located on the lateral aspect of the calf and the dorsal surface of the ankle, mainly when he was sitting or walking. The

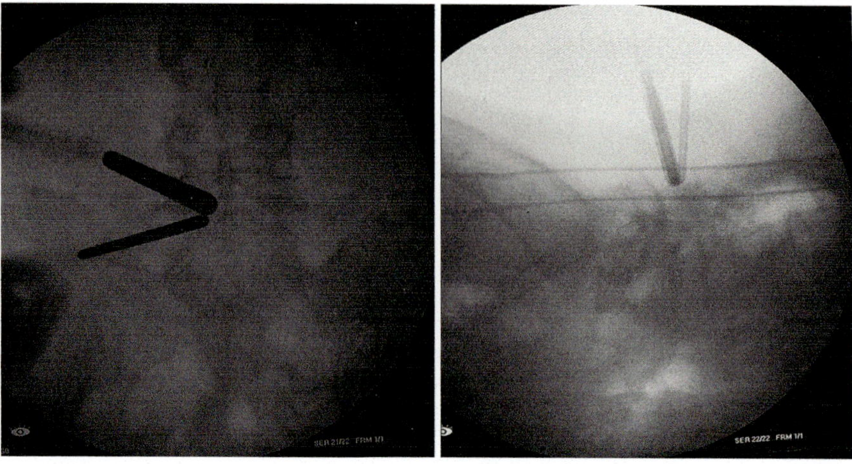

Fig. 15.13 Paramedian approach addressed to the lower part of the L4–L5 interlaminar space on the right side

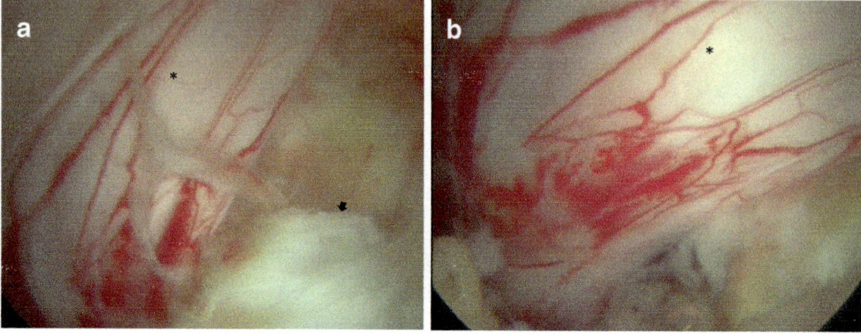

Fig. 15.14 Intraoperative images under endoscopic visualization from Case 2. (**a**) The right L5 nerve root (*) was released, and the disc herniation was exposed (black arrow). (**b**) L5 nerve root (*) after discectomy

neurological examination revealed a significant 4−/5 weakness in the dorsiflexion of the ankle and the great toe of the right foot. Also, the Achillean reflex on the same side was diminished compared to the left side.

Preoperative MRI demonstrated a high-grade upward-migrated HLD at L5–S1 with subligamentous sequestered fragments, the lesion compressing the right L5 nerve root. Anatomical features were observed such as a wide laminar angle in L5 and an interlaminar space accessible for any posterior approach (Fig. 15.16).

A lumbar inclinatory approach was performed, addressed to the laminofacet junction in L5–S1 on the right side. A mediolateral and caudocranial trajectory was

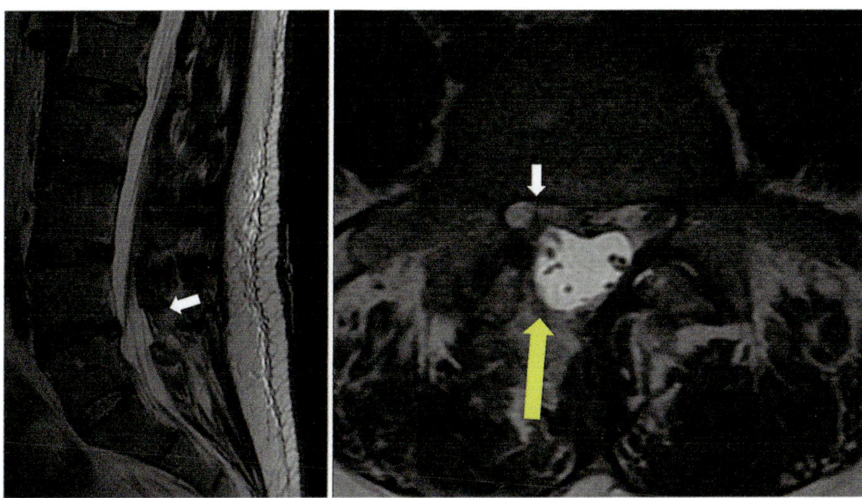

Fig. 15.15 Case 2: postoperative lumbar MRI. The white arrows point to L4–L5 after complete disc migrated removal. The yellow arrow indicates the trans-flavum approach at L4–L5 on the right side

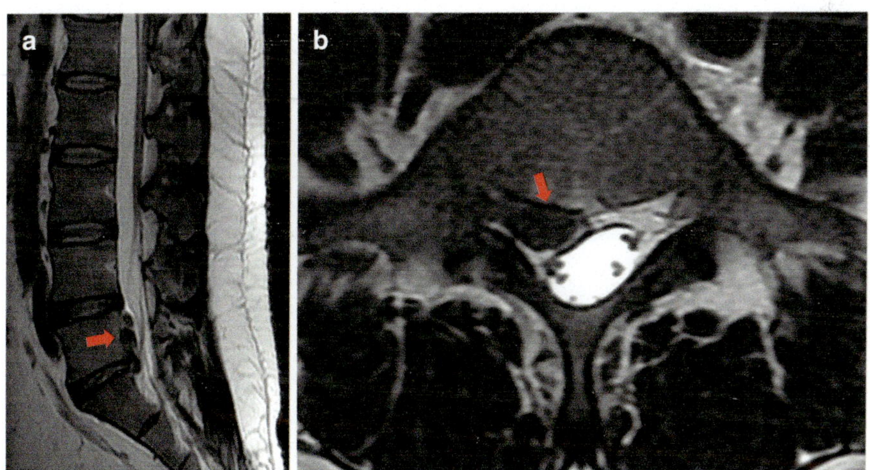

Fig. 15.16 Case 3: preoperative lumbar MRI. (**a**) Two retrocorporeal sequestered disc fragments were observed at L5 from the L5–S1 intervertebral disc (red arrow). (**b**) The L5 axial view demonstrated a parapedicular disc particle located medial to the L5 traversing nerve on the right side (red arrow)

planned to access the epidural space, preserving the flavum ligament and the facet joint (Fig. 15.17).

The mediolateral and caudocranial trajectory of the approach and the 30° lens angulation were helpful to reach the lateral recess (Fig. 15.18) and the inferior part

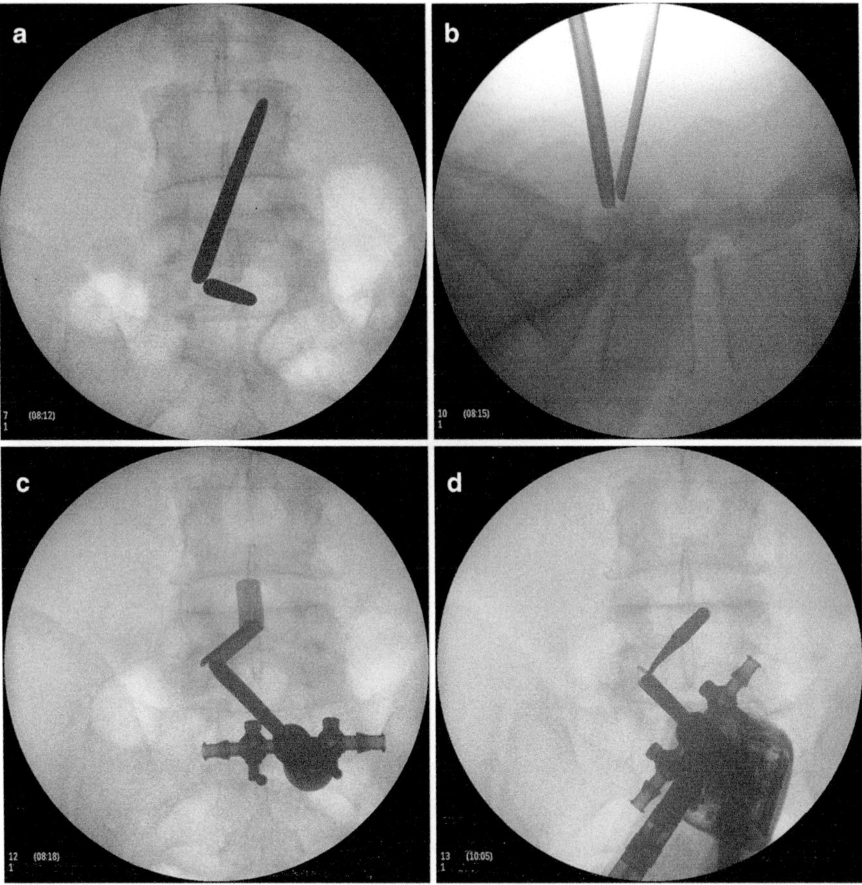

Fig. 15.17 Biportal endoscopic posterior lumbar inclinatory approach at L5–S1 on the right side through the C-arm. (**a**) AP view showing the triangular approach addressed to laminofacet junction. (**b**) Lateral view showing the triangular approach. (**c**) Both portals were placed. (**d**) The nerve hook and the endoscope in a mediolateral inclinatory trajectory

of the intervertebral foramen (Fig. 15.19) of L5–S1. Thanks to this, it was possible to remove three fragments sequestered in the epidural space, the last one located in the right L5–S1 proximal foraminal area (Video 15.3).

The patient was discharged the next day with paracetamol and general measures, and the radicular pain in the right leg disappeared after surgery. Immediate postoperative lumbar MRI demonstrated complete decompression of the neural elements at L5–S1 (Fig. 15.20). A lumbar CT scan confirmed the preservation of the lamina and L5–S1 facet joint on the right side (Fig. 15.21). Two weeks after surgery, a complete improvement in dorsiflexion weakness of the ankle and the great toe of the right foot was observed.

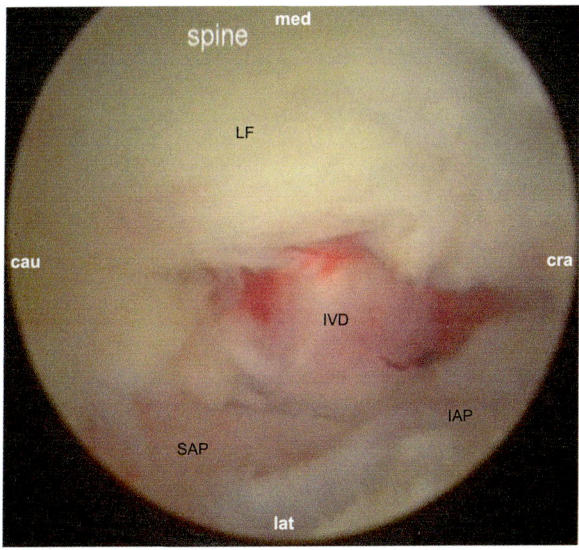

Fig. 15.18 L5–S1 right lateral recess. *IAP* inferior articular process, *SAP* superior articular process, *LF* ligamentum flavum, *IVD* intervertebral disc, *cra* cranial, *cau* caudal, *med* medial, *lat* lateral

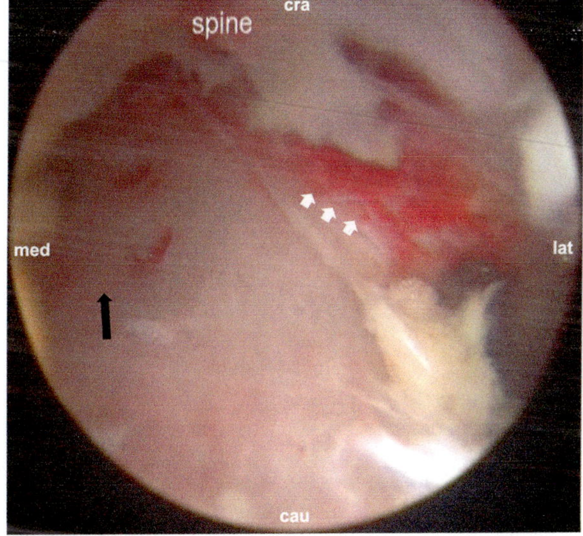

Fig. 15.19 Caudocranial view through the endoscope. The L5 posterior wall (black arrow) and the perineural tissue into the foramen of the right L5 exiting nerve (white arrows) were exposed

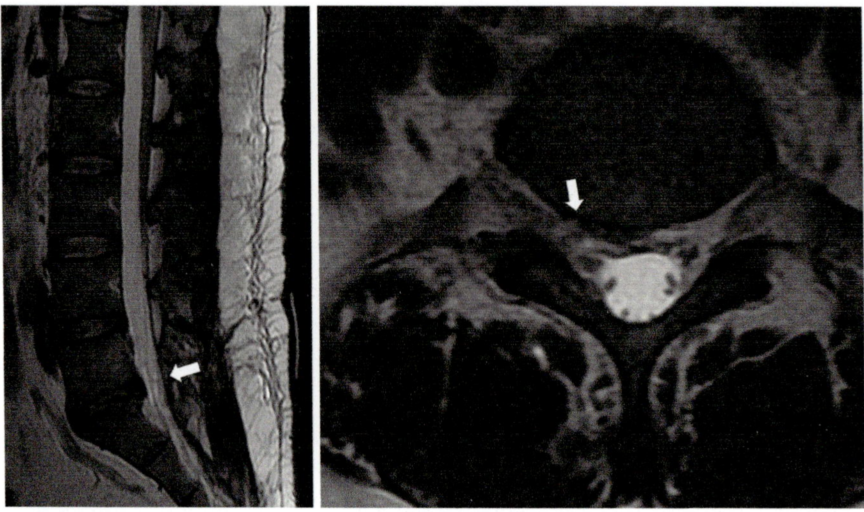

Fig. 15.20 Case 3: postoperative lumbar MRI. The sagittal and axial views show complete neural decompression and HLD removal at L5–S1 on the right side (white arrows)

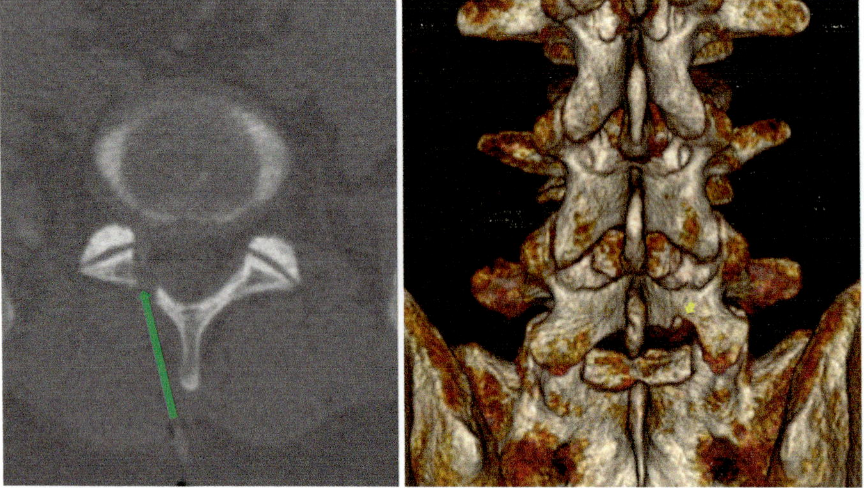

Fig. 15.21 Case 3: postoperative lumbar CT scan. The axial view of L5 shows the mediolateral trajectory of the approach (green arrow), and a small bone defect in the right L5 lamina is identified in the 3D reconstructed view (yellow arrow)

Discussion

Preservation of the anatomy is one of the advantages associated with minimally invasive techniques in spinal surgery. It has been observed mainly in water-based endoscopic procedures (uniportal and biportal) [2, 21, 22]. This benefits the patient in many ways, including a rapid return to daily living activities. In addition, due to the minimal aggression to stabilizing paraspinal structures such as muscles, ligaments, and facet joints, iatrogenic instability can be avoided [16, 23].

However, in cases of HLD with high-grade migration, open surgery is still a feasible option to attempt to remove the disc entirely and has been recommended in most cases due to the complex and intricate anatomy that the herniated and migrated fragment has with the epidural space and other anatomical barriers that hide it [24]. Most high-grade migrated HLDs will require broad bone removal, including the lamina, pars, and facet joints, with the potential risk of segmental instability. Furthermore, these disc herniations can migrate to the epidural space even below the posterior longitudinal ligament (PLL). This situation requires that the access chosen to treat them also allows the surgeon to have enough space to mobilize the neural elements and remove the ventral epidural fragment. Therefore, the risk of dural injury and the same neural structures will exist.

It is clear that migrated HLDs, particularly high-grade ones, represent a challenge for the surgeon. In this situation, uniportal endoscopy (transforaminal and interlaminar) is a feasible option but has the disadvantage of having a steeper learning curve and requires experience from the surgeon. Also, there is a concern of insufficient decompression through conventional uniportal endoscopic approaches; that is why it is necessary to combine them with special maneuvers such as foraminotomy, foraminoplasty, or pediculectomy, among others, in addition to the fact that highly specialized surgical instruments are necessary as curved and flexible grasps or drill systems with deflector tips, etc. [25, 26].

Biportal endoscopic surgery can fill in the gaps left by uniportal endoscopic surgery due to the following:

1. Biportal endoscopy is like uniportal, a water-based technique, which means that it is used through continuous irrigation during the surgical procedure, allowing adequate visibility through an endoscopic lens.
2. The surgical tools are usually those of a standard set of lumbar spine surgery. That is why any spine surgeon can more easily access biportal endoscopy.
3. The anatomy through the endoscope in the biportal technique is similar to the anatomy seen through microsurgery. Both methods are posterior approaches.
4. The essential feature of this technique is that the surgeon uses the working instrument independently of the endoscopic lens, which means a certain degree of freedom with the tool during the surgery.

Concerning invasiveness, biportal endoscopic surgery remains one of the least invasive techniques compared with open surgery and microsurgery. A study evaluated the invasiveness of four surgical methods: (1) microdiscectomy (MD), (2) transforaminal lumbar endoscopic discectomy (TELD), (3) interlaminar endoscopic lumbar discectomy (IELD), and (4) unilateral biportal endoscopy (UBE). The study included 20 patients in each group and demonstrated that UBE is between uniportal endoscopy and microsurgery regarding invasiveness. It was shown by measuring the inflammatory response after surgery in the different groups. Creatine phosphokinase and C-reactive protein levels in the UBE group were significantly lower than MD group. Also, the postoperative high-intensity cross-sectional area of paraspinal muscle in the UBE group was lower than that in the MD group [27].

Several series have reported acceptable outcomes regarding the effectiveness of the UBE technique for HLD. For example, Kim et al. [14] reported results from a series of 81 patients treated for discectomy through UBE and MD. The estimated blood loss (EBL) and hospitalization time were 34.7 mL and 2.77 days in patients treated with UBE, respectively. In the MD group, it was 140 mL and 6.4 days, respectively, even though the operative time in both groups was similar (70.2 min in UBE and 60.4 min in MD). Also, the clinical results were encouraging, observing a satisfaction rate in the group treated through UBE of 73.4%, while in the MD group, it was 68.5%.

Kang et al. [16] evaluated the results obtained in 262 patients diagnosed with migrated HLD and operated with UBE. There were 208 patients with low-grade migration and 54 with high-grade migration. Of those with high-grade migration, 10 patients had high-grade up and 44 high-grade down. The mean follow-up was 16 ± 2.5 months. The mean age of the high-grade group was 53.74 years, while the low-grade group was 50.72 years.

The most frequent level involved in both groups was L4–L5. In addition, a post-operative lumbar MRI was performed in 98% of the operated patients (258/262), in which a successful decompression was found.

The operative time in the high-grade group was 65.63 ± 16.5 min, while in the low-grade group, 60.74 ± 18.1 min. The hospital stay was 3.48 ± 2.8 days in the high-grade group, while it was 3.65 ± 2.5 days in the low-grade group. Only one patient in the low-grade group had a postoperative hematoma, and three more patients underwent revision surgery with UBE in the same group. In the high-grade group, no complications or revisions were reported.

The mean preoperative VAS score in the low-grade group was 8.4 ± 1.3, and at the end of the follow-up, it was 1.4 ± 0.7, while in the high-grade group, it was 8.2 ± 1.2 at the beginning of the follow-up and 1.5 ± 0.7 at the end. The mean preoperative ODI in the low-grade group was 42 ± 5.1, and at the end of follow-up, it improved to 9 ± 2.2, while in the high-grade group, it was 41 ± 5.5 at the start of follow-up and 10 ± 2.5 at the end. 70.2% of patients reported excellent satisfaction at the end of follow-up in both groups.

Tips and Pearls

- Although the UBE technique has a shorter learning curve than uniportal endoscopy, it is important to have experience in microsurgery before trying it, especially in migrated herniated discs.
- The general steps of the UBE technique are a correct triangulation of the ports, the creation of the epiperiosteal workspace, an adequate inflow and outflow of the irrigated solution, and the location of the working instrument with the endoscope, which should always be completed before starting the biportal endoscopic procedure.
- The surgeon must remember that the triangulation must be target-addressed, which means that each herniated disc has its specific considerations. Therefore, there are different approaches to remove them: the contralateral, ipsilateral paramedian, and in particular cases inclinatory route.

- There is inevitably no bleeding during the procedure. However, bleeding may arise from bone drilling, flavectomy, or epidural space exploration, especially when removing the subligamentous disc. The surgeon will have several options, such as temporarily increasing the irrigation pressure to identify the source of bleeding. In addition, it is advised to locate the endoscopic lens as close as possible to the bleeding site so as not to lose it in the surgical field and to be able to perform correct hemostasis. Hemostasis can be achieved using the RF coagulation tip, bone wax, hemostatic sponges, or different fibrin matrices available on the market. After successfully achieving hemostasis, the surgeon should return to baseline 30 mmHg to continue the procedure.
- Precisely, migrated HLDs are hindered behind anatomical barriers. Therefore, in biportal endoscopic surgery, the surgeon should not perform extensive bone removal. In this technique, handling the endoscope and the surgical tools independently allows more freedom with the movements in the surgical field. Thus, it is advantageous for working in reduced spaces. Furthermore, a deeper visual field obtained with the 30° lens is crucial, especially during the exploration of the epidural space.
- Dissection of the flavum ligament should be gentle since there may be meningovertebral ligaments or tight adhesions between the ventral aspect of the flavum ligament and the dorsal dural sac. It will prevent dural tears during flavectomy.
- Excessive bone removal should always be avoided, especially the facet joints. This can be achieved by planning a suitable trajectory of the approach. For example, the more perpendicular to the bone element, the more bone removal is required to visualize a structure below it.
- It will not always be necessary to remove the flavum ligament altogether; in patients with minimal degenerative changes, removing only the lateral part of the ligament will be enough to access the lateral aspect of the epidural space.
- There are various options to treat dural tears, but the surgeon should always identify them to avoid a possible cerebrospinal fluid leak after the procedure.
- It is important to always observe the surgical instrument with the endoscope; never perform blind maneuvers, especially in the epidural space.

Conclusion

The proper application of unilateral biportal endoscopy (UBE) in cases of migrated lumbar disc herniations will allow the surgeon to obtain satisfactory clinical and radiological outcomes with the advantages observed in other minimally invasive spinal procedures. The principles used for any spinal surgery procedure must be applied when trying UBE. For example, the diagnosis, location, and extent of migration; the anatomy to be overcome; and the patient's safety are factors that the surgeon must consider before deciding on any technique.

References

1. Ebeling U, Reulen HJ. Are there typical localisations of lumbar disc herniations? A prospective study. Acta Neurochir (Wien). 1992;117:143–8.
2. Choi KC, Lee DC, Shim HK, Shin SH, Park CK. A strategy of percutaneous endoscopic lumbar discectomy for migrated disc herniation. World Neurosurg. 2017;99:259–66.
3. Oppenheim H, Krause F. Ueber Einklemmung bzw. Strangulation der Cauda equina. Dtsch Med Wochenschr. 1909;35:697–700.
4. Goldthwait JE. The lumbosacral articulation: an explanation of many cases of lumbago, sciatica and paraplegia. N Engl J Med. 1911;164:365–72.
5. Middleton GS, Teacher JH. Injury of the spinal cord due to rupture of the intervertebral disc during muscular effort. Glasgow Med J. 1911;76:1–6.
6. Mixter WJ, Barr JS. Rupture of the intervertebral disc with involvement of the spinal canal. N Engl J Med. 1934;211:210–4.
7. Yasargil MG. Microsurgical operation of herniated lumbar disc. In: Lumbar disc adult hydrocephalus, Advances in neurosurgery, vol. 4. Berlin: Springer; 1977. p. 81.
8. Caspar W. A new surgical procedure for lumbar disc herniation causing less tissue damage through a microsurgical approach. In: Lumbar disc adult hydrocephalus, Advances in neurosurgery, vol. 4. Berlin: Springer; 1977. p. 74–80.
9. Williams RW. Microlumbar discectomy. A conservative surgical approach to the virgin herniated lumbar disc. Spine J. 1978;3:175–82.
10. McCulloch JA, Young PH, editors. Essentials of spinal microsurgery. Philadelphia: Lippincott Raven; 1998.
11. Hijikata S. A method of percutaneous nuclear extraction. J Toden Hosp. 1975;5:39–42.
12. Kambin P, Sampson S. Posterolateral percutaneous suction-excision of herniated lumbar intervertebral discs. Report of interim results. Clin Orthop Relat Res. 1986;207:37–43.
13. Schreiber A, Suezawa Y, Leu H. Does percutaneous nucleotomy with discoscopy replace conventional discectomy? Eight years of experience and results in treatment of herniated lumbar disc. Clin Orthop Relat Res. 1989;238:35–42.
14. Kim SK, Kang SS, Hong YH, Park SW, Lee SC. Clinical comparison of unilateral biportal endoscopic technique versus open microdiscectomy for single-level lumbar discectomy: a multicenter, retrospective analysis. J Orthop Surg Res. 2018;13:22.
15. Wei FL, Zhou CP, Zhu KL, et al. Comparison of different operative approaches for lumbar disc herniation: a network meta-analysis and systematic review. Pain Physician. 2021;24:E381–92.
16. Kang T, Park SY, Park GW, Lee SH, Park JH, Suh SW. Biportal endoscopic discectomy for high-grade migrated lumbar disc herniation. J Neurosurg Spine. 2020:1–6. https://doi.org/10.3171/2020.2.SPINE191452.
17. Fardon DF, Milette PC, Combined Task Forces of the North American Spine Society, American Society of Spine Radiology, American Society of Neuroradiology. Nomenclature and classification of lumbar disc pathology. Recommendations of the combined task forces of the North American Spine Society, American Society of Spine Radiology, and American Society of Neuroradiology. Spine (Phila Pa 1976). 2001;26(5):E93–E113.
18. Kim JY, Heo DH. Contralateral sublaminar approach for decompression of the combined lateral recess, foraminal, and extraforaminal lesions using biportal endoscopy: a technical report. Acta Neurochir (Wien). 2021;163:2783–7.
19. Heo DH, Lee N, Park CW, Kim HS, Chung HJ. Endoscopic unilateral laminotomy with bilateral discectomy using biportal endoscopic approach: technical report and preliminary clinical results. World Neurosurg. 2020;137:31–7.
20. Heo DH, Kim JS, Park CW, Quillo-Olvera J, Park CK. Contralateral sublaminar endoscopic approach for removal of lumbar juxtafacet cysts using percutaneous biportal endoscopic surgery: technical report and preliminary results. World Neurosurg. 2019;122:474–9.

21. Choi KC, Kim JS, Park CK. Percutaneous endoscopic lumbar discectomy as an alternative to open lumbar microdiscectomy for large lumbar disc herniation. Pain Physician. 2016;19:E291–300.
22. Ruetten S, Komp M, Merk H, Godolias G. Full-endoscopic interlaminar and transforaminal lumbar discectomy versus conventional microsurgical technique: a prospective, randomized, controlled study. Spine (Phila Pa 1976). 2008;33:931–9.
23. Yeung AT, Tsou PM. Posterolateral endoscopic excision for lumbar disc herniation: surgical technique, outcome, and complications in 307 consecutive cases. Spine (Phila Pa 1976). 2002;27:722–31.
24. Lee S, Kim SK, Lee SH, et al. Percutaneous endoscopic lumbar discectomy for migrated disc herniation: classification of disc migration and surgical approaches. Eur Spine J. 2007;16:431–7.
25. Choi KC, Lee JH, Kim JS, Sabal LA, Lee S, Kim H, et al. Unsuccessful percutaneous endoscopic lumbar discectomy: a single-center experience of 10,228 cases. Neurosurgery. 2015;76:372–80.
26. Choi G, Lee SH, Lokhande P, Kong BJ, Shim CS, Jung B, et al. Percutaneous endoscopic approach for highly migrated intracanal disc herniations by foraminoplastic technique using rigid working channel endoscope. Spine (Phila Pa 1976). 2008;33:E508–15.
27. Choi KC, Shim HK, Hwang JS, et al. Comparison of surgical invasiveness between microdiscectomy and 3 different endoscopic discectomy techniques for lumbar disc herniation. World Neurosurg. 2018;116:e750–8.

Chapter 16
Unilateral Laminotomy for Bilateral Decompression (ULBD) Through Biportal Endoscopy for Lumbar Spinal Stenosis

Weibing Xu, Da-Sheng Tian, Wang Qi-Fei, and Javier Quillo-Olvera

Abbreviations

CRP	C-reactive protein
CSF	Cerebrospinal fluid
CT	Computed tomography
EBL	Estimated blood loss
FJ	Facet joint
IAP	Inferior articular process
LF	Ligamentum flavum
LSS	Lumbar spinal stenosis
MISS	Minimally invasive spine surgery
MRI	Magnetic resonance imaging
ODI	Oswestry Disability Index

Supplementary Information The online version contains supplementary material available at [https://doi.org/10.1007/978-3-031-14736-4_16].

W. Xu
Spinal Surgery Department, Dalian Central Hospital Affiliated to Dalian Medical University, Dalian, Liaoning, China
e-mail: xuweibingsmmu@163.com

D.-S. Tian · W. Qi-Fei
Spine Surgery Department, The Second Affiliated Hospital of Anhui Medical University, Hefei, China
e-mail: tiandasheng@ahmu.edu.com; wqfcn@qq.com

J. Quillo-Olvera (✉)
The Brain and Spine Care, Minimally Invasive Spine Surgery Group, Hospital H+ Querétaro, Spine Clinic, Querétaro, México
e-mail: neuroqomd@gmail.com

J. Quillo-Olvera et al. (eds.), *Unilateral Biportal Endoscopy of the Spine*,
https://doi.org/10.1007/978-3-031-14736-4_16

RCT	Randomized controlled trial
RF	Radiofrequency
SAP	Superior articular process
SLIP	Spinal Laminectomy versus Instrumented Pedicle screw
SP	Spinous process
SPORTS	Spine Patient Outcomes Research Trial
SSSS	Swedish Spinal Stenosis Study
UBE	Unilateral biportal endoscopy
UE	Uniportal endoscopy
ULBD	Unilateral laminotomy for bilateral decompression
VAS	Visual analog scale

Introduction

Lumbar spinal stenosis (LSS) is a narrowing of the spinal canal in its transverse or anteroposterior axis, causing clinical symptoms secondary to radicular compromise. However, anatomical findings could not be congruent with the severity of clinical symptoms since an anatomically narrow canal is often asymptomatic. Spinal stenosis can be classified according to its etiology or anatomy. Regarding spinal stenosis etiology, two types have been described: congenital and, more frequently, acquired. The anatomical classification refers to which compartment the stenosis is happening, for example, the central canal, lateral recess, or foramina. Most patients will have acquired lumbar canal stenosis, often due to degenerative causes. Lumbar spinal stenosis is a degenerative process that counts for 5 cases per 100,000 habitats, and some degree of stenosis is present in up to 80% of individuals over 70 years old. It happens because the lumbar spine's bony, ligamentous, and synovial elements degenerate and overgrow, progressively compressing the neural and vascular components of epidural space [1]. Surgery for spinal stenosis is performed in 3–11.5 cases per 100,000 inhabitants per year, and it is the most common indication for spinal surgery in elderly patients over 65s. In 2007, more than 37,500 operations for spinal stenosis were performed in Medicare patients in the United States, with a total cost of almost $1.65 billion [2–4].

Rationale

Surgical intervention is generally recommended for patients who do not improve with conservative management or have severe symptoms and thecal sac compression at presentation. A systematic review showed that a surgical procedure for spinal stenosis is more effective after trying nonoperative treatment for 6 months and failing [5]. The Spine Patient Outcomes Research Trial (SPORTS) is the most extensive study that compared standard posterior decompressive laminectomy with nonoperative management in patients with lumbar spinal stenosis without spondylolisthesis. The study concluded that patients treated surgically had substantially more significant improvement in pain and function at 2 years [6]. The 4-year follow-up same study outcome reported sustained improvement in pain and function in favor of surgery [7].

Concerning if fusion is required to treat LSS in the setting of degenerative spondylolisthesis, in the 90s, two small trials showed better outcomes in patients with LSS and degenerative spondylolisthesis when fusion and laminectomy were performed at the same stage [8, 9]. However, in 2016, the Swedish Spinal Stenosis Study (SSSS), a large randomized controlled trial (RCT) that compared decompression plus fusion versus decompression alone in patients with LSS and degenerative spondylolisthesis, found no significant difference in clinical outcome or reoperation rates between the two groups at 2 and 5 years of follow-up [10]. Therefore, the authors in this chapter believe that each patient deserves a tailored and specific surgical plan covering all aspects of lumbar spinal pathology. Based on the EBM, only decompression or decompression plus fusion can be beneficial options for treating LSS. The Spinal Laminectomy versus Instrumented Pedicle screw (SLIP) RCT study demonstrated an improved physical health-related quality of life and lower rates of reoperation in patients treated with decompression plus fusion in a setting of LSS and spondylolisthesis. However, higher costs increased estimated blood loss (EBL), and longer hospital stays were also observed in those patients [11].

However, other decompression options in patients with LSS have made it possible to reduce the collateral effect of surgery on the patient. This series of so-called minimally invasive spine surgery (MISS) techniques allow for less aggressive treatment of the paraspinal tissues, preserving the stability of the spinal segment and allowing the patient to return to essential life activities sooner than with conventional surgical procedures, even in challenging cases such as obese patients or degenerative scoliosis and spondylolisthesis [12, 13].

The traditional laminectomy with partial or even complete facet joint (FJ) resection was proved to be an effective treatment. However, this extensive resection of the posterior stabilizing structure has led to a favorable outcome in early stage postoperatively but may lead to instability later. The recurrence rate is as high as 30% [14–16]. Given this, Young et al. [17] and Aryanpur et al. [18] simultaneously proposed a new decompression technique in 1988 called "bilateral subarticular fenestration" under a microscope to perform a more accurate decompression. They used a drill to undercut the FJs hypertrophied and the thickened ligamentum flavum (LF) only and at the same time preserve the posterior stabilizing structures, like spinous process (SP), interspinous ligaments, and most of the lamina and FJs.

Poletti [19] introduced the term unilateral laminotomy for bilateral ligamentectomy in 1995. However, the term "unilateral laminotomy for bilateral decompression or ULBD" was formally coined by Spetzger et al. [20] in 1997. The authors claimed that decompression via ULBD could minimize postoperative instability because only the compressive part of FJ was resected. The same authors concluded that preserving paraspinal muscle attachment and posterior tension band midline structures were associated with better clinical experience outcomes [21]. A bit later,

Guiot et al. [22] reported the feasibility of ULBD under micro-endoscopy in a cadaver study in 2002. With the application of full endoscopy in spine surgery, the traditional aggressive surgical concept of decompressive laminectomy and facetectomy gradually became more selective. In 2011, Komp et al. [23] reported encouraging clinical results with the full-endoscopic ULBD technique in LSS. The authors also concluded that the capacity to decompress the neural elements bilaterally through one-side access is feasible through the uniportal endoscope, in addition to observing all the advantages associated with MISS, such as reduced EBL, shorter hospital stay, minor invasiveness, and a decreased injury to stabilizing structures of the lumbar spine. However, in some cases of LSS where a grander bony work is anticipated, the uniportal endoscopic technique may not be sufficient.

Recently, the growing acceptance of unilateral biportal endoscopy (UBE) has allowed performing addressed decompressions to a specific target, associated with the same advantages observed in MISS, but with the high-quality visualization obtained through uniportal endoscopy, with an addition: the ability to introduce standard working tools for lumbar surgery through an independent port of the endoscope.

After Soliman [24] and Eun et al. [25] reported their respective clinical experience with UBE-ULBD, it has become a more suitable option to deal with LSS. With the mutually independent working and viewing portal, UBE has several specific advantages:

- Wider surgical motion range
- Direct visualization of neural structures
- Versatility
- More instrument choices

And these advantages help surgeons perform ULBD more easily and sufficiently.

Surgical Procedure

Incision Planning and Portal Building

After general anesthesia, the patient was placed in the prone position. If only an ipsilateral decompression is planned, the skin incision should be close to the spinous process (SP). Yet, for contralateral decompression, the skin incision location should be moved 5 mm (left side) to 10 mm (right side) outward depending on the surgeon's side (Fig. 16.1).

Take the left-side procedure as an example. The working portal incision was ideally set at 1/3 to 1/2 of the lower pedicle to facilitate decompression for the upper edge of the lower lamina. At the same time, the viewing portal (cranial incision) was at 2.5–3 cm (depending on the patient's fat thickness) to the working portal. It is suggested to do a crosscut through facia to facilitate smooth water flow. With the

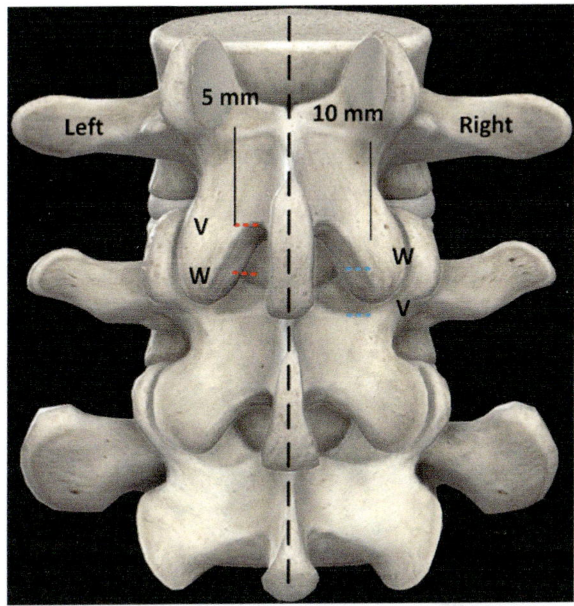

Fig. 16.1 The skin incision in UBE-ULBD in different operation sides

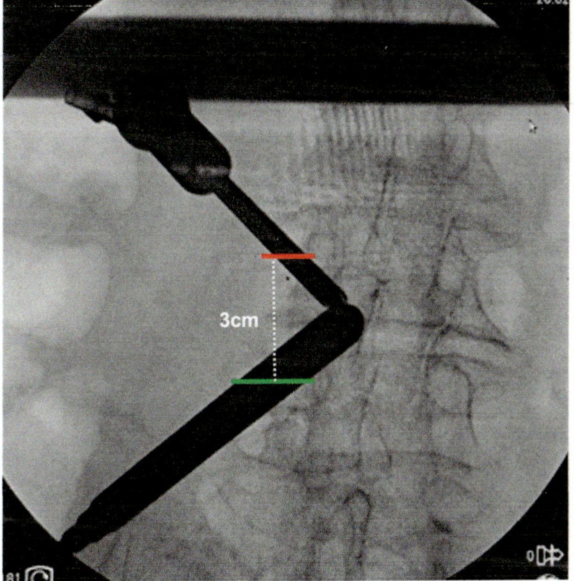

Fig. 16.2 The initial docking site of the two portals under an AP view of the C-arm

inserted dilators addressed to the upper SP base, the attachment of the multifidus muscle is stripped to reach the spinolaminar junction (Fig. 16.2).

Ipsilateral Decompression

After identifying the spinolaminar junction, dissect the soft tissue around the interlaminar window to create a working space (Fig. 16.3a). Herein, the external layer of ligamentum flavum (LF) is removed to expose the bony margin of the SP base, the inferior edge of the upper lamina, the ipsilateral inferior articular process (IAP), and the superior border of the inferior lamina (Fig. 16.3b, c).

Bone removal can be performed following this sequence:

1. Bone removal begins in the spinolaminar junction. The surgeon requires to undercut the base of the SP and the inferior border of the upper lamina to detach

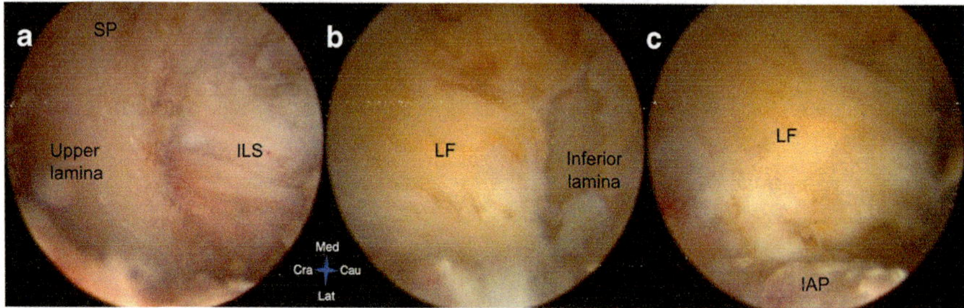

Fig. 16.3 Landmarks of working space. (**a**) The upper lamina and the spinous process (SP) bordering the cranial interlaminar space (ILS). (**b**, **c**) After outer layer removal of LF, the IAP and inferior lamina are identified. *Cra* cranial, *Cau* caudal, *Med* medial, *Lat* lateral, *LF* ligamentum flavum, *IAP* inferior articular process

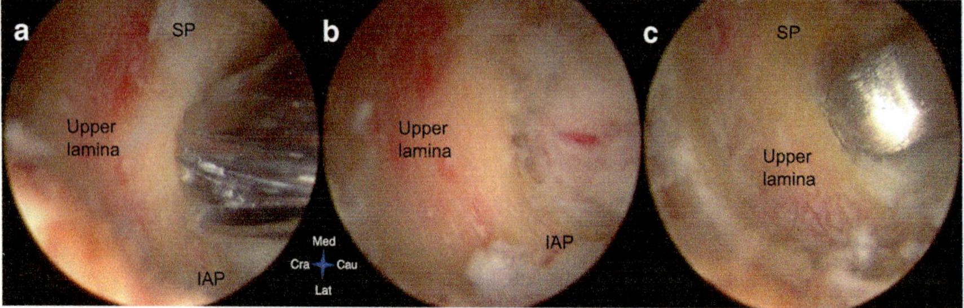

Fig. 16.4 Spinolaminar junction undercut. (**a**) The upper lamina and the base of the spinous process (SP) are drilled out. (**b**) The medial aspect of the IAP is also removed. (**c**) The cranial attachment of LF is released. *Cra* cranial, *Cau* caudal, *Med* medial, *Lat* lateral, *LF* ligamentum flavum, *IAP* inferior articular process

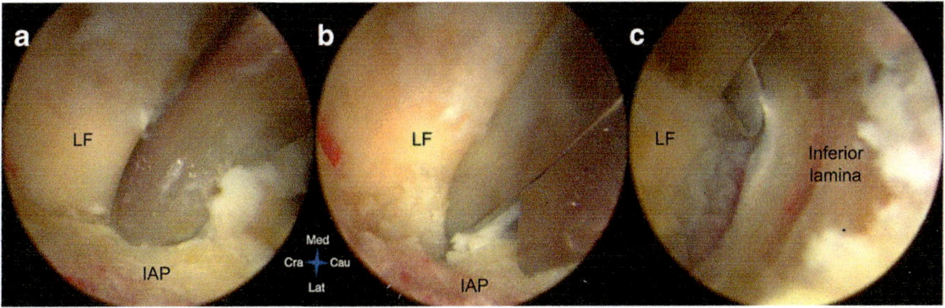

Fig. 16.5 Circumferential bone removal sequence. (**a**) The lateral extension of LF is detached. (**b**) The IAP is undercut. (**c**) The superior border of the inferior lamina is removed, and the LF is detached from it. *Cra* cranial, *Cau* caudal, *Med* medial, *Lat* lateral, *LF* ligamentum flavum, *IAP* inferior articular process

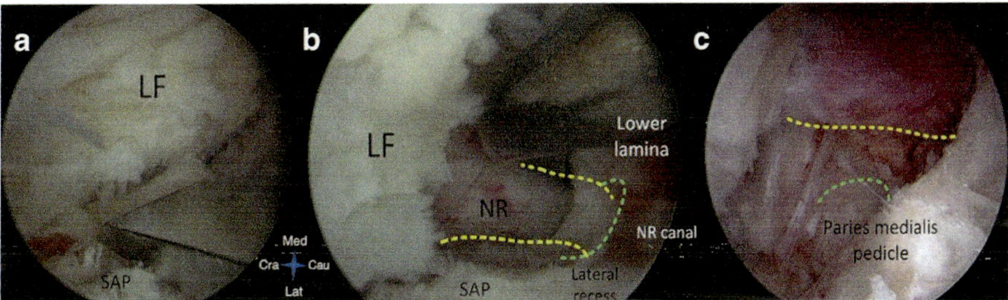

Fig. 16.6 Ipsilateral subarticular decompression. (**a**) The ipsilateral SAP is removed medially. (**b**) The traversing nerve (NR) is identified. (**c**) Lateral recess decompression is concluded, and the paries medialis pedicle (medial wall of the pedicle) is observed. *Cra* cranial, *Cau* caudal, *Med* medial, *Lat* lateral, *LF* ligamentum flavum, *SAP* superior articular process

the cranial insertion of LF. A curved-ending-tip dissector could be used in this step (Fig. 16.4).

2. Then, the medial aspect of the ipsilateral IAP is undercut. After lateral extension detachment of LF, a Kerrison rongeur could be helpful to remove the IAP medially. However, care must be taken not to excessively remove the IAP to avoid the risk of iatrogenic instability (Fig. 16.5).
3. The ipsilateral superior articular process (SAP) undercutting can be completed with different tools to achieve lateral recess decompression. The bone should be removed enough to expose the transversing nerve root, not only the dural sac's lateral border. Different landmarks could be used as endpoints of the lateral recess decompression, such as identifying the "paries medialis pedicle" (medial wall of the pedicle) or freely mobilizing the traversing nerve root (Fig. 16.6).
4. For the following "over-the-top" manipulation, the LF must be preserved intact as much as possible since it protects the neural elements during bone removal.

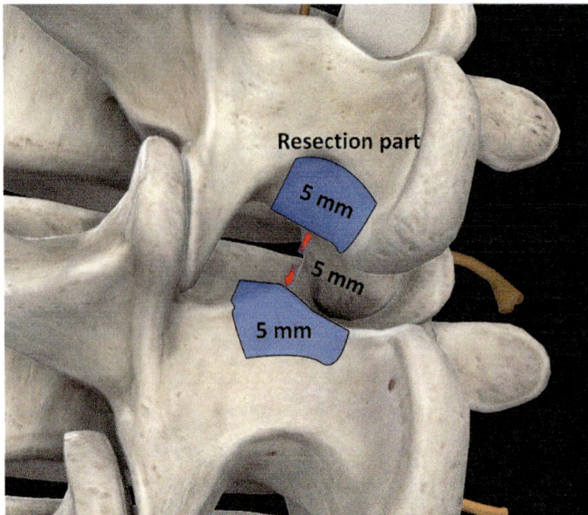

Fig. 16.7 Suggested bone removal area to address the contralateral side in a sublaminar trajectory. The blue highlighted area below the superior and inferior spinous processes should be removed

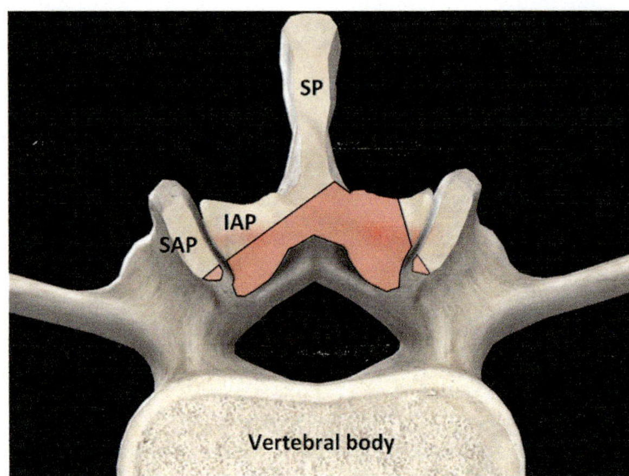

Fig. 16.8 The cross-sectional area of the anatomical scheme is highlighted in orange as the bone resection extent during a UBE-ULBD procedure. *IAP* inferior articular process, *SAP* superior articular process, *SP* spinous process

Contralateral Decompression

Undercutting the base of the spinous process to reach the contralateral side and decompressing it with a sublaminar trajectory are suggested. For this reason, the authors recommend removing at least 5 mm of the base of the superior and inferior spinous processes (Fig. 16.7) at the index level. This will allow access to the contralateral side and removal of the ventral aspect of the upper and lower laminae. The advantage of preserving the dorsal surface of both laminae is that it is not necessary to detach the muscles that adhere to them; it also avoids performing total laminectomies, which allows a direct view of the contralateral IAP and SAP.

A wider laminectomy is unnecessary to cross the midline (Fig. 16.8). About 3–4 mm sublaminar bone removal is enough. Passing over the LF, it is easy to find the medial part of the contralateral IAP. In addition, tight fibrous connections between LF and capsular ligament can be found during dissection of the medial surface of the IAP. Therefore, we recommend detaching the LF from the bony IAP surface with a blunt-tip dissector and reaching its ventral aspect. With the LF separated from the IAP, the surgeon could use a high-speed drill, Kerrison of different sizes and tips, and chisels to undercut the IAP.

The curve chisel may be more efficient but has a higher possibility of causing neural elements' injury. The medial border and the tip of the SAP will be exposed after appropriate IAP resection. Here, use a curette to detach the deep layer of the LF insertion underneath the SAP. And cut off the tip of the SAP until the contralateral "paries medialis pedicle" is observed.

Undercut the SAP further to reveal the shoulder, and the axilla of the transversing root means sufficient decompression. Ensure that the transversing nerve root canal is unobstructed by using a curette or a nerve hook. If not, perform the decompression again. The deep layer of the LF is suggested to be maintained intact until all bone work is done.

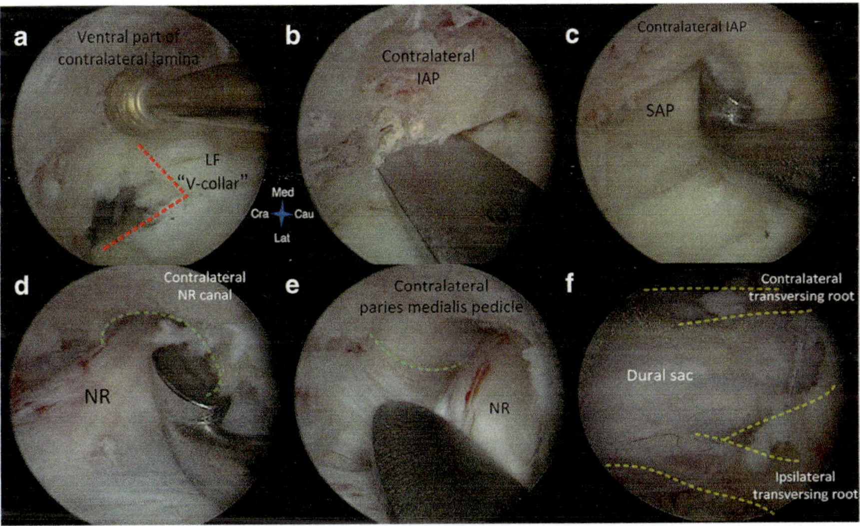

Fig. 16.9 A sequence of contralateral lumbar decompression during a UBE-ULBD. (**a**) Undercutting the contralateral lamina. (**b**) Undercutting the contralateral IAP. (**c**) Ventral SAP removal and decompressing the traversing nerve root (NR). (**d**) Completing the contralateral traversing NR decompression. (**e**) The contralateral paries medial pedicle (medial wall of the pedicle) is identified. (**f**) Side-to-side decompression with both traversing nerves and the dural sac exposed. *Cra* cranial, *Cau* caudal, *Med* medial, *Lat* lateral, *IAP* inferior articular process, *SAP* superior articular process, *LF* ligamentum flavum, *NR* nerve root

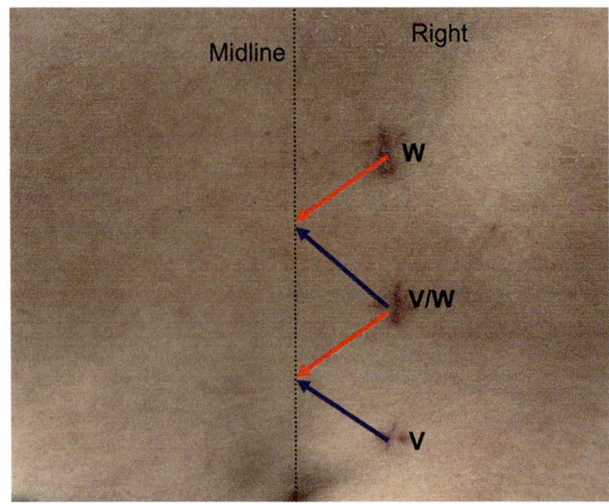

Fig. 16.10 Picture of the surgical wounds on the tenth day postoperatively. A UBE-ULBD L4–L5 and L5–S1 was performed on this patient on the right side. A black dotted line represents the midline. On the right side, the purpose of wounds is illustrated with arrows and capitals (W; working portal—red arrow, V; viewing portal—blue arrow)

Finally, the LF can be removed. First, it is suggested to explore and detach the epidural space between LF and dural sac with a nerve hook. In most of the cases, between both, there is a fat tissue layer; however, sometimes meningovertebral tight adhesions or ligaments can be found, especially in the midline. The surgeon can also distinguish the midline in the ligamentum flavum, identifying a "V-shape." It is also called a "V-collar." So, before flavectomy, dissect the flavum carefully and then remove it with the Kerrison punch (Fig. 16.9).

The steps to perform bilateral decompression through a unilateral laminotomy (ULBD) are exemplified in Video 16.1. The surgeon must remember that this procedure is intended to preserve stabilizing structures (facet joints, lamina, interspinous ligaments, paraspinal muscles) as much as possible. The biportal endoscopic technique or UBE also allows us to have a sublaminar trajectory by undercutting the contralateral lamina avoiding the total laminectomy or facetectomy for neural decompression, thus preventing further iatrogenic instability. The UBE-ULBD is a powerful option for decompressing the neural elements in the lumbar region for central and subarticular stenosis.

In cases where multilevel decompression is required, it is suggested to use the caudal incision as a portal to the next level. For example, the caudal incision will be used for the next level's working portal on the right side. The same incision will be used as a viewing portal on the left side (Fig. 16.10).

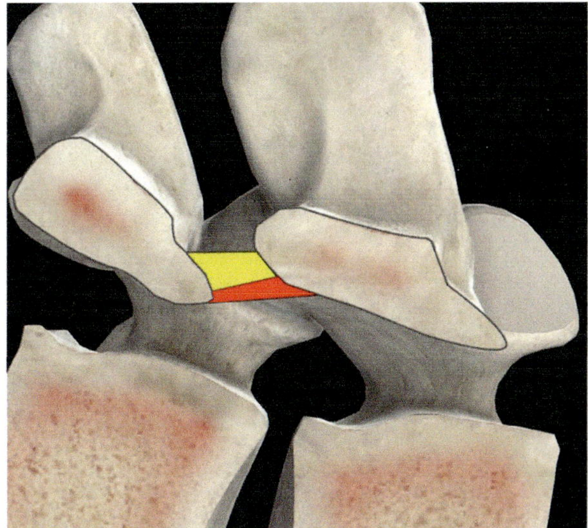

Fig. 16.11 The attachments of LF to the laminae (sagittal section). The yellow area represents the external layer of LF. The red area, the deeper

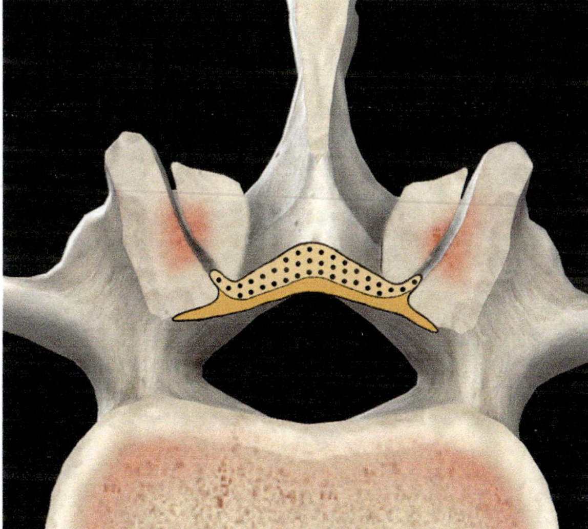

Fig. 16.12 The attachment of LF to the lamina (cross section). The black dotted yellow area represents the external layer of LF. The yellow area below represents the deeper

Surgical Anatomy of Ligamentum Flavum Applied to Biportal Endoscopy

The anatomy of the ligamentum flavum is essential, especially in endoscopic procedures, including UBE. According to the previous studies, the LF has been interpreted as a ligament divided into two layers—external and deep layers. However, Viejo-Fuertes et al. [26] defined the two layers based on the fiber's orientation. Other studies [27, 28] have found that external and deep LF layers are divided

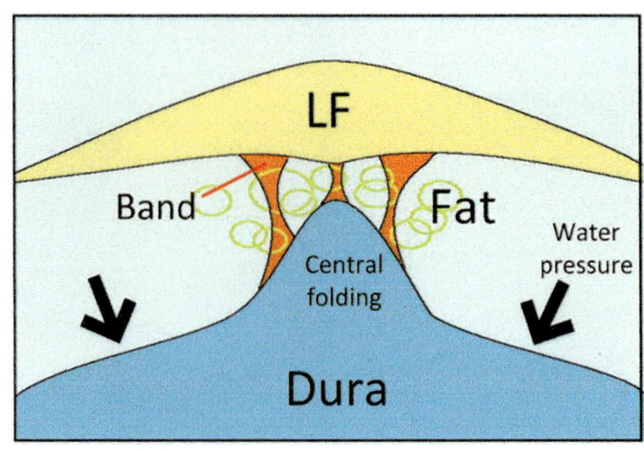

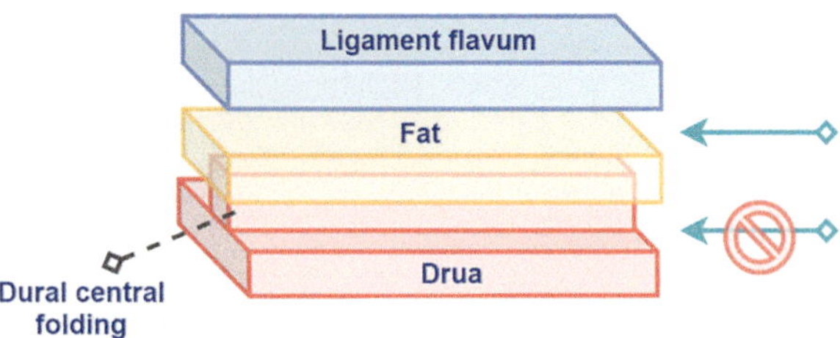

Fig. 16.13 "Sandwich theory" for safe resection of LF

according to their bony insertions. The external layer fills the dorsal aspect of the interlaminar space, and it extends from the anteroinferior edge of the cranial lamina to the posterosuperior edge of the caudal lamina. At the same time, the deep layer extends from the ridge of the cranial lamina to the anterosuperior and anteroinferior part of the caudal lamina (Figs. 16.11 and 16.12).

A recent study [29] suggested a distinct conclusion indicating that the so-called superficial or external layer of the LF may be the extension of the interspinous ligament; despite the controversial issue regarding the two-layer structure, the LF should be well identified in UBE-ULBD.

A proper dissection of the external LF layer leads to correctly identifying the edge of bone structures, such as the laminae, the base of the SP, and the medial surface of the IAP and SAP, and at the same time, the over-drilling of bone structures could be avoided by observing directly the bony landmarks.

Furthermore, as already mentioned, the dissection of the deep layer of the LF must be careful due to the fibrous bands and meningovertebral ligaments connecting the LF to the dura, and the intermediate fold forms precisely in the midline. In addition, there is epidural fat covering this central fold and these ligamentous structures; therefore, it can be easy to cause a dural tear at this site.

According to the author's "sandwich theory" (Fig. 16.13), the dorsal surface of LF, epidural fat tissue, and dura form a three-tiered structure that must be identified. The Kerrison rongeur is supposed to enter the upper-middle layer (over the fat tissue) to avoid dura injury.

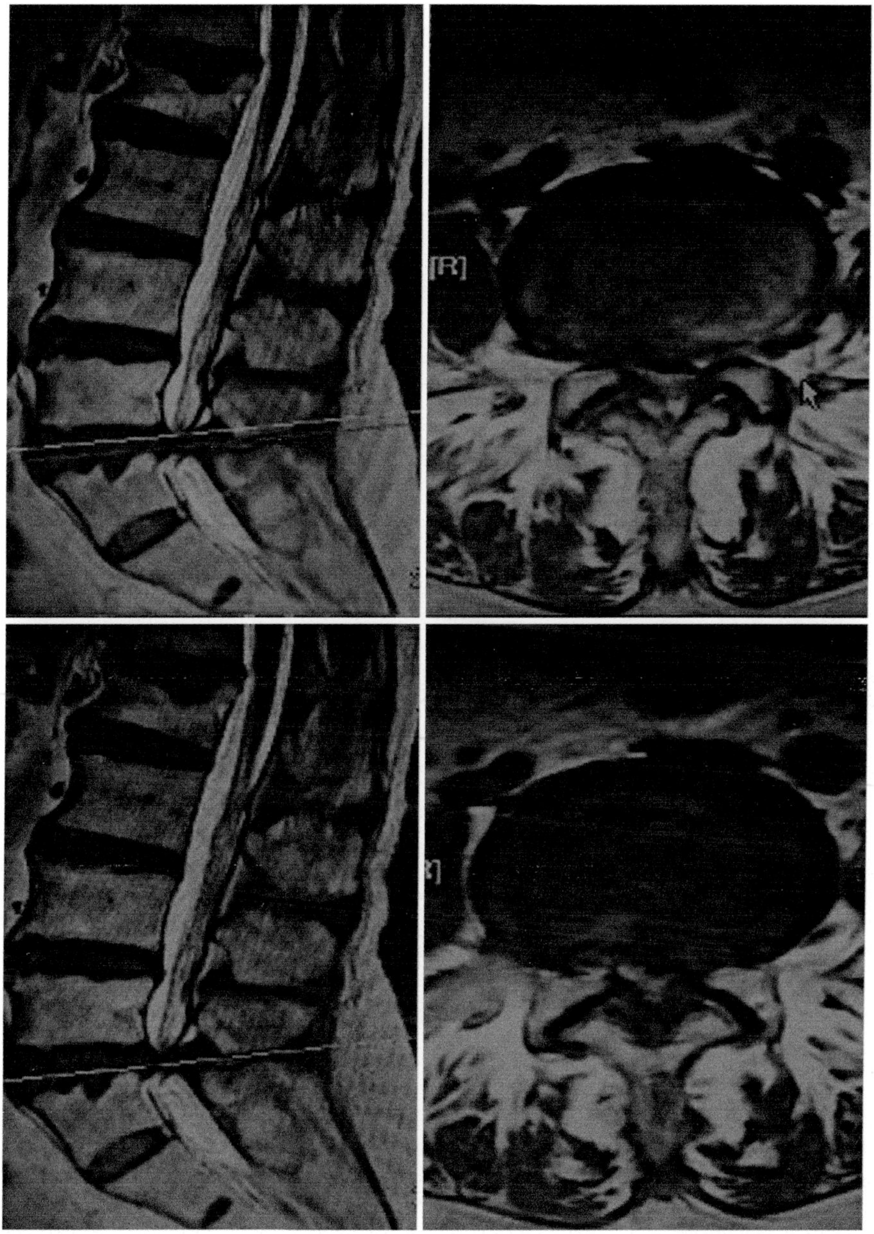

Fig. 16.14 Preoperative lumbar MRI from Case 1. A severe central spinal stenosis involving both lateral recesses can be observed at L4–L5

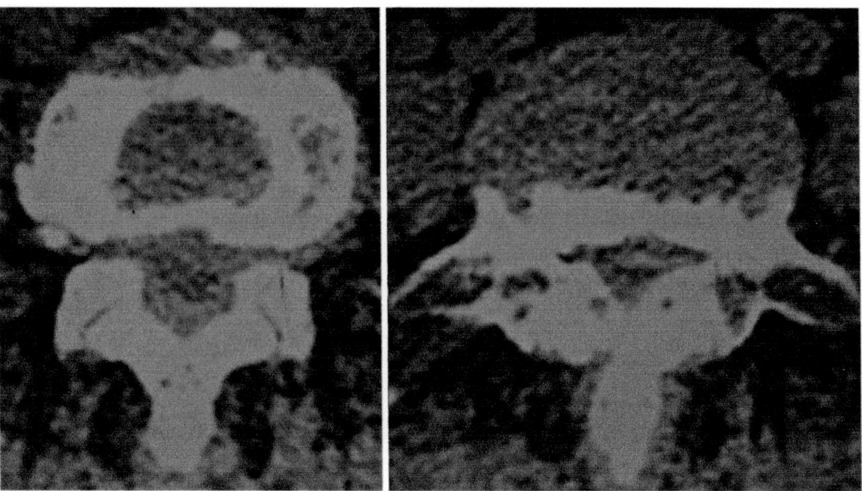

Fig. 16.15 Preoperative lumbar CT scan from Case 1. Overgrowth of facet joints and resulting stenosis of the lateral recesses from both sides are noted at L4–L5

Illustrated Cases

Case 1

A 78-year-old female complains of severe radicular pain radiating down her right leg. The pain in the right leg goes down along the anterior thigh and lateral surface of the calf. However, the patient feels sensitivity disturbances such as numbness in both legs. The neurologic examination demonstrated bilateral great toe dorsiflexion and plantar flexion weakness (4/5), and bilateral ankle reflex was absent. Preoperative lumbar MRI revealed severe central spinal stenosis at L4–L5, with bilateral narrowing of both lateral recesses (Fig. 16.14). The CT scan confirmed the finding (Fig. 16.15). The following procedure was planned because symptoms on the right side also included the ones from the L4 nerve root: UBE-ULBD L4–L5 on the left side to decompress the ipsilateral L5 nerve root, and a contralateral approach (left to right) to release the right-sided L4 and L5 nerve roots (Fig. 16.16). The postoperative immediate lumbar CT scan corroborated sufficient decompression ipsilaterally and a proper undercutting of the lateral recess and foramen on the right side at L4–L5 (Fig. 16.17). No intraoperative and postoperative complications were reported. The patient was discharged on the second day after the surgery. The radicular pain on the right leg improved immediately after the procedure. At the 6-week follow-up visit, we noted normal strength in the dorsiflexion of the great toe and plantar flexion bilaterally.

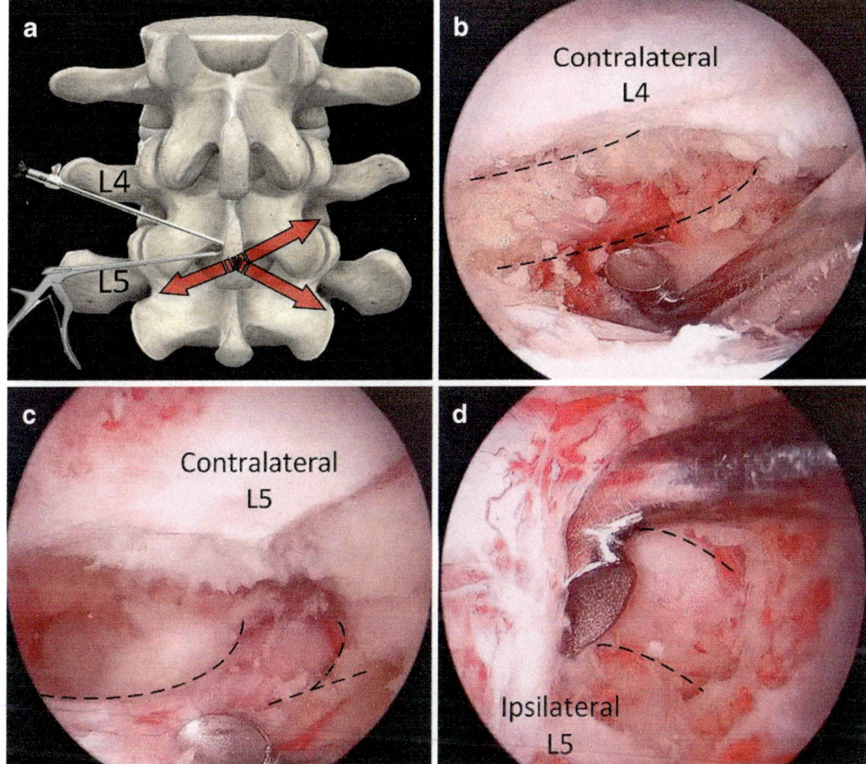

Fig. 16.16 Intraoperative images through the endoscope from Case 1. (**a**) Anatomical scheme showing the surgical planning at L4–L5; the red arrows point the trajectories to follow for decompressing the neural structures involved in the pathology. The intermittent black lines on (**b**, **c**) represent the nerves decompressed. (**b**) L4 exiting nerve root decompressed on the right side contralateral to the UBE-ULBD approach. (**c**) The L5 traversing nerve root decompressed on the right side. (**d**) The curette palps the ipsilateral L5 traversing nerve root (left side). The intermittent black line shows the intervertebral disc

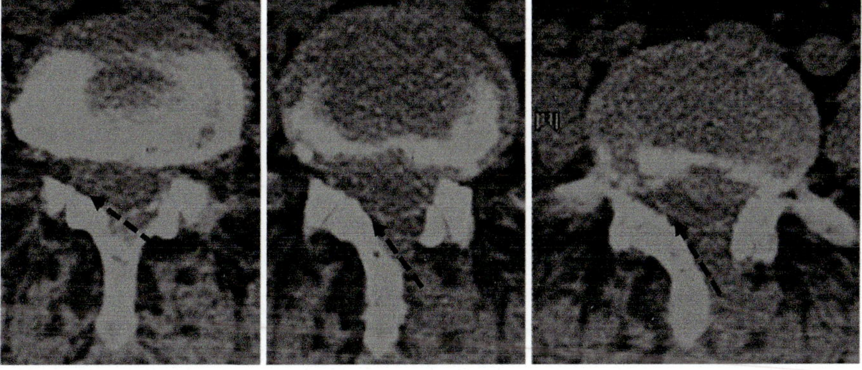

Fig. 16.17 Postoperative lumbar CT scan from Case 1. Sufficient bilateral decompression was achieved through the UBE-ULBD procedure at L4–L5 (three cross-sectional cuts). The intermittent black arrow shows the approach trajectory in the three axial views

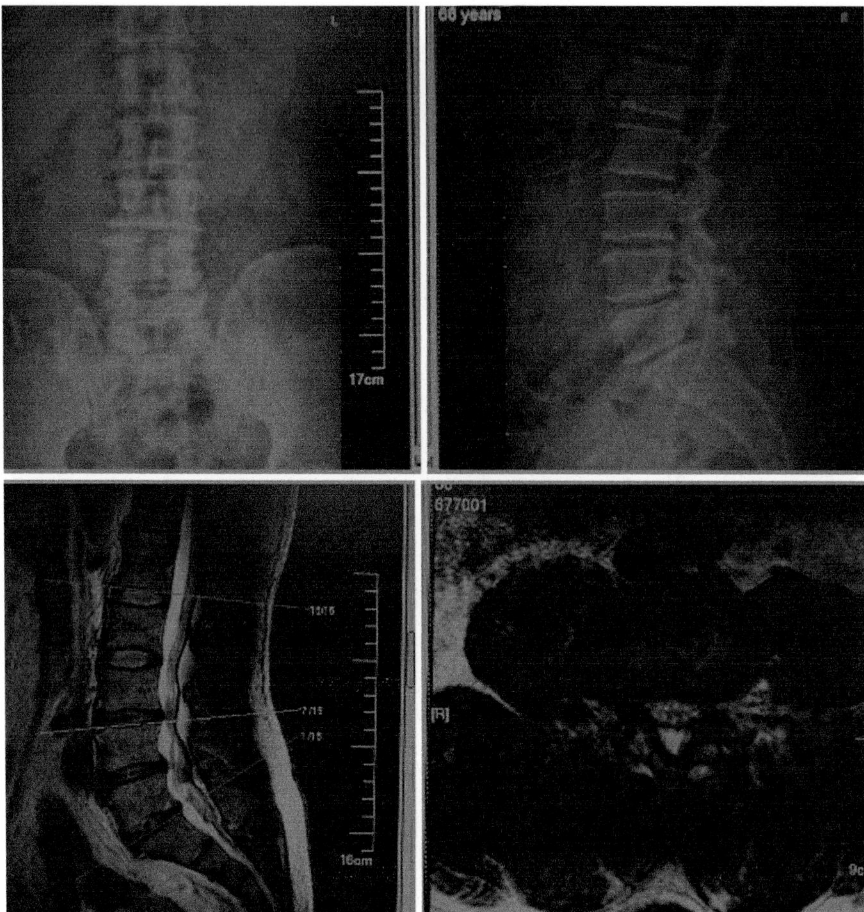

Fig. 16.18 Preoperative lumbar X-rays and MRI from Case 2. The superior panel shows the lumbar X-rays. The inferior panel shows the lumbar MRI. The axial view on T2-weighted image at L3–L4 (right side) demonstrated lateral lumbar stenosis

Case 2

A 66-year-old male patient complained of severe electric shock-like pain in his right leg for 8 weeks, which did not subside with conservative measures or the use of opioids. The pain radiates to the anterior aspect of the thigh and lateral surface of the calf of the right leg. Also, numbness on the right leg was felt by the patient. Neurological examination revealed weakness (4/5) in dorsiflexion and plantar flexion of the right ankle and an absent patellar reflex on the right side. Preoperative X-ray images did not demonstrate sagittal or coronal balance disorders. However, lumbar MRI showed proximal foraminal stenosis at L3–L4 on the right side

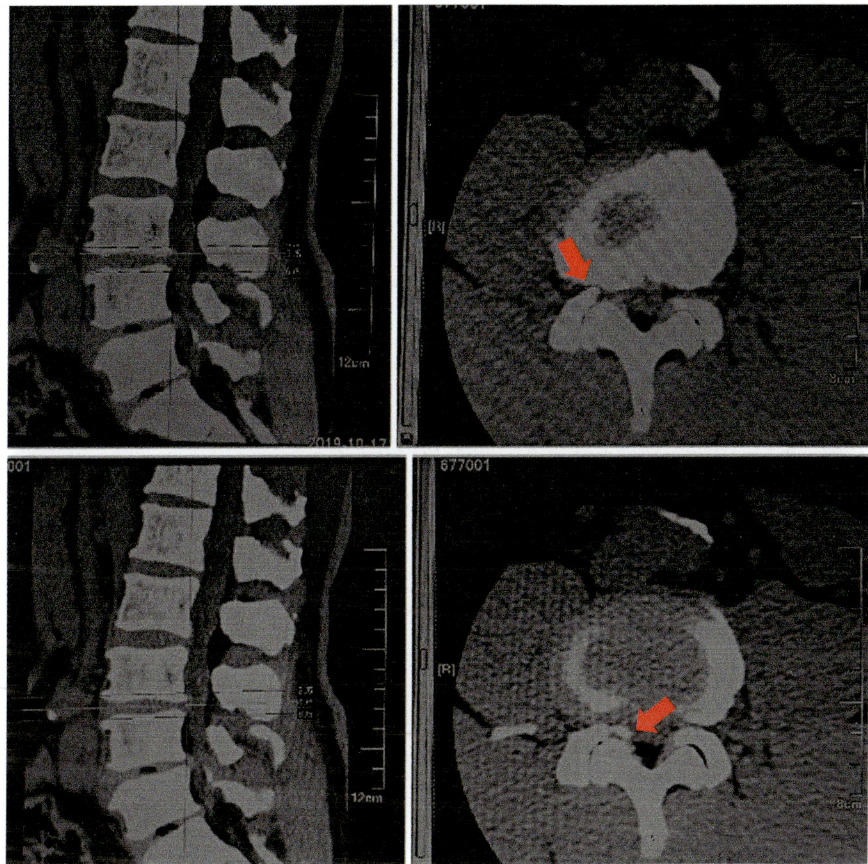

Fig. 16.19 Preoperative lumbar CT scan from Case 2. The superior panel shows the cross-sectional view of L3–L4 at the inferior height of foramen. Hypertrophy of the L4 SAP on the right side is noted (red arrow). The inferior panel shows the cross-sectional view of L3–L4 at the lateral recess height. The red arrow points to the flavum osteophyte on the right side

(Fig. 16.18). The preoperative lumbar CT scan showed medial facet bone osteophyte, probably associated with calcification at the lateral insertion of the flavum (Fig. 16.19). The surgical planning was a UBE-ULBD from the left side to address the approach to the contralateral side and decompress the L3 and L4 nerves on the right side. The initial landmark was the spinolaminar junction at L3–L4 on the left side (Fig. 16.20a); then through a sublaminar trajectory, the L3 exiting nerve was reached (Fig. 16.20b); and caudally, the L4 traversing nerve along its course in the lateral recess was decompressed (Fig. 16.20c, d). The procedure turned out to be successful, being able to adequately decompress the contralateral L3 and L4 roots on the right side, in addition to the central canal (Fig. 16.21). Postoperative CT scan

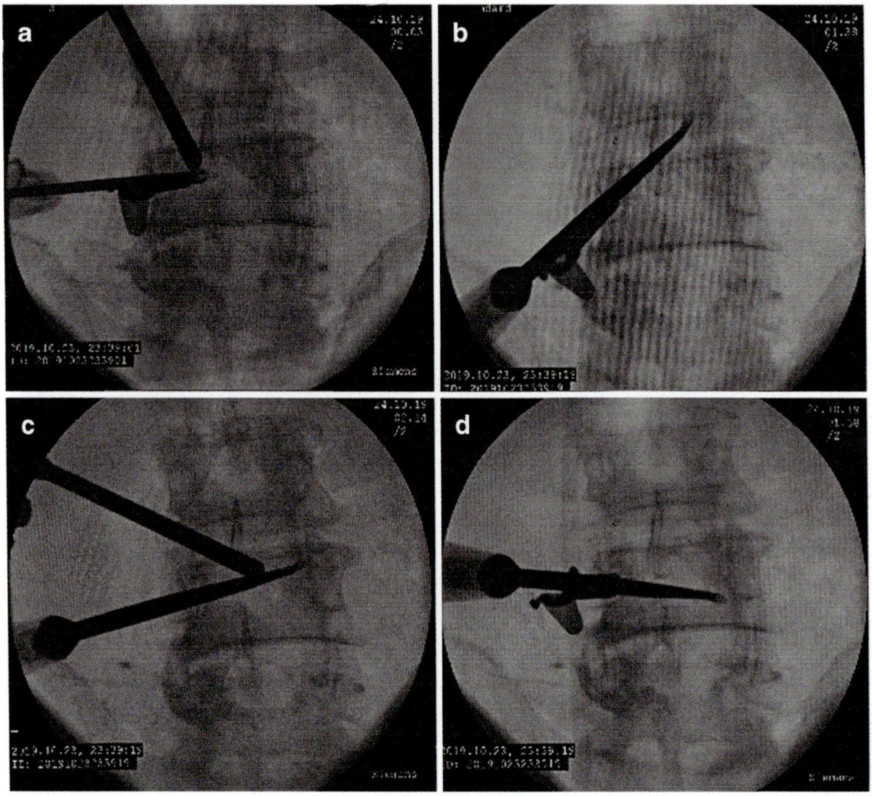

Fig. 16.20 Intraoperative images from the C-arm during the UBE-ULBD with contralateral decompression at L3–L4. (**a**) The triangulation is addressed to the spinolaminar junction on the left side. (**b**) The midline is crossed, and the contralateral decompression of the L3 exiting nerve is performed. (**c**) The contralateral undercutting of the lamina and medial facet joint is done. (**d**) The L4 traversing nerve is released through its entire course

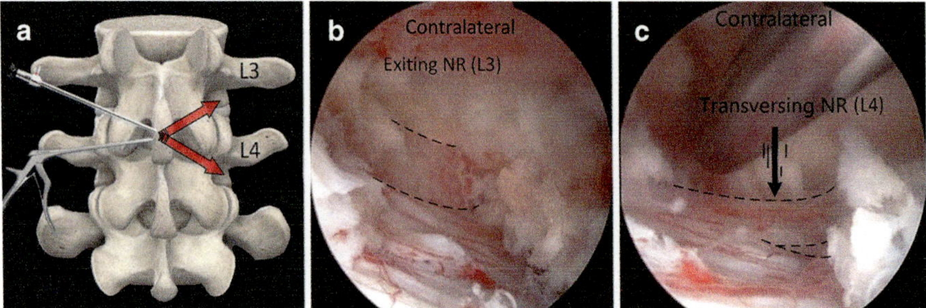

Fig. 16.21 Intraoperative images through the endoscope from Case 2. (**a**) Anatomical scheme showing the surgical planning at L3–L4 on the left side; the red arrows point the trajectories to follow during the contralateral decompression. The intermittent black lines on (**b**, **c**) represent the nerves decompressed. (**b**) L3 exiting nerve root (NR) decompressed on the right side contralateral to the UBE-ULBD approach. (**c**) The L4 traversing nerve root decompressed on the right side. The dural sac medial to the nerves is also released from the central stenosis

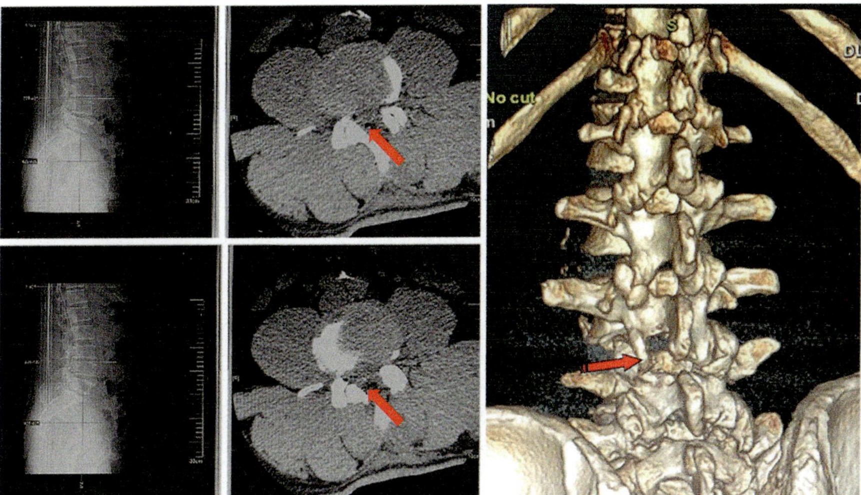

Fig. 16.22 Postoperative lumbar CT scan from Case 2. The red arrows point out to the decompression sites and the contralateral trajectory. Left side: special attention should be put on the proximal foramen and lateral recess decompression on the right side. The 3D reconstructed CT scan (right side) shows the interlaminar bone defect after the UBE-ULBD at L3–L4. But the preservation of the facet joint on the approach side can be noted

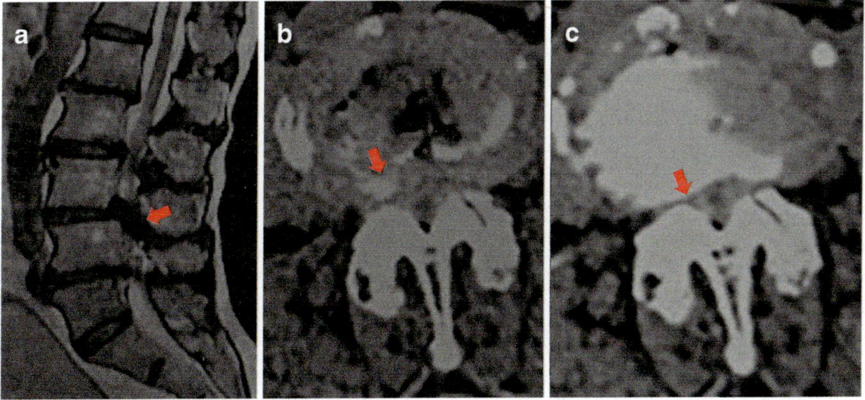

Fig. 16.23 Preoperative images from Case 3. (**a**) The T2-weighted sagittal view of the lumbar MRI demonstrated central canal stenosis at L3–L4. (**b**) The axial view of the lumbar CT scan shows stenosis on the foraminal area (red arrow) at L3–L4 on the right side. (**c**) The axial view at the height of lateral recesses shows bilateral stenosis of the subarticular area at L3–L4 predominantly on the right side (red arrow)

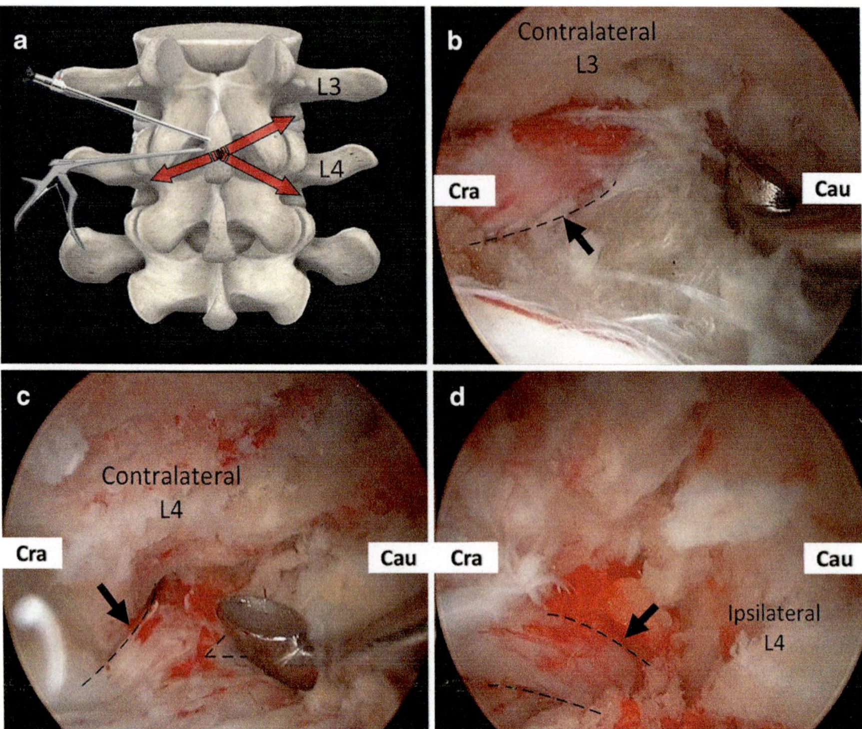

Fig. 16.24 Intraoperative images through the endoscope from Case 3. (**a**) Anatomical scheme showing the surgical planning at L3–L4 on the left side; the red arrows point the trajectories to follow during the ipsilateral and contralateral decompression. (**b**) The decompressed exiting L3 nerve root (black arrow) can be observed. (**c**) The L4 traversing nerve root on the right side is pointed by the black arrow, while on the ipsilateral side (**d**) the other L4 nerve is observed (black arrow)

demonstrated sufficient bone decompression and joint preservation on both sides at L3–L4 (Fig. 16.22). The patient immediately improved his right leg's pain and sensory disorders and was discharged on day 2 after surgery with mild analgesics such as paracetamol. At the 12-day postoperative visit, a complete improvement in the strength of the right ankle was observed.

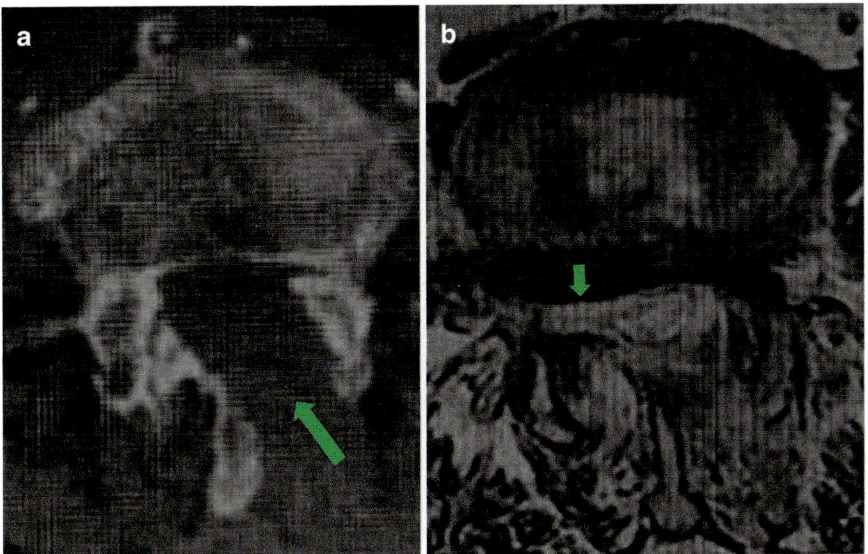

Fig. 16.25 Postoperative images from Case 3. (**a**) The axial view of the lumbar CT scan at L3–L4 shows sufficient central and bilateral subarticular decompression (green arrow). (**b**) The T2-weighted axial view of the lumbar MRI confirmed a foraminal decompression (green arrow) at L3–L4 on the right side

Case 3

A 70-year-old female patient complains of radicular pain radiating to her right leg. The pain descends through the anterior thigh and the medial aspect of the calf until it reaches the right ankle. Moreover, the patient also reports numbness in both legs. These symptoms make it hard for her to walk. The neurological examination showed significant 3/5 weakness in dorsiflexion of both ankles, in addition to bilateral abolition of the patellar reflex. Preoperative lumbar MRI demonstrated significant central narrowing canal at L3–L4 (Fig. 16.23a), while a predominantly right-sided lateral recess and proximal foraminal stenosis due to significant spondylosis were seen on preoperative CT scan at L3–L4 (Fig. 16.23b, c). Therefore, a UBE-ULBD for L3–L4 on the left side was planned (Fig. 16.24a) with a contralateral extended approach to reach the L3 and L4 nerves (Fig. 16.24b–d). Immediate postoperative lumbar MRI and CT images demonstrated adequate central and lateral decompression at L3–L4, consistent with the patient's considerable immediate postoperative clinical improvement (Fig. 16.25).

Discussion

Throughout this chapter, we have highlighted the potential benefits of the biportal endoscopy to decompress the neural elements in cases of lumbar spinal stenosis (LSS). In addition, the authors have noted the following particular advantages associated with the UBE:

1. The high-quality imaging obtained with the arthroscope and the continuous saline irrigated throughout the procedure make the UBE technique a genuine water-based endoscopic procedure.
2. The surgeon's ability to handle the instrument and the endoscope independently provides versatility to the UBE technique, safety during manipulation of critical anatomy, and confidence during the surgery.
3. The surgeon's familiarity with standard instruments for spinal surgery.
4. Minimal muscle damage compared with open surgery and less intraoperative radiation than other full-endoscopic techniques.
5. Surgeons with experience in other minimally invasive decompression procedures such as tubular or full endoscopy could shorten the learning curve in biportal endoscopy.
6. Other spine regions like the cervical or thoracic can be decompressed through UBE.
7. Besides, in the unilateral laminotomy for bilateral decompression (ULBD) procedure, we consider that biportal endoscopy compensates for the shortcomings observed in uniportal endoscopy (UE). For example, in interlaminar UE, the instrument can only be used through the same trajectory as the endoscope; the point is that if the surgeon requires to reach a specific location, the endoscopic system needs to be also mobilized together with the tool, and sometimes it is not possible because of intricated spaces within the spinal canal. Moreover, the surgeon could damage the expensive spinal endoscope if forced levering is done. However, in UBE, the instrument and the endoscope have some degree of freedom, and if needed, reorganization of both can be done to reach enough visibility of complex anatomy and the surgical instrument.

Unilateral laminotomy with bilateral decompression (ULBD) through MISS procedures is associated with less damage to important paraspinal tissues with a biomechanical role, such as paravertebral muscles, interspinous and supraspinous ligaments, and of course facet joints. Therefore, this procedure in a minimally invasive fashion is associated with a lower risk of iatrogenic postoperative instability [19, 30, 31].

In addition, several studies have shown that UBE-ULBD for the treatment of LSS can get sufficient and adequate decompression of the neural elements similar to open or microsurgical techniques [32–34].

UBE-ULBD aims to achieve the same or similar enlargement of epidural space for decompressing the neural elements than UE or microsurgery. The bony structures removed through UBE-ULBD are the ipsilateral partial laminotomy, the undercutting of the base of the spinous process, and the medial facet, but all the techniques for performing ULBD can get the same. The main differences that make UBE-ULBD special among the other methods are the high-quality vision under a water environment and the versatility of using the technique through two ports. The endpoint of the UBE-ULBD is to observe the neural elements free. Bilateral decompression of the lateral recess is confirmed by observing the medial wall of both inferior pedicles at the index level.

In addition, an extra advantage associated with endoscopic techniques (uniportal or biportal) concerning open or microsurgery is the preservation of the facet joint and minor damage to the paravertebral muscles related to the approach [34].

A concern in ULBD is decompression of the ipsilateral lateral recess. However, in UBE, the surgeon can reorganize the endoscope and the instrument in the surgical field so that the attack trajectory on the ipsilateral facet joint could be compelling, with less restriction than in the UE, and using a lens of 30°, by rotating it, the undercutting of the IAP and SAP can be performed preserving the FJ as much as possible.

Eum et al. [35] were the first to report encouraging clinical outcomes in patients with LSS treated with UBE-ULBD. The authors included 58 patients in their study, all of whom achieved sufficient decompression of the neural elements. According to the Macnab satisfaction criteria, 47 patients rated the procedure excellent or good. The complications presented were three cases with postoperative headache, durotomy noted in two patients, postoperative numbness in two patients, and epidural hematoma in one patient.

Li et al. [36] reported the results of a systematic review comparing the clinical effectiveness and safety between UBE-ULBD and microsurgery for LSS. The authors included seven articles that met the methodological quality. Allocation of the groups was as follows: 288 patients were included in the UBE group and 234 in the microsurgery group. The authors found no superiority between any of the groups concerning hospital stay. UBE was found to require less operative time than microsurgery. Patients in the UBE group had a better postoperative VAS score for back pain than those in the microsurgery group.

UBE was superior to microsurgery only on the first postoperative day regarding the postoperative leg VAS score. In addition, the authors found no differences in postoperative ODI, complications, revision rate, or cross-sectional area of the dura between the two groups. Finally, the authors reported that the UBE group had lower C-reactive protein (CRP) levels only on the first day than the microsurgery group. However, the authors conclude that the most important difference between UBE and microsurgery remains technical, considering image quality, ability to use two independent ports, and ability to use tools familiar to the surgeon as the most important advantages of UBE over microsurgery.

Also, an RCT from 2019 focused on UBE versus microscopic lumbar decompressive laminectomy included 64 patients divided into two groups (UBE versus microscopic) with 32 patients in each group. The study reported no significant difference in postoperative clinical outcomes at 1-year follow-up between the two groups. Therefore, no inferiority was demonstrated in the clinical effectiveness of the UBE technique compared to microscopy in the decompression of the LLS [37].

Another systematic review by Pao [38] from 2021 found that the most frequent complication in UBE-ULBD was a dural tear, with an incidence that varies from 1.5% to 9.7%. Most of these tears were small and could be treated without converting the procedure. However, a tear greater than 10 mm requires direct repair to prevent cerebrospinal fluid (CSF) leakage [39]. This chapter discussed how the surgeon must be careful when performing the flavectomy and how the intermediate dural fold usually has a higher risk of being damaged due to its anatomical characteristics.

Other complications are epidural hematoma, which can be prevented by performing adequate hemostasis with the radiofrequency (RF), bone wax, hemostatic matrices, and leaving postoperative epidural drainage. In addition, neurological disorders associated with increased hydrostatic pressure in the epidural space, such as postoperative headaches or chronic subdural hematoma following lumbar UBE-ULBD, have been reported [40, 41].

Conclusions

Based on the most recent evidence on biportal endoscopy for the treatment of lumbar spinal stenosis, unilateral laminotomy with bilateral decompression is usually effective and associated with encouraging clinical outcomes with a lower complication profile. In addition, the same advantages related to other minimally invasive procedures, such as a shorter hospital stay and a faster return to daily activities, are perceived with biportal endoscopy. However, it is recommended that the surgeon interested in this technique consider the systematized process discussed in this chapter to decompress the lumbar spinal stenosis to ensure similar results.

References

1. Kalichman L, Cole R, Kim DH, et al. Spinal stenosis prevalence and association with symptoms: the Framingham Study. Spine J. 2009;9(7):545–50.
2. Deyo RA, Mirza SK, Martin BI, Kreuter W, Goodman DC, Jarvik JG. Trends, major medical complications, and charges associated with surgery for lumbar spinal stenosis in older adults. JAMA. 2010;303(13):1259–65.

3. Bagley C, MacAllister M, Dosselman L, Moreno J, Aoun SG, El Ahmadieh TY. Current concepts and recent advances in understanding and managing lumbar spine stenosis. F1000Res. 2019;8:F1000 Faculty Rev-137.
4. Melancia JL, Francisco AF, Antunes JL. Spinal stenosis. Handb Clin Neurol. 2014;119:541–9.
5. Kovacs FM, Urrútia G, Alarcón JD. Surgery versus conservative treatment for symptomatic lumbar spinal stenosis: a systematic review of randomized controlled trials. Spine (Phila Pa 1976). 2011;36(20):E1335–51.
6. Weinstein JN, Tosteson TD, Lurie JD, et al. Surgical versus nonsurgical therapy for lumbar spinal stenosis. N Engl J Med. 2008;358(8):794–810.
7. Weinstein JN, Tosteson TD, Lurie JD, et al. Surgical versus nonoperative treatment for lumbar spinal stenosis four-year results of the Spine Patient Outcomes Research Trial. Spine (Phila Pa 1976). 2010;35(14):1329–38.
8. Bridwell KH, Sedgewick TA, O'Brien MF, Lenke LG, Baldus C. The role of fusion and instrumentation in the treatment of degenerative spondylolisthesis with spinal stenosis. J Spinal Disord. 1993;6(6):461–72.
9. Herkowitz HN, Kurz LT. Degenerative lumbar spondylolisthesis with spinal stenosis. A prospective study comparing decompression with decompression and intertransverse process arthrodesis. J Bone Joint Surg Am. 1991;73(6):802–8.
10. Försth P, Ólafsson G, Carlsson T, et al. A randomized, controlled trial of fusion surgery for lumbar spinal stenosis. N Engl J Med. 2016;374(15):1413–23.
11. Ghogawala Z, Dziura J, Butler WE, et al. Laminectomy plus fusion versus laminectomy alone for lumbar spondylolisthesis. N Engl J Med. 2016;374(15):1424–34.
12. Hudak EM, Perry MW. Outpatient minimally invasive spine surgery using endoscopy for the treatment of lumbar spinal stenosis among obese patients. J Orthop. 2015;12(3):156–9.
13. Hasan S, McGrath LB, Sen RD, Barber JK, Hofstetter CP. Comparison of full-endoscopic and minimally invasive decompression for lumbar spinal stenosis in the setting of degenerative scoliosis and spondylolisthesis. Neurosurg Focus. 2019;46(5):E16.
14. Rosomoff HL. Neural arch resection for lumbar spinal stenosis. Clin Orthop Relat Res. 1981;154:83–9.
15. Johnsson KE, Willner S, Johnsson K. Postoperative instability after decompression for lumbar spinal stenosis. Spine (Phila Pa 1976). 1986;11(2):107–10.
16. Lee CK. Lumbar spinal instability (olisthesis) after extensive posterior spinal decompression. Spine (Phila Pa 1976). 1983;8(4):429–33.
17. Young S, Veerapen R, O'Laoire SA. Relief of lumbar canal stenosis using multilevel subarticular fenestrations as an alternative to wide laminectomy: preliminary report. Neurosurgery. 1988;23(5):628–33.
18. Aryanpur J, Ducker T. Multilevel lumbar laminotomies for focal spinal stenosis: case report. Neurosurgery. 1988;23(1):111–5.
19. Poletti CE. Central lumbar stenosis caused by ligamentum flavum: unilateral laminotomy for bilateral ligamentectomy: preliminary report of two cases. Neurosurgery. 1995;37(2):343–7.
20. Spetzger U, Bertalanffy H, Naujokat C, von Keyserlingk DG, Gilsbach JM. Unilateral laminotomy for bilateral decompression of lumbar spinal stenosis. Part I: anatomical and surgical considerations. Acta Neurochir. 1997;139(5):392–6.
21. Spetzger U, Bertalanffy H, Reinges MH, Gilsbach JM. Unilateral laminotomy for bilateral decompression of lumbar spinal stenosis. Part II: clinical experiences. Acta Neurochir (Wien). 1997;139(5):397–403.
22. Guiot BH, Khoo LT, Fessler RG. A minimally invasive technique for decompression of the lumbar spine. Spine (Phila Pa 1976). 2002;27(4):432–8.
23. Komp M, Hahn P, Merk H, Godolias G, Ruetten S. Bilateral operation of lumbar degenerative central spinal stenosis in full-endoscopic interlaminar technique with unilateral approach: prospective 2-year results of 74 patients. J Spinal Disord Tech. 2011;24(5):281–7.
24. Soliman HM. Irrigation endoscopic decompressive laminotomy. A new endoscopic approach for spinal stenosis decompression. Spine J. 2015;15(10):2282–9.

25. Eun SS, Eum JH, Lee SH, Sabal LA. Biportal endoscopic lumbar decompression for lumbar disk herniation and spinal canal stenosis: a technical note. J Neurol Surg A Cent Eur Neurosurg. 2017;78(4):390–6.
26. Viejo-Fuertes D, Liguoro D, Rivel J, Midy D, Guerin J. Morphologic and histologic study of the ligamentum flavum in the thoraco-lumbar region. Surg Radiol Anat. 1998;20(3):171–6.
27. Olszewski AD, Yaszemski MJ, White AA 3rd. The anatomy of the human lumbar ligamentum flavum. New observations and their surgical importance. Spine (Phila Pa 1976). 1996;21(20):2307–12.
28. Chau AM, Pelzer NR, Hampton J, et al. Lateral extent and ventral laminar attachments of the lumbar ligamentum flavum: cadaveric study. Spine J. 2014;14(10):2467–71.
29. Iwanaga J, Ishak B, Saga T, et al. The lumbar ligamentum flavum does not have two layers and is confluent with the interspinous ligament: anatomical study with application to surgical and interventional pain procedures. Clin Anat. 2020;33(1):34–40.
30. Bresnahan LE, Smith JS, Ogden AT, et al. Assessment of paraspinal muscle cross-sectional area after lumbar decompression: minimally invasive versus open approaches. Clin Spine Surg. 2017;30(3):E162–8.
31. Storzer B, Schnake KJ. Microscopic bilateral decompression by unilateral approach in spinal stenosis. Eur Spine J. 2016;25(Suppl 2):270–1.
32. Heo DH, Quillo-Olvera J, Park CK. Can percutaneous biportal endoscopic surgery achieve enough canal decompression for degenerative lumbar stenosis? Prospective case-control study. World Neurosurg. 2018;120:e684–9.
33. Kim SK, Kang SS, Hong YH, Park SW, Lee SC. Clinical comparison of unilateral biportal endoscopic technique versus open microdiscectomy for single-level lumbar discectomy: a multicenter, retrospective analysis. J Orthop Surg Res. 2018;13(1):22.
34. Heo DH, Lee DC, Park CK. Comparative analysis of three types of minimally invasive decompressive surgery for lumbar central stenosis: biportal endoscopy, uniportal endoscopy, and microsurgery. Neurosurg Focus. 2019;46(5):E9.
35. Hwa Eum J, Hwa Heo D, Son SK, Park CK. Percutaneous biportal endoscopic decompression for lumbar spinal stenosis: a technical note and preliminary clinical results. J Neurosurg Spine. 2016;24(4):602–7.
36. Li C, Ju F, Li W, et al. Efficacy and safety of unilateral biportal endoscopy compared with microscopic decompression in the treatment of lumbar spinal stenosis: a protocol for systematic review and meta-analysis. Medicine (Baltimore). 2021;100(50):e27970.
37. Park SM, Park J, Jang HS, et al. Biportal endoscopic versus microscopic lumbar decompressive laminectomy in patients with spinal stenosis: a randomized controlled trial. Spine J. 2020;20(2):156–65.
38. Pao JL. A review of unilateral biportal endoscopic decompression for degenerative lumbar canal stenosis. Int J Spine Surg. 2021;15(suppl 3):S65–71.
39. Kim JE, Choi DJ, Park EJ. Risk factors and options of management for an incidental dural tear in biportal endoscopic spine surgery. Asian Spine J. 2020;14(6):790–800.
40. Lin GX, Chen CM, Kim JS, Song KS. The transformation of intracranial subdural hygroma to chronic subdural hematoma following endoscopic spinal surgery: a case report. J Neurol Surg A Cent Eur Neurosurg. 2021; https://doi.org/10.1055/s-0041-1723812.
41. Lee KH, Kim GL, Park J, Lee HB, Hong SY, Kim TH. Retinal hemorrhage and transient consciousness disturbance after biportal endoscopic lumbar discectomy: a case report and literature review [published online ahead of print, 2021 May 31]. J Orthop Sci. 2021. pii: S0949-2658(21)00150-0.

Chapter 17
The Unilateral Biportal Endoscopic Paraspinal Approach for Lumbar Foraminal Pathology

Javier Quillo-Olvera, Diego Quillo-Olvera, Javier Quillo-Reséndiz, and Michelle Barrera-Arreola

Abbreviations

BESS	Biportal endoscopic spinal surgery
Cau	Caudal
Cra	Cranial
CSF	Cerebrospinal fluid
CT	Computed tomography
ExF	Extraforaminal area
FL	Foraminal ligament
IAP	Inferior articular process
IONM	Intraoperative neuromonitoring
IST	Isthmus
Lat	Lateral
LFS	Lumbar foraminal stenosis
Med	Medial
MRI	Magnetic resonance imaging
NSAID	Nonsteroidal anti-inflammatory drug
RF	Radiofrequency
SAP	Superior articular process
TP	Transverse process

Supplementary Information The online version contains supplementary material available at [https://doi.org/10.1007/978-3-031-14736-4_17].

J. Quillo-Olvera (✉) · D. Quillo-Olvera · J. Quillo-Reséndiz · M. Barrera-Arreola
The Brain and Spine Care, Minimally Invasive Spine Surgery Group, Hospital H+ Querétaro, Spine Clinic, Querétaro, México
e-mail: neuroqomd@gmail.com; drquilloolvera86@gmail.com; kitnoz@hotmail.com; michelle.barrera@anahuac.mx

J. Quillo-Olvera et al. (eds.), *Unilateral Biportal Endoscopy of the Spine*,
https://doi.org/10.1007/978-3-031-14736-4_17

UBE	Unilateral biportal endoscopy
UBE-TLIF	Unilateral biportal endoscopic transforaminal lumbar interbody fusion
VAS	Visual analog scale

Introduction

Lumbar foraminal stenosis (LFS) is a common cause of compressive radiculopathy. It is estimated that the incidence of this lumbar degenerative pathology is 8–11%, with 75% of these cases from L5–S1 [1–3].

The narrowing lumbar foramen and the subsequent compression of the exiting nerve can cause symptoms of radicular pain. Even this pathology has been implicated as a cause of failed-back surgery syndrome when it goes unnoticed in diagnosing patients with lumbar spinal stenosis [4–6].

The age-related degeneration is admitted as a triggering factor for foraminal stenosis since the deterioration of the intervertebral disc will cause segmental instability in most cases, and hypermobility will be associated with thickening of foraminal soft tissues and facet hypertrophy, mainly of the superior articular process (SAP) [7]. These events will trigger radiculopathy symptoms eventually.

Conventional surgical options for treating lumbar foraminal stenosis may include open facetectomy with or without lumbar fusion or facet-sparing microforaminotomy. However, the more disruptive the facet joint is, the more risk of segmental instability and postoperative back pain will exist [1, 4, 8, 9].

The paraspinal route has been considered the gold standard for lumbar foraminal and extraforaminal lesions. This route was reported by Wiltse et al. [10] in 1968 and updated in 1988 by Wiltse and Spencer [11]. The anatomical principle of this approach is to use a corridor between the multifidus and longissimus muscle. Since then, it has been modified to be performed laterally between the longissimus and iliocostalis muscles to have more oblique access to the lateral aspect of the facet joint and the intervertebral disc.

The success rate reported for open paraspinal foraminotomies in different studies is 72–83%. However, the limited visibility through an open approach and intricate anatomy can lead to an incomplete decompression with unsatisfactory clinical results [2, 4, 12–18].

The optimization of visualization in spinal surgery improved with various tools. One was the microscope, but currently, the implementation of endoscopic lenses and the continuous irrigation of fluid during the procedure enhance the surgeon's visual experience, allowing a more targeted surgery [19].

In addition, spinal endoscopy has been associated with minimal damage to the paraspinal muscles, shorter hospital stay, reduced recovery times, and less intraoperative bleeding, and recently several studies have reported encouraging outcomes in patients who underwent unilateral biportal endoscopy (UBE) through a paraspinal approach for the treatment of foraminal stenosis at various levels of the lumbar spine [20–24]. This chapter summarizes the step-by-step biportal endoscopic paraspinal technique.

Relevant Anatomy

Although the paraspinal route is known to the spine surgeon, the way of looking at the anatomy is slightly different in biportal endoscopy than in an open or microsurgery, because in biportal endoscopy, we can use a 30° endoscope. Angulation of this lens will allow us to observe the structures of the foramen from a posterolateral perspective (Fig. 17.1).

There are three bone landmarks to guide the surgeon in biportal endoscopic transforaminal decompression through a paraspinal approach (Fig. 17.2):

1. Transverse and accessory process
2. Isthmus (IST)
3. Superior articular process (SAP)

The transverse and accessory processes are accurate references for the exiting nerve root. After drilling, the foraminal ligament can be identified (Fig. 17.3). In

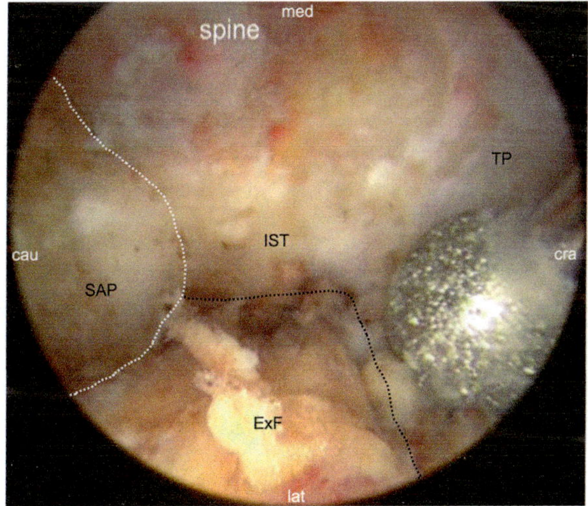

Fig. 17.1 UBE paraspinal approach for an L4–L5 right-sided decompressive foraminotomy. The SAP was outlined (white dotted line). The isthmus (IST) and transverse process (TP) are delineated by a black dotted line. *ExF* extraforaminal area, *Cau* caudal, *cra* cranial, *med* medial, *lat* lateral

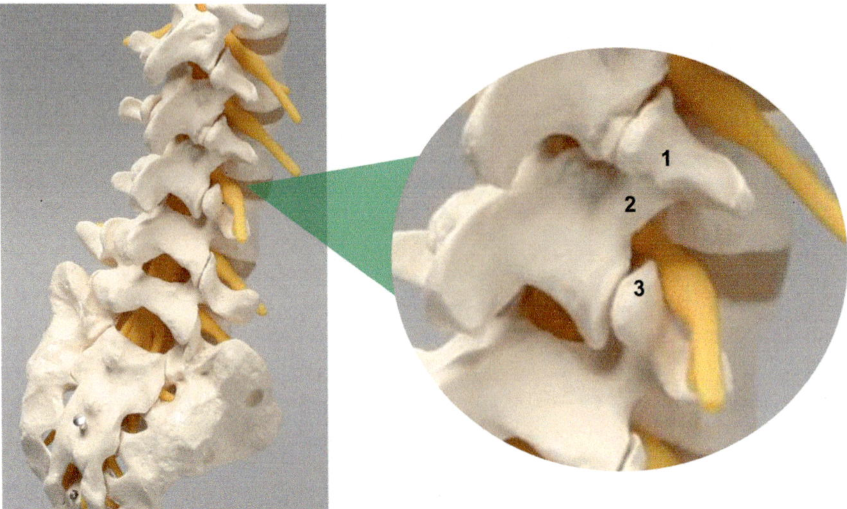

Fig. 17.2 Anatomical model of the lumbar spine showing the following: (1) transverse and accessory processes, (2) isthmus, (3) superior articular process (SAP)

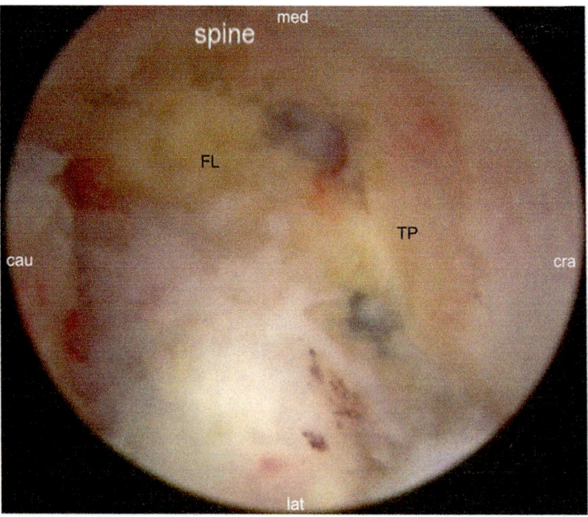

Fig. 17.3 Intraoperative view with a 30° angulated lens. The lateral aspect of the isthmus was drilled out, and the foraminal ligament (FL) has been exposed. The inferior edge of the transverse process (TP) was also removed

addition, the lateral aspect of the SAP can also be prepared for a more ventral decompression, respecting the isthmus.

The trans-isthmus approach is also precise for the exiting nerve root and has the advantage of immediate access to the SAP tip. Therefore, we can remove it if the case requires it.

The trans-SAP approach has also been described for uniportal endoscopy [25]. Here, the ventral aspect of the SAP is removed to decompress the lateral recess and

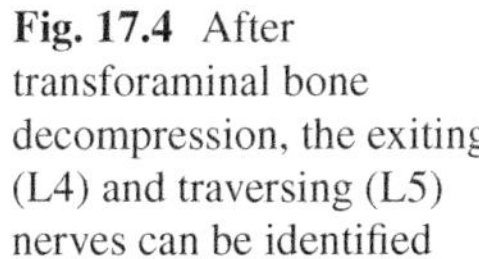

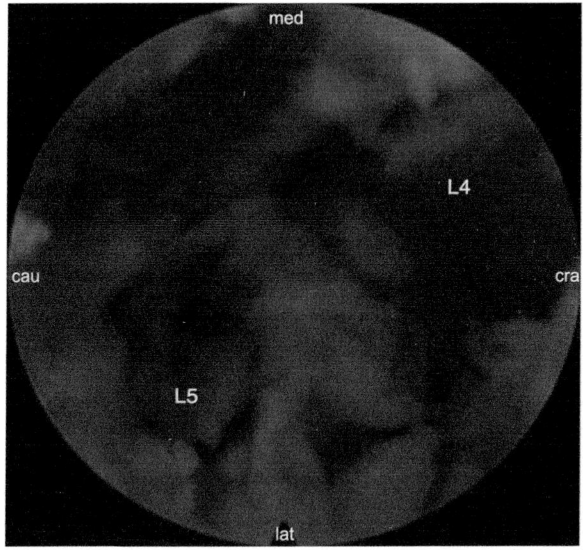

Fig. 17.4 After transforaminal bone decompression, the exiting (L4) and traversing (L5) nerves can be identified

the traversing nerve root. Furthermore, this landmark is used for biportal endoscopic lumbar transforaminal fusion (UBE-TLIF) [26].

The neural elements (Fig. 17.4) are the final landmarks that confirm decompression and surgical endpoint. The free mobilization of the exiting nerve root, in addition to the pulse of the traversing nerve, ensures adequate decompression.

Indications and Contraindications

The following are indications for UBE paraspinal approach:

1. Lumbar foraminal stenosis (LFS)
2. Lumbar extraforaminal degenerative pathology (extraforaminal lumbar disc herniation)
3. Far-lateral degenerative pathologies (far-lateral lumbar disc herniation, far-out syndrome at L5–S1)
4. Biportal endoscopic transforaminal lumbar interbody fusion
5. Symptomatic lumbar facet joint syndrome (biportal endoscopic facet medial branch rhizotomy)
6. Revision surgery requiring a paraspinal entry (repositioning transpedicular screws under direct biportal endoscopic vision, foraminal restenosis in a fused segment, and foraminal stenosis due to adjacent segment disease)

Contraindications

1. Segmental instability
2. Bilateral foraminal stenosis (however, if the patient is elderly with high-risk comorbidities and pure both-sided radiculopathy, a trial with paraspinal UBE foraminal decompression can be performed)
3. Mild symptoms that respond to conservative measures
4. Systemic conditions such as infection, tumor, or trauma require other reasonable treatments

Surgical Procedure

Step 1: Patient Positioning and Anesthesia

The patient is placed prone on an abdominal support frame to enable venous return and indirectly reduce epidural venous congestion. The use of IONM is at the surgeon's discretion, but anesthetic considerations should be taken into account if it is used. Anesthesia can be general, epidural, or sedation with local anesthesia. The surgeon is sided ipsilateral to the pathology. A regular workout for sterile patient cleaning and drape is done (Fig. 17.5).

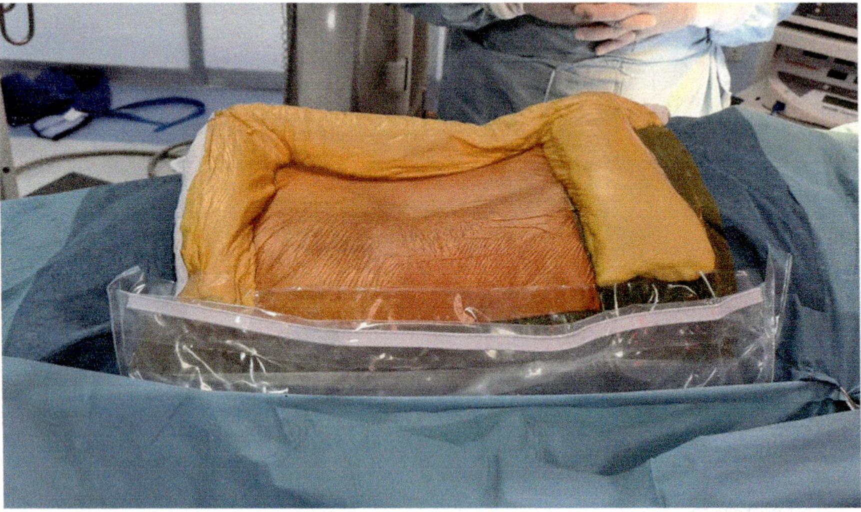

Fig. 17.5 Patient draped before starting the surgical procedure

Step 2: Entry Point Planning

It is advisable to orient yourself with bone anatomical landmarks. Therefore, identifying the midline, the lateral pedicle line, and the index level's interpedicular area is the first step (Fig. 17.6) to mark the entry points.

In the right paraspinal approach, the cranial incision will be used by right-handed surgeons to create the working channel while the caudal one for the endoscope. On the left side, this will be the opposite. According to the original description of the paraspinal approach reported by Wiltse [10, 11], intermuscular dissection is performed between the multifidus and longissimus muscle. For this reason, the incisions can be planned 1 cm lateral to the external pedicle line. A distance of 3 cm is left between both skin incisions to properly triangulate the biportal endoscopic approach (Fig. 17.7a). The extraforaminal area can be accessed through this paraspinal approach, and it is usually convenient for cases in L5–S1.

However, other cases require more lateral access, including between the longissimus and the iliocostalis muscles. In this situation, the entry points can be planned similarly but 3–4 cm lateral to the lateral pedicle line (Fig. 17.7b). This more lateral entry will allow the surgeon to work ventral with the facet joint (Fig. 17.8). In the patient, the planning will be carried out with orthogonal projections in AP and lateral of the fluoroscope.

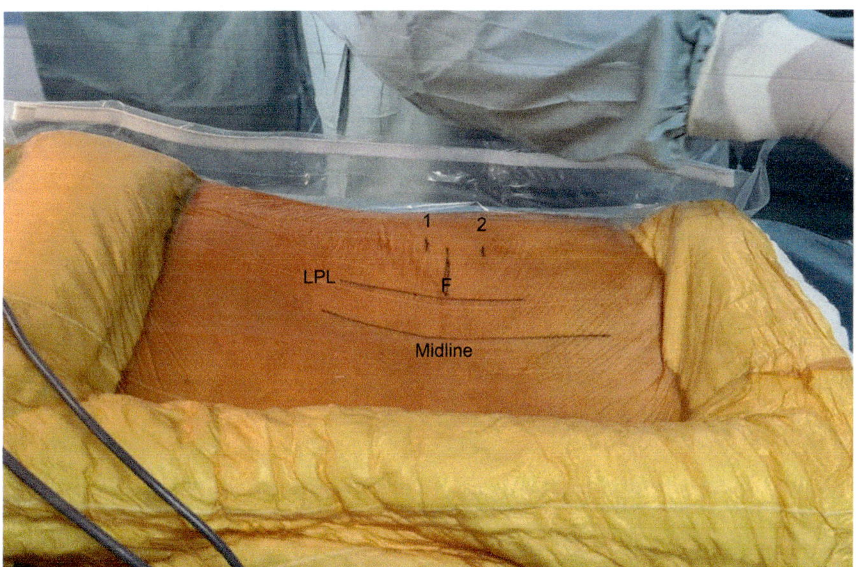

Fig. 17.6 Guided lines marked in the surgical field on the right side. Midline, lateral pedicular line (LPL), index-level foramen (F), and skin entries (1, 2)

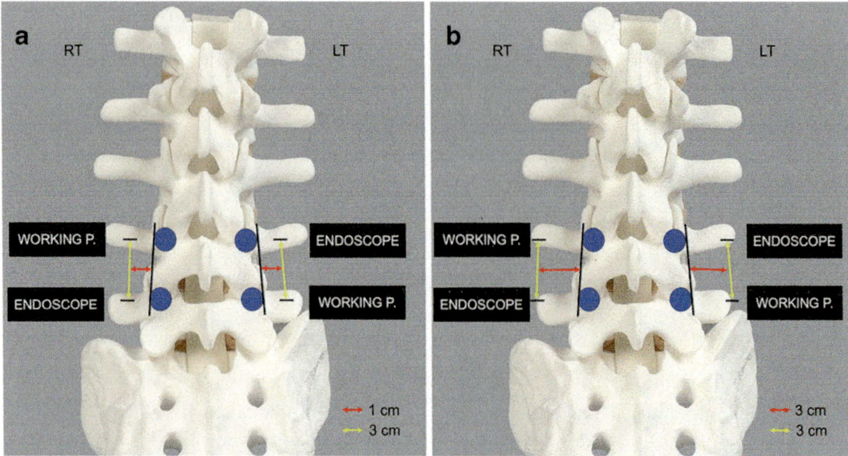

Fig. 17.7 Anatomical model of the lumbar region exemplifying the accesses in the biportal endoscopic paraspinal approach. (**a**) The approach was planned 1 cm lateral to the external pedicle line. (**b**) Planning done 3 cm lateral to the external pedicle line. The blue circles represent the pedicles at the index level. The bi-arrow red line is the lateral distance, while the yellow represents the distance between the skin incisions

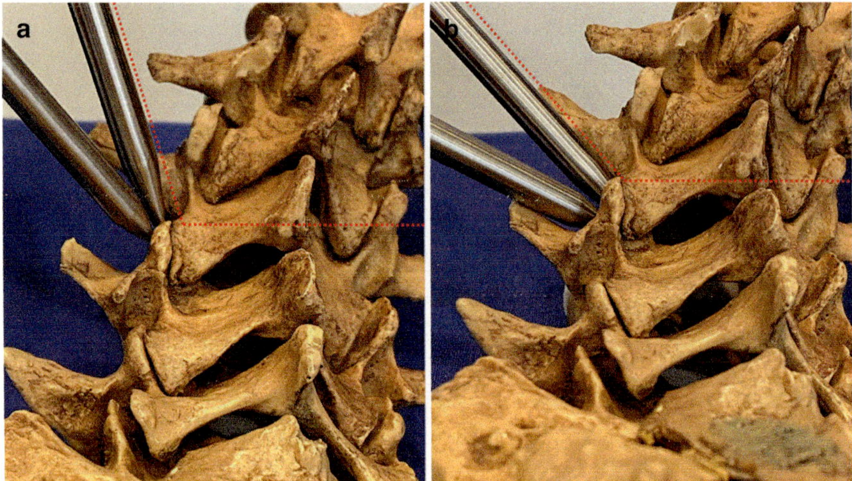

Fig. 17.8 Different paraspinal entries in the anatomical model. (**a**) Medial paraspinal. (**b**) Lateral paraspinal. The dotted red lines represent the angulation of both concerning the horizontal plane

Step 3: Triangular Paraspinal Approach

After the entry points have been rightly planned, a pair of approximately 6–8 mm transverse incisions will be made. The thoracolumbar fascia must also be adequately incised to facilitate the outflow of irrigated fluid during the procedure.

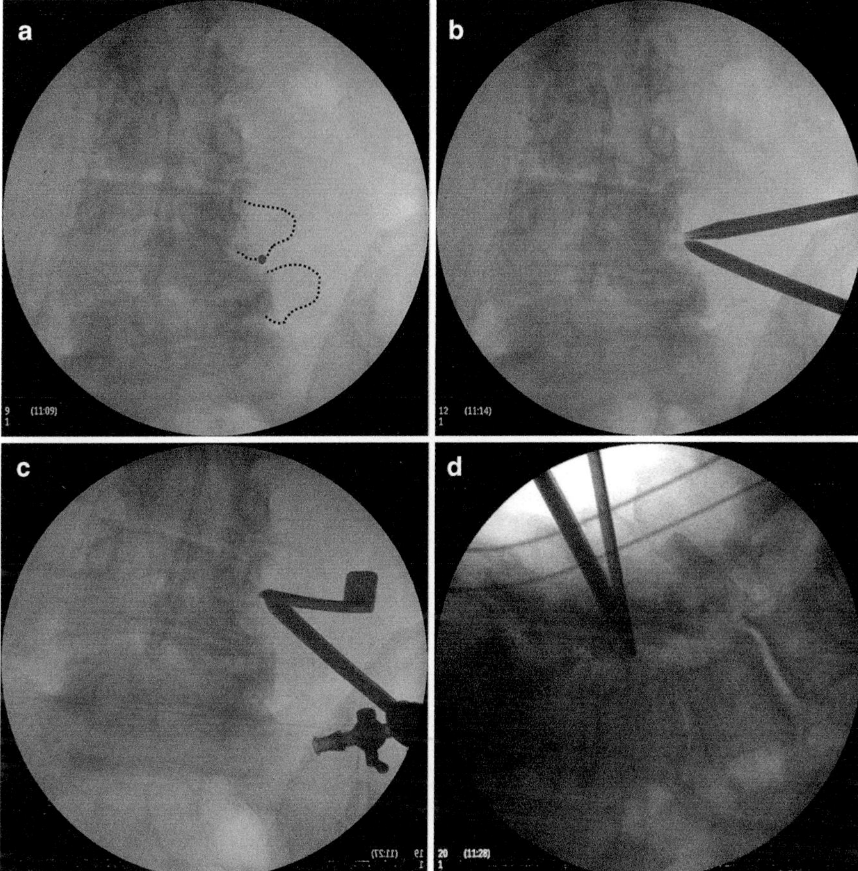

Fig. 17.9 Unilateral biportal endoscopic L4–L5 paraspinal approach on the right side addressed to the L4 transverse process. (**a**) Lumbar AP view. The black dotted lines represent the L4 and L5 transverse processes. The red circle is the target. (**b**) Both dilators were docked in the lower edge of the L4 transverse process. (**c**) Both ports were created: the working channel and the endoscope port. (**d**) The lateral view of the C-arm confirmed the triangular approach docked in the lower edge of the L4 transverse process

Subsequently, the dilators will be introduced. The dilation sequence includes introducing the dilator first to create the working channel and addressing it to the chosen bone landmark to start the approach. This landmark can be the index level's accessory or upper transverse process, the isthmus, or the SAP. The authors perform this step with progressive dilation of 6–8 mm. Then, a semi-tubular, customized working sheet is inserted along the dilator. Next, the endoscopic port is created similarly, but it will be addressed to the working sheet. This maneuver makes it possible to triangulate both ports simply and safely. This process is confirmed by AP and lateral views of the C-arm (Fig. 17.9). Then, the endoscope will be introduced, the working instrument will be located in the surgical field, and the bone landmark will be identified. Before starting the endoscopic procedure, the surgeon must always confirm the proper inflow and outflow of continuous irrigation.

Step 4: Identifying the Bone Landmarks

The biportal endoscopic procedure begins by creating a workspace. This step involves removing the soft tissue adhered to the bone surfaces to identify them. Next, the surgeon can use the radiofrequency (RF) probe and pituitary forceps for the same purpose. After surgical field clearance, the bony landmarks such as the lower part of the transverse process, the isthmus, or the tip of the SAP can be identified (Fig. 17.10).

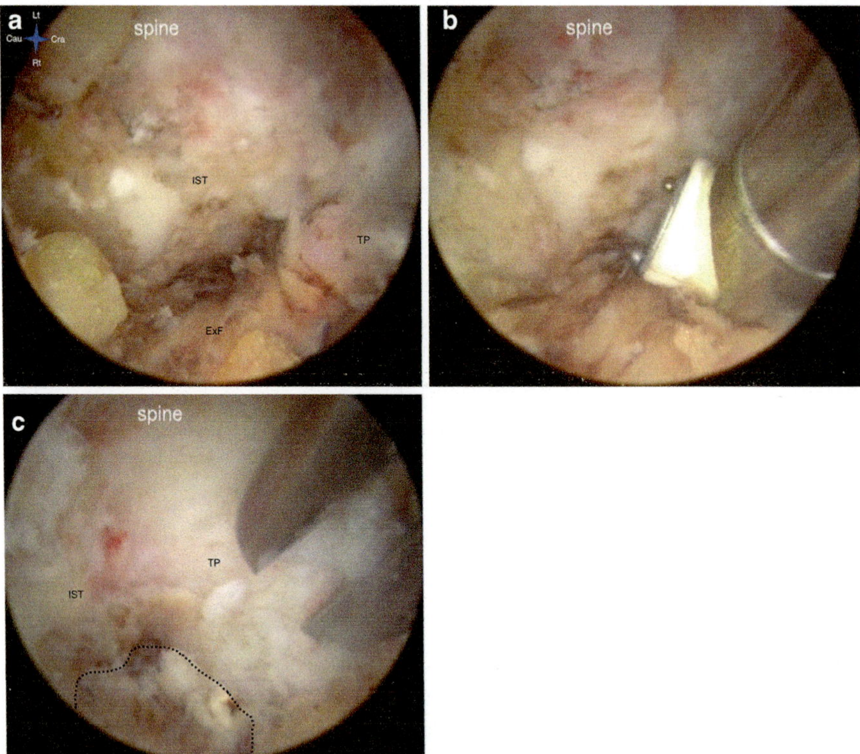

Fig. 17.10 Sequence to identify bone landmarks in the biportal endoscopic paraspinal approach addressed to the isthmus on the right side. (**a**) Intraoperative image through the endoscope showing soft tissue over the bone landmarks. (**b**) Use of the RF probe in the surgical field. (**c**) Clean surgical field with clear bone landmarks outlined by a black dotted line. *Cra* cranial, *Cau* caudal, *Rt* right, *Lt* lateral, *IST* isthmus, *TP* transverse process, *ExF* extraforaminal area

Step 5: Bone Decompression

This procedure aims to enlarge the foramen and decompress the exiting nerve. That is why extraforaminal injuries such as herniated discs or bone spurs impinging the nerve are suitable for paraspinal biportal endoscopy.

The surgeon will use various surgical tools such as a drill with a 3 mm diamond tip, chisels, and Kerrison rongeur of different sizes and angles to remove the bone. Bone removal can include the lower part of the transverse process, from medial to lateral. However, transverse process dimensions could be considerable, and sometimes depth drilling is needed; this aims to detach the cranial part of the foraminal ligament. The lateral aspect of the isthmus can be removed until identifying the proximal attachment of the foraminal ligament.

The SAP can be observed posteriorly with a steeper paraspinal oblique view, or its lateral aspect can be identified with a more shallow trajectory. The surgeon could remove the tip of the SAP or its ventral aspect depending on the surgery goals. After proper bone removal, the following landmark to identify is the foraminal ligament (FL). This anatomical structure should be preserved during bone decompression since it acts like a barrier protecting the exiting nerve. Therefore, after bone removal, the foraminal ligament exposed is removed (Fig. 17.11).

Step 6: Release of the Exiting Nerve

After exposing the foraminal ligament, direct decompression of the exiting nerve can be concluded by removing the ligament mentioned above. However, sometimes other components that cause ventral compression of the nerve can be found. For example, we can have a herniated disc or ventral osteophytes that must be removed so that the exiting nerve can be mobilized without restriction. The surgeon can perform these maneuvers with chisels, drill with a diamond tip, and pituitary forceps. Subsequently, the adequate mobilization of the nerve root will be confirmed, and finally, it is possible to leave a drain in the area of the foraminotomy to prevent an epidural hematoma. Then, the skin incisions can be closed with a single stitch, and the procedure can be concluded (Fig. 17.12).

A resume of the stepwise technique can be found in Table 17.1.

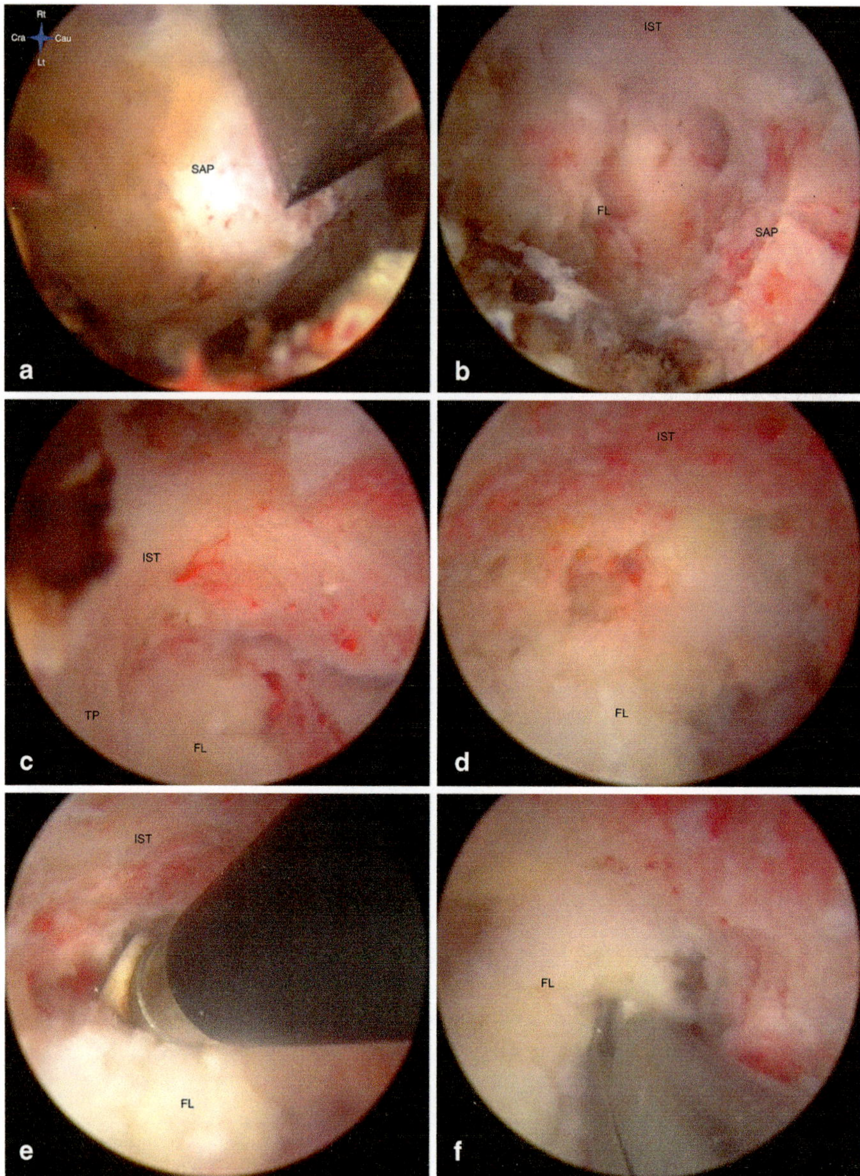

Fig. 17.11 Sequence of bone decompression during a paraspinal endoscopic biportal foraminotomy addressed to the tip of SAP at L4–L5 on the left side. (**a**) The SAP has been exposed, and the tip will be removed with a chisel. (**b**) The tip of the SAP has been removed, and its base is showing (SAP). The lateral surface of the isthmus (IST) and the proximal part of the foraminal ligament (FL) can be observed. (**c**) Foraminal ligament (FL) exposed. (**d**) The base of the transverse process has been removed, and the cranial attachment of the foraminal ligament (FL) is observed. (**e**) Foraminal ligament (FL) detached. (**f**) Foraminal ligament removal with curved Kerrison punch. *Cra* cranial, *Cau* caudal, *Rt* right, *Lt* left, *SAP* superior articular process, *IST* isthmus, *FL* foraminal ligament, *TP* transverse process

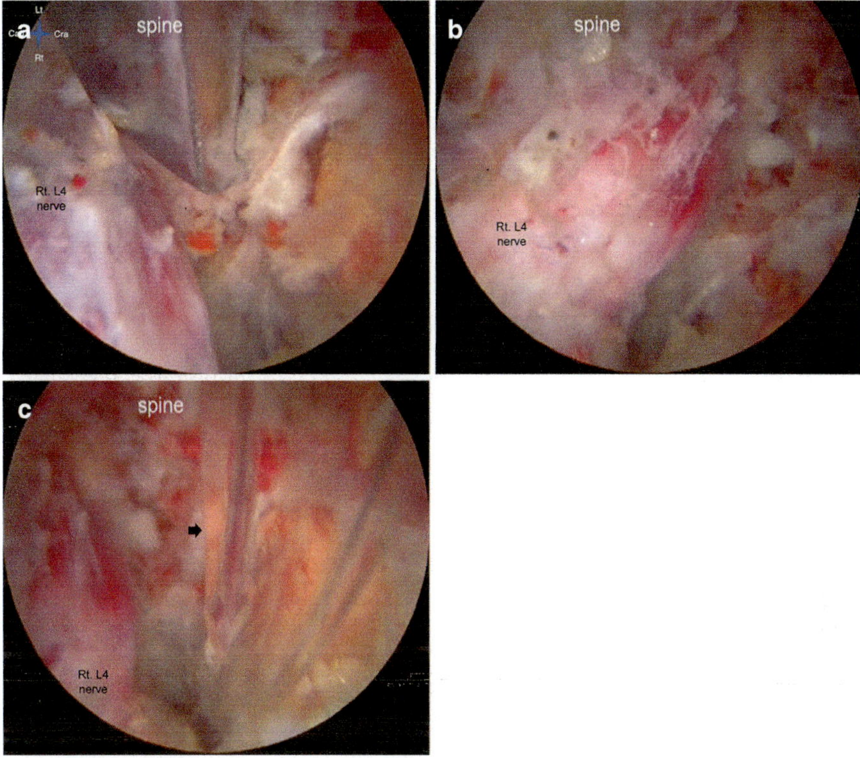

Fig. 17.12 Realizing the exiting nerve root at L4–L5 on the right side through a paraspinal biportal endoscopic foraminotomy. (**a**) A small angulated-tip chisel has been introduced to remove a bony spur ventrally. (**b**) The nerve has been decompressed and released. (**c**) An epidural drain is left (black arrow)

Table 17.1 Summary of paraspinal unilateral biportal endoscopic (UBE) approach

1. Identify the pedicles and transverse processes of the index level
2. There are two trajectories: (a) Wiltse paraspinal approach (multifidus—longissimus) (b) Modified extraforaminal approach (longissimus—iliocostalis)
3. Incisions: 1.5–2 cm lateral to the pedicles as usual Wiltse trajectory or 4 cm in a modified far-lateral Wiltse approach
4. Both sides: Address the dilator to the starting bone reference: (a) Transverse process—isthmic junction: address superior foraminal area (b) SAP (dorsal or lateral aspect) (c) SAP base—transverse process junction (UBE-TLIF)
5. The viewing incision could be located 3 cm far from the working channel incision. Address the dilator to the same landmark independently and meet with the first dilator (working channel dilator)
6. Introduce the complete system

UBE-TLIF unilateral biportal endoscopic transforaminal lumbar interbody fusion

Illustrated Cases

Case 1

A 76-year-old male with a history of multiple myeloma in remission and chronic mild sciatic pain treated by several foraminal blocks at L5–S1 on the left side complained of severe (VAS 10/10) electric shock-type pain radiating down his left leg. Neurologic examination demonstrated left-leg claudication at the beginning of the walking and paresthesia in the lateral aspect of the left calf. In addition, a decreased strength in left-ankle dorsiflexion (3/5) was noted. Preoperative imaging studies demonstrated severe foraminal stenosis at L5–S1 on the left side (Fig. 17.13). After signed informed consent, the patient underwent a paraspinal unilateral biportal endoscopic (UBE) foraminal decompression. The procedure started creating a working space in the extraforaminal area. A 30° arthroscope and standard surgical tools for the lumbar spine were used. The paraspinal approach addressed the left L5 transverse process (TP).

Then, craniocaudal decompression was performed. First, the base of TP was drilled out until the foraminal ligament (FL) was reached. After that, the lateral surface and the tip of the SAP were removed. Next, the FL was cleared and the L5 exiting nerve exposed. The SAP bone spurs were also removed with chisels. Finally, a complete decompression of the L5 exiting nerve root was confirmed through the endoscope (Fig. 17.14) (Video 17.1). The lumbar spine's immediate postoperative MRI and CT scan showed sufficient bone removal (Fig. 17.15). The patient was discharged one day after surgery. The pain improved to VAS 1/10 immediately, and on day 14 of the follow-up, the strength in the left-ankle dorsiflexion improved to 4/5. No claudication was noted after surgery.

Case 2

A 68-year-old woman complained of severe (8/10) radicular pain in her right leg. She also complains of severe numbness in the right leg and claudication during walking. In addition, the neurologic examination demonstrated decreased patellar

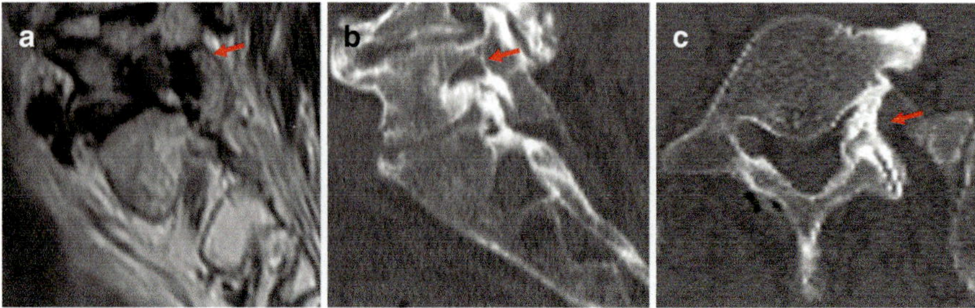

Fig. 17.13 Preoperative imaging studies from Case 1. (**a**) Sagittal view of lumbar MRI showing foraminal stenosis at L5–S1 on the left side (red arrow). (**b**, **c**) The lumbar CT scan confirmed the pathology (red arrow)

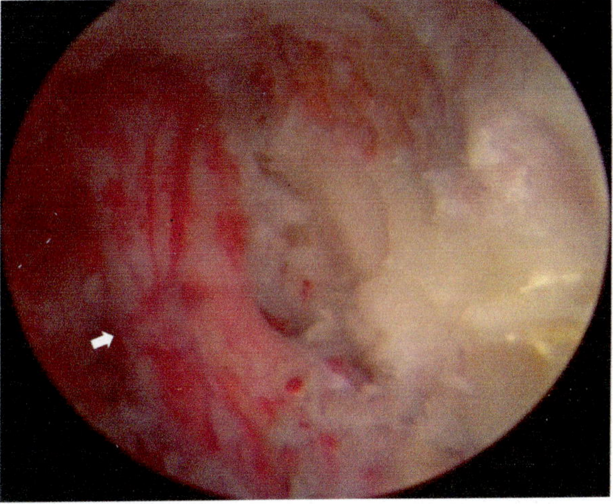

Fig. 17.14 Intraoperative image through the endoscope showing the left L5 exiting nerve (white arrow) decompressed

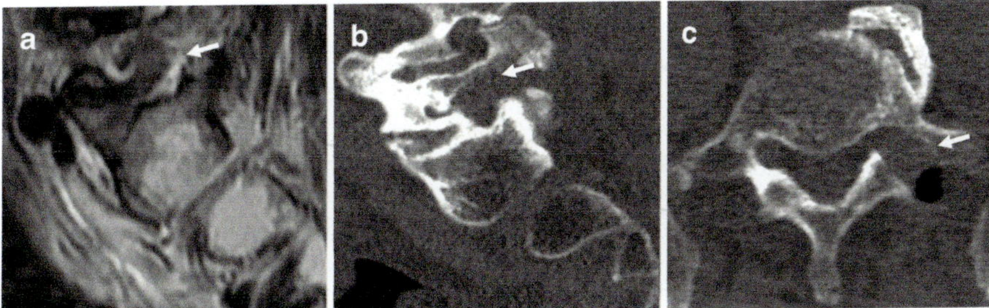

Fig. 17.15 Postoperative imaging studies from Case 1. (**a**) Sagittal view of lumbar MRI. The white arrow points to the enlarged foraminal area at L5–S1 on the left side after paraspinal UBE foraminotomy. (**b**, **c**) The lumbar CT scan shows the bone removal (white arrows) achieved

and Achillean reflexes on the right side. Hypoesthesia in the calf and dorsal surface of the right foot was noted. The preoperative lumbar MRI revealed foraminal and subarticular (lateral recess) degenerative stenosis at L4–L5 on the right side (Fig. 17.16). A right L4–L5 paraspinal approach with the UBE technique was planned (Video 17.2). Both transverse processes (TP) of L4–L5 were identified during the surgery. Then, the drilling started on the lateral surface of the SAP. First, the tip and medial aspect of the SAP were removed with a diamond burr tip. Then, the base of the L4 TP was drilling out. After bone removal of mentioned anatomical landmarks, the foraminal ligament was observed. Undercutting the facet joint was necessary for decompressing the lateral recess at L4–L5. Finally, the traversing L5 nerve root and the L4 exiting nerve on the right side were directly decompressed (Fig. 17.17). The patient was discharged on the next day of the surgery with minimal analgesia, paracetamol, and an NSAID. The pain and numbness on the right leg improved to VAS 0/10 immediately after surgery. The postoperative lumbar MRI

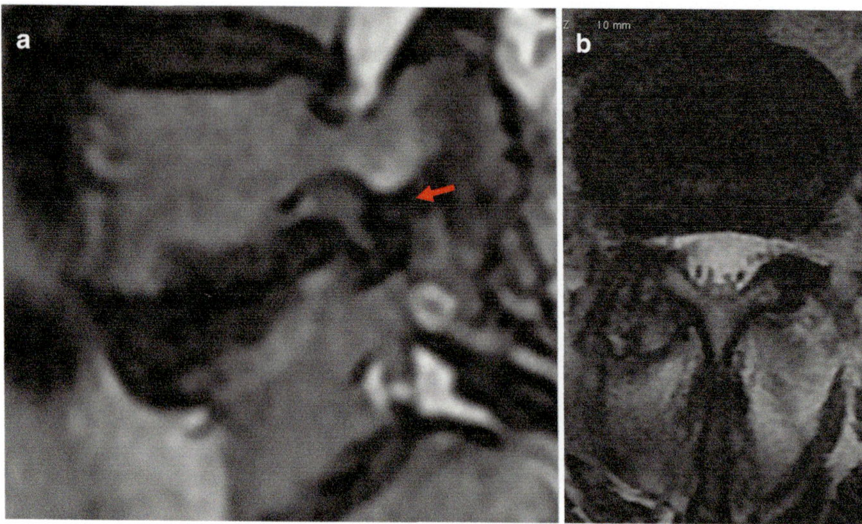

Fig. 17.16 Preoperative lumbar MRI from Case 2. (**a**) The sagittal view shows severe foraminal stenosis at L4–L5 on the right side (red arrow). (**b**) Significant facet joint degeneration and lateral recess stenosis at L4–L5 on the right side are observed in the axial view

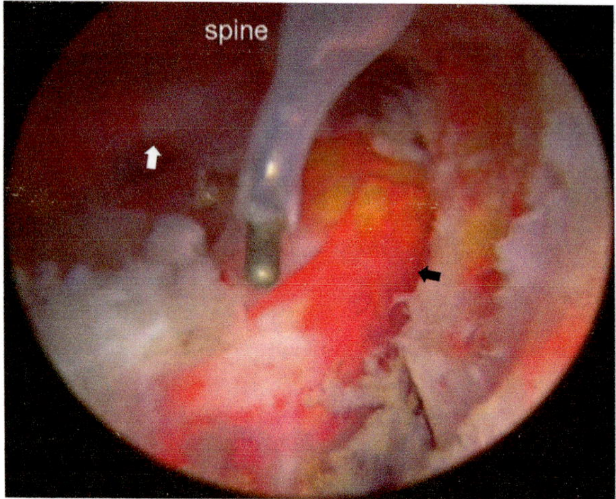

Fig. 17.17 Intraoperative image through the endoscope. The white arrow points to the Rt. L5 traversing nerve, while the black arrow shows the Rt. L4 exiting nerve

showed sufficient decompression of the foramen and lateral recess of L4–L5 on the right side (Fig. 17.18).

Case 3

A 48-year-old male complained of severe pain (VAS 9/10) in the left leg, radiating from the buttock to the calf. The pain is electric shock type and is associated with numbness and claudication of the impaired leg—history of lumbar surgery 3 years

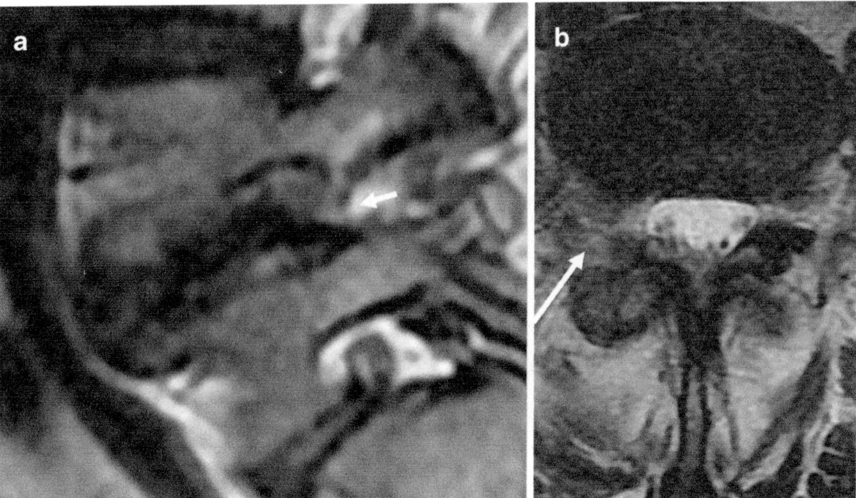

Fig. 17.18 Postoperative lumbar MRI from Case 2. (**a**) Enlarged foraminal area (white arrow) is observed in the sagittal view at L4–L5 on the right side. (**b**) The trajectory of the approach is represented by the white arrow. Undercutting of the facet joint is observed on the right side

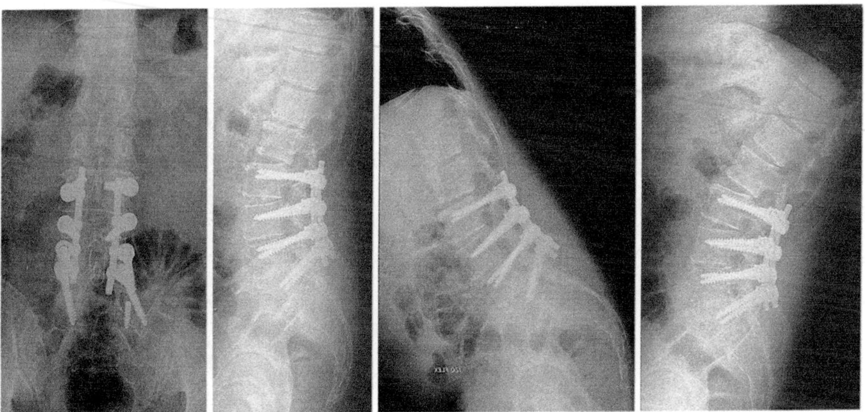

Fig. 17.19 Preoperative lumbar X-ray films of Case 3

ago with transpedicular fixation of L2–L5. Neurological examination revealed decreased strength in dorsiflexion of the left ankle and left great toe (4/5). In addition, the left Achillean reflex was absent. X-rays of the lumbar spine show instability at L1–L2 due to adjacent segment disease. In S1 on the left side, a broken screw was observed, and an interspinous stabilization was also in L4–L5 (Fig. 17.19). In the preoperative lumbar MRI, significant foraminal stenosis at L5–S1 on the left side was noted (Fig. 17.20). While the lumbar spine CT demonstrated left L5–S1 foraminal stenosis due to heterotopic ossification within the foramen (Fig. 17.21). It

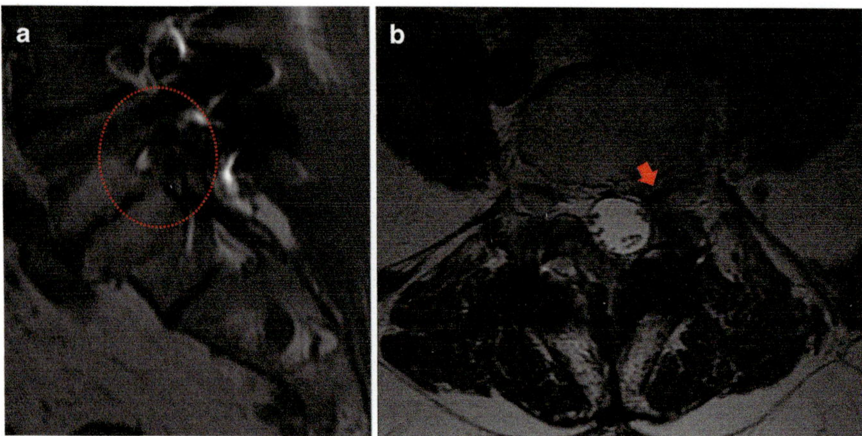

Fig. 17.20 Preoperative lumbar MRI of Case 3. (**a**) The sagittal view at L5–S1 shows foraminal stenosis on the left side (red dotted circle). (**b**) The red arrow points to the nerve entrapment in its course through the foramen at L5–S1 on the left side in the axial view

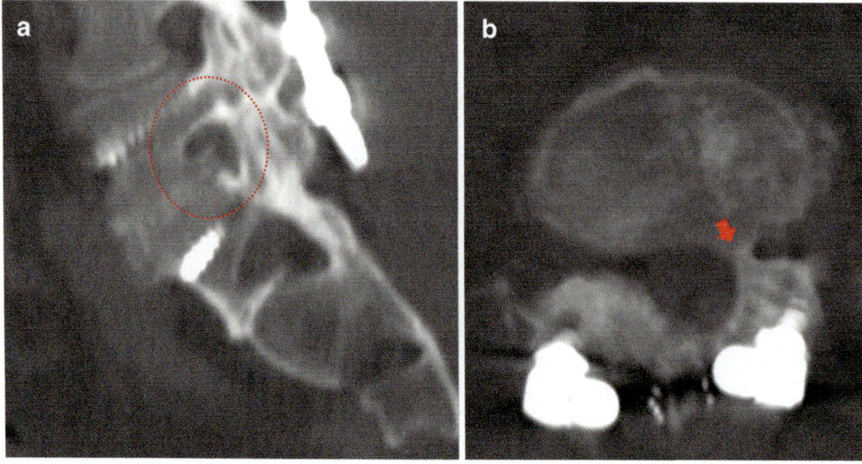

Fig. 17.21 Preoperative lumbar CT of Case 3. (**a**) An osteophyte within the L5–S1 left foramen is observed on the sagittal view. (**b**) A heterotopic bone within the foramen can be noted on the left foraminal space at L5–S1 (red arrow)

was decided to perform a biportal endoscopic foraminotomy through a left paraspinal approach at L5–S1. It was possible to remove the heterotopic bone formation in the foramen during surgery and decompress the exiting L5 nerve root on the left side (Fig. 17.22). Satisfactory foraminal decompression was accomplished and demonstrated on immediate postoperative lumbar spine CT (Fig. 17.23). The patient improved his pain (VAS 0/10) immediately after surgery. The weakness in the left ankle and big toe of the left foot improved 1 month after surgery.

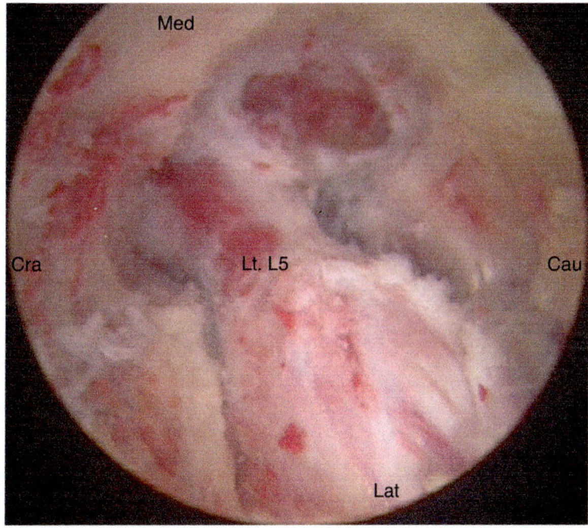

Fig. 17.22 Intraoperative view through the endoscope. The L5 exiting nerve root is in the center of the image after complete decompression

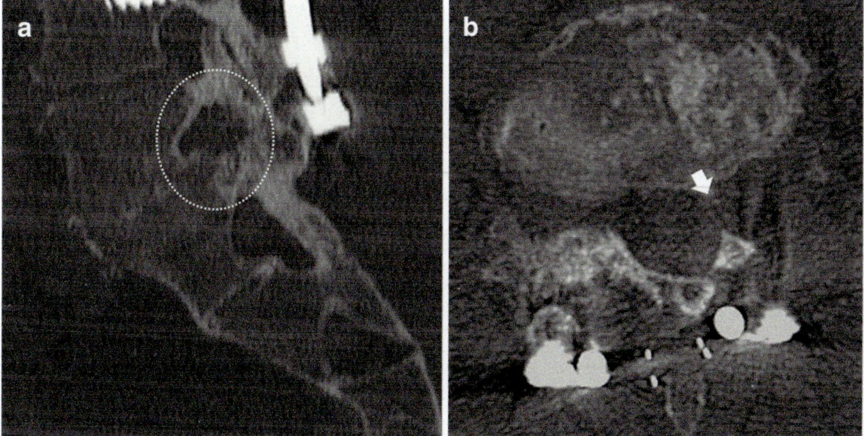

Fig. 17.23 The immediate postoperative lumbar CT of Case 3. (**a**) The osteophyte was removed (white circle), and it is shown in the left-sided foraminal space at L5–S1 on the sagittal view. (**b**) The axial view demonstrated enough decompression at L5–S1 on the left side (white arrow)

Discussion

The indications for biportal endoscopic spine surgery (BESS) have expanded since De Antoni et al. [27] in 1996 described the procedure to remove soft lumbar disc herniation at a single level. However, it should be noted that from the beginning, the authors of this manuscript identified advantages associated with the use of biportal endoscopy in the spine, such as the ability to explore the epidural space and remove extruded or intradiscal disc fragments under outstanding visualization thanks to the use of an arthroscope with continuous fluid irrigation throughout the procedure. It can allow easier identifying of the anatomy and driving of a safer surgery.

However, there is an advantage that the authors noted since 1996 and that laid the foundations for other approaches: "The potential to complement the paralateral spinal endoscopic technique and thereby increase the power of and indications for minimally invasive spine surgery" [27]. That meant the possibility of planning other routes through biportal endoscopy.

This chapter has detailed how to perform lumbar foraminal decompressions through a paraspinal route using the biportal endoscopic technique. However, the spine surgeon must first determine a lumbar foraminal injury and treat it later.

Lee et al. [28], in 1988, classified the LFS in three areas according to the location of narrowing. The first is the entrance zone, the most cephalad part of the lateral lumbar canal, and is located medial to or underneath the superior articular process. This zone has only anterior and posterior walls—the posterior surface of the disc bordered anteriorly and posteriorly the facet joint. The neural structure contained in this zone is the lumbar nerve root covered by the dura. The mid-zone is located under the pars interarticularis and below the pedicle. The anterior border is the posterior wall of the vertebral body. The posterior border is the pars. The neural structure in this zone is the dorsal root ganglion and ventral motor nerve root covered by fibrous connective tissue extension of the dura. The exit zone is the area surrounding the intervertebral foramen. The posterior border is the lateral aspect of the facet joint. The anterior wall is the disc. The neural structure contained here is the exiting nerve covered by perineurium.

An MRI-based LFS classification determines the severity of narrowing as follows: grade 0 or a normal foramen; grade 1 or mild foraminal stenosis refers to fat obliteration in two opposing directions; in grade 2 or moderate foraminal stenosis, there is fat obliteration in four directions; and in grade 3 or severe foraminal stenosis, morphological changes are already found in the exiting nerve root [29].

Something concerning about lumbar foraminotomy is the possibility of developing segmental instability. Although studies warn of postoperative increased segmental motion after removing between 50% and 75% of the facet joint, others report the same finding with a total facetectomy [30–33].

However, it is crucial to clarify that a complete facetectomy is not performed in a biportal endoscopic lumbar foraminotomy through a paraspinal route. The SAP is removed only in its most cephalic or ventral portion, the inferior articular process in its most ventral part, and the pars only in its most lateral aspect. Therefore, the intention to perform a total facetectomy is not considered. For this reason, iatrogenic instability after a biportal endoscopic foraminotomy through a paraspinal approach is not common; however, it is also important to note that there are no biomechanical or long-term studies that demonstrate this possible iatrogenic side effect in UBE.

Various clinical studies [22, 24, 34] have reported encouraging outcomes after biportal endoscopic lumbar foraminotomy. Kim et al. [22] retrospectively studied

31 patients diagnosed with foraminal stenosis and treated with a biportal endoscopic foraminotomy. In this study, the authors used 0° and 30° endoscopes. They reported that 50% of the SAP was removed in all subjects. From 31 patients included in the study, 14 were male and 17 females, with a mean age of 70.5 ± 8.9 years (range, 51–89 years), and the mean follow-up was 14.8 ± 1.6 months. The back pain was assessed by VAS score, and it improved from 5.13 ± 0.8 preoperatively to 1.52 ± 1.02 at the annual follow-up. The same was noted after comparing the VAS for leg pain. It improved from 7.87 ± 0.88 preoperatively to 1.45 ± 1.28 at 1 year of follow-up; 80% of the patients reported improvement according to the Macnab criteria. Of those with clinical improvement, 42% reported excellent results, 39% good, 13% fair, and 6% poor. No complications were reported, and only 1 patient with lithic spondylolisthesis experienced a recurrence of the symptoms requiring lumbar fusion. The authors also informed that no definite postoperative instability occurred or progressed in this study at the last follow-up. It could be associated with less muscle and ligament destruction through minimally invasive techniques such as UBE.

Another study carried out by Ahn et al. [24] included 21 patients (10 men and 11 women) and 27 treated segments. The patients presented foraminal lesions and were treated using the paraspinal UBE approach. The authors also used 0° and 30° endoscopes. 52.4% of the patients were diagnosed with foraminal stenosis, 42.8% with herniated discs with or without stenosis, and only 4.8% with adjacent segment disease. The mean age of the patients was 64.2 ± 10.7 years. The mean follow-up was 14.8 ± 2.96 months. The clinical outcomes reported by the authors included VAS for leg pain that decreased from 7.5 ± 0.9 preoperatively to 2.5 ± 1.2 at the last follow-up. According to Macnab criteria, an 80.9% satisfaction rate was obtained, from which 5 patients reported excellent, 12 good, and 4 fair results. The authors reported a dural tear in a single patient managed with shielding material and fibrin glue. No CSF leakage was seen later.

Regarding the use of 0° or 30° angulated arthroscopes for paraspinal UBE lumbar foraminotomy, a study by Kim and Choi [34] with 12 patients treated for L5–S1 foraminal stenosis with a 30° angled lens pointed out that the advantage of using this type of arthroscopy, particularly in L5–S1 or for intraforaminal lesions, is the perception of a more profound or lateral image obtained when the arthroscope is rotated, allowing to see deeper into the foramen.

Therefore, the advantages associated with the UBE paraspinal approach for lumbar foraminotomy can be summarized as follows:

1. Unlike open surgery, microsurgery, or tubular surgery, where the depth to work is challenging, biportal endoscopy is a targeted technique, so the depth of the approach is not relevant because the surgeon is working precisely on the target.
2. The imaging quality is superior to that obtained in open surgery or even through the microscope. In biportal endoscopy, the game-changer is the continuous irrigation of fluid throughout the procedure leading to a better illumination of the surgical field, and the magnification of the anatomy is outstanding. These advantages give accuracy to the endoscopic procedure.

3. Unlike uniportal endoscopy, in biportal endoscopic surgery, we use the working instrument in a port independent from the viewing channel. Therefore, our surgical tools have no motion restriction compared with full endoscopy, where any device must pass through the integrated endoscopic working channel in the same trajectory of the endoscope. For this reason, less manipulation to the exiting nerve root can be expected with the UBE technique.
4. Another advantage observed in UBE is that the triangular approach is a floating technique; we do not require to dock any working cannula into the foramen. For example, in full endoscopy, a bevel-ending-tip cannula anchored into a narrowing foramen could damage the exiting nerve or the dorsal root ganglion, causing dysesthesia. We do not expect this in UBE.
5. Reaching the L5–S1 foraminal and extraforaminal spaces is feasible through biportal endoscopic surgery because a more vertical approach is performed with UBE. That trajectory can overcome the iliac crest. In addition, the use of conventional surgical tools such as chisels and curettes allows for overcoming bone barriers such as the transverse process or the sacral ala.

Tips, Pearls, and Pitfalls

- Be aware of the intertransverse space and muscles since it is the edge of the retroperitoneal area.
- It is imperative to plan and locate the entry points to create the viewing and working ports; therefore, the radiological anatomy through the C-arm must be clear. In addition, the location of the triangular approach must always be confirmed with an AP and lateral projection to prevent catastrophe before starting the procedure.
- Be cautious with the exiting nerve root; always dock the triangulation over a bone surface (transverse process, isthmus, SAP). Care must be taken during the creation of the workspace, as the arterial vessels supplying the facet joint and the exiting nerve root come directly from the segmental lumbar artery. Thus, the dissection must always be performed starting from a bone element, particularly the superior articular process or the base of the transverse process. In addition, radiofrequency (RF) dissection should be in a medial-to-lateral direction.
- Plan your paraspinal approach regarding your pathological target: foraminal or extraforaminal pathology.
- Always confirm with the C-arm before further maneuvers.
- Bone drilling should never be started if bone landmarks are not identified first. It can be easy to remove excessive or wrong-site bone if you lose your orientation.
- It is unnecessary to remove the transverse process entirely. Particularly in L5, which can be broad and deep, an adequate decompression must be confirmed through the free mobilization of the exiting nerve root. This advice is essential because if we damage the intertransverse membrane, the risk of causing hydro-retroperitoneum is high.
- As pointed out in each chapter, before starting the biportal endoscopic surgery, the surgeon must confirm the correct inflow and outflow of the fluid irrigated

throughout the procedure. An altered flow circuit can lead to blurred surgical view and muscle edema.

- Although durotomy is not common in this approach, it can occur in addition to injury to the exiting nerve root. Therefore, it is recommended to complete the bone decompression before removing the foraminal ligament (FL) and exposing the nerve root. This ligament will serve as a protective barrier for the neural element.
- Finally, if the goals of surgery include intraforaminal decompression or lateral recess, it is necessary to perform a more ventral undercutting of the IAP and SAP. For this reason, it is recommended that the paraspinal approach be more lateral and use a 30° lens.

Conclusion

The biportal endoscopic paraspinal approach for foraminal and extraforaminal lesions of the lumbar spine is a minimally invasive and feasible option to treat this pathology with acceptable clinical outcomes. Furthermore, based on previous studies that have shown that endoscopic foraminotomy with partial resection of the SAP does not result in an increased risk of instability, compared to open surgery, it is probable that biportal endoscopic surgery also does not due to the preservation of muscular structures and spinal and paraspinal ligaments. However, this approach requires experience in biportal endoscopic surgery.

References

1. Jenis LG, An HS. Spine update. Lumbar foraminal stenosis. Spine (Phila Pa 1976). 2000;25:389–94.
2. Kunogi J, Hasue M. Diagnosis and operative treatment of intraforaminal and extraforaminal nerve root compression. Spine (Phila Pa 1976). 1991;16(11):1312–20.
3. Ahn Y, Oh HK, Kim H, Lee SH, Lee HN. Percutaneous endoscopic lumbar foraminotomy: an advanced surgical technique and clinical outcomes. Neurosurgery. 2014;75(2):124–33.
4. Epstein NE. Foraminal and far lateral lumbar disc herniations: surgical alternatives and outcome measures. Spinal Cord. 2002;40:491–500.
5. Burton CV, Kirkaldy-Willis WH, Yong-Hing K, Heithoff KB. Causes of failure of surgery on the lumbar spine. Clin Orthop Relat Res. 1981;157:191–9.
6. Macnab I. Negative disc exploration. An analysis of the causes of nerve-root involvement in sixty-eight patients. J Bone Joint Surg Am. 1971;53:891–903.
7. Rauschning W. Pathoanatomy of lumbar disc degeneration and stenosis. Acta Orthop Scand. 1993;64:3–12.
8. Reulen HJ, Pfaundler S, Ebeling U. The lateral microsurgical approach to the "extracanalicular" lumbar disc herniation. I: a technical note. Acta Neurochir (Wien). 1987;84(1–2):64–7.
9. Garrido E, Connaughton PN. Unilateral facetectomy approach for lateral lumbar disc herniation. J Neurosurg. 1991;74(5):754–6.

10. Wiltse LL, Bateman JG, Hutchinson RH, Nelson WE. The paraspinal sacrospinalis-splitting approach to the lumbar spine. J Bone Joint Surg. 1968;50A:921.
11. Wiltse LL, Spencer CW. New uses and refinements of the paraspinal approach to the lumbar spine. Spine (Phila Pa 1976). 1988;13(6):696–706.
12. Donaldson WF III, Star MJ, Thorne RP. Surgical treatment for the far lateral herniated lumbar disc. Spine (Phila Pa 1976). 1993;18(10):1263–7.
13. Lejeune JP, Hladky JP, Cotten A, Vinchon M, Christiaens JL. Foraminal lumbar disc herniation. Experience with 83 patients. Spine (Phila Pa 1976). 1994;19(17):1905–8.
14. Darden BV II, Wade JF, Alexander R, Wood KE, Rhyne AL III, Hicks JR. Far lateral disc herniations treated by microscopic fragment excision. Techniques and results. Spine (Phila Pa 1976). 1995;20(13):1500–5.
15. Baba H, Uchida K, Maezawa Y, Furusawa N, Okumura Y, Imura S. Microsurgical nerve root canal widening without fusion for lumbosacral intervertebral foraminal stenosis: technical notes and early results. Spinal Cord. 1996;34(11):644–50.
16. Hodges SD, Humphreys SC, Eck JC, Covington LA. The surgical treatment of far lateral L3-L4 and L4-L5 disc herniations. A modified technique and outcomes analysis of 25 patients. Spine (Phila Pa 1976). 1999;24(12):1243–6.
17. Gioia G, Mandelli D, Capaccioni B, Randelli F, Tessari L. Surgical treatment of far lateral lumbar disc herniation. Identification of compressed root and discectomy by lateral approach. Spine (Phila Pa 1976). 1999;24(18):1952–7.
18. Chang HS, Zidan I, Fujisawa N, Matsui T. Microsurgical posterolateral transmuscular approach for lumbar foraminal stenosis. J Spinal Disord Tech. 2011;24(5):302–7.
19. Mayer HM. A history of endoscopic lumbar spine surgery: what have we learnt? Biomed Res Int. 2019;2019:4583943.
20. Park JH, Jung JT, Lee SJ. How I do it: L5/S1 foraminal stenosis and far-lateral lumbar disc herniation with unilateral bi-portal endoscopy. Acta Neurochir. 2018;160(10):1899–903.
21. Choi DJ, Kim JE, Jung JT, et al. Biportal endoscopic spine surgery for various foraminal lesions at the lumbosacral lesion. Asian Spine J. 2018;12(3):569–73.
22. Kim JE, Choi DJ, Park EJ. Clinical and radiological outcomes of foraminal decompression using unilateral biportal endoscopic spine surgery for lumbar foraminal stenosis. Clin Orthop Surg. 2018;10(4):439–47.
23. Kim JE, Choi DJ. Unilateral biportal endoscopic spinal surgery using a 30° arthroscope for L5-S1 foraminal decompression. Clin Orthop Surg. 2018;10(4):508–12.
24. Ahn JS, Lee HJ, Choi DJ, Lee KY, Hwang SJ. Extraforaminal approach of biportal endoscopic spinal surgery: a new endoscopic technique for transforaminal decompression and discectomy. J Neurosurg Spine. 2018;28(5):492–8.
25. Hasan S, White-Dzuro B, Barber JK, Wagner R, Hofstetter CP. The endoscopic trans-superior articular process approach: a novel minimally invasive surgical corridor to the lateral recess. Oper Neurosurg (Hagerstown). 2020;19(1):E1–E10.
26. Quillo-Olvera J, Quillo-Reséndiz J, Quillo-Olvera D, Barrera-Arreola M, Kim JS. Ten-step biportal endoscopic transforaminal lumbar interbody fusion under computed tomography-based intraoperative navigation: technical report and preliminary outcomes in Mexico. Oper Neurosurg (Hagerstown). 2020;19(5):608–18.
27. De Antoni DJ, Claro ML, Poehling GG, Hughes SS. Translaminar lumbar epidural endoscopy: anatomy, technique, and indications. Arthroscopy. 1996;12(3):330–4.
28. Lee CK, Rauschning W, Glenn W. Lateral lumbar spinal canal stenosis: classification, pathologic anatomy and surgical decompression. Spine (Phila Pa 1976). 1988;13(3):313–20.
29. Lee S, Lee JW, Yeom JS, et al. A practical MRI grading system for lumbar foraminal stenosis. AJR Am J Roentgenol. 2010;194(4):1095–8.
30. Abumi K, Panjabi MM, Kramer KM, Duranceau J, Oxland T, Crisco JJ. Biomechanical evaluation of lumbar spinal stability after graded facetectomies. Spine (Phila Pa 1976). 1990;15(11):1142–7.

31. Haufe SM, Mork AR. Effects of unilateral endoscopic facetectomy on spinal stability. J Spinal Disord Tech. 2007;20(2):146–8.
32. Kiapour A, Ambati D, Hoy RW, Goel VK. Effect of graded facetectomy on biomechanics of Dynesys dynamic stabilization system. Spine (Phila Pa 1976). 2012;37(10):E581–9.
33. Teo EC, Lee KK, Qiu TX, Ng HW, Yang K. The biomechanics of lumbar graded facetectomy under anterior-shear load. IEEE Trans Biomed Eng. 2004;51(3):443–9.
34. Kim JE, Choi DJ. Bi-portal arthroscopic spinal surgery (BASS) with 30° arthroscopy for far lateral approach of L5-S1—technical note. J Orthop. 2018;15(2):354–8.

Chapter 18
Challenging Cases Treated with UBE: The Far-Out Syndrome

Javier Quillo-Olvera, Diego Quillo-Olvera, Javier Quillo-Reséndiz, and Michelle Barrera-Arreola

Abbreviations

ADS	Adult degenerative scoliosis
AP	Anteroposterior
BESS	Biportal endoscopic spinal surgery
CT	Computed tomography
FBSS	Failed back surgery syndrome
FOB	Far-out band
FOS	Far-out syndrome
IAA	Inferior articular artery
IAA	Interarticular artery
ITA	Intertransverse artery
IVS	Intervertebral space
LBP	Lower back pain
LSJ	Lumbosacral junction
LSL	Lumbosacral ligament
LSTV	Lumbosacral transitional vertebrae
MRI	Magnetic resonance imaging
NR	Nerve root
NSAIDs	Nonsteroidal anti-inflammatory drugs

Supplementary Information The online version contains supplementary material available at [https://doi.org/10.1007/978-3-031-14736-4_18].

J. Quillo-Olvera (✉) · D. Quillo-Olvera · J. Quillo-Reséndiz · M. Barrera-Arreola
The Brain and Spine Care, Minimally Invasive Spine Surgery Group, Hospital H+ Querétaro, Spine Clinic, Querétaro, México
e-mail: neuroqomd@gmail.com; drquilloolvera86@gmail.com; kitnoz@hotmail.com; michelle.barrera@anahuac.mx

J. Quillo-Olvera et al. (eds.), *Unilateral Biportal Endoscopy of the Spine*, https://doi.org/10.1007/978-3-031-14736-4_18

PI	Pelvic incidence
RF	Radiofrequency
SA	Sacral ala
SAA	Superior articular artery
SAP	Superior articular process
SLA	Segmental lumbar artery
SPECT	Single-photon emission computed tomography
SSN	Superior sacral notch
T2W	T2-weighted
TP	Transverse process
UBE	Unilateral biportal endoscopy
UE	Uniportal endoscopy
XR	X-rays

Introduction

Wiltse et al. [1], in 1984, described the far-out syndrome (FOS), referring to the entrapment and compression of the fifth lumbar nerve beyond the foramen and between the L5 transverse process (TP) and the sacral ala (SA), at the lumbosacral junction (LSJ). According to the authors, this entrapment syndrome could be present clinically in elderly individuals with degenerative diseases such as scoliosis or asymmetric degeneration in the L5–S1 intervertebral disc that causes the TP to tilt towards the SA. Besides, an extraforaminal disc herniation or even a disc bulge at L5–S1 in the setting of TP hypertrophy, a prominent accessory process, TP degeneration with osteophytes, or lumbosacral transitional vertebrae (LSTV) anomalies could displace the L5 exiting nerve root posteriorly and force it to have a more lateral course outside the foramen, resulting in the passage through the reduced intermediate space between TP and sacral ala leading to entrapment and compression of the fifth lumbar nerve.

Other causes that may contribute to diminished extraforaminal space at the LSJ are spondylolisthesis and the well-known LSTV anomalies [2]. This set of congenital anatomical variations is characterized by fusion or pseudoarthrosis of the TP with the first sacral segment in various degrees that can range from a partial/complete sacralization of L5 to a partial/complete lumbarization of S1. The modern classification of LSTVs was introduced by Castellvi et al. [3] in 1984. The authors classified LSTVs into four types and additionally defined whether the anomaly is unilateral (a) or bilateral (b) (Table 18.1).

Among LSTVs, Castellvi's type 1 is usually the most commonly observed in imaging studies, while type 1 and type 2 together account for 40% of the total

Table 18.1 Castellvi classification system of lumbosacral transitional vertebrae (LSTVs) [3]

Type	Description	Unilateral (a)	Bilateral (b)
1	A TP height is greater than or equal to 19 mm	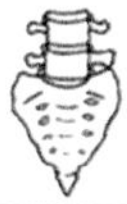	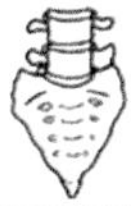
2	Presence of articulation between the TP and the sacrum	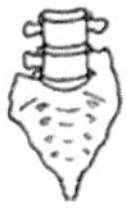	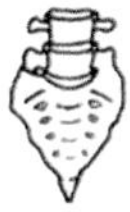
3	Fusion of the TP and the sacrum	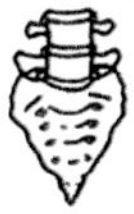	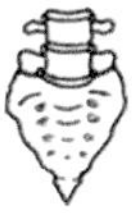
4	Unilateral type 2 transition (articulation) with a type 3 (fusion) on the contralateral side	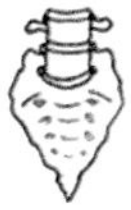	

TP transverse process

anomalies found radiologically [4]. In general, LSTVs have an estimated prevalence of 4–35% in the general population, with an overall average of 12.3% [3, 5–8].

Lower back pain (LBP) in a setting of LSTV was initially reported by Mario Bertolotti in 1917, who coined the term "Bertolotti's syndrome" [9]. This symptom is still the most common form of presentation of LSTV, especially in young people, due to its congenital nature [7, 10, 11]. However, other sources of pain associated with the congenital anomaly include arthritic changes on the side of the pseudoarthrosis, facet and disc degeneration, and extraforaminal compression and entrapment of the fifth lumbar nerve root (far-out syndrome). In addition, FOS as Bertolotti's syndrome manifestation has been reported by various authors [5, 10, 12–21].

Symptomatic LSTVs or Bertolotti's syndrome can be initially treated with conservative measures. Analgesics, NSAIDs, physical therapy, chiropractic, and steroid or anesthetic injections are just some conventional treatment options. However, if these fail, surgical treatment is warranted. FOS may be present in 13% of patients with LSTV and become symptomatic in more than 70% of those patients [22]. Surgical options aim at extraforaminal decompression of the fifth lumbar root in symptomatic patients who fail conservative treatment [1, 23].

Surgical options to decompress the L5 exiting nerve in FOS include microsurgery [24], uniportal endoscopy (UE) [25], and recently unilateral biportal endoscopy (UBE) [26–28] through a paraspinal route, which has been attempted with encouraging outcomes. The UBE technique for treating FOS is the focus of this chapter.

Diagnosis

Lumbar spine X-rays allow the identification of LSTVs in patients with clinical suspicion of FOS. In particular, the AP view (Fig. 18.1) is commonly used for this purpose. The sensitivity to identify LSTVs by X-ray is 76–84%, while the accuracy to classify LSTV according to the Castellvi type is 53–58% [29–31]. However, MRI and CT scan allow identification and classification of an LSTV with more precision than traditional X-ray films and provide additional information on other possible findings associated with the disease (Fig. 18.2). MRI has demonstrated more than 80% sensitivity in identifying LSTVs (Fig. 18.3) [14, 29–31]. Furthermore, Chalain et al. [32] proposed measuring two angles on the T2-weighted (T2W) MRI to predict the presence of an LSTV. Angle 1 is measured between a line parallel to the superior surface of the sacrum and a line perpendicular to the table's axis. If the angle is ≥40°, it predicts the presence of LSTV with 80% sensitivity and specificity.

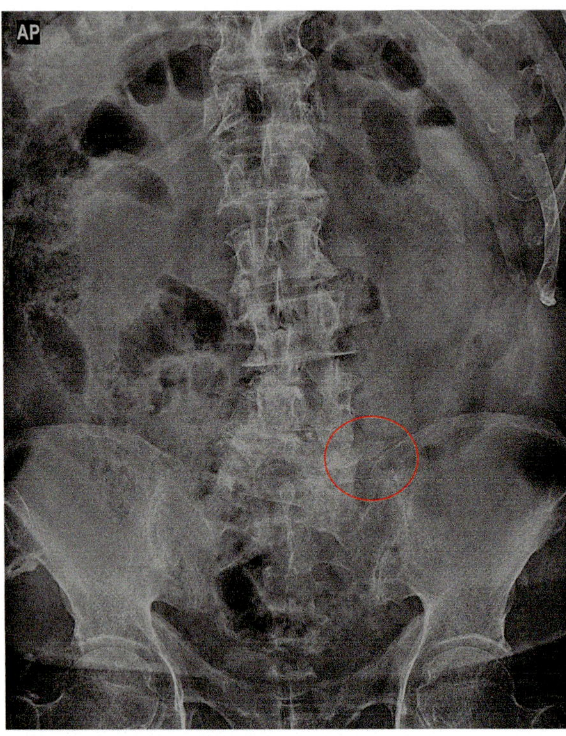

Fig. 18.1 Lumbar X-ray film on AP showing an LSTV on the left side (red circle)

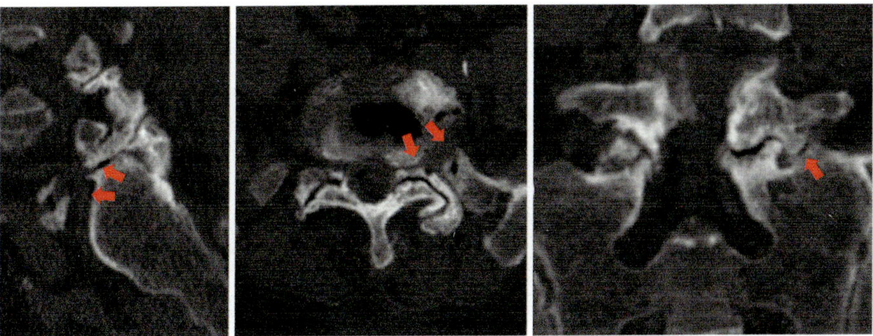

Fig. 18.2 Lumbar CT scan of Fig. 18.1. The red arrows point to an LSTV Castellvi's type 2, leading to symptomatic FOS on the left side

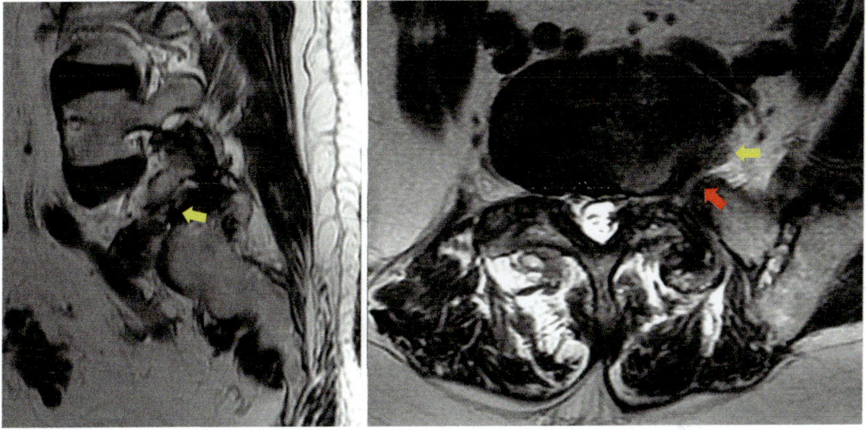

Fig. 18.3 Lumbar MRI of Fig. 18.1. The T2W sagittal view (right) shows the L5 exiting nerve root (yellow arrow) compressed on the left side. The T2W axial view demonstrated compression of the L5 exiting nerve (yellow arrow) caused by the LSTV Castellvi's type 2 (red arrow)

Angle 2 is measured between the line parallel to the superior endplate of L3 and a line parallel to the superior surface of the sacrum. A result ≥36° predicts the presence of an LSTV with 80% sensitivity and 54% specificity (Fig. 18.4). Another imaging modality, such as SPECT bone scintigraphy based on the metabolic changes of the pseudo-articulation in LSTVs, allows finding the possible focus of LBP in patients with Bertolotti's syndrome [33].

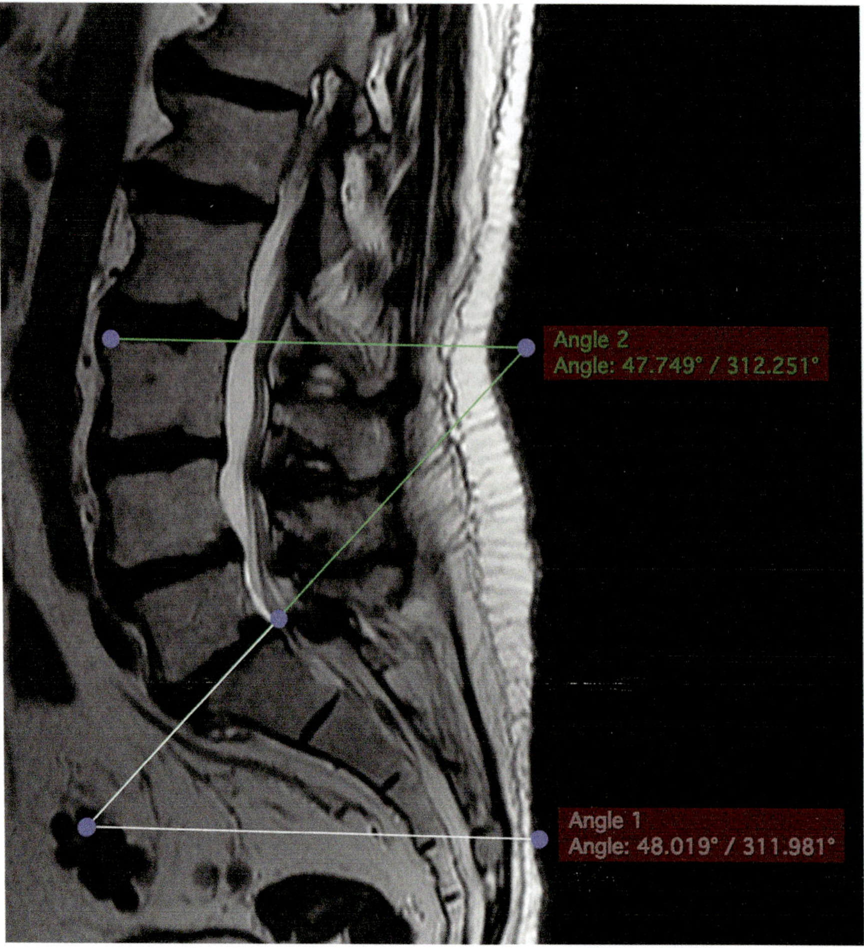

Fig. 18.4 Midsagittal view on T2W of the lumbar MRI showing Angle 1 (48.019°) and Angle 2 (47.749°)

Biportal Endoscopic Decompression of Far-Out Syndrome

Rationale

In elderly patients with adult degenerative scoliosis (ADS) and symptoms of L5 radiculopathy, or those with radicular symptoms of the fifth lumbar nerve root (NR) in whom findings at L5–S1 (central canal or foraminal) have been ruled out, it is necessary to exclude FOS since extraforaminal stenosis in the lumbosacral junction may be a cause of failed back surgery syndrome (FBSS) or poor outcomes after posterior decompression by any technique [34–36].

If FOS is confirmed, direct decompression is recommended and associated with acceptable results. Surgical options for this condition, in addition to posterior decompression, include posterolateral fusion and transforaminal interbody fusion. However, the anatomical features of Bertolotti's syndrome with manifestations of FOS are usually complex, so minimally invasive techniques are feasible and assertive with minor collateral effects than conventional techniques [37].

Paraspinal access has been the gold standard for FOS treatment since Wiltse et al. [38] described it in 1968. Various authors have reported minimally invasive microsurgical techniques through this approach to achieve lumbosacral extraforaminal decompression [24, 39, 40].

However, the intricate anatomy of the extraforaminal space in patients with FOS can make docking the tubular retractor in that region harsh. The iliac crest can hide and hinder direct access to that space. In addition, it may be challenging to tilt the tube during the procedure due to the narrow space left by the iliac crest laterally and the facet joint medially. Furthermore, in the case of redo surgery, in patients with previous screwing and an unnoticed FOS, it is improbable to reach the extraforaminal space properly because the implants limit access.

Another concern is targeted bony structures' depth in the extraforaminal space. It is important to consider the pelvic incidence (PI) in patients with FOS. The more horizontal the sacrum disposition is, the deeper the location of the TP and exiting nerve root. This is even more marked in patients with spondylolisthesis since the TP will be mounted anteriorly in the SA. Working in deep space with the tubular retractor makes it fixed between the iliac bone and the facet joint. But also, the depth not just affects the maneuverability of the tubular retractor, but is also a technical factor that impacts the visibility and illumination of the surgical field through a reduced and deep tubular space. This circumstance could limit correctly identifying the pathological bony structures and the soft tissues above the exiting nerve.

And last but not least, the use of long tools and the maneuverability of surgical instruments with two hands require the surgeon's skills, tolerance, and precision. For example, in cases of FOS, the use of drill for bone removal of the TP, SA, and pseudoarthrosis can tire the surgeon's hands and favor a complex environment through the tubular retractor requiring more extraordinary skills or tolerance to avoid fatigue and shaking hands. In addition, the assistance to irrigate, aspirate, or retract by the surgical assistant makes the visibility through the tube even more difficult. These circumstances are relevant because they can lead to insufficient decompression or excessive manipulation of the dorsal root ganglion of the exiting nerve and trigger postoperative dysesthesia or radiculitis [39, 41–44].

Recently, water-based endoscopic techniques have expanded their indications. In the case of uniportal endoscopy (UE), some authors have reported encouraging results in lumbosacral extraforaminal neural decompression. However, the vast majority are related to extraforaminal disc herniations without an LSTV [45, 46]. Wu et al. [25] reported the direct UE technique for decompression of the exiting nerve root in a patient with Bertolotti's syndrome and a Castellvi type 2a pseudoarthrosis. Nevertheless, since it is only a technical report, more future evidence is required to establish it as a standard reference in FOS treatment.

We found certain drawbacks in UE for FOS, the first being the high level of skills required [47]. If to this critical point we add that FOS is a complex pathology for being treated with any technique, to employ UE to resolve it can be a challenge. Second, the surgeon can only use specialized surgical instruments built just for the particular endoscopic system, which is expensive. Third, in cases where different angles of attack are required to approach the targets (TP, SAP, SA, pseudoarthrosis, and various extraforaminal ligamentous structures) involved in the pathology, the UE technique may be insufficient due to the null maneuverability of the surgical instruments outside the working channel integrated to the endoscope. Fourth, the pathology may exceed the UE technique scope. FOS cases require the use of different surgical tools appropriated to deal with complex anatomy in the extraforaminal region of the LSJ. Unfortunately, through the UE, only fine tools can be introduced, designed exclusively for a given system, wasting many standard surgical instruments such as Kerrison punches of different measurements and angles, chisels, curettes, pituitary forceps, and various tips for the drilling system to overcome the pathological anatomy.

However, it is also necessary to highlight the excellent visibility, lighting, and magnification achieved through the UE, enhanced by the water environment through continuous fluid irrigation during the procedure. And all the clinical advantages associated with minimally invasive procedures include reduced estimated blood loss (EBL), less aggressiveness to the paraspinal tissues, decreased postoperative pain, minor consumption of postoperative analgesics and opioids, shorter hospital stay, and ability to get mobility outside of the bed earlier compared with open or conventional procedures.

Therefore, it is possible to have a water-based endoscopic technique with the advantages related to high-quality visibility and at the same time those associated with a minimally invasive surgical procedure of the spine, but with the ability to have versatility in its performance through the use of more powerful surgical instruments, used independently, especially for complex pathologies such as FOS. The answer is unilateral biportal endoscopic surgery (UBE) [26–28].

Indications and Contraindications

The indications for FOS treatment by biportal endoscopy are the same as an open surgery or other minimally invasive techniques.

1. Patients with Bertolotti's syndrome and radicular manifestations derived from extraforaminal neural entrapment and compression (FOS) due to any of the following causes:

   (a) Spondylosis of the transverse process (TP)
   (b) Pseudoarthrosis of the TP and the sacral ala
   (c) Extraforaminal lumbar disc herniation
   (d) Spondylolisthesis associated with LSTVs

2. Radicular symptoms irradiated to one or both legs derived from the fifth lumbar nerve.
3. Failed to conservative measures for at least 4–6 weeks.
4. LSTVs and other causes of lumbosacral extraforaminal stenosis confirmed by imaging studies such as XR, MRI, or CT of the lumbar spine consistent with the patient's symptoms.
5. Exclusions of other sources of L5 compression in the lumbar spine.
6. Positive response after an L5–S1 foraminal block on the symptomatic side provides more certainty to the diagnosis [48].

The following circumstances could contraindicate a paraspinal lumbar UBE decompression of FOS: (1) infection, (2) tumor, (3) trauma, (4) inexperience with the UBE technique; first is recommended to try with other UBE procedures. (5) The previous screwing of the spine is a relative contraindication. (6) The height of the iliac bone is not a contraindication for a paraspinal UBE procedure because of the posterior nature of the approach.

Relevant Surgical Anatomy

The anatomical landmarks that should be recognized as compression factors [26] and the surgeon must identify through the endoscope to drive the procedure properly are the following (Fig. 18.5):

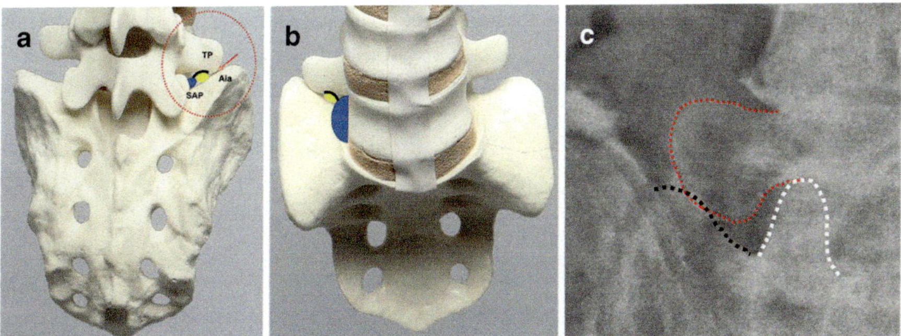

Fig. 18.5 Compressive landmarks in far-out syndrome (FOS). (**a**) Posterior view of the lumbosacral junction in an anatomical model. The most important anatomical structures are circled in red. The transverse process (TP) forms a pseudoarthrosis (red arrow) with the sacral ala (Ala). A concomitant factor such as an extraforaminal disc herniation or a marginal osteophyte ventrally (blue semicircle) displaces the exiting nerve root (yellow circle) more dorsal and lateral being entrapped and impinged in the narrow space left by the TP and Ala. Tight ligaments called extraforaminal and lumbosacral (black curved line) fixed the nerve, resulting in a Bertolotti's syndrome with FOS manifestations. (**b**) Anterior view of (**a**). (**c**) Lumbar X-ray on AP view showing Castellvi 2a type LSTVs. The bony compressive landmarks in the FOS have been highlighted with dotted lines of different colors. The red line represents the TP, the black one is the sacral ala, and the white line is the SAP

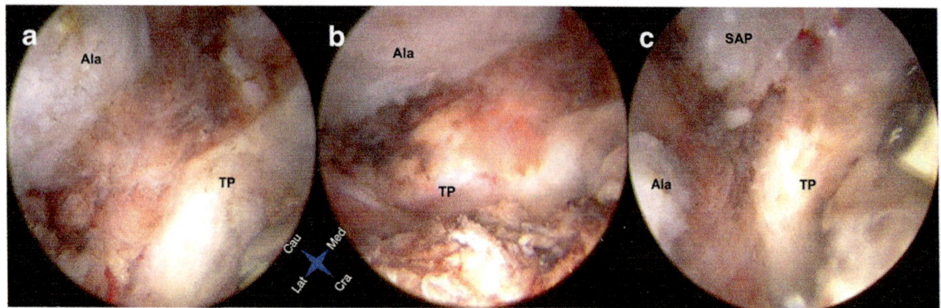

Fig. 18.6 Endoscopic view through a paraspinal UBE FOS decompression. (**a**) The bony elements have been cleaned during the preparation of the working space. (**b**) Panoramic view of pseudoarthrosis between the TP and sacral ala. (**c**) Extraforaminal view of the SAP, TP, and sacral ala. *Cra* cranial, *Cau* caudal, *Lat* lateral, *Med* medial, *FOS* far-out syndrome, *TP* transverse process, *Ala* sacral ala, *SAP* superior articular process

1. The hypertrophied transverse process (TP) of the L5 vertebra
2. The sacral wing with which the TP forms a pseudoarthrosis or fusion in Bertolotti's syndrome
3. The superior articular process (SAP) of S1

A correct dissection of these structures must be carried out before performing decompression. It will avoid removing excessive bone or transgressing the boundaries to the retroperitoneum, among other adverse situations (Fig. 18.6).

However, FOS may have other associated compression components, such as an extraforaminal herniated disc or marginal spondylosis with osteophytes. These findings should be noted in the preoperative lumbar MRI or CT scan. The extraforaminal ventral compression is because these degenerative changes cause the posterior and lateral displacement of the exiting nerve root, which is entrapped between the TP and the SA that are fused or with pseudoarthrosis in patients with Bertolotti's syndrome causing radicular symptoms which feature the FOS.

Surgical Technique

As mentioned, the paraspinal approach is ideal for reaching the extraforaminal space in the LSJ [1, 38]. However, performing neural decompression through a biportal endoscopic approach requires experience, which could have been acquired by performing other paraspinal procedures such as microsurgery with tubular retractors or uniportal endoscopy (UE). Either way, this will allow the surgeon to be more confident with the anatomy of the extraforaminal space.

On the other hand, biportal endoscopic spinal surgery (BESS) consists of the correct triangulation of two ports to create a working space above the target. This allows the proper inflow and outflow of fluid irrigated, which will provide advantages such as clear visualization of the surgical field, easier recognition of bleeding source for correct hemostasis, and keeping the surgical field free of debris, which will reduce the risk of infection.

Proper triangulation of both ports is based on adequate preoperative planning. The biportal approach on the right side will use the cranial portal as the working channel, while the caudal will be used as the viewing channel when performed by a right-handed surgeon. On the left side, it will be the opposite. The cranial portal will be used for the endoscope and the caudal for the instruments. The general aspects of the UBE lumbar paraspinal approach have been discussed in the first chapters of this book. However, some principles should never go unnoticed by the surgeon, which include the following:

1. Correct preoperative planning: All water-based endoscopic techniques have the advantage of being minimally invasive procedures because they are specifically targeted, which decreases tissue damage around the surgical target. BESS is no exception.
2. The correct triangulation of both ports favors the proper performance of the technique. It allows the dissection of soft tissues (fat, connective tissue) above pathological bone surfaces. It facilitates the location of the working instruments with the endoscope. And it prevents both portals from becoming obstructed during the procedure. Finally, it ensures the correct continuous irrigation during the surgery.
3. Triangulation should be confirmed by palpating the same bone structure with both dilators, feeling both dilators touching, and ensuring with AP and lateral views obtained with the C-arm.
4. Before starting the endoscopic stage of UBE, the surgeon must always ensure that the fluid irrigated through the endoscope exits through the working port. This is of particular interest in paraspinal approaches due to the risk of transgressing the limit to the retroperitoneum and causing a collection in the retroperitoneal space with significant repercussions.

Step 1: Anesthesia and Patient Position

This procedure can be performed under general anesthesia, epidural anesthesia, or conscious sedation. This should be considered based on an in-depth pre-anesthetic assessment that guarantees that the surgery will be done with the highest safety standards for the patient, who will be placed prone on an abdominal support frame. Subsequently, the cleaning of the surgical area and drapes will be carried out.

Step 2: Skin Incision Planning

The biportal approach requires a pair of incisions to access the L5–S1 extraforaminal space. First, the following radiological landmarks will be located in the AP view of the C-arm (Fig. 18.7):

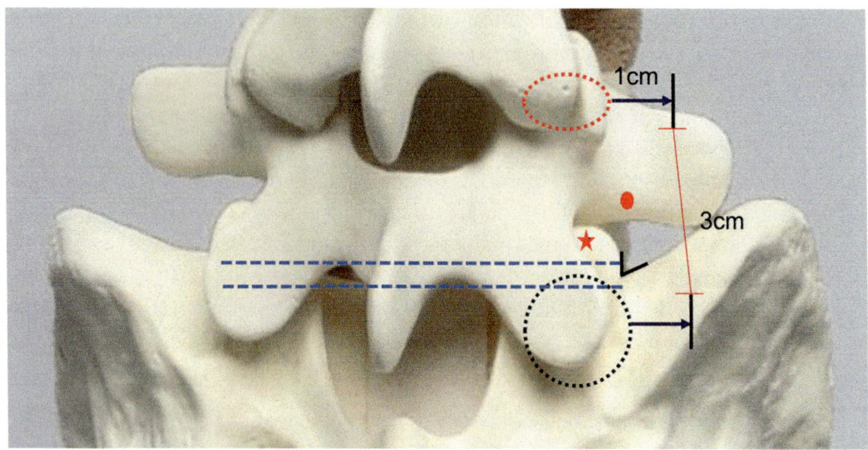

Fig. 18.7 An anteroposterior view of an anatomical model exemplifies the location of skin incisions in a biportal approach to the extraforaminal space at the lumbosacral junction. The red dotted circle represents the L5 pedicle while the black one the S1 pedicle. The intermittent blue lines show the IVS. In addition, the SAP (red star) and the TP (red circle) can be observed. The SSN (V) below the TP is also noted. The skin incisions are placed 1 cm lateral to L5 and S1 pedicles. A 3 cm of distance between both incisions is left. *SAP* superior articular process, *TP* transverse process, *SSN* superior sacral notch

1. L5 and S1 pedicles
2. S1 SAP
3. L5-S1 intervertebral space (IVS)
4. L5 transverse process
5. The superior sacral notch (SSN)

Subsequently, the skin incisions (cranial and caudal) will be planned 1 cm lateral to the L5 and S1 pedicles (or from the LSJ depending on whether the LSTV has a lumbarized or sacralized variant, for example, an L6–S1 level). Both incisions will have a separation of 3 cm. Next, it is recommended that the surgeon incise the skin and fascia to introduce the dilators and allow the proper flow of continuous irrigation.

At the beginning of this section, it was commented that if the side of the pathology is right, and the surgeon is right-handed, then the cranial incision will be used for the working channel, while the caudal will be used as the viewing channel. On the left side, it will be the opposite. On some occasions, the iliac bone can obstruct the caudal portal. Therefore, it is suggested to make the caudal incision slightly more medial (0.5 cm) to the S1 pedicle.

Step 3: Biportal (Triangular) Approach

In this step, the surgeon must introduce the dilators through both incisions to reach a specific target in a triangular fashion. A dilator placed on each incision should be addressed to the same target independently. Depending on surgeon preferences, the

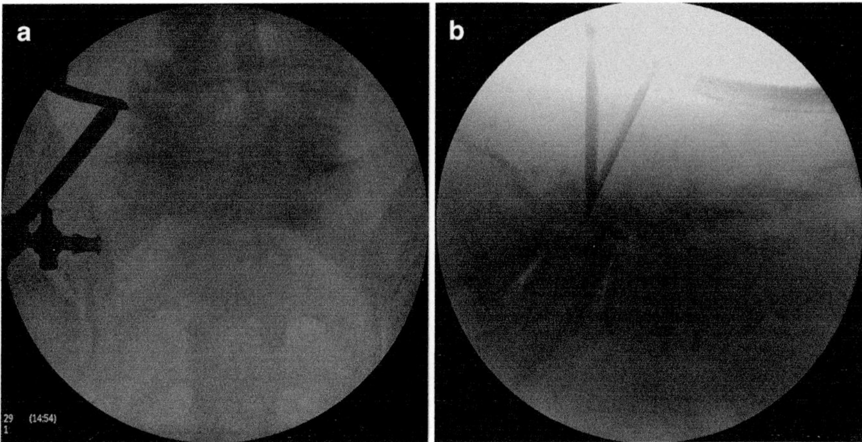

Fig. 18.8 UBE lumbar paraspinal approach at L5–S1 on the right side. The approach was confirmed under the AP (**a**) and lateral (**b**) views. The triangular approach is addressed to the transverse process (TP)

triangular approach can be addressed to TP, SAP, or SSN. We recommend docking both dilators over the base of TP. The surgeon should palpate the landmark with each dilator's tip and dissect the bony surface. Feeling that both dilators meet at the bony landmark is the goal of the triangular approach. Then, the dilator in the working portal is replaced by the customized semicircular working cannula and the other one placed in the viewing portal by the endoscopic system. The surgeon must confirm the triangular approach and the proper creation of both ports with an AP and lateral views of the C-arm (Fig. 18.8).

Step 4: Completing the Working Space to Identify the Bone Landmarks

The endoscope is introduced through the viewing portal, and the radiofrequency (RF) probe through the working channel. The surgeon must locate it in the surgical field with the endoscope and confirm that the inflow and outflow of irrigated fluid are continuous. Subsequently, dissection of the proximal and lower portion of the L5 TP, the lateral aspect of the facet joint, and the sacral ala is performed with the RF probe. After identifying these anatomical structures, the surgeon could start with decompression (Fig. 18.9; Video 18.1).

Step 5: Bone Removal and Nerve Root Decompression

The lower part of the TP proximal third is removed from proximal to lateral. The same is performed with the superomedial portion of the sacral ala and the lateral surface of the SAP. This step is usually done with the drilling system. It should be kept in mind that in some cases of Bertolotti's syndrome, the TP may be fused or

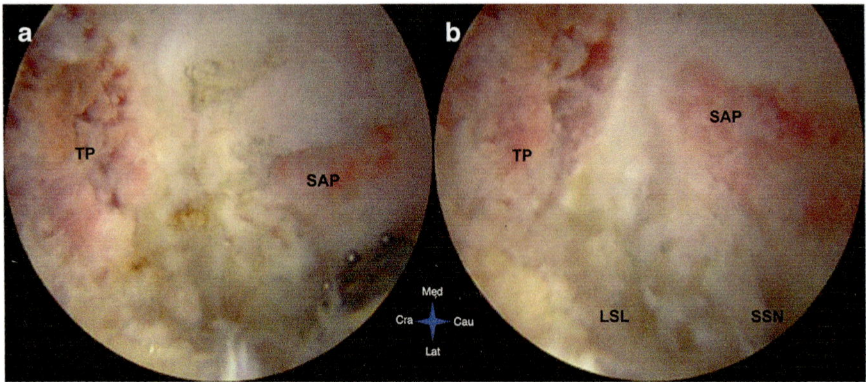

Fig. 18.9 Intraoperative images through the endoscope showing the working space (**a**) and the bony references (**b**). *Cra* cranial, *Cau* caudal, *Lat* lateral, *Med* medial, *TP* transverse process, *SAP* superior articular process, *SSN* superior sacral notch, *LSL* lumbosacral ligament

have pseudoarthrosis with the sacral ala; therefore, the surgeon should complete the nerve root decompression laterally as necessary, even if a total removal of the pseudoarthrosis or fusion between the TP and the sacral wing is needed.

After removing the lower part of the TP and the superomedial sacral ala, the cranial and caudal attachments of a tight and thickened ligament are observed between both bony structures (TP and sacral wing). This ligament is called the lumbosacral ligament (LSL) (Video 18.2). The LSL should be removed with a deeper and more distal extraforaminal ligament called the far-out band (FOB). Both the LSL and FOB usually fix the exiting L5 nerve root. Therefore, they must be removed to complete extraforaminal decompression of the L5 exiting root. Decompression can be confirmed when the surgeon can freely mobilize the exiting nerve root (Fig. 18.10; Video 18.3).

Step 6: Other Maneuvers

An extraforaminal disc herniation associated with the compression may be found in some patients. Other significant degenerative changes include marginal osteophytes and foraminal stenosis. Because of this, the surgeon can perform, in addition to direct root decompression, extraforaminal discectomy or foraminal and extraforaminal decompression through the same biportal endoscopic paraspinal approach (Fig. 18.11).

Step 7: Final Suggestions and Wound Closure

After decompression, the surgeon must ensure adequate hemostasis. The bone or soft tissue can cause perineural hematoma leading to radiculitis. A drain can be left for 12 h to evacuate residual collection and avoid nerve root inflammation. It is

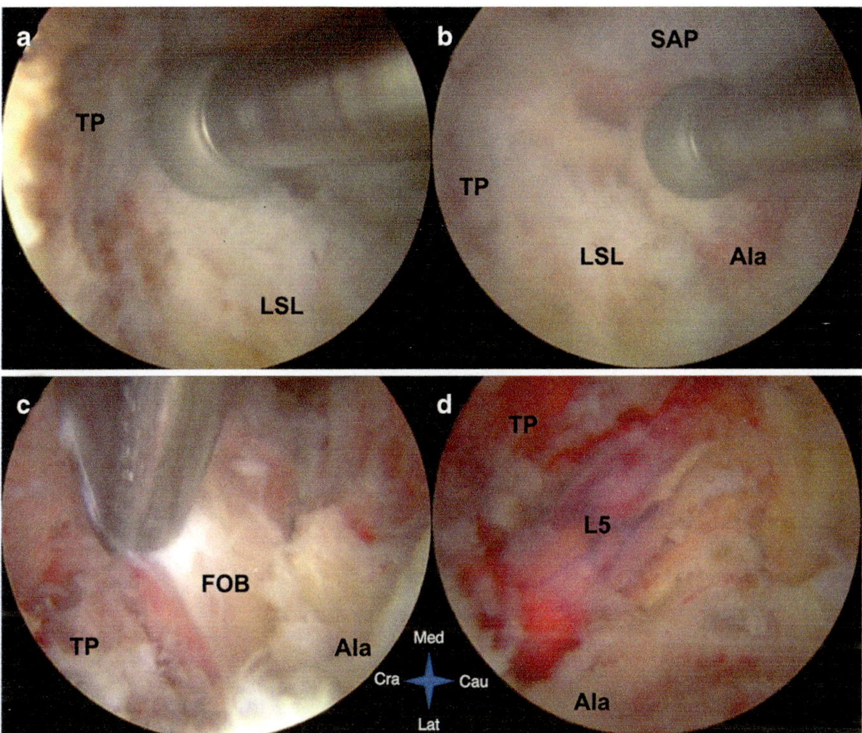

Fig. 18.10 Decompression of the extraforaminal part of exiting L5 nerve root. (**a**) Drilling out the lower part of TP. (**b**) Sacral and SAP lateral surface removal by using the drill. (**c**) The extraforaminal ligament (ExFL) is removed. (**d**) The L5 exiting nerve is decompressed. *Cra* cranial, *Cau* caudal, *Lat* lateral, *Med* medial, *TP* transverse process, *LSL* lumbosacral ligament, *Ala* sacral ala, *SAP* superior articular process, *ExFL* extraforaminal ligament

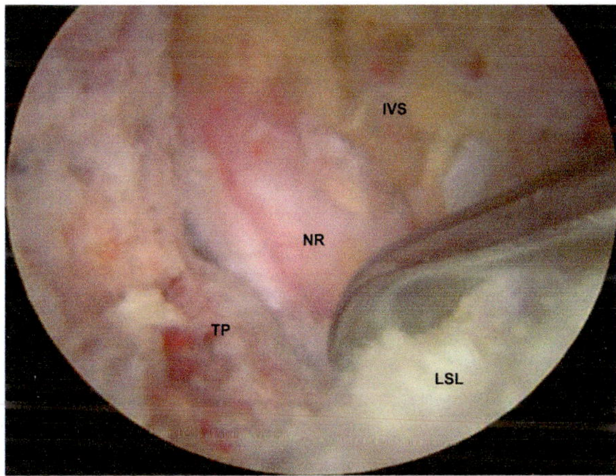

Fig. 18.11 The nerve root can be compressed ventrally by an extraforaminal lumbar disc herniation, which can be reached through the same paraspinal UBE approach. This imaging shows the intervertebral space (IVS) below the nerve root (NR) and, distally, the lumbosacral ligament (LSL). *TP* transverse process

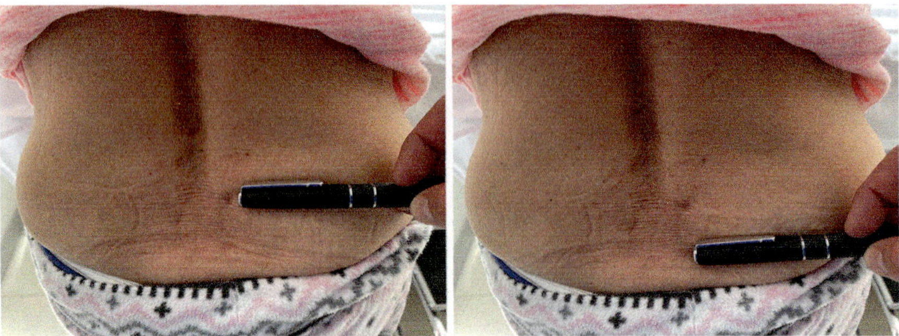

Fig. 18.12 Wounds after 4 weeks

recommended to confirm that the same volume of fluid irrigated throughout the procedure was also evacuated to prevent hydro-retroperitoneum or paravertebral soft-tissue edema. Finally, both wounds are closed with a single stitch (Fig. 18.12).

Illustrated Cases

Case 1

A 67-year-old male with a history of Parkinson's and prior spine surgery at L5–S1 (interspinous device) complains of severe pain radiating down his right leg until the lateral surface of his calf. The pain does not improve with physical therapy, NSAIDs, or opioids. A foraminal block at L5–S1 on the right side improved the pain for only 3 weeks, but currently, the pain is intense VAS 8/10. X-ray studies revealed an adult degenerative scoliosis with findings of Castellvi type 2b LSTVs (Fig. 18.13a). An extraforaminal disc herniation at L5–S1 on the right side, compressing the L5 exiting nerve root, was found in the lumbar MRI (Fig. 18.13b). In addition, the precise extraforaminal entrapment of the right-sided L5 nerve was noted on the CT scan of the lumbar spine (Fig. 18.14). A right-sided unilateral biportal endoscopic (UBE) paraspinal approach was carried out at L5–S1 (Video 18.4). Decompression of the extraforaminal course of the L5 nerve was accomplished. Also, the extraforaminal disc was removed (Fig. 18.15). Postoperative imaging studies confirmed proper decompression at the site of pathology (Fig. 18.16). The patient was discharged the following day of the surgery with no pain (VAS 0/10) of his right leg.

Case 2

A 78-year-old male complains of radicular pain and numbness in his right leg and dysesthesias in the lateral aspect of the right calf VAS 8/10. On physical examination, the patient had 4/5 weakness in dorsiflexion of the right ankle and decreased Achilles reflex on the right side. The X-ray AP view of the lumbar spine showed an adult degenerative scoliosis and an L5 transverse process (TP) on the right side with a height of 19 mm (Fig. 18.17a). Lumbar spine MRI

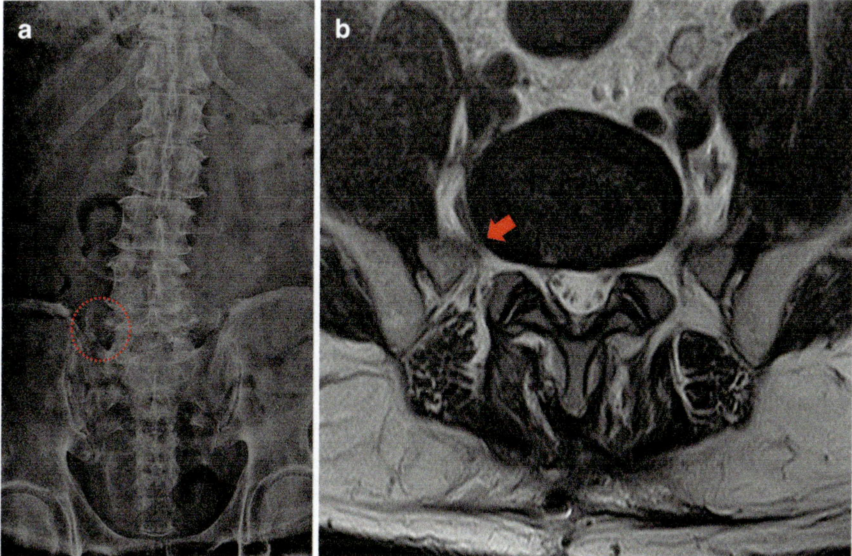

Fig. 18.13 Preoperative lumbar X-ray and MRI imaging of Case 1. (**a**) A pseudoarthrosis (red dotted circle) between the L5 transverse process (TP) and sacral ala at L5–S1 on the right side is noted. (**b**) The red arrow points to the extraforaminal entrapment of the L5 nerve on the right side and the far-lateral disc in the axial view of the lumbar MRI

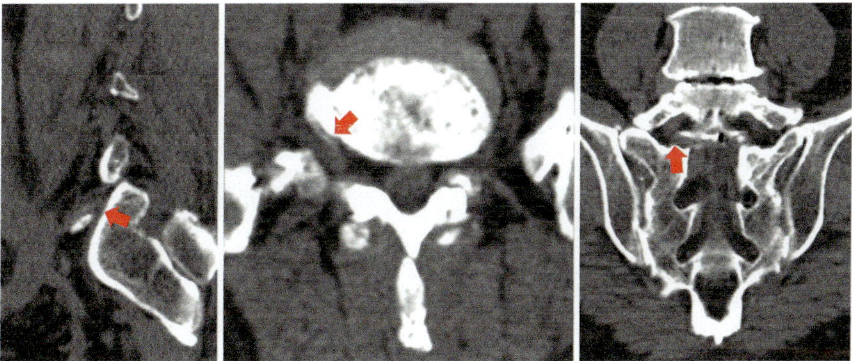

Fig. 18.14 Lumbar CT scan of Case 1. The red arrows show the extraforaminal compression at L5–S1 on the right side

revealed extraforaminal stenosis associated with spondylosis at L5–S1 on the right side (Fig. 18.17b–d). A lumbar biportal endoscopic paraspinal approach was performed at L5–S1 on the right side to decompress the L5 root in its extraforaminal course (Video 18.5). It was possible to remove the lower part of the TP and the superomedial part of the sacral ala to enlarge the extraforaminal space and release the L5 nerve root without intraoperative complications

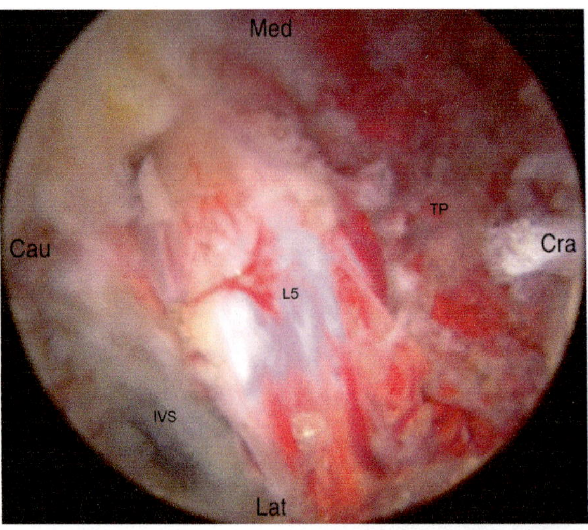

Fig. 18.15 The L5 exiting nerve decompressed. *Cra* crania, *Cau* caudal, *Lat* lateral, *Med* medial, *IVS* intervertebral space, *TP* transverse process

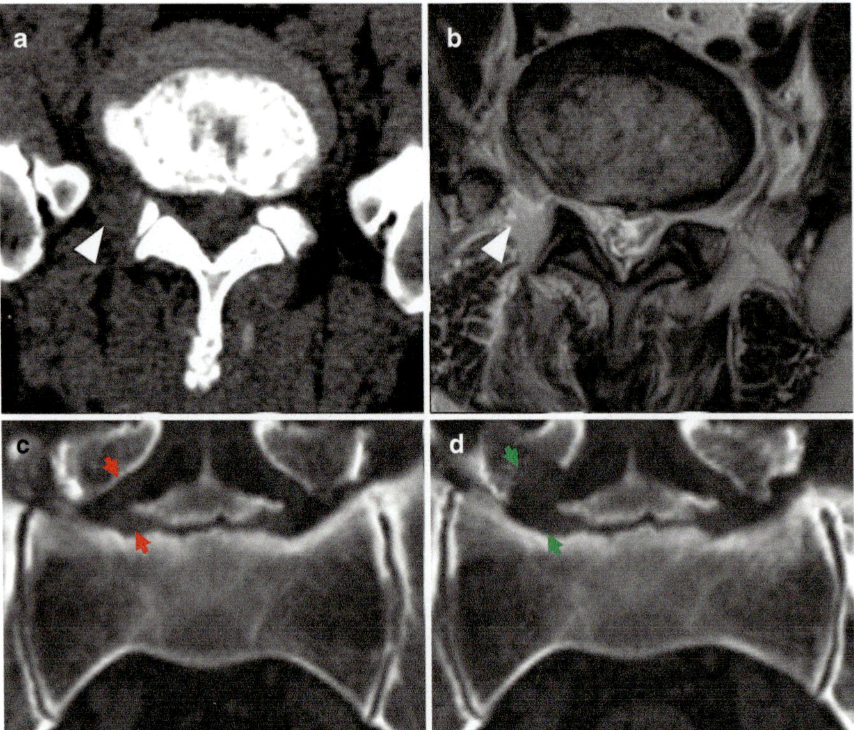

Fig. 18.16 Postoperative imaging studies of Case 1. (**a**) Axial view of the CT at L5–S1. The bone removal included the lateral aspect of the SAP, the sacral ala, and the transverse process (TP) on the right side (**d**). The white arrowheads in (**a**) and (**b**) show the paraspinal route. (**b**) Axial view of the lumbar MRI at L5–S1. The extraforaminal course of the L5 nerve root on the right side is observed (white arrowhead). (**c**) Preoperative coronal view of L5–S1 on the CT scan; the red arrows show the extraforaminal entrapment of the L5 nerve root on the right side. (**d**) Postoperative coronal view of L5–S1 on the CT scan. The green arrows demonstrate the TP removal after the procedure

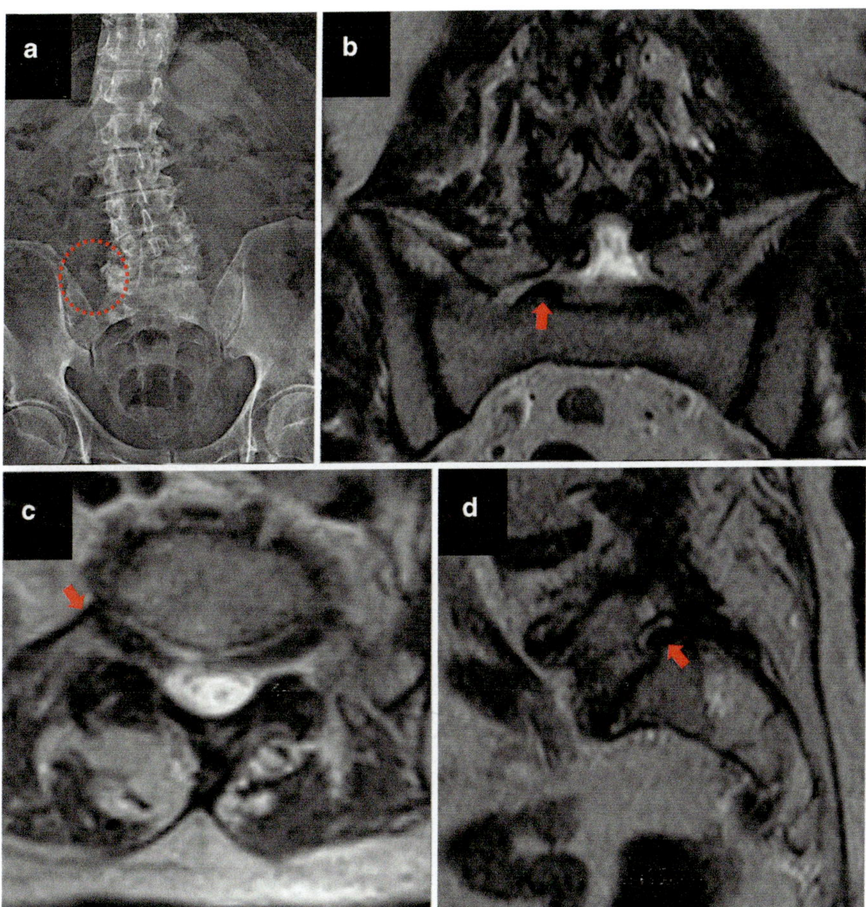

Fig. 18.17 Preoperative imaging from Case 2. (**a**) The X-ray on AP view of the lumbar spine shows degenerative scoliosis. In this case, the big-sized TPs are located anteriorly. In addition, a calcified disc and marginal spondylosis at L5–S1 on the right side (red arrows on **b**, **c**, and **d**) were noted on the lumbar MRI. These findings displace the L5 nerve root posterior and lateral, causing entrapment and compression of the extraforaminal course of the nerve root between the TP and sacral ala (red arrow on **b** and **c**)

(Fig. 18.18). Immediate postoperative lumbar CT scan demonstrated satisfactory decompression (Fig. 18.19). The patient was discharged 24 h after surgery with minimal analgesia, the dysesthesia in the lateral aspect of the calf disappeared, and the radicular pain in his right leg and the numbness improved to VAS 1/10. In his clinical follow-up at 1 month, the dorsiflexion weakness of the right ankle improved to 5/5, at which time the VAS was 0/10 in the right leg.

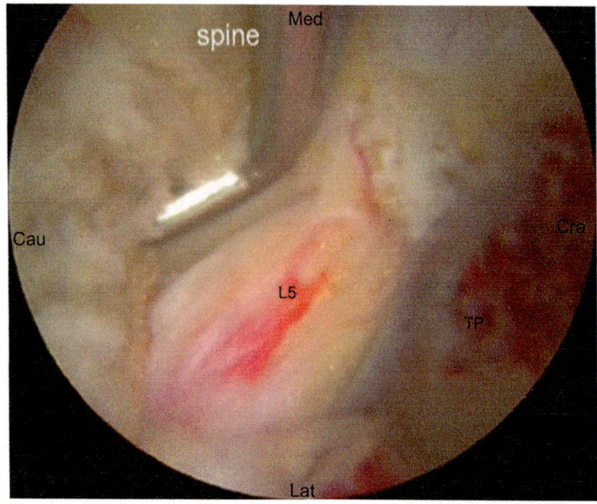

Fig. 18.18 Intraoperative view through the endoscope of the L5 nerve root in the extraforaminal space after decompression. *Cra* cranial, *Cau* caudal, *Lat* lateral, *Med* medial, *TP* transverse process

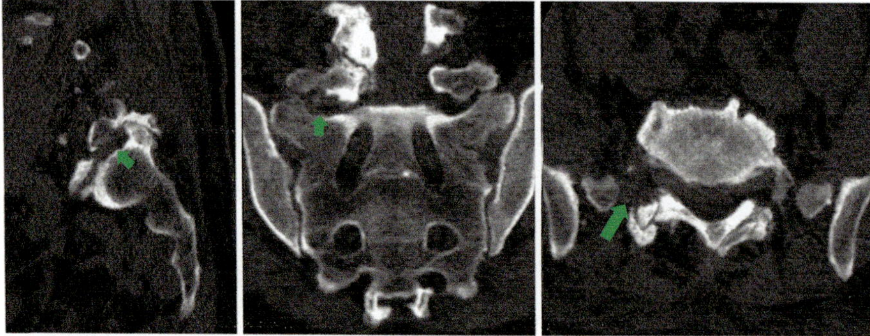

Fig. 18.19 Postoperative CT scan of Case 1. The green arrows point to the extraforaminal decompression at L5–S1 on the right side

Discussion

The far-out syndrome (FOS) is the radicular manifestation associated with entrapment and compression of the fifth lumbar nerve root (NR) in its extraforaminal course between the L5 transverse process (TP) and the sacral ala (SA), especially in the circumstances such as LSTV anomalies or patients with Bertolotti's syndrome [1, 2].

The basis of FOS is anatomical since an enlarged TP that causes pseudoarthrosis or fusion with the SA restricts the extraforaminal space. In addition, the caudal and medial-to-lateral course of the fifth lumbar nerve root in the extraforaminal area makes it susceptible to entrapment as it passes below the TP. In addition, marginal spondylotic changes at L5–S1 will displace the L5 NR laterally and posteriorly, causing it to compress against the bone, as mentioned earlier.

The lumbosacral ligament (LSL) attached to the TP cranially and SA caudally, as well as deep ligamentous bands that attach to the intervertebral disc and the TP or the facet joint and that in normal situations do not have a compressive effect, can fix the L5 NR in the extraforaminal space when they undergo degenerative changes producing radicular symptoms [49–51].

For this reason, surgical treatment should include bone decompression (SAP, TP, SA), L5 NR release, removal of the LSL as laterally as necessary, and deep ligamentous bands that prevent free mobilization of the L5 NR, and in some cases the herniated extraforaminal disc or marginal osteophytes if necessary.

It is important to note that extraforaminal access to L5–S1 can be challenging. Spinopelvic parameters such as pelvic incidence (PI) are relevant. Patients with low-grade spondylolisthesis associated with a high PI can cause the TP to move anterior to the SA, generating intricate anatomy and arduous bone remodeling. In addition, a prominent iliac crest can make paraspinal access to the L5–S1 complex [26, 34, 37, 39, 52].

The paraspinal approach for extraforaminal lesions at L5–S1 (far-out syndrome) using unilateral biportal endoscopy (UBE) has been recently introduced [26–28]. Park et al. [26] reported the results obtained by applying this technique in 35 patients (16 males and 19 females) with a mean age of 68.4 ± 6.6 years and a clinical follow-up of 14.9 months. In addition, 10 patients had concomitant foraminal stenosis. Preoperatively, the average VAS for back pain was 3.7 ± 1.8 and a year after 2.3 ± 1.2. However, the clinical improvement was better appreciated when analyzing the VAS for leg pain, which in the preoperative period was an average of 7.2 ± 1.1 and 2.3 ± 1.2 at 1-year follow-up. The ODI score was 61.5 before surgery and 28.6 after 1 year. The authors in this study reported no postoperative complications. In addition, in 19 patients (51.4%), LSL and other tight and thickened ligamentous bands associated with compression were found.

Heo et al. [28] reported the results of 14 patients (4 males and 10 females) who underwent paraspinal UBE decompression for FOS at L5–S1. The average age was 59.5 ± 7.2 years, and the follow-up period was 11 ± 5 months. The VAS for leg pain improved from 8.4 ± 1.1 to 2.8 ± 1.4 and the ODI from 60.2 ± 5.5 preoperatively to 22.1 ± 3.4 at the end of follow-up. Of the 14 cases, 7 patients had an associated extraforaminal disc herniation. The authors reported immediate postoperative abdominal pain in 2 patients because of hydro-retroperitoneum that resolved 3 h later with conservative management.

UBE specifically for FOS is associated with relevant technical advantages, such as the ability to access deep anatomy in the extraforaminal space of L5–S1 with excellent visualization, minimal damage to paraspinal tissues, less postoperative pain, and prompt mobilization out of bed. However, there are also significant risks associated with this approach, such as dural injury, root injury, postoperative dysesthesia, postoperative hematoma, infection, and insufficient decompression. Moreover, the retroperitoneal collection caused by the fluid irrigated by the endoscope has been reported [26, 28]. However, this can be avoided if the decompression does not extend laterally more than necessary. Also, the surgeon must be careful when using the working instruments to prevent injury to the common iliac vessels anterior to the spine, mainly when extraforaminal discectomy is performed [53].

Tips and Pearls

- In-depth knowledge of lumbosacral anatomy and experience with microsurgery and uniportal and biportal endoscopy are required to perform FOS cases confidently.
- Dissection of the TP and the SA must be careful since we can injure any vascular structure coming from the segmental lumbar artery (SLA) and cause significant intraoperative bleeding challenging to control, forcing to convert the surgery. In addition, correct hemostasis must be confirmed due to the high risk of retroperitoneal hematoma, mainly due to a poor technique in the coagulation of the following arteries such as intertransverse (ITA), interarticular (IAA), and superior and inferior articular (SAA and IAA).
- The LSL should be removed as lateral as necessary to meet the decompression objective and confirm it with the free mobilization of the fifth lumbar nerve. However, care must be taken when removing the most distal portion of the LSL due to the risk of hydro-retroperitoneum.
- Traction of the root should be avoided, especially when deciding to remove an extraforaminal disc fragment or a marginal osteophyte. Bone decompression (TP, SA, and SAP) must first be completed until the nerve is identified, then the LSL and deep bands must be removed, and finally, special maneuvers must be performed to complete ventral decompression. This may prevent postoperative iatrogenic radiculitis or dysesthesia.

Conclusions

Paraspinal access using the unilateral biportal endoscopic technique (UBE) can be an alternative to microsurgery, tubular surgery, and uniportal endoscopy for extraforaminal decompression of lumbosacral junction. Acceptable results have been published in the literature, and technically this procedure is associated with advantages, the main one being excellent visualization in intricate and deep anatomy such as the extraforaminal space at L5–S1. However, this technique requires skills acquired with experience in other methods first. Therefore, more studies with adequate samples and methodology would confirm the potentials and shortcomings of this technique in the FOS.

References

1. Wiltse LL, Guyer RD, Spencer CW, Glenn WV, Porter IS. Alar transverse process impingement of the L5 spinal nerve: the far-out syndrome. Spine (Phila Pa 1976). 1984;9(1):31–41.
2. Mahato NK. Redefining lumbosacral transitional vertebrae (LSTV) classification: integrating the full spectrum of morphological alterations in a biomechanical continuum. Med Hypotheses. 2013;81(1):76–81.

3. Castellvi AE, Goldstein LA, Chan DP. Lumbosacral transitional vertebrae and their relationship with lumbar extradural defects. Spine (Phila Pa 1976). 1984;9(5):493–5.
4. Nardo L, Alizai H, Virayavanich W, et al. Lumbosacral transitional vertebrae: association with low back pain. Radiology. 2012;265(2):497–503.
5. Alonzo F, Cobar A, Cahueque M, Prieto JA. Bertolotti's syndrome: an underdiagnosed cause for lower back pain. J Surg Case Rep. 2018;2018(10):rjy276.
6. Otani K, Konno S, Kikuchi S. Lumbosacral transitional vertebrae and nerve-root symptoms. J Bone Joint Surg Br. 2001;83(8):1137–40.
7. Kapetanakis S, Chaniotakis C, Paraskevopoulos C, Pavlidis P. An unusual case report of Bertolotti's syndrome: extraforaminal stenosis and L5 unilateral root compression (Castellvi type III an LSTV). J Orthop Case Rep. 2017;7(3):9–12.
8. Hughes RJ, Saifuddin A. Numbering of lumbosacral transitional vertebrae on MRI: role of the iliolumbar ligaments. AJR Am J Roentgenol. 2006;187(1):W59–65.
9. Bertolotti M. Contributo alla conoscenza dei vizi di differenzazione regionale del rachide con speciale reguardo all assimilazione sacrale della V. lombare. Radiol Med. 1917;4:113–44.
10. Adams R, Herrera-Nicol S, Jenkins AL III. Surgical treatment of a rare presentation of Bertolotti's syndrome from Castellvi type IV lumbosacral transitional vertebra: case report and review of the literature. J Neurol Surg Rep. 2018;79(3):e70–4.
11. Quinlan JF, Duke D, Eustace S. Bertolotti's syndrome. A cause of back pain in young people. J Bone Joint Surg Br. 2006;88(9):1183–6.
12. Mahato NK. Morphological traits in sacra associated with complete and partial lumbarization of first sacral segment. Spine J. 2010;10(10):910–5.
13. Vergauwen S, Parizel PM, van Breusegem L, et al. Distribution and incidence of degenerative spine changes in patients with a lumbo-sacral transitional vertebra. Eur Spine J. 1997;6(3):168–72.
14. Hashimoto M, Watanabe O, Hirano H. Extraforaminal stenosis in the lumbosacral spine. Efficacy of MR imaging in the coronal plane. Acta Radiol. 1996;37(5):610–3.
15. Paik NC, Lim CS, Jang HS. Numeric and morphological verification of lumbosacral segments in 8280 consecutive patients. Spine (Phila Pa 1976). 2013;38(10):E573–8.
16. Brault JS, Smith J, Currier BL. Partial lumbosacral transitional vertebra resection for contralateral facetogenic pain. Spine (Phila Pa 1976). 2001;26(2):226–9.
17. Marks RC, Thulbourne T. Infiltration of anomalous lumbosacral articulations. Steroid and anesthetic injections in 10 back-pain patients. Acta Orthop Scand. 1991;62(2):139–41.
18. Jancuska JM, Spivak JM, Bendo JA. A review of symptomatic lumbosacral transitional vertebrae: Bertolotti's syndrome. Int J Spine Surg. 2015;9:42.
19. Weber J, Ernestus RI. Transitional lumbosacral segment with unilateral transverse process anomaly (Castellvi type 2A) resulting in extraforaminal impingement of the spinal nerve: a pathoanatomical study of four specimens and report of two clinical cases. Neurosurg Rev. 2010;34(2):143–50.
20. Abe E, Sato K, Shimada Y, Okada K, Yan K, Mizutani Y. Anterior decompression of foraminal stenosis below a lumbosacral transitional vertebra. A case report. Spine (Phila Pa 1976). 1997;22(7):823–6.
21. Ichihara K, Taguchi T, Hashida T, Ochi Y, Murakami T, Kawai S. The treatment of far-out foraminal stenosis below a lumbosacral transitional vertebra: a report of two cases. J Spinal Disord Tech. 2004;17(2):154–7.
22. Porter NA, Lalam RK, Tins BJ, Tyrrell PN, Singh J, Cassar-Pullicino VN. Prevalence of extraforaminal nerve root compression below lumbosacral transitional vertebrae. Skelet Radiol. 2014;43(1):55–60.
23. McGrath K, Schmidt E, Rabah N, Abubakr M, Steinmetz M. Clinical assessment and management of Bertolotti syndrome: a review of the literature. Spine J. 2021;21(8):1286–96.
24. Sasaki M, Aoki M, Matsumoto K, Tsuruzono K, Akiyama C, Yoshimine T. Middle-term surgical outcomes of microscopic posterior decompression for far-out syndrome. J Neurol Surg A Cent Eur Neurosurg. 2014;75(2):79–83.

25. Wu PH, Sebastian M, Kim HS, Heng GTY. How I do it? Uniportal full endoscopic pseudoarthrosis release of left L5/S1 Bertolotti's syndrome under intraoperative computer tomographic guidance in an ambulatory setting. Acta Neurochir. 2021;163(10):2789–95.
26. Park MK, Son SK, Park WW, Choi SH, Jung DY, Kim DH. Unilateral biportal endoscopy for decompression of extraforaminal stenosis at the lumbosacral junction: surgical techniques and clinical outcomes. Neurospine. 2021;18(4):871–9.
27. Lee CK, Kim I. Commentary on "Unilateral biportal endoscopy for decompression of extraforaminal stenosis at the lumbosacral junction: surgical techniques and clinical outcomes". Neurospine. 2021;18(4):880–1.
28. Heo DH, Sharma S, Park CK. Endoscopic treatment of extraforaminal entrapment of L5 nerve root (far out syndrome) by unilateral biportal endoscopic approach: technical report and preliminary clinical results. Neurospine. 2019;16(1):130–7.
29. Farshad-Amacker NA, Herzog RJ, Hughes AP, Aichmair A, Farshad M. Associations between lumbosacral transitional anatomy types and degeneration at the transitional and adjacent segments. Spine J. 2015;15(6):1210–6.
30. Neelakantan S, Anandarajan R, Shyam K, Philip B. Multimodality imaging in Bertolotti's syndrome: an important cause of low back pain in young adults. BMJ Case Rep. 2016;2016:bcr2016217121.
31. Konin GP, Walz DM. Lumbosacral transitional vertebrae: classification, imaging findings, and clinical relevance. AJNR Am J Neuroradiol. 2010;31(10):1778–86.
32. Chalian M, Soldatos T, Carrino JA, Belzberg AJ, Khanna J, Chhabra A. Prediction of transitional lumbosacral anatomy on magnetic resonance imaging of the lumbar spine. World J Radiol. 2012;4(3):97–101.
33. Pekindil G, Sarikaya A, Pekindil Y, Gültekin A, Kokino S. Lumbosacral transitional vertebral articulation: evaluation by planar and SPECT bone scintigraphy. Nucl Med Commun. 2004;25(1):29–37.
34. Matsumoto M, Watanabe K, Ishii K, et al. Posterior decompression surgery for extraforaminal entrapment of the fifth lumbar spinal nerve at the lumbosacral junction. J Neurosurg Spine. 2010;12(1):72–81.
35. Tubbs RS, Iwanaga J, Aly I, et al. Extraforaminal compression of the L5 nerve: an anatomical study with application to failed posterior decompressive procedures. J Clin Neurosci. 2017;41:139–43.
36. Shibayama M, Ito F, Miura Y, Nakamura S, Ikeda S, Fujiwara K. Unsuspected reason for sciatica in Bertolotti's syndrome. J Bone Joint Surg Br. 2011;93(5):705–7.
37. Matsumoto M, Chiba K, Ishii K, Watanabe K, Nakamura M, Toyama Y. Microendoscopic partial resection of the sacral ala to relieve extraforaminal entrapment of the L-5 spinal nerve at the lumbosacral tunnel. Technical note. J Neurosurg Spine. 2006;4(4):342–6.
38. Wiltse LL, Bateman JG, Hutchinson RH, Nelson WE. The paraspinal sacrospinalis-splitting approach to the lumbar spine. J Bone Joint Surg Am. 1968;50(5):919–26.
39. O'Toole JE, Eichholz KM, Fessler RG. Minimally invasive far lateral microendoscopic discectomy for extraforaminal disc herniation at the lumbosacral junction: cadaveric dissection and technical case report. Spine J. 2007;7(4):414–21.
40. Ikuta K, Kitamura T, Masuda K, Hotta K, Senba H, Shidahara S. Minimally invasive transtubular endoscopic decompression for L5 radiculopathy induced by lumbosacral extraforaminal lesions. Asian Spine J. 2018;12(2):246–55.
41. Lee S, Kang JH, Srikantha U, Jang IT, Oh SH. Extraforaminal compression of the L-5 nerve root at the lumbosacral junction: clinical analysis, decompression technique, and outcome. J Neurosurg Spine. 2014;20(4):371–9.
42. Pirris SM, Dhall S, Mummaneni PV, Kanter AS. Minimally invasive approach to extraforaminal disc herniations at the lumbosacral junction using an operating microscope: case series and review of the literature. Neurosurg Focus. 2008;25(2):E10.
43. Kotil K, Akcetin M, Bilge T. A minimally invasive transmuscular approach to far-lateral L5-S1 level disc herniations: a prospective study. J Spinal Disord Tech. 2007;20(2):132–8.

44. Voyadzis JM, Gala VC, Sandhu FA, Fessler RG. Minimally invasive approach for far lateral disc herniations: results from 20 patients. Minim Invasive Neurosurg. 2010;53(3):122–6.
45. Yang D, Wu X, Zheng M, Wang J. A modified percutaneous endoscopic technique to remove extraforaminal disk herniation at the L5-S1 segment. World Neurosurg. 2018;119:e671–8.
46. Lübbers T, Abuamona R, Elsharkawy AE. Percutaneous endoscopic treatment of foraminal and extraforaminal disc herniation at the L5-S1 level. Acta Neurochir. 2012;154(10):1789–95.
47. Hsu HT, Chang SJ, Yang SS, Chai CL. Learning curve of full-endoscopic lumbar discectomy. Eur Spine J. 2013;22(4):727–33.
48. Golubovsky JL, Momin A, Thompson NR, Steinmetz MP. Understanding quality of life and treatment history of patients with Bertolotti syndrome compared with lumbosacral radiculopathy. J Neurosurg Spine. 2019; https://doi.org/10.3171/2019.2.SPINE1953.
49. Nathan H, Weizenbluth M, Halperin N. The lumbosacral ligament (LSL), with special emphasis on the "lumbosacral tunnel" and the entrapment of the 5th lumbar nerve. Int Orthop. 1982;6(3):197–202.
50. Qian Y, Qin A, Zheng MH. Transforaminal ligament may play a role in lumbar nerve root compression of foraminal stenosis. Med Hypotheses. 2011;77(6):1148–9.
51. Kraan GA, Smit TH, Hoogland PV, Snijders CJ. Lumbar extraforaminal ligaments act as a traction relief and prevent spinal nerve compression [published correction appears in Clin Biomech (Bristol, Avon). 2012 Dec;27(10):1087]. Clin Biomech (Bristol, Avon). 2010;25(1):10–5.
52. Yamada H, Yoshida M, Hashizume H, et al. Efficacy of novel minimally invasive surgery using spinal microendoscope for treating extraforaminal stenosis at the lumbosacral junction. J Spinal Disord Tech. 2012;25(5):268–76.
53. Busardò FP, Frati P, Carbone I, Pugnetti P, Fineschi V. Iatrogenic left common iliac artery and vein perforation during lumbar discectomy: a fatal case. Forensic Sci Int. 2015;246:e7–e11.

Chapter 19
The Biportal Endoscopic Contralateral Approach for Juxtafacet Cystic Lesions of the Lumbar Spine

Javier Quillo-Olvera, Diego Quillo-Olvera, Javier Quillo-Reséndiz, and Michelle Barrera-Arreola

Abbreviations

AP	Anteroposterior
CSF	Cerebrospinal fluid
DVT	Deep venous thrombosis
EBL	Estimated blood loss
FJ	Facet joint
FL	Flavum ligament
IAP	Inferior articular process
ILS	Interlaminar space
IVS	Intervertebral space
JFCs	Juxtafacetary cysts
LBP	Low back pain
LSS	Lumbar spinal stenosis
LSTV	Lumbosacral transitional vertebra
MISS	Minimally invasive spine surgery
MRI	Magnetic resonance imaging
ODI	Oswestry Disability Index
RF	Radiofrequency
SAP	Superior articular process

Supplementary Information The online version contains supplementary material available at [https://doi.org/10.1007/978-3-031-14736-4_19].

J. Quillo-Olvera (✉) · D. Quillo-Olvera · J. Quillo-Reséndiz · M. Barrera-Arreola
The Brain and Spine Care, Minimally Invasive Spine Surgery Group, Hospital H+ Querétaro, Spine Clinic, Querétaro, México
e-mail: neuroqomd@gmail.com; drquilloolvera86@gmail.com; kitnoz@hotmail.com; michelle.barrera@anahuac.mx

J. Quillo-Olvera et al. (eds.), *Unilateral Biportal Endoscopy of the Spine*,
https://doi.org/10.1007/978-3-031-14736-4_19

SP	Spinous process
T1W	T1-weighted
T2W	T2-weighted
UBE	Unilateral biportal endoscopy
ULBD	Unilateral laminotomy for bilateral decompression
VAS	Visual analog scale

Introduction

It is estimated that the prevalence of synovial cysts (those arising from the zygapophyseal joint capsule of the lumbar spine) is around 7.5–9.6% [1, 2]. However, synovial, ganglion, and flavum ligament (FL) cysts make up a group of juxtafacetary cystic (JFC) lesions that, despite their histological differences, represent distinct endpoints of the same lumbar degenerative process [3, 4]. Synovial cysts are associated with a degenerative process in the facet joint (FJ) that results in increased pressure within it and protrusion of the synovial membrane through defects in the joint capsule; this herniation causes the formation of a para-articular cavity filled with synovial fluid that has the potential to compress the neural elements [5–7].

These JFCs arise more frequently at L4–L5 because it is the single-most mobile level of the spine, and they also have a strong association with lumbar spondylolisthesis (43.4%), either favoring it or as part of the degenerative instability disease [8, 9]. Furthermore, trauma has been considered another predisponent factor due to hemosiderin found in different cystic lesions with a history of traumatic spine injuries [10, 11]. In addition, various factors such as the degenerative process of the intervertebral disc (13.2%) and osteoarthritis (40.5%), spinal stenosis (1.4%), and scoliosis (1.4%) are also associated with lumbar JFCs [9].

JFCs share a similar clinical presentation, treatment options, and clinical outcomes [12, 13]. The most common clinical manifestations of these lesions are radiculopathy in 70% of cases, low back pain (LBP) in 48%, sensory deficits in 35%, neurogenic claudication in 28%, and paresis in 21% [5]. Symptoms will depend on the size, location, and structures adjacent to the cyst. MRI is usually the ideal study for diagnosing JFCs with 90% sensitivity compared to 70% in the lumbar CT [6, 9, 14]. They are typically lesions with a low-intensity signal in T1-weighted views and a high-intensity signal in T2-weighted (T2W) sequences, although sometimes these features may vary due to the amount of protein and blood in the cyst [15, 16]. Treatment of JFCs may include conservative measures such as bed rest, analgesic and anti-inflammatory medications, bracing, transcutaneous electrical stimulation, physical therapy, epidural and intra-articular steroid injections, and cyst aspiration [8, 15, 17, 18]. However, in about 60% of patients, surgical treatment will be chosen due to the failure of conservative medical treatment [16].

Surgical treatment may be recommended when conservative measures show persistent failure or intolerant symptoms associated with a neurological deficit

[9]. In a review published by Boviatitis et al. [9], the outcomes related to surgical treatment were excellent in 75% of 413 patients, good in 14%, and fair/poor in 11%. However, the proposed hemilaminectomy and facetectomy to remove juxtafacet cystic lesions [16], through microsurgical technique, despite being associated with low recurrence and complete resection of the cyst, may risk segmental stability while more joint is removed. Another surgical alternative is decompression and lumbar fusion; however, this can be associated with increased costs for the patient and other particular risks. This chapter reviews the biportal endoscopic sublaminar contralateral approach for resection of JFCs. This surgical option appears as a minimally invasive alternative that, in addition to having the objective of achieving adequate decompression of the traversing nerve root and the dural sac, also allows maximum preservation of the FJ, reducing the bone work necessary to reach the cyst [19].

Indications and Contraindications of the Biportal Endoscopic Contralateral Approach

1. Unilateral radicular pain congruent with radiological findings observed in the MRI.
2. Symptoms of radiculopathy such as tingling, numbness, cramps, or other sensitivity disturbances associated with the radiological finding on the MRI.
3. Neurogenic claudication and cauda equina.
4. Motor deficit (absolute indication).
5. Symptoms refractory to conservative treatment attempted for at least 6 weeks.
6. Segmental instability at the site of the cystic lesion, infection, or suspicion of neoplasia must be treated independently with the broad spectrum of spinal surgical techniques.

Surgical Technique

Step 1: Patient Position and Anesthesia

The patient is placed on an abdominal support frame on the operating table in prone. The hips, knees, and ankles are protected with soft pads, and the knees are semiflexed to avoid venous stasis in the limbs. The arms are abducted with the elbows flexed at 90°, avoiding stretching the cervical plexus or hurting the shoulder joint. The face is protected to prevent compression injuries. Maximum attention must be paid to the eyes to prevent any damage associated with the surgical position. The anesthesia used could be general or epidural. Waterproof draping is used due to the continuous irrigation of fluid during the procedure.

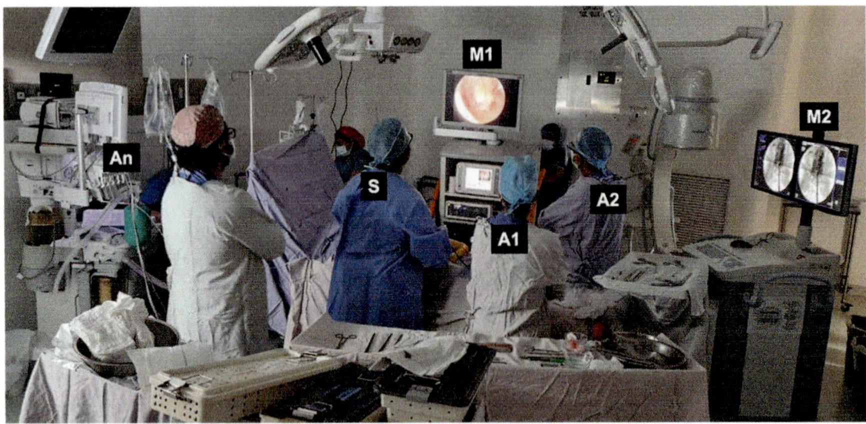

Fig. 19.1 Usual organization of the operating room in a biportal endoscopic procedure. *S* surgeon, *A1* surgical assistant 1, *A2* surgical assistant 2, *An* anesthesiologist, *M1* endoscopic display, *M2* C-arm display

Step 2: Organization of Surgical Staff

The surgeon should be positioned on the contralateral side of the pathology. If the cyst is on the right side, the approach will be planned on the left side and vice versa. The endoscope and C-arm displays should be located facing the surgeon. A surgical assistant stays next to the surgeon, and the other could be in front of him or her. The anesthesiology team will be at the head of the patient (Fig. 19.1).

Step 3: Location of Entry Points

The C-arm is necessary to locate the radiological references that will allow us to identify the entry points and create the portals for the contralateral biportal endoscopic approach. Generally, the cranial entry will be used as a viewing portal and the caudal as a working portal by a right-handed surgeon in a left-sided procedure.

The following references will be located on the AP view of the C-arm (Fig. 19.2):

1. The pedicles of the superior and inferior vertebra
2. The intervertebral space (IVS)
3. The interlaminar space (ILS)
4. The middle line

The surgeon will draw a line on the skin medial to both pedicles under the AP view (Fig. 19.3a). Subsequently, in the lateral view, the surgeon will identify the FJ

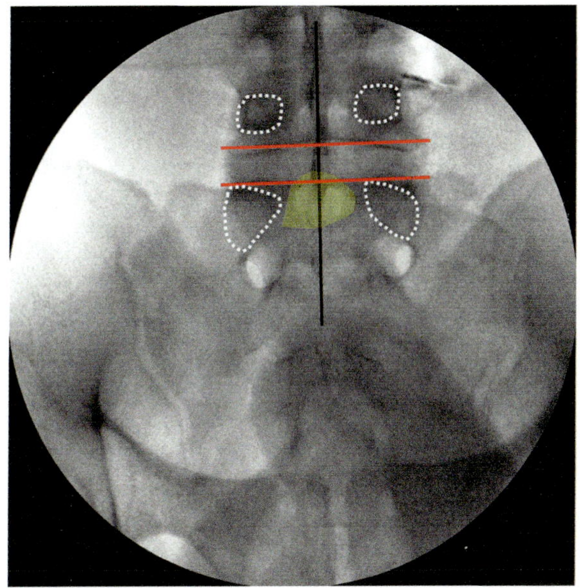

Fig. 19.2 AP projection of the C-arm where the radiological references were highlighted to guide the location of the entries in the contralateral biportal endoscopic approach. The dotted white circles represent the pedicles of L5/S1. The red lines are the L5–S1 intervertebral space, and the black line is the midline. The L5–S1 interlaminar space is highlighted in yellow

and the IVS and draw a line through these references that intersect the previous one (Fig. 19.3b). The cranial and caudal entry points for the biportal approach will be located 15 mm above and below the intersection of both lines (Fig. 19.3b, c). Finally, this will be confirmed in a lateral view and the simulation of the triangular approach using two needles placed on the entries (Fig. 19.3d).

Step 4: Contralateral Biportal Approach—Triangulation

The term triangulation refers to creating both portals towards the same anatomical reference, in this case, the spinolaminar junction. First, the surgeon will make a pair of 7 mm incisions. These could be transverse or stab at the previously planned cranial and caudal entries. Then, a 5 mm outer diameter dilator should be introduced through each incision to create both portals. In the caudal incision, the dilator will have a lateral-to-medial and caudal-to-cranial trajectory to palpate the spinolaminar junction; once the surgeon feels this, he or she will perform a subperiosteal dissection in the same place that will facilitate the creation of the working space later. The same process will be repeated in the cranial incision with a lateral-to-medial and cranial-to-caudal trajectory. After creating both portals with the 5 mm dilators, it is advised to confirm the proper triangulation of both addressed to the spinolaminar junction with the C-arm (Fig. 19.4).

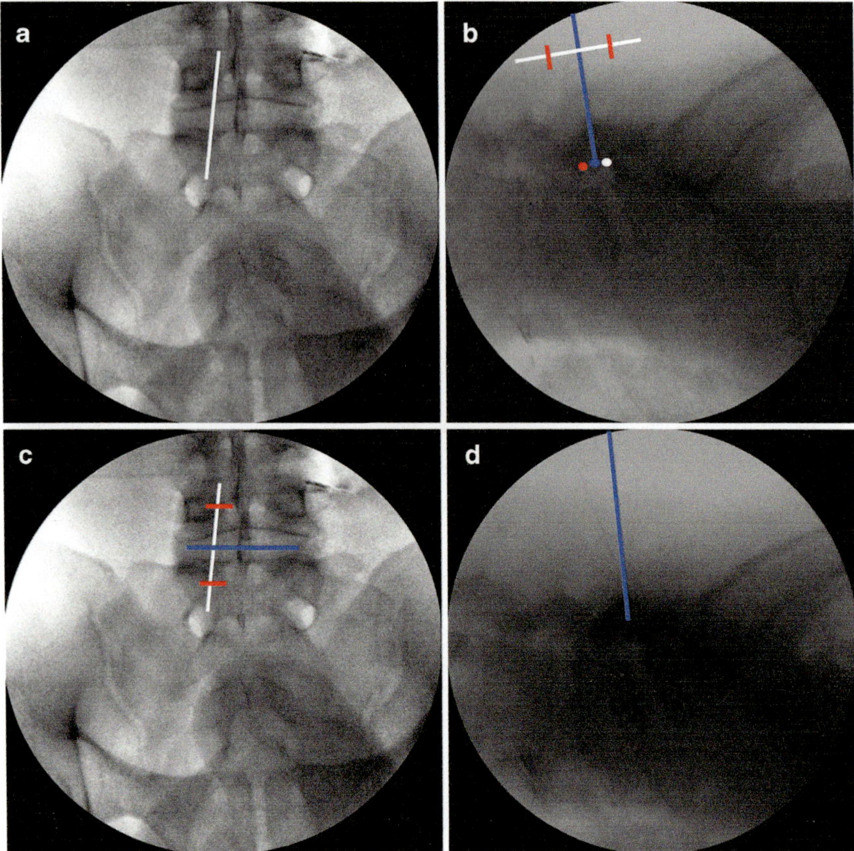

Fig. 19.3 Process for planning the skin incisions during the contralateral biportal endoscopic approach. (**a**) AP view, a white line passes medial to the L5 and S1 pedicles. (**b**) In the lateral view, it has been marked to which part of the facet joint (red, blue, and white circles) the contralateral approach will be addressed (blue line), depending on the location of the juxtafacet cyst. The intersection of that line with the medial-to-pedicle line represents the center of the triangular approach. (**c**) The incisions (horizontal red lines) will be located 15 mm above and below that intersection. (**d**) Simulation of the biportal endoscopic approach with two needles addressed to the planned target

Step 5: Contralateral Biportal Endoscopic Approach Through a Sublaminar Route

The following steps include the biportal endoscopic procedure to remove the contralaterally located JFC and, if necessary, perform bilateral decompression of the neural elements through a unilateral approach (ULBD). The endoscope will be

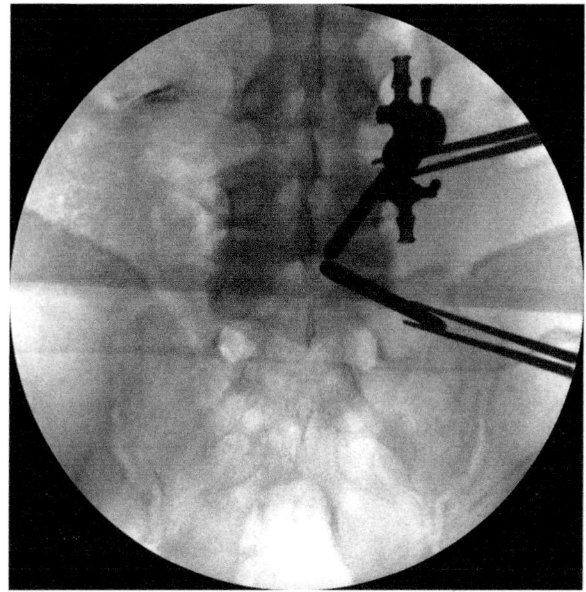

Fig. 19.4 Biportal triangular approach for contralateral sublaminar decompression from left to right. Note how the viewing portal has been introduced through the cranial entry and handled with the left hand by a right-handed surgeon

introduced through the viewing portal (on the left-sided approach placed in the cranial entry, the contrary on the right side), and the radiofrequency (RF) through the working portal (on the right-sided approach set in the cranial access, the opposite on the left side). There are two situations that the surgeon must verify before proceeding with the endoscopic procedure; the first is to check that the continuous fluid irrigation is working, the inflow of saline through the endoscope, and the outflow through the working portal, preventing the stagnation of the saline in the tissues and improving the quality of the image through the endoscope. The other situation is to locate the working tool with the endoscope, confirming that the triangular approach was correct.

Step 6: Creating the Working Space

In this step, the surgical field will be delimited. As mentioned in the earlier chapters of this book, the working area lies medial to the multifidus muscle, in a space usually filled with fat and loose connective tissue. This space is called epiperiosteal (Fig. 19.5). Next, the surgeon will use various surgical tools, including the RF probe and pituitary forceps, to clean the working space (epiperiosteal), identify the bony landmarks (lamina, spinous process, interlaminar space), and continue the decompression (Fig. 19.6).

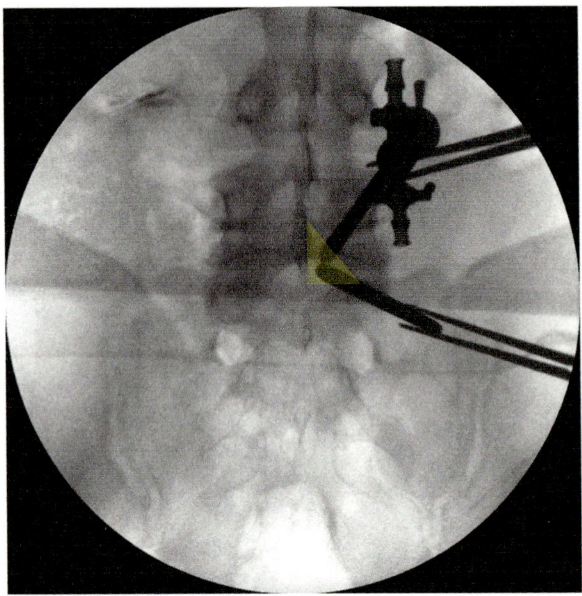

Fig. 19.5 The triangle medial to the multifidus has been highlighted in yellow

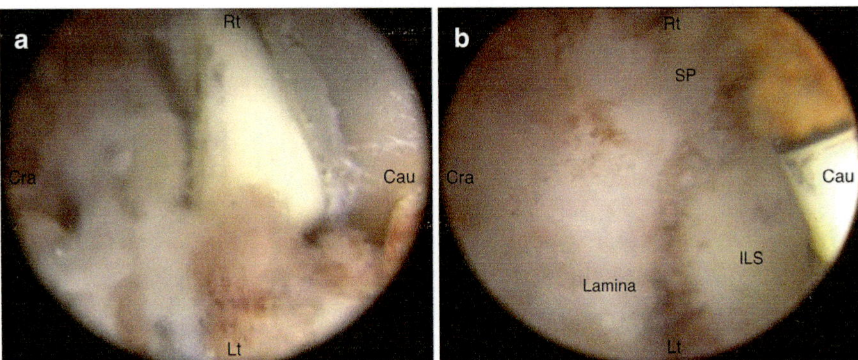

Fig. 19.6 Intraoperative endoscopic images where the RF probe has been located by the endoscope. The working space (**a**) is created to identify the anatomical landmarks (**b**) in L5–S1 on the left side. *Cra* cranial, *Cau* caudal, *Rt* right, *Lt* left, *SP* spinous process, *ILS* interlaminar space

Step 7: Bone Removal

The unilateral biportal endoscopic (UBE) technique allows rapid access to the contralateral side through a sublaminar approach, removing the base of the spinous process (SP) (Fig. 19.7). A high-speed drilling system with a protected cutting tip will be used. The ventral aspect of the contralateral lamina will be undercut with the

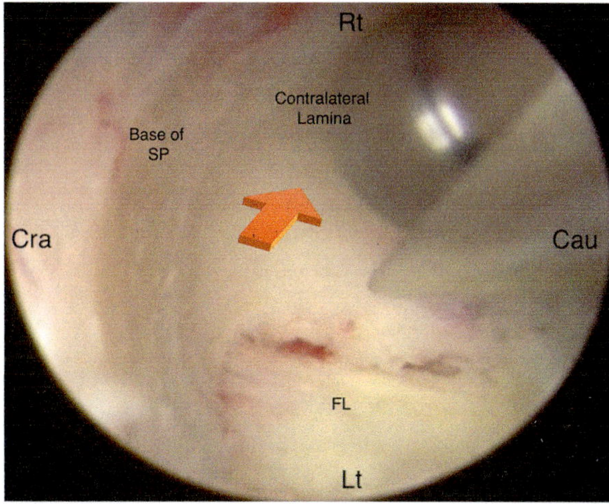

Fig. 19.7 Left L5–S1 contralateral sublaminar biportal endoscopic approach. The drill is used to cross the midline by undercutting the base of the SP. *Cra* cranial, *Cau* caudal, *Med* medial, *SP* spinous process, *FL* flavum ligament

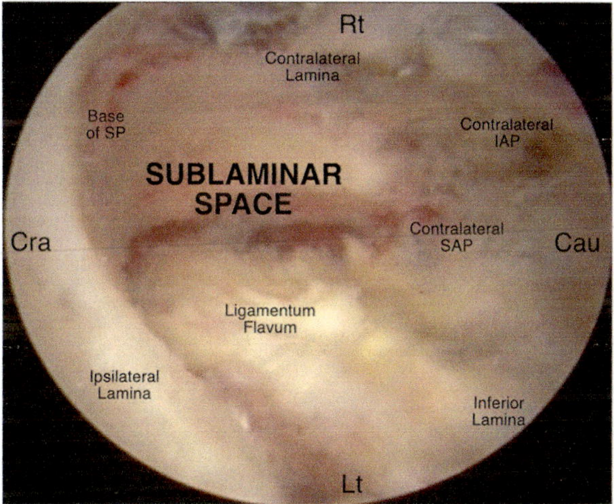

Fig. 19.8 Various bone landmarks were exposed through a left biportal endoscopic sublaminar contralateral approach at L5–S1. The sublaminar space is referred to with a legend on capitals. *Cra* cranial, *Cau* caudal, *Rt* right, *Lt* left, *SP* spinous process, *IAP* inferior articular process, *SAP* superior articular process

drill. The endpoint of bone removal is achieved when the FL attachments are identified. The medial part of the inferior articular process (IAP), the superior articular process (SAP), and the inferior lamina will be recognized during contralateral bone decompression. The surgeon may perform an ipsilateral superior and inferior laminotomy if the case was also planned for a unilateral laminotomy for bilateral decompression (ULBD) in addition to cyst removal. It is recommended that the bone work with the drilling system and the use of Kerrison rongeur be carried out in an over-the-top fashion to use the FL as a protective barrier of the neural elements (Fig. 19.8).

Step 8: Cyst Removal and Flavectomy

It is essential to consider that patients with JFCs may experience incidental dural tears during cyst dissection or flavectomy in the side of pathology [20] due to the tight adhesions between the ventral surface of the FL or the cyst and the dural sac or another neural element. Therefore, this step is crucial since an adequate and meticulous dissection will decrease the risk of an incidental durotomy. It is suggested that the flavectomy is started ipsilaterally on the non-pathological side and from the midline, where the medial fold of the dural sac can be identified. Flavectomy can be performed with Kerrison rongeur of different sizes. The authors recommend dissecting the dorsal epidural space with a nerve hook before biting the FL with Kerrison punches. The surgeon must release the medial fold of the dura from the FL. It will allow recognition of a plane between the contralateral FL and the dural sac, and following that plane, it could be easier to dissect the cyst. After complete dissection of the ventral wall of the cyst, it can be removed with Kerrison punches as the contralateral FL (Fig. 19.9). Sometimes, firm adhesions can be found between the ventral wall of the cyst and the dural sac or traversing nerve root. In that situation, it is advised only to detach the cyst from the FL or leave the wall adhered to the dura floating. Aggressive dissection of the cyst can lead to durotomy.

Step 9: Direct Decompression of the Traversing Nerve Root

Once the contralateral traversing nerve root is identified, its proper decompression must be confirmed (Fig. 19.10). That means after removing the cyst, it should be checked whether the SAP does not pinch the nerve as it passes through the lateral recess, and if so, medial undercutting of the FJ should be performed. Precisely, the

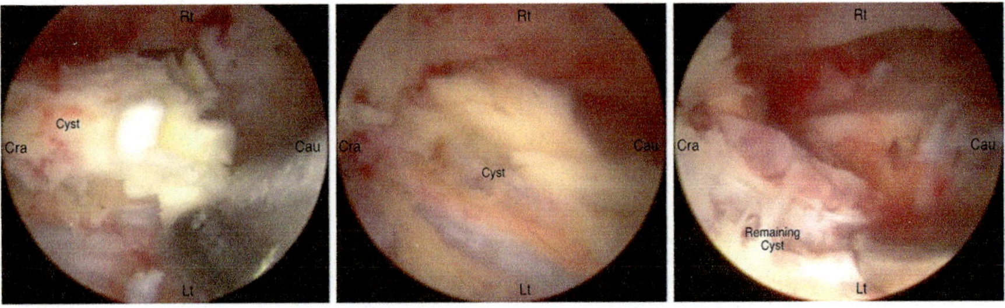

Fig. 19.9 Endoscopic images show a right juxtafacet cyst resection reached by a left biportal endoscopic contralateral sublaminar approach at L5–S1. *Cra* cranial, *Cau* caudal, *Rt* right, *Lt* left

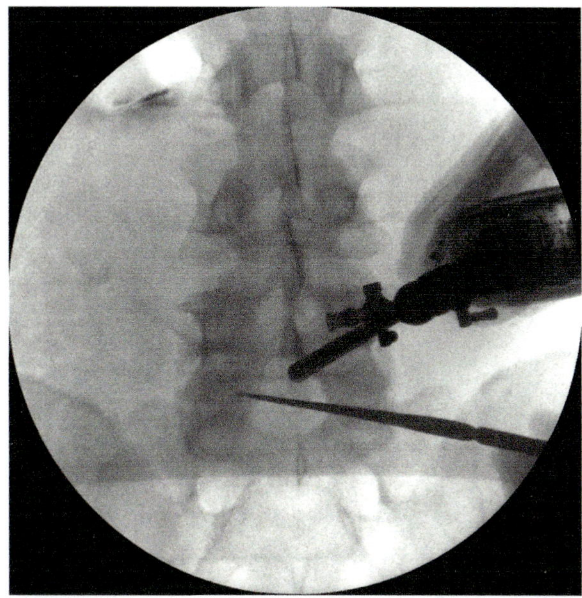

Fig. 19.10 AP view of the C-arm from a left sublaminar contralateral biportal endoscopic approach at L5–S1

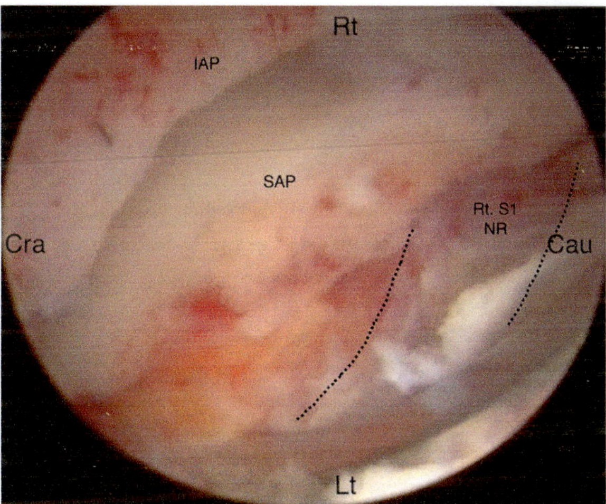

Fig. 19.11 The right S1 nerve root (black dotted lines) has been decompressed in its subarticular course, completely removing the juxtafacet cystic lesion and partially the ventral SAP. *Cra* cranial, *Cau* caudal, *Rt* right, *Lt* left, *IAP* inferior articular process, *SAP* superior articular process, *NR* nerve root

contralateral approach facilitates this procedure since bone remodeling of the most ventral portion of the SAP can be selectively performed without the need to remove a larger volume of the FJ. Finally, proper decompression of the traversing nerve root will be confirmed by free mobilization of the nerve and direct observation of the dural pulse (Fig. 19.11).

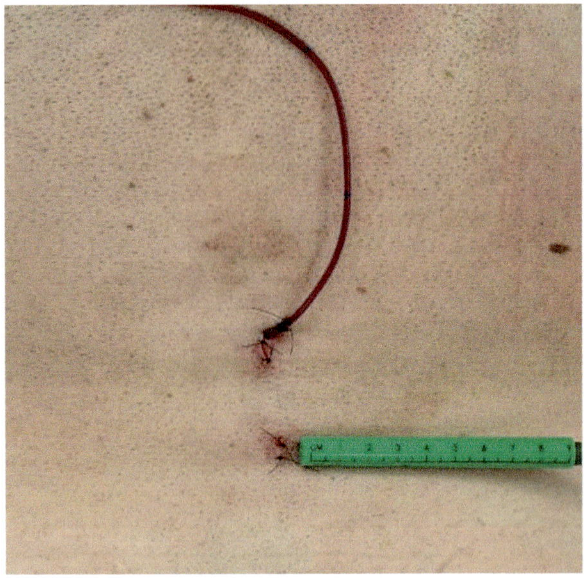

Fig. 19.12 Surgical wounds after a contralateral UBE sublaminar approach

Step 10: Hemostasis and Closure

After a successful neural decompression, the surgeon will confirm hemostasis, reducing the irrigation pressure to identify bleeding sources or ensuring none, especially those that come from the bone. Hemostasis can be performed with the RF probe, bone wax, or use of various hemostatic matrices on the market. Subsequently, the neural elements will be checked for any incidental dural tears that may have occurred inadvertently during the procedure. Lastly, an epidural drain will be left to prevent any epidural collection, including a hematoma, and the incisions will be closed to finish the surgery (Fig. 19.12).

Illustrated Cases

Case 1

A 54-year-old male had progressive radicular pain of 3 months on evolution, ultimately severe and located in the right leg. He also complained of numbness in his leg and a tingling sensation in his calf and right foot. Neurological examination demonstrated weakness in the right ankle's plantar flexion and flexion of the great toe. Physical therapy and various medications, including opioids, failed. Lumbar X-ray images identified a Meyerding grade 1 spondylolisthesis with no instability observed on lateral projections in flexion and extension of the lumbar spine (Fig. 19.13). Nonetheless, the patient did not complain of LBP. A juxtafacet cyst at L5–S1 on the right side with compressive effect on the dural sac and the S1 nerve

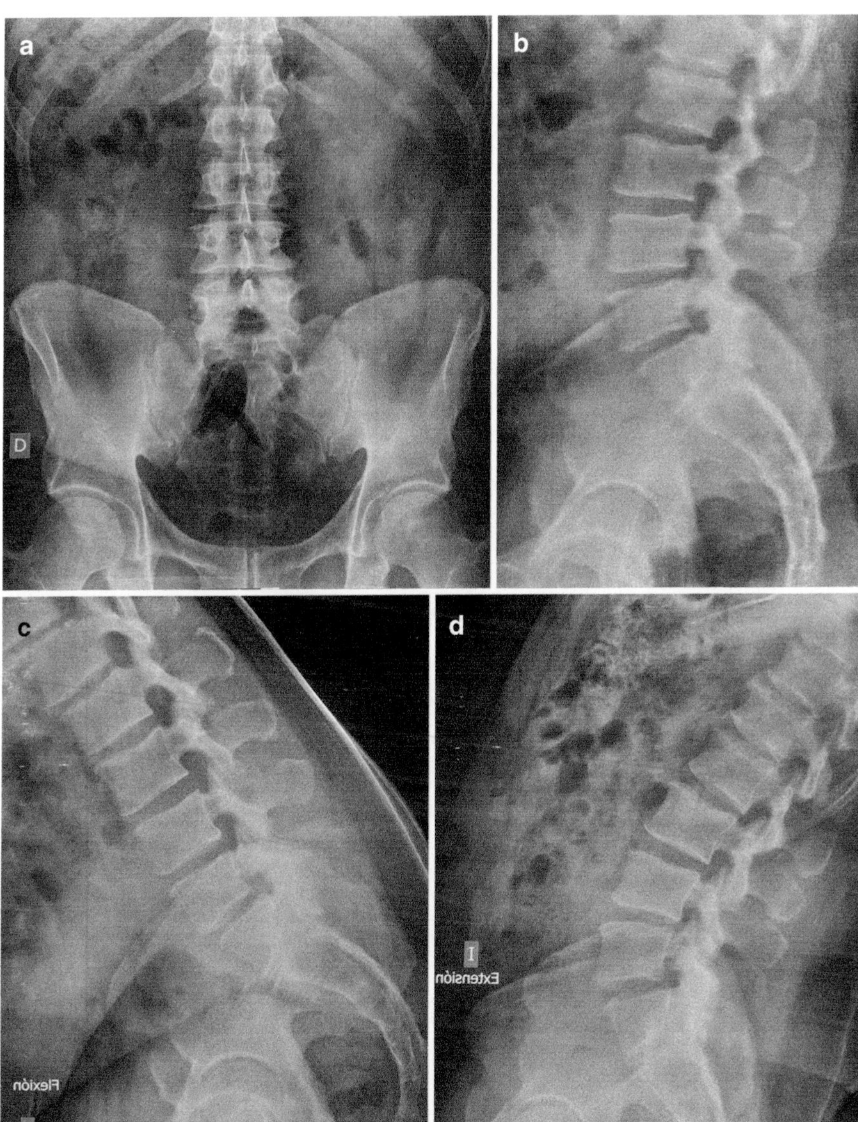

Fig. 19.13 Preoperative X-rays of the lumbar spine of Case 1. (**a**) AP. (**b**) Neutral lateral. (**c**) Lateral flexion. (**d**) Lateral in extension

root was identified on preoperative lumbar MRI. The finding was consistent with the patient's symptoms (Fig. 19.14). The surgical options presented to the patient were multiple; however, he opted for a contralateral sublaminar decompression with UBE in the affected segment. At the surgery, tight adhesions were identified between the ventral wall of the cyst and the neural elements, especially with the dural sac and

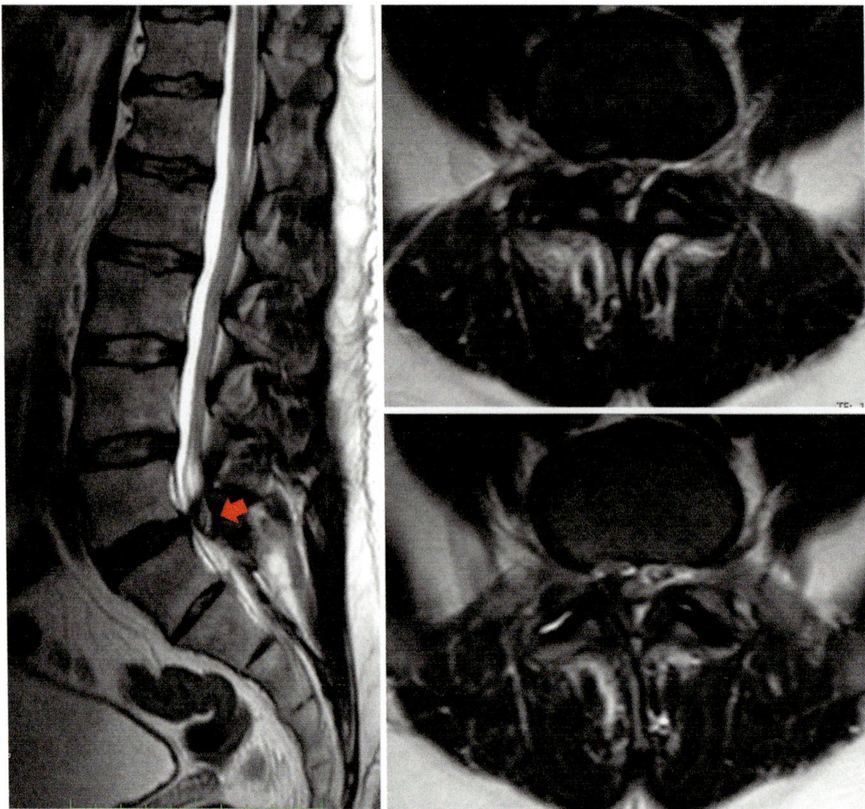

Fig. 19.14 Preoperative lumbar MRI of Case 1. On the left, the T2W sagittal view showed a cyst in L5–S1 (red arrow). On the right, two representative T2W axial views of L5–S1 in which severe right central and lateral stenosis associated with the juxtafacet cystic lesion can be observed

the S1 traversing nerve root; however, it was possible to remove the cystic lesion altogether without incident (Video 19.1). Immediate postoperative MRI demonstrated encouraging results concerning decompression of the neural elements (Fig. 19.15). In addition, the patient was discharged the day after his surgery with no pain in his leg and minimal paresthesia compared to what he had preoperatively. At the 2-week visit, the weakness in the ankle's plantar flexion and the great toe flexion on the right side had disappeared.

Case 2

A 58-year-old man was treated for significant pain in his right leg and progressive weakness in walking of 7 weeks on evolution. The pain began in the right buttock and radiated through the posterior aspect of the thigh and calf until it reached the lateral edge of the right foot. Recently, this pain was severe in intensity and related

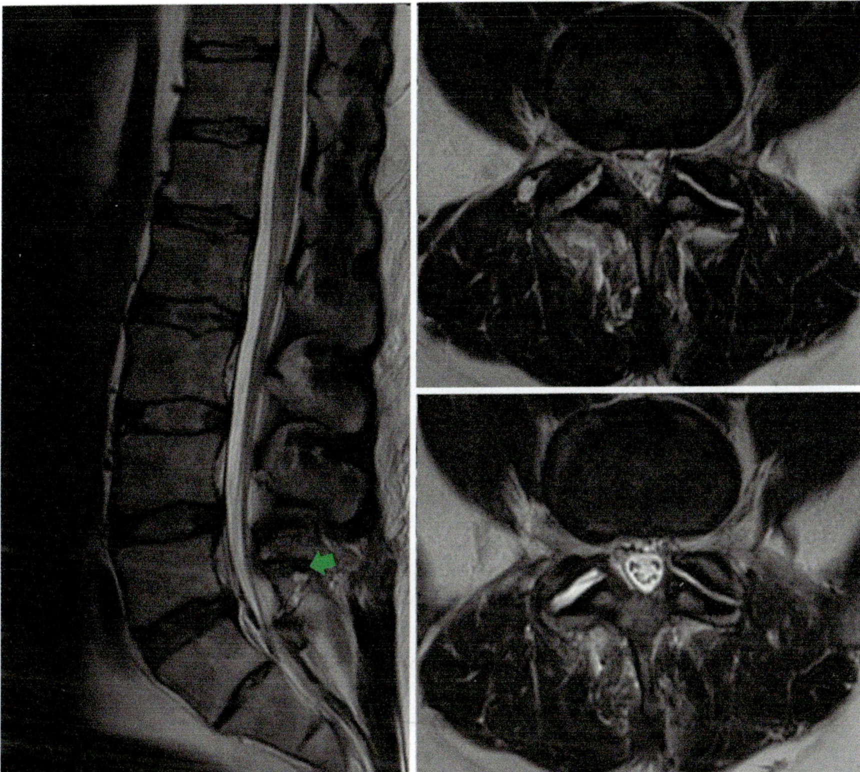

Fig. 19.15 Postoperative lumbar MRI of Case 1. On the left, the T2W sagittal view confirmed a complete decompression of the dural sac. On the right, two representative T2W axial views of L5–S1 show adequate decompression of the dural sac and the right S1 transverse root. In addition, intrafacet fluid is observed after biportal endoscopic decompression associated with continuous saline irrigation

to numbness in both legs. Furthermore, the neurological examination revealed neurogenic claudication and weakness in plantar flexion of both ankles. The patient was previously treated with epidural steroids without success. An LSTV anomaly was identified on lumbar radiographs (Fig. 19.16). The lumbar spine MRI showed a cystic lesion on the right side, coming from the FL associated with segmental degenerative changes leading to central and bilateral subarticular LSS (Fig. 19.17). The imaging findings corresponded with the patient's symptoms. A left contralateral biportal endoscopic approach was performed at L5–L6 (S1) to remove the cystic lesion and decompress the neural elements on both sides (Fig. 19.18; Video 19.2). Postoperative lumbar MRI demonstrated successful decompression (Fig. 19.19). The patient was discharged 16 h after the procedure with no pain in the right leg and no numbness in his legs. The follow-up at 1 month showed a clear improvement in the patient's gait.

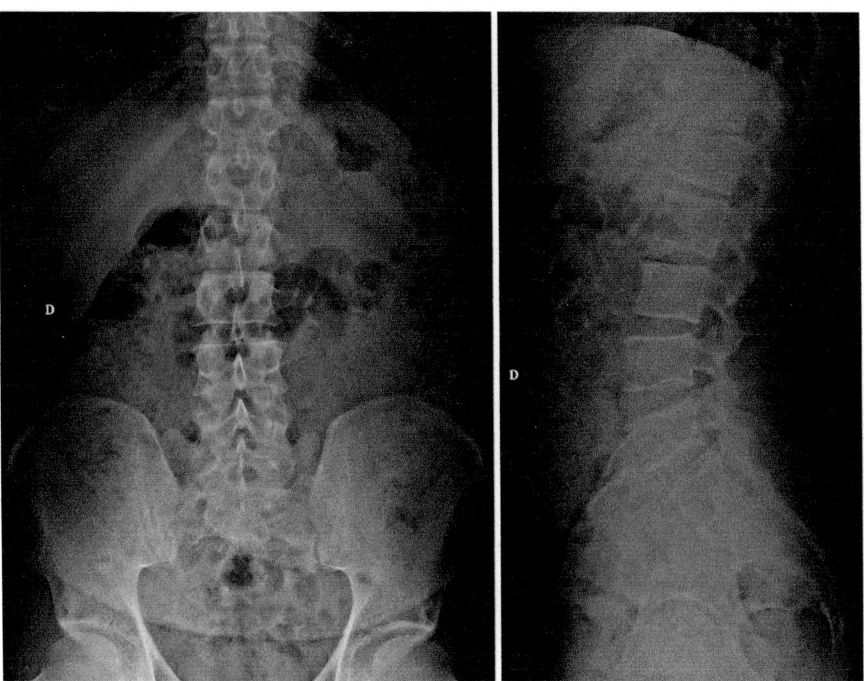

Fig. 19.16 Preoperative X-ray on AP (left) and lateral (right) views of Case 2 shows an LSTV anomaly

Case 3

A 62-year-old male complained of sciatica pain in both legs, particularly when sitting and walking. The pain was severe, VAS (8/10), and associated with spasms in both calves. In addition, neurological examination revealed weakness in the left-ankle dorsiflexion. The patient had a history of several epidural steroid injections, foraminal blocks, and physical therapy, with no improvement of his symptoms. Preoperative lumbar MRI demonstrated a juxtafacet cyst at L4–L5 on the left side associated with significant degenerative changes in the facet joints and hypertrophy of FL leading to LSS (Fig. 19.20). A lumbar fusion procedure was offered; however, the patient opted for selective segmental decompression of findings associated with his symptoms. Therefore, a right contralateral UBE was performed to remove the cyst and, simultaneously, a ULBD; both were successfully achieved (Fig. 19.21). Immediate postoperative lumbar MRI demonstrated adequate central and subarticular decompression at L4–L5 (Fig. 19.22). The patient was discharged without radicular pain and substantially improved neurogenic claudication on the following day.

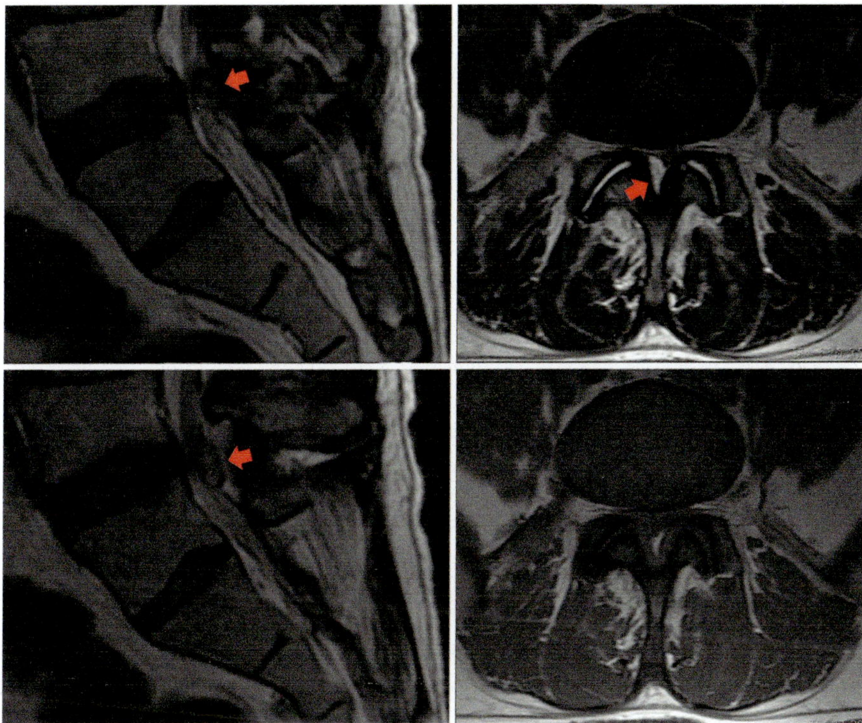

Fig. 19.17 Preoperative lumbar MRI of Case 2. On the left, the representative T2W sagittal views demonstrated a cyst that affects the lateral recess and the central spinal canal (red arrows). On the left, and superior: a T2W axial view shows a severe narrowing of the central spinal canal at L5–L6 (S1) with a cyst (red arrow) adhered to the FL wall on the right side. On the left, and down: the same axial view as above but in T1W confirms the finding

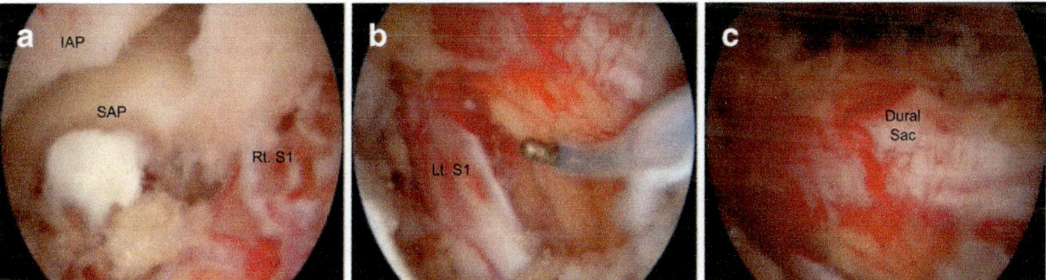

Fig. 19.18 Intraoperative endoscopic pictures of Case 2. (**a**) The right S1 root has been decompressed using a contralateral approach at L5–L6 (S1). Through the same UBE procedure, a ULBD was also performed in which the left S1 root (**b**) and the dural sac (**c**) were also decompressed. *IAP* inferior articular process, *SAP* superior articular process

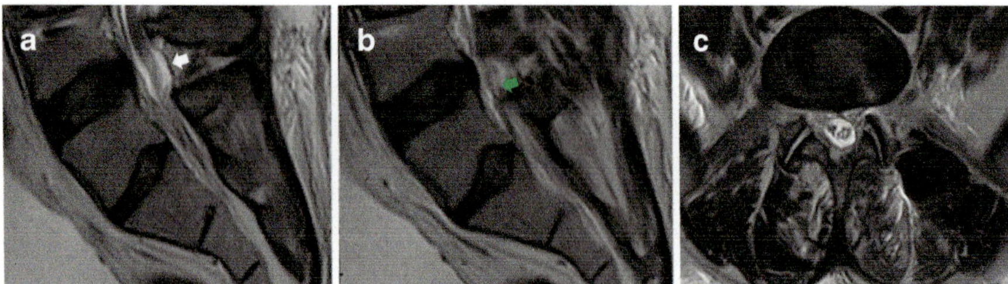

Fig. 19.19 Postoperative lumbar MRI of Case 2. (**a**, **b**) show the sagittal T2W views after decompression and cyst resection. In (**a**), the dural sac (white arrow) is expanded, and in (**b**), the right S1 traversing nerve root (green arrow) is observed free. (**c**) T2W axial view of L5–L6 (S1) demonstrates adequate central and subarticular decompression

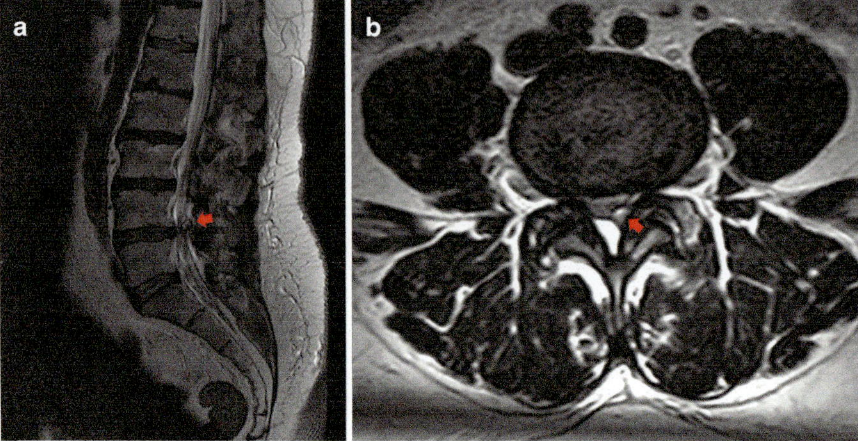

Fig. 19.20 Preoperative lumbar MRI of Case 3. (**a**) T2W sagittal view showed a left cyst at L4–L5 (red arrow). (**b**) Degenerative changes of both facet joints, hypertrophy of the FL, and a left juxtafacet cyst were identified in the T2W axial view at L4–L5

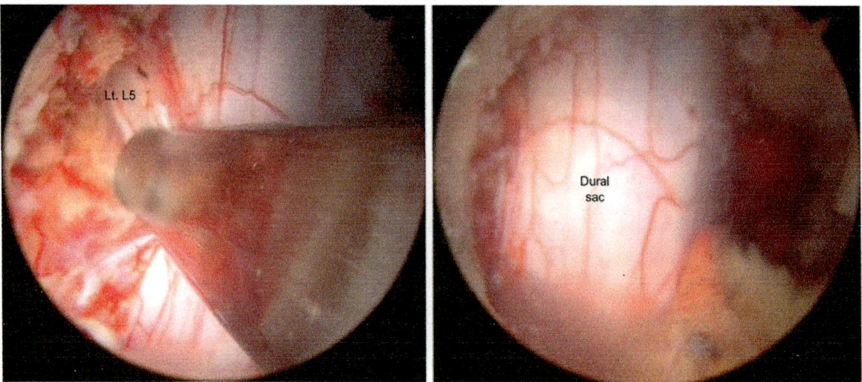

Fig. 19.21 Intraoperative endoscopic images of Case 3. The left L5 nerve root was successfully released through the biportal endoscopic sublaminar contralateral approach. The ipsilateral neural elements were also decompressed

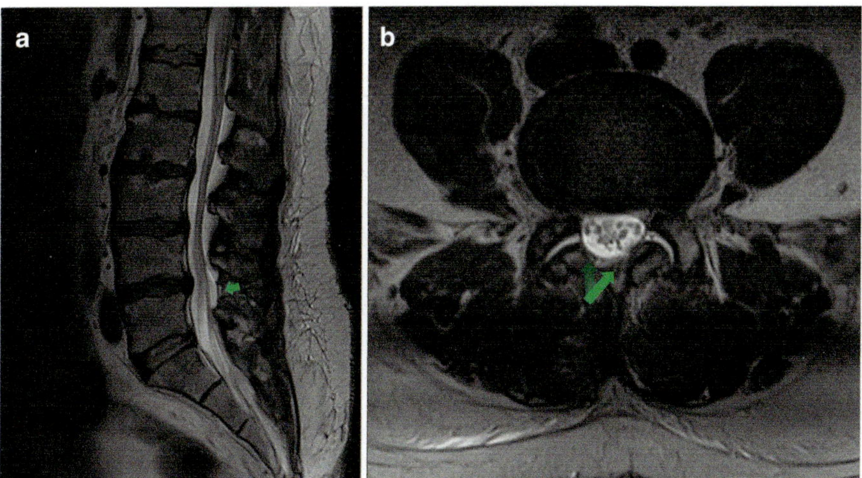

Fig. 19.22 Postoperative lumbar MRI of Case 3. (**a**) T2W sagittal view showing complete resection of the cyst in L4–L5. (**b**) T2W axial view of L4–L5 showing bilateral decompression with adequate re-expansion of the dural sac through the contralateral approach

Discussion

Surgical treatment of JFCs is an option with acceptable clinical results [9]. However, there is no ideal surgical technique, and the proper selection of any depends on factors such as the cyst features, those of the patient, and the surgeon's personal experience. Any surgical decision must prioritize patient safety. It is also important to point out that complications, although considered infrequent, do exist. In a systematic review [9] that included 499 patients, 15 cases (3%) with complications were reported. CSF leak was the most frequently seen complication, 6/499, followed by epidural hematoma with 2 cases, seroma 2, discitis 1, nonunion after fusion 1, DVT 1, wound dehiscence 1, and perioperative death 1. It should be noted that none of the study included in this review dealt with biportal endoscopy as a surgical option.

Heo et al. [19], in 2018, reported clinical results in a series of 10 cases with JFCs treated with biportal endoscopic contralateral sublaminar approach. The mean age of the patients was 57.3 ± 14.7 years; 7 cases were synovial cysts, 1 calcified synovial cyst, 1 ligamentum flavum cyst, and 1 disc cyst. The most affected lumbar level was L4–L5 (6 cases), followed by L3–L4 (4 cases), which corresponds to the current literature. The surgical time was 60.1 ± 23.4 min, and the reported postoperative complications were one patient with transient hypoesthesia and one patient with postoperative epidural hematoma; both complications did not require surgical management. In addition, the authors reported a complete resection of the lesion in all patients confirmed by postoperative MRI. At the end of follow-up, the clinical results were satisfactory, the mean VAS for leg and back improved from 7.64 ± 0.71 to 1.63 ± 1.28, and the ODI changed from 45.35 ± 16.15 to 15.82 ± 10.21.

There are certain advantages of UBE observed by various authors: the use of standard spinal surgery surgical instruments, excellent maneuverability of the surgical instruments in a working portal independent of the endoscopic lens, and high quality of the image obtained through the endoscopic lens with continuous saline irrigation. In addition, biportal endoscopy is considered a minimally invasive technique due to its capacity to preserve the paravertebral anatomical structures during the procedure. That means, it is not required to remove important ligaments such as the intra- and supraspinous ligaments, or it is avoided to perform laminectomies or complete facetectomies to achieve the surgical objective of decompression of the peripheral nervous system. This leads to a reduced EBL, less iatrogenic transgression to stabilizing structures, less postoperative pain and consumption of narcotics, rapid return to activity out of bed, and less hospital stay [21–23].

Some advantages associated with the contralateral sublaminar endoscopic biportal approach are the following: The surgeon avoids dealing with the affected side initially; this means that the normal anatomical structures will first be identified on the ipsilateral side. It is highly relevant considering that cysts present firm adhesions to the dural sac or other neural elements. In these cases, the surgeon will be able to identify and dissect normal anatomical structures and later on the contralateral side where the pathology is found, reducing the risk of dural injuries. This can be seen in the cases presented in this chapter, mainly in Cases 1 and 2, in which a first ipsilateral and later contralateral dissection is evidenced (Videos 19.1 and 19.2). Another critical situation is the maximum preservation of the FJ. In the ipsilateral decompression of the cystic lesion, the medial facetectomy can be extensive, leading to a risk of unnecessary instability. However, through the contralateral approach, the surgeon can see the structures that make up the joint from the front and perform tailored undercutting concerning the cyst and what is required to decompress the traversing nerve root.

The limitations of the contralateral sublaminar endoscopic biportal approach are as follows: (1) If the triangular approach is not performed correctly, the surgeon will not be able to access the lesion with both portals. It can happen due to a short learning curve or the lack of recognition of the initial landmark, the spinolaminar junction. (2) The biportal endoscopic contralateral approach requires experience in microsurgery and endoscopy. (3) The same anatomical foundation as in microsurgery and other MISS techniques is applied to UBE, which performs bone remodeling in an over-the-top fashion to protect the neural elements. The risk of a dural or neural injury with the working instruments can be significant if the surgeon does not use the FL as a protective barrier against the nerves. (4) It should be considered that the most common complication in cases of JFCs is incidental durotomy; therefore, in UBE, this is no different and even more so when dissection of the cyst and the dural sac is performed. It is recommended that the surgeon be patient in removing the cyst, first dissecting a normal anatomical plane between the FL and the dural sac ipsilaterally, and then moving to the contralateral side to identify the interface between the cyst and the neural element. If a dural tear occurs and is punctiform, the course of action may be to place a patch of material similar to the dura mater or fibrin sealant, but if the defect is more significant and there is herniation or incarceration of the nerve roots through the dural tear, it is suggested to convert the procedure and conclude it with microsurgery.

Conclusion

Biportal endoscopy via contralateral and sublaminar route allows removal of lumbar juxtafacet cystic lesions with minimal collateral effect on the paraspinal muscles, axial and capsular lumbar ligaments, and facet joints, thus reducing the risk of iatrogenic instability. However, this approach requires experience, deep knowledge, and familiarity with the epidural space at the lumbar level.

References

1. Charest DR, Kenny BG. Radicular pain caused by synovial cyst: an underdiagnosed entity in the elderly? J Neurosurg. 2000;92(1 Suppl):57–60.
2. Doyle AJ, Merrilees M. Synovial cysts of the lumbar facet joints in a symptomatic population: prevalence on magnetic resonance imaging. Spine (Phila Pa 1976). 2004;29(8):874–8.
3. Hagen T, Daschner H, Lensch T. Juxtafacettenzysten: Magnetresonanztomographische Diagnostik [Juxta-facet cysts: magnetic resonance tomography diagnosis]. Radiologe. 2001;41(12):1056–62.
4. Kao CC, Winkler SS, Turner JH. Synovial cyst of spinal facet. Case report. J Neurosurg. 1974;41(3):372–6.
5. Bydon A, Xu R, Parker SL, et al. Recurrent back and leg pain and cyst reformation after surgical resection of spinal synovial cysts: systematic review of reported postoperative outcomes. Spine J. 2010;10(9):820–6.
6. Hemminghytt S, Daniels DL, Williams AL, Haughton VM. Intraspinal synovial cysts: natural history and diagnosis by CT. Radiology. 1982;145(2):375–6.
7. Kirkaldy-Willis WH, Farfan HF. Instability of the lumbar spine. Clin Orthop Relat Res. 1982;165:110–23.
8. Shah RV, Lutz GE. Lumbar intraspinal synovial cysts: conservative management and review of the world's literature. Spine J. 2003;3(6):479–88.
9. Boviatsis EJ, Stavrinou LC, Kouyialis AT, et al. Spinal synovial cysts: pathogenesis, diagnosis and surgical treatment in a series of seven cases and literature review. Eur Spine J. 2008;17(6):831–7.
10. Howington JU, Connolly ES, Voorhies RM. Intraspinal synovial cysts: 10-year experience at the Ochsner Clinic. J Neurosurg. 1999;91(2 Suppl):193–9.
11. Yarde WL, Arnold PM, Kepes JJ, O'Boynick PL, Wilkinson SB, Batnitzky S. Synovial cysts of the lumbar spine: diagnosis, surgical management, and pathogenesis. Report of eight cases. Surg Neurol. 1995;43(5):459–65.
12. Finkelstein SD, Sayegh R, Watson P, Knuckey N. Juxta-facet cysts. Report of two cases and review of clinicopathologic features. Spine (Phila Pa 1976). 1993;18(6):779–82.
13. Rosenberg AE, Schiller AL. Tumors and tumor-like lesions of joints and related structures. In: Kelley WN, editor. Textbook of rheumatology, vol. 2. 5th ed. Philadelphia: WB Saunders; 1997. p. 1593–5.
14. Kao CC, Uihlein A, Bickel WH, Soule EH. Lumbar intraspinal extradural ganglion cyst. J Neurosurg. 1968;29(2):168–72.

15. Mercader J, Muñoz Gomez J, Cardenal C. Intraspinal synovial cyst: diagnosis by CT. Follow-up and spontaneous remission. Neuroradiology. 1985;27(4):346–8.
16. Métellus P, Fuentes S, Adetchessi T, et al. Retrospective study of 77 patients harbouring lumbar synovial cysts: functional and neurological outcome. Acta Neurochir. 2006;148(1):47–54.
17. Hsu KY, Zucherman JF, Shea WJ, Jeffrey RA. Lumbar intraspinal synovial and ganglion cysts (facet cysts). Ten-year experience in evaluation and treatment. Spine (Phila Pa 1976). 1995;20(1):80–9.
18. Sauvage P, Grimault L, Ben Salem D, Roussin I, Huguenin M, Falconnet M. Kystes synoviaux intraspinaux lombaires: imagerie et traitement par infiltration [Lumbar intraspinal synovial cysts: imaging and treatment by percutaneous injection. Report of thirteen cases]. J Radiol. 2000;81(1):33–8.
19. Heo DH, Kim JS, Park CW, Quillo-Olvera J, Park CK. Contralateral sublaminar endoscopic approach for removal of lumbar juxtafacet cysts using percutaneous biportal endoscopic surgery: technical report and preliminary results. World Neurosurg. 2019;122:474–9.
20. Takahashi Y, Sato T, Hyodo H, et al. Incidental durotomy during lumbar spine surgery: risk factors and anatomic locations: clinical article. J Neurosurg Spine. 2013;18(2):165–9.
21. Kim CW. Scientific basis of minimally invasive spine surgery: prevention of multifidus muscle injury during posterior lumbar surgery. Spine (Phila Pa 1976). 2010;35(26 Suppl):S281–6.
22. Mobbs RJ, Li J, Sivabalan P, Raley D, Rao PJ. Outcomes after decompressive laminectomy for lumbar spinal stenosis: comparison between minimally invasive unilateral laminectomy for bilateral decompression and open laminectomy: clinical article. J Neurosurg Spine. 2014;21(2):179–86.
23. Kim JS, Park CW, Yeung YK, Suen TK, Jun SG, Park JH. Unilateral bi-portal endoscopic decompression via the contralateral approach in asymmetric spinal stenosis: a technical note. Asian Spine J. 2021;15(5):688–700.

Chapter 20
The Contralateral Sublaminar Approach to Decompress the Lateral Recess and Foramen of the Lumbar Spine at the Same Stage

Javier Quillo-Olvera, Diego Quillo-Olvera, Javier Quillo-Reséndiz, and Michelle Barrera-Arreola

Abbreviations

BESS	Biportal endoscopic spinal surgery
CSF	Cerebrospinal fluid leak
DRG	Dorsal root ganglion
ENR	Exiting nerve root
FJ	Facet joint
IAP	Inferior articular process
ILS	Interlaminar space
IVD	Intervertebral disc
LF	Ligamentum flavum
LIF	Lumbar intervertebral foramen
MRI	Magnetic resonance imaging
NRS	Numeric rating scale
RF	Radiofrequency
SAP	Superior articular process
UBE	Unilateral biportal endoscopy

J. Quillo-Olvera (✉) · D. Quillo-Olvera · J. Quillo-Reséndiz · M. Barrera-Arreola
The Brain and Spine Care, Minimally Invasive Spine Surgery Group,
Hospital H+ Querétaro, Spine Clinic, Querétaro, México
e-mail: neuroqomd@gmail.com; drquilloolvera86@gmail.com; kitnoz@hotmail.com; michelle.barrera@anahuac.mx

J. Quillo-Olvera et al. (eds.), *Unilateral Biportal Endoscopy of the Spine*,
https://doi.org/10.1007/978-3-031-14736-4_20

Introduction

The lumbar intervertebral foramen (LIF) is a space that contains the spinal nerve and the dorsal root ganglia (DRG). Lee et al. [1] subdivided the lumbar intervertebral lateral region into the lateral recess (entrance) zone, foraminal (vertical interpedicular) zone, and extraforaminal zone (Fig. 20.1). Therefore, the exiting nerve root (ENR) can be pinched in any of these three zones. The reported prevalence of foraminal stenosis ranges from 8% to 11%. In addition, this diagnosis represents 60% of cases associated with failed back surgery [2–5].

Anatomically, the LIF is bounded by the adjacent superior-inferior vertebral pedicles, the posteroinferior margin of the superior vertebral body, the intervertebral disc (IVD), and the posterosuperior margin of the inferior vertebral body as the anterior boundaries. The ligamentum flavum (LF) and the superior and inferior articular processes act as the posterior boundaries (Fig. 20.2) [6].

Under normal conditions, the foraminal area can vary between 40 and 160 mm^2 and the foraminal height from 20 to 23 mm, ranging at each level [6]. The exiting

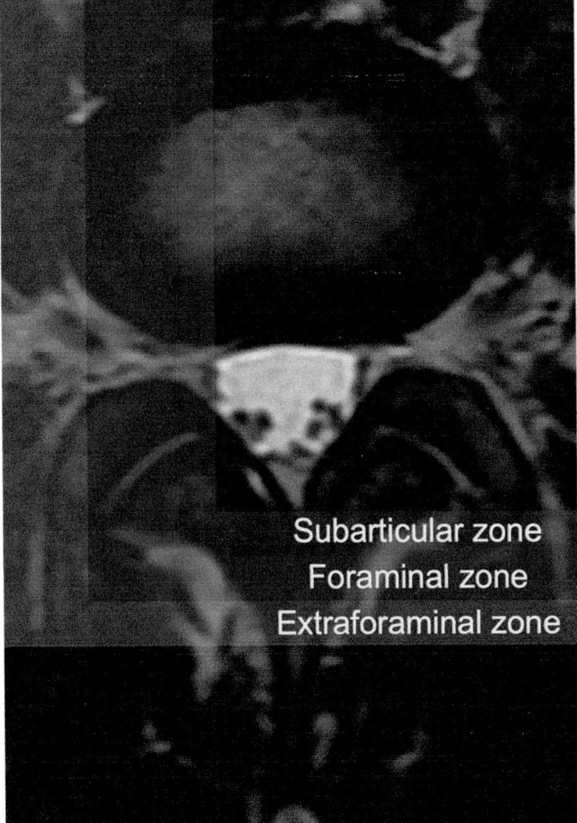

Fig. 20.1 According to Lee's classification of foraminal stenosis [1], there are three different zones where the exiting nerve root could impinge. It is represented in a typical axial view of lumbar magnetic resonance imaging (MRI)

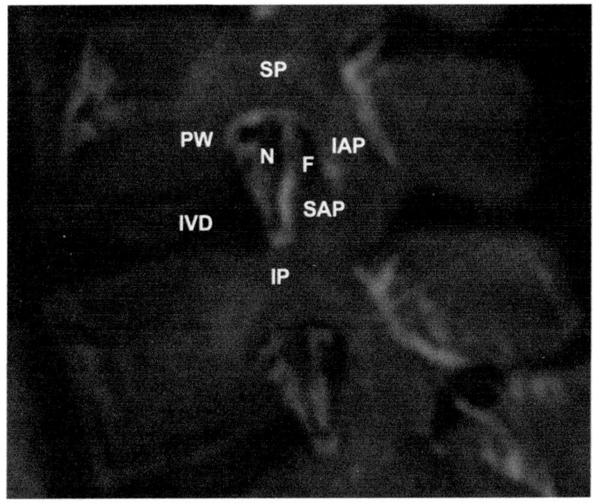

Fig. 20.2 Foraminal boundaries. *SP* superior pedicle, *IP* inferior pedicle, *PW* vertebral body's posterior wall, *IVD* intervertebral disc, *IAP* inferior articular process, *SAP* superior articular process, *F* ligamentum flavum, *N* exiting nerve root

nerve root (ENR) and the DRG are usually surrounded by epidural fat and radicular vessels generally located in the superior and anterior regions of the foramen or subpedicular notch, occupying approximately 30% of the available foraminal area [7].

The surgeon must consider the location of the DRG. This neural structure is part of the ENR and can be intraforaminal or intraspinal. An anatomical study of the lumbar region showed that the more caudal the level, the greater the distance between the medial edge of the pedicle and the DRG, being 1.77 mm in L1, 2.79 mm in L2, 3.23 mm in L3, 7.28 mm in L4, and 8.31 mm in L5 [8–11].

Foraminal stenosis derives from a cascade of degenerative changes related to the collapse of the disc height triggering a disorder in the facet joint (FJ) function, leading to articular hypertrophy, LF buckling, calcification, and hypertrophy, and the resulting spondylosis [6]. The ENR can be entrapped within the LIF differently depending on the vector that exerts compression. Vertical foraminal stenosis occurs due to a decrease in the height of the foramen itself associated with severe degenerative changes in the IVD. Also, the ENR can be compressed within the foramen transversely. This is usually associated with FL hypertrophy or buckling and anterior subluxation of the superior articular process (SAP). Finally, circumferential stenosis represents a combination of both types of stenosis discussed. In this last type of stenosis, the foraminal volume is highly reduced, and the patient usually requires treatment to release the nerve [12].

In addition, other anatomical features are associated with lumbar foraminal stenosis, such as the dynamic behavior of the foramen itself concerning lumbar motion. For example, one study showed that lumbar extension significantly reduced foraminal area by up to 15%, while flexion increased dramatically by up to 12%. Compression of the ENR in neutral position was observed in up to 21%, while 15.4% in flexion and 33% in extension [13].

Patients with LFS are initially treated with conservative measures. However, refractory symptoms will require a surgical option. The surgical strategy to decompress the vertebral nerve will depend on the pathology. Direct decompression of the neural elements is possible through different techniques, among which minimally invasive procedures such as endoscopic surgery stand out. Water-based endoscopic methods, specifically full endoscopy, have been related to successful outcomes in treating different types of lumbar spinal stenosis [14]. An important reason why these procedures are advantageous compared with microsurgery is the high-quality image that the surgeon obtains throughout the surgery with the endoscopic system based on continuous irrigation fluid. In addition to keeping the surgical field clear, it also assists the surgeon in controlling hemostasis, and although it has not yet been possible to confirm its relationship with a lower incidence of postoperative infections, clinicians have noted this. Other procedure-related benefits are decreased operative bleeding, shorter hospital stay, lower rate of postoperative infections and consumption of opioids, and a rapid return to basic activities of daily living [14, 15].

Some authors have successfully decompressed the trapped exiting nerve root in the lateral recess, foramen, or extraforaminal area through full-endoscopic interlaminar procedures [16–18]. The technique uses the space between both laminae to access the contralateral side and has a direct view of the lateral recess, foramen, and extraforaminal space. However, the standardized and generalized implementation of these procedures has not been possible due to various factors such as a steeper learning curve, the elevated costs of highly specialized technology to perform this type of spinal endoscopy, and the multiple causes and presentations of stenosis of the lateral compartment of the lumbar region having other available methods different to endoscopy to solve the problem [12]. To overcome these impediments, biportal endoscopic spinal surgery (BESS) has recently emerged as a new water-based endoscopic option. BESS achieves clinical and radiological results equal to or better than those obtained with open and microscopic surgery standards for treating different types of lumbar spinal stenosis [19, 20]. And recently, this has been used in lateral stenosis of the lumbar region achieving adequate decompression of the neural elements in the lateral recess, foramen, and extraforaminal zones [21–23]. This chapter describes the contralateral biportal endoscopic technique through a sublaminar route for lumbar subarticular and foraminal decompression.

Indications and Contraindications

Indications

This approach allows ipsilateral decompression of the lateral recess and the contralateral subarticular and foraminal space. Therefore, asymmetric stenosis or a combination of different types of stenosis (asymmetric and central) that have unilateral radicular symptoms may be the ideal indication for this approach.

1. Unilateral lumbar radiculopathy explained by stenosis of the lateral or foraminal recess.
2. Symptoms of lumbar narrowing canal and unilateral radicular pain in the leg explained by central stenosis combined with bilateral subarticular stenosis, unilateral foraminal stenosis, or both.
3. In cases of foraminal or extraforaminal stenosis without the involvement of the lateral recess, it is preferable to resolve with a paraspinal approach discussed in another chapter.

Contraindications

1. Symptomatic bilateral subarticular and foraminal stenosis, since these cases may benefit from techniques other than endoscopy.
2. Clinical presentations where lower or axial back pain prevails.
3. Lumbar lateral stenosis associated with unstable spondylolisthesis: A relative contraindication is in patients with low-grade spondylolisthesis (Meyerding I and II), in whom the clinical presentation is unilateral radiculopathy with no or minimal back pain and instability.
4. Far-out syndrome.

Surgical Technique

Incision Planning

It is imperative to remember that triangulation in biportal endoscopic surgery must be tailored to the pathology. When a contralateral decompression towards the right side is planned, the triangular approach will be located on the left side. The surgeon must plan the trajectory of his or her working channel based on the area that requires decompression. The viewing portal will only accompany the working channel and follow it to complete the triangle. Laterally, the incisions may be 10 mm from the spinous process. The foraminal region will determine the craniocaudal location of both skin incision portals, taking the intervertebral space as the intermediate point. Both skin incisions should be separated by 2.5–3 cm and can be made longitudinally or stab. A 6 mm skin incision for the viewing portal and 8 mm for the working channel is sufficient (Fig. 20.3). For a right-handed surgeon working on the left side, the upper incision will be used for the viewing portal and the inferior incision for the surgical instruments.

In the right-to-left approach, the working channel will use the upper incision; for this reason, it must be planned with a slightly more caudocranial trajectory. The same values to locate the incisions are applied in the right contralateral approach (Fig. 20.4).

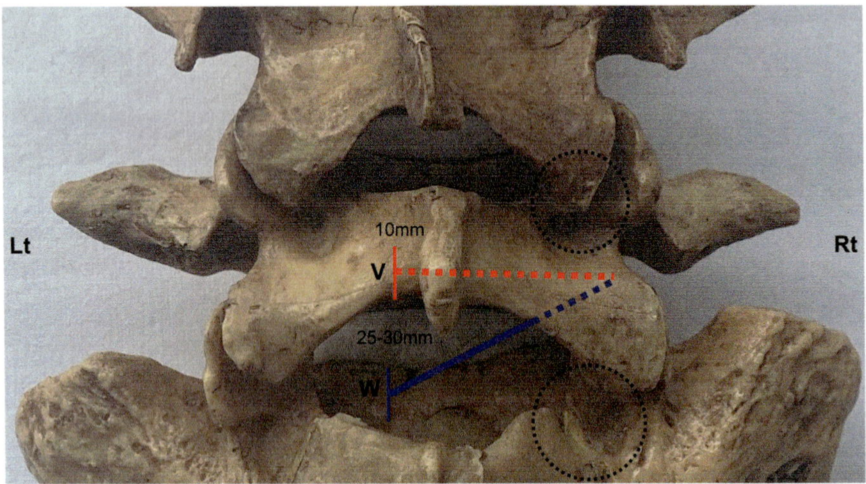

Fig. 20.3 Planning for a left-to-right contralateral sublaminar approach to the lateral recess and foramen. The black dotted circles represent both pedicles. *Lt* left, *Rt* right, *V* viewing portal, *W* working portal

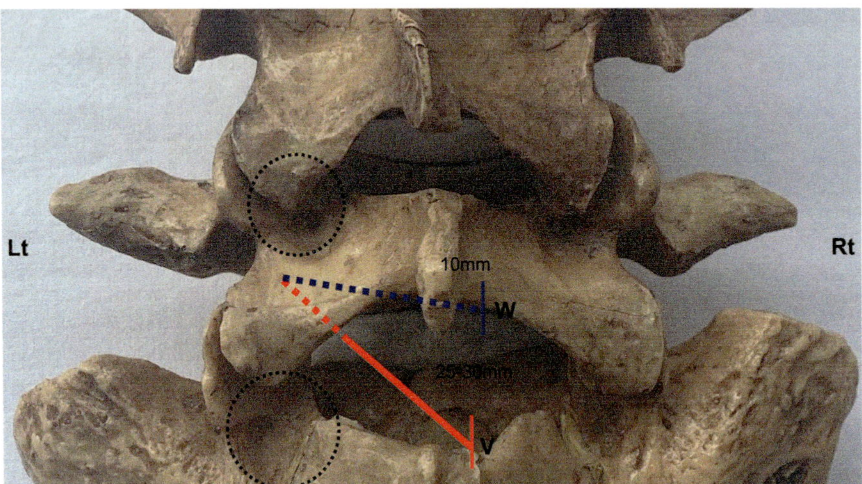

Fig. 20.4 Planning for a right-to-left contralateral sublaminar approach to the lateral recess and foramen. The black dotted circles represent both pedicles. *Lt* left, *Rt* right, *V* viewing portal, *W* working portal

Triangular Approach

The approach begins by introducing the 6 mm dilator through the incision for the working channel. It should be addressed at the base of the spinous process. Then, a 7 mm cannulated dilator is inserted through the previous one to dilate the muscle

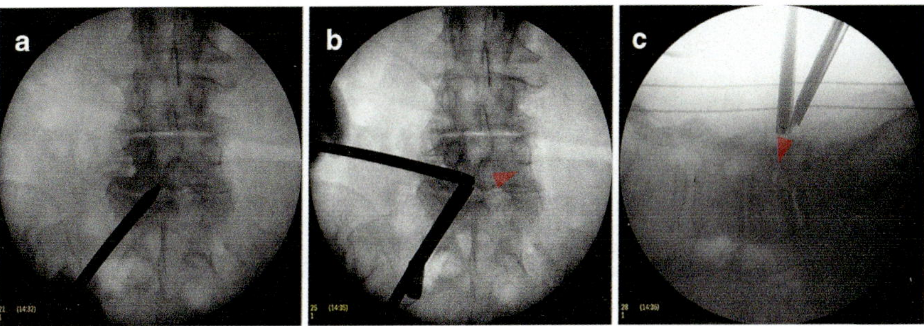

Fig. 20.5 Left-to-right unilateral biportal endoscopic (UBE) contralateral sublaminar approach to decompress the lateral recess and foramen. (**a**) AP view of the C-arm showing the working channel. (**b**) AP view showing the appropriate triangulation between the working and the viewing channels. The triangle is addressed towards the foramen (red triangle). (**c**) The triangular approach towards the foramen (red triangle) is confirmed in the lateral view of the C-arm

trajectory. The thoracolumbar fascia must be opened with the knife before dilation. After that, the working cannula will be docked. Next, a 6 mm dilator addressed to the lateral aspect of the spinous process will be introduced into the incision used for the viewing portal. Finally, the endoscopic system should be introduced through the viewing portal, and continuous inflow and outflow of saline should be confirmed (Fig. 20.5). The authors commonly use a 30° arthroscopic lens and a customized working semi-tubular sheet.

Creating the Working Space

After achieving the co-location of both instruments in the place where the endoscope and the surgical instrument meet, cleaning the area to identify the bone references will allow orientation to start with bone remodeling. It is essential to properly recognize the base of the spinous process (SP), the proximal portion of the ipsilateral lamina, and the interlaminar space (ILS). After identifying them, the surgeon can start with bone removal (Fig. 20.6).

Contralateral Sublaminar Decompression of the Lateral Recess and Foramen

The next thing is to create a space below the contralateral lamina that allows the accessible introduction of instruments into the lateral recess and foramen. In this way, the surgeon can efficiently work in that location (Fig. 20.7). However, it depends on adequate undercutting of the spinous process base and the contralateral lamina. It could be done by using a high-speed drill with a 3 mm diamond burr to

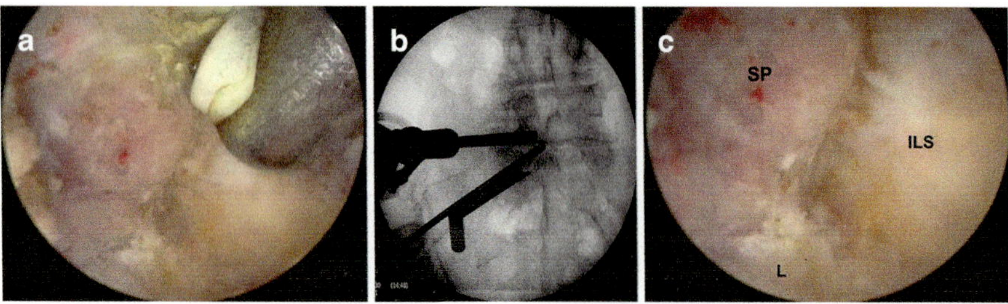

Fig. 20.6 The working space and bone surfaces. (**a**) The radiofrequency (RF) probe is used to clean the working space and identify the bone landmarks for starting with the bone removal. (**b**) It is confirmed with an AP view of the C-arm. The RF is located below and lateral of the spinous process (SP). (**c**) The area is prepared for starting with bone removal. The SP, lamina (L), and interlaminar space (ILS) can be identified

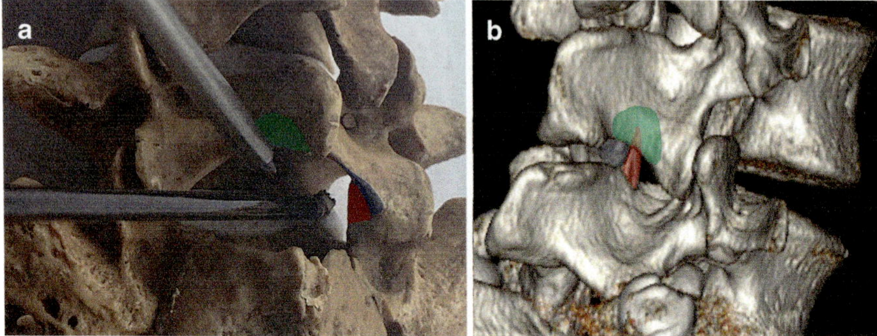

Fig. 20.7 Identification of bone landmarks. (**a**) The surgeon should identify the bone references highlighted with different colors in the anatomic model during a contralateral sublaminar left-to-right approach. The green color represents the spinous process base that must be removed, the blue color is the sublaminar undercut area that favors the pass of both portals to the lateral recess and foramen, and the red color is the superior articular process tip. (**b**) A lumbar 3D reconstructed CT in an oblique right-to-left view used for planning shows the bone references highlighted with the same colors in a real clinical scenario

access the lateral region of the lumbar spine (Fig. 20.8). During this step and depending on the patient's bone quality, there is usually bleeding from the bone that is easily controlled with coagulation using the RF probe or applying bone wax.

Enlarging the space in the lateral recess is achieved by removing the IAP's medial aspect until the FL's lateral insertion is reached. It must be done with caution to avoid excessive removal of the IAP. After releasing the FL with a dissector, more ventral structures should be identified, particularly the superior pedicle, SAP, and intervertebral disc. These references vertically delimit the lumbar intervertebral foramen. Between them, the most lateral or foraminal ligamentum flavum will be observed. In this step, chisels can be used to easily remove the tip of the SAP and enlarge the

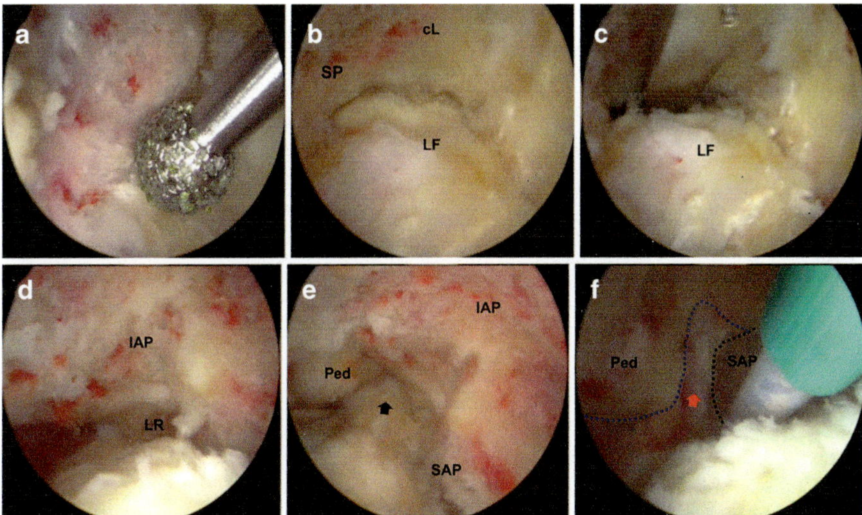

Fig. 20.8 Contralateral sublaminar lateral recess and foramen decompression. (**a**) The bone drilling starts at the base of the spinous process (SP). (**b**) The contralateral (cL) lamina is undercut until identifying the lateral attachment of LF. (**c**) The LF is detached with a dissector to obtain space and continue drilling the IAP's medial surface. (**d**) The IAP is undercut to achieve the SAP and enlarge the lateral recess. (**e**) The superior pedicle (Ped) and the SAP are identified, and between them, the foraminal ligament (black arrow) is observed. (**f**) The surgeon needs to remove the tip of the SAP to enlarge the foraminal area and release the ENR (red arrow). *IAP* inferior articular process, *SAP* superior articular process

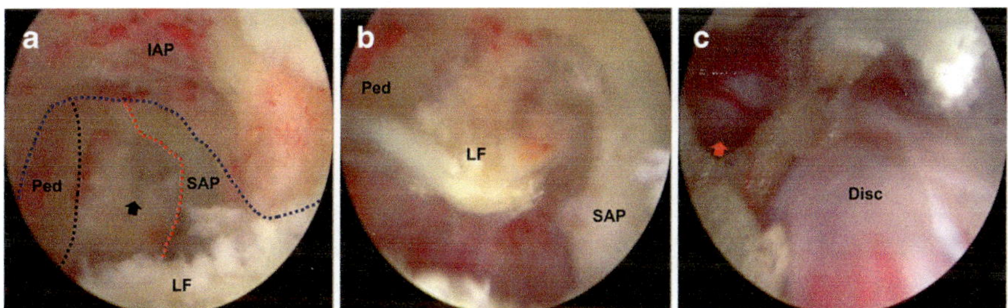

Fig. 20.9 Foraminotomy and direct visualization of the exiting nerve root. (**a**) Foraminotomy is completed with chisels to remove the tip of the SAP (red dotted line). The foraminal ligament (black arrow) is observed and the pedicle (Ped) (black dotted line) bounded the narrowing lumbar foramen vertically. The most ventral part of IAP is observed (blue dotted line). (**b**) The foraminal ligament is removed. (**c**) The ENR (red arrow) can be mobilized and observed

vertical foraminal area. The intervertebral disc is a structure that can be observed ventrally. If it is part of the compression, the discectomy could be performed (Fig. 20.9). The contralateral foraminotomy is completed when the nerve can be mobilized and confirmed with intraoperative fluoroscope images (Fig. 20.10).

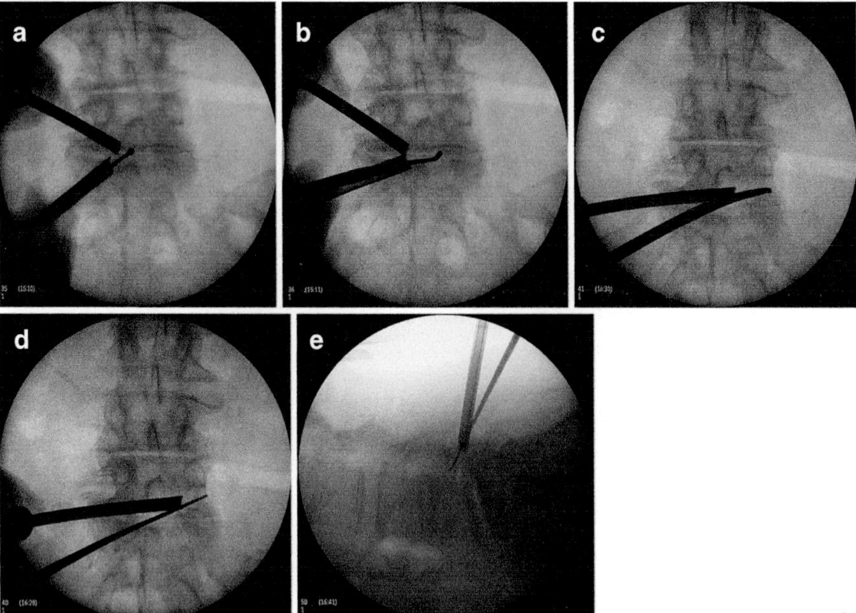

Fig. 20.10 Contralateral sublaminar decompression confirmed with intraoperative fluoroscopy. (**a**) The base of the spinous process is drilled. (**b**) The contralateral access is confirmed. (**c**) Lateral recess and foraminotomy using different instruments. (**d**, **e**) Confirmation of the endpoint of surgery. The decompression of the exiting nerve root

Surgical Tips

Surgeons who decide to use this technique should consider the following:

1. The radiological and clinical findings must be congruent.
2. Lumbar levels with a larger interlaminar space are usually more accessible due to the ease with which the instruments can be introduced into the surgical area and the less bone work required. Levels L4–L5 and L5–S1 without anomalies of the lumbosacral junction are accessible for this technique.
3. The upper lumbar levels require more bone work due to the thickness and width of the lamina. However, the surgeon must be careful at these levels because the lamina is shorter, and the inferior articular process (IAP) is more accessible. Therefore, complete IAP removal and iatrogenic instability must be avoided.
4. The ligamentum flavum (LF) can be spared since only its most lateral insertion must be removed, but its central part can be preserved in cases where only lateral decompression of the lumbar canal is required.
5. The trajectory of the decompression is fundamental. It is determined that since the triangular approach is planned, it will facilitate the introduction of both

ports to the surgical field and the freedom to use them. In addition, it will allow proper orientation and recognition of bone landmarks such as the suprapedicular notch, the SAP, and the intervertebral disc. An inadequate trajectory will cause long surgical times, more significant bleeding, and extensive bone removal. The trajectory of the triangular approach is defined by the direction in which the triangulation is addressed.

6. The base of the spinous process must be adequately removed since this is the key to crossing over to the contralateral side.
7. The joint capsule must be respected to the maximum. Therefore, bone remodeling must be addressed to the most ventral structures, easily identified when removing the LF.
8. It is recommended to access the lateral recess and intervertebral foramen over the top, using the central LF as a protective barrier of the dural sac.
9. Identifying the disc space is important because it could be a compression source. But the disc at the foraminal or extraforaminal zones should not always be removed. The surgery was successful if the exiting nerve could be mobilized free and the foramen was enlarged.
10. If decompression of the foramen or extraforaminal area is not achieved, a paraspinal approach should be performed to accomplish an appropriate exiting nerve root decompression.
11. The surgeon should never lose the tip of his or her instrument due to the high risk of vascular and neural damage.

Possible Complications

1. Dural sac injury.
2. Cerebrospinal fluid (CSF) leak.
3. Ventral epidural bleeding due to inadequate hemostasis in the venous plexuses. Surgery should never be continued if bleeding has not been controlled due to the high risk of injury to the ENR.
4. ENR injury during foraminal decompression: The surgeon must be cautious in removing the SAP since the nerve can even tear with this structure when trying to remove it.
5. Thermal injury due to using the RF probe near the ENR or for long periods.
6. Excessive bone remodeling or injury to the facet joint leads to segmental instability.
7. Despite the low risk of infection, you should always ensure that all protocols are taken to avoid it.
8. Insufficient decompression requiring a procedure other than endoscopic.

Illustrated Cases

Case 1

A 77-year-old female complained of severe radicular pain in her left leg. Preoperative lumbar MRI showed severe foraminal and extraforaminal stenosis due to an osteophyte on the left SAP. Right-to-left sublaminar biportal endoscopic foraminal and extraforaminal decompression was performed. Postoperative lumbar MRI demonstrated complete decompression of the exiting nerve root (Fig. 20.11).

Case 2

An 84-year-old male complained of severe pain in his right leg and bilateral neurogenic claudication. The patient also reported a 4−/5 dorsiflexion paresis of the right ankle. Lateral and foraminal recess stenosis on the right side at L5–S1 was identified on preoperative lumbar MRI, in addition to a central narrowing of the lumbar canal at the same level. The patient underwent surgery using a left-to-right contralateral sublaminar approach and ipsilateral and central decompression of the spinal canal using biportal endoscopy at L5–S1. Immediately after surgery, the patient's pain in his right leg decreased by more than 90%. Two weeks after the procedure,

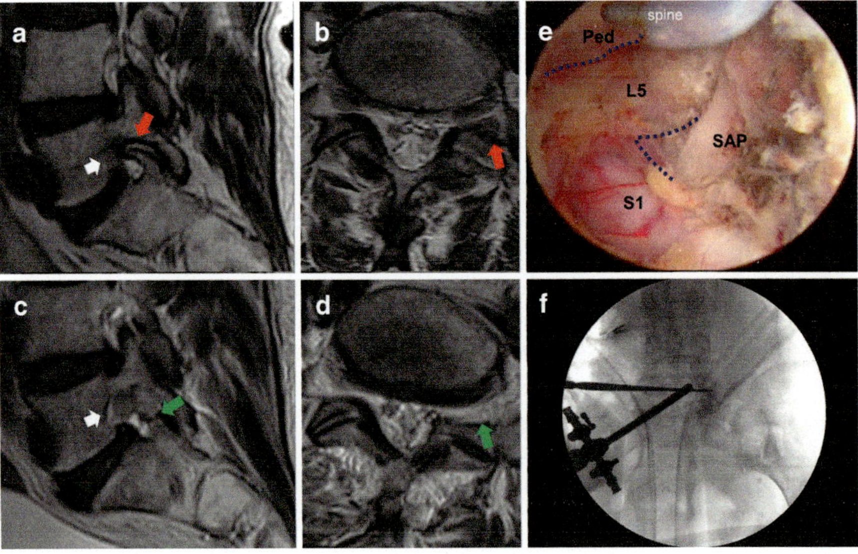

Fig. 20.11 Images from Case 1. (**a**) Sagittal view of preoperative lumbar MRI showing a severe horizontal foraminal stenosis (red arrow) on the left side at L5–S1. The nerve is compressed against the L5 posterior wall (white arrow). (**b**) Pre-op axial view of lumbar MRI showing a severe foraminal and extraforaminal stenosis on the left side at L5–S1. The red arrow points to a bone spur. (**c**) Sagittal view of postoperative lumbar MRI. The tip of the SAP has been removed (green arrow), and the foraminal area is enlarged after the biportal endoscopic decompression. The exiting nerve root is completely free within the foramen (white arrow). (**d**) The bone spur was removed (green arrow) confirmed in the axial view of the post-op lumbar MRI. (**e**) Intraoperative endoscopic view after decompression. The exiting nerve L5 is identified (blue dotted lines), and the pedicle (Ped), SAP, and S1 nerve can be observed. (**f**) The nerve hook's location confirms the appropriate foraminal decompression at L5–S1 on the left side

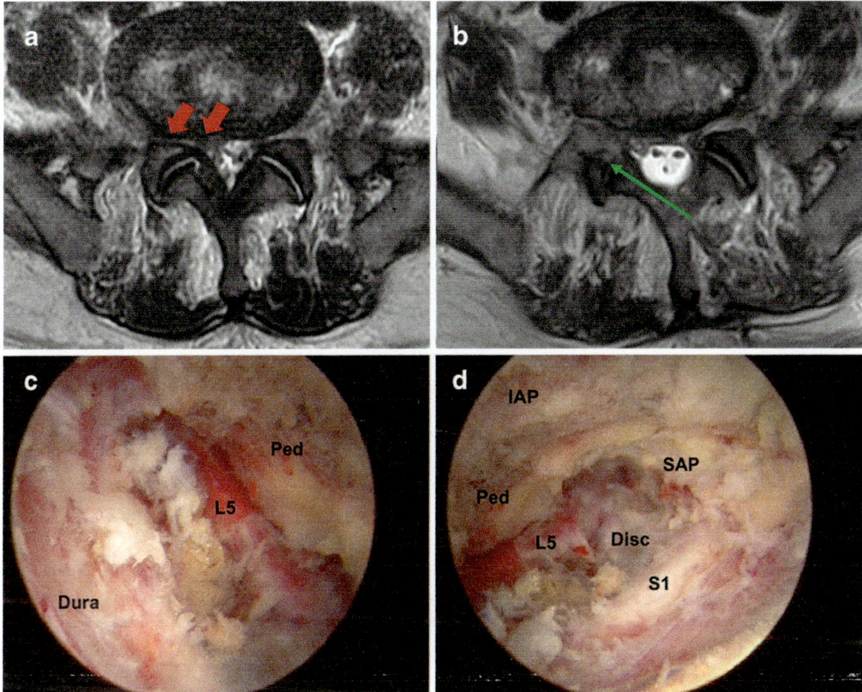

Fig. 20.12 Images from Case 2. (**a**) Sagittal view of lumbar MRI at L5–S1 showing a severe lateral recess and foraminal stenosis (red arrows) on the left side. Also, central spinal stenosis at the same level can be noted. (**b**) Postoperative lumbar MRI shows the lateral recess decompression and foramen on the right side at L5–S1. The trajectory of the contralateral sublaminar approach is highlighted with a green arrow. The cross-sectional area of the dural sac also increased after central and ipsilateral decompression. (**c**) Intraoperative endoscopic view after decompression of the contralateral L5 nerve root. (**d**) Panoramic view with the endoscope at L5–S1. The lateral recess has been decompressed, and the S1 nerve is free. The tip of the SAP was removed to expose the L5 nerve on the right side. The bone references observed included the pedicle (Ped), inferior articular process (IAP), superior articular process (SAP), disc, and exiting and traversing nerves L5 and S1, respectively

the patient had improved the strength in his right ankle to 4+/5, and the neurogenic claudication disappeared. Immediate postoperative MRI confirmed decompression of the lateral and foraminal recesses on the right side and central canal with re-expansion of the dural sac (Fig. 20.12).

Case 3

A 62-year-old male complained of severe pain in his right leg VAS 9/10 of 5 months' evolution, treated in the last month with opioids, and an L4–L5 foraminal block on the right side without improvement of his symptoms. The patient also presented decreased strength in dorsiflexion of the right ankle 4−/5 and marked neurogenic claudication. Preoperative imaging studies included CT and MRI of the lumbar spine. In them, a severe narrowing of the lumbar spinal canal was found at L3–L4 and L4–L5, the latter associated with significant lateral and foraminal recess stenosis on the right side. The patient underwent bilateral decompression through a

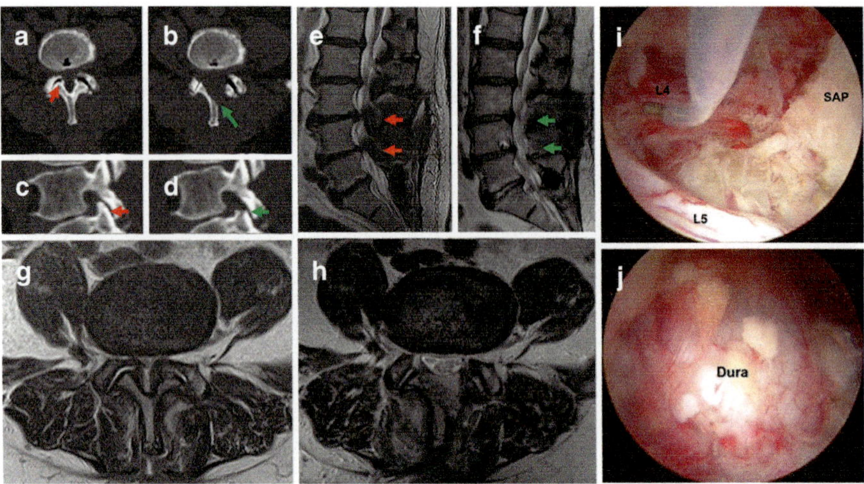

Fig. 20.13 Images from Case 3. (**a**) Preoperative lumbar CT on the axial view of L4–L5 showing facet joint arthrosis and spurs predominantly on the right side. (**b**) Postoperative axial view at L4–L5 confirmed an outstanding left-to-right contralateral sublaminar decompression. The green arrow shows the trajectory of the contralateral approach. (**c**) Preoperative axial view of the foraminal area at L4–L5 (red arrow) on the right side in the lumbar CT scan. (**d**) Postoperative sagittal view of the lumbar CT at L4–L5 on the right side demonstrating the SAP tip removal and an enlarged foraminal area. (**e**) Preoperative sagittal view of the lumbar MRI. The red arrows point to L3–L4 and L4–L5 with central stenosis. (**f**) The postoperative sagittal view of the same case demonstrated a sufficient central decompression through a UBE-ULBD procedure at both levels (green arrows). (**g**) Preoperative axial view of the lumbar MRI at L4–L5. Severe central stenosis and symptomatic radiculopathy related to right-side lateral recess and foraminal stenosis. (**h**) Postoperative axial view of the lumbar MRI showing an L4–L5 decompression with re-expansion of the dural sac after the surgery. (**i**) Intraoperative endoscopic view of the lateral recess and foraminal decompression at L4–L5 on the right side. The exiting and traversing L4 and L5 nerves, respectively, can be observed in the image. The tip of the SAP was removed to accomplish the decompression of the foraminal area. (**j**) Dural sac at L4–L5 after central decompression

unilateral laminotomy (ULBD) through biportal endoscopy at L3–L4 and a left-to-right contralateral sublaminar approach at L4–L5 and ULBD through biportal endoscopy. The patient's pain in his right leg improved to VAS 0/10 postoperatively, in addition to improving the neurogenic claudication. The right-ankle dorsiflexion paresis required physical therapy for 4 weeks and improved considerably. Postoperative lumbar spine CT and MRI demonstrated excellent central decompression at L3–L4 and L4–L5, in addition to lateral and foraminal recess decompression on the right side that was performed using a left-to-right sublaminar contralateral biportal endoscopic approach at L4–L5 (Fig. 20.13).

Case 4

A 78-year-old female complained of mild lower back pain VAS 3/5 associated with severe lumbar radiculopathy in the right leg VAS 8/10. The patient also presented bilateral neurogenic claudication at 40 steps and reported continuous paresthesia in both legs since 3 months ago. Preoperative lumbar MRI demonstrated narrowing of

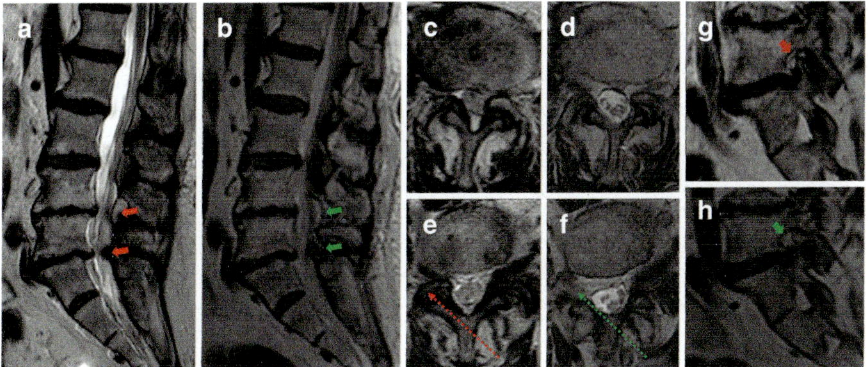

Fig. 20.14 Images from Case 4. (**a**) Preoperative lumbar MRI on sagittal view. The red arrows point to lumbar spinal stenosis at L4–L5 and L5–S1. (**b**) Postoperative sagittal view of the same patient showing sufficient central decompression through a UBE-ULBD in both levels (green arrows). (**c**) Preoperative axial view on the MRI at L4–L5 with central canal and bilateral lumbar subarticular stenosis. (**d**) Postoperative axial view of the MRI with an increased dural sac cross-sectional area at L4–L5. (**e**) Preoperative MRI on the axial view at L5–S1. The red arrow points to the right side's severe lateral recess and foraminal stenosis. (**f**) The postoperative lumbar MRI showed on the axial view at L5–S1 the decompression of both lateral recess and foramen on the right side. The green arrow represents the trajectory of the left-to-right contralateral sublaminar biportal endoscopic approach. Also, the ipsilateral approach achieved sufficient decompression, and the dural sac was expanded regarding the preoperative image. (**g**) Lumbar sagittal view of the preoperative MRI demonstrating a right-side foraminal stenosis at L5–S1 (red arrow). (**h**) The postoperative imaging of the same patient confirmed the increased foraminal area at L5–S1 on the right side (green arrow)

the central and bilateral subarticular lumbar canal at L4–L5 and right foraminal and subarticular stenosis at L5–S1. Therefore, a UBE-ULBD was performed at L4–L5 and a left-to-right contralateral sublaminar approach at L5–S1. The patient was discharged the following day without pain in her right leg and with minimal changes in gait associated with the disease, which disappeared 1 month after surgery. Postoperative MRI showed adequate central decompression obtained by the UBE-ULBD procedure at L4–L5 and L5–S1 and an enlarged foraminal area at L5–S1 on the right side after the contralateral biportal endoscopic approach (Fig. 20.14).

Discussion

Different authors have reported encouraging results using the biportal endoscopic sublaminar contralateral lumbar approach for decompression of the lateral recess and foraminal and extraforaminal areas. Akbary et al. [21] reported the clinical results obtained from 30 decompressed levels using the same technique without any adverse events. The NRS leg pain and ODI scores improved from 7.5 ± 0.86 and 67.9 ± 9.7 preoperatively to 1.53 ± 0.86 and 15.7 ± 6.6 at the last follow-up, respectively. The cross-sectional area of the spinal canal improved from 99.34 ± 34.01 to 186.83 ± 41.41, indicating good canal decompression. The cross-sectional area of the intervertebral foramen improved from 56.40 ± 19.28 to 97.60 ± 28.46, indicating adequate foraminal decompression, and the cross-sectional area of the facet joint improved from 231.37 ± 62.53 to 194.96 ± 50.56, indicating satisfactory foraminal decompression with lesser damage to facet joints. All morphometric changes were statistically significant ($P < 0.05$).

Park et al. [22] reported the clinical outcomes from 27 patients with lumbar disc herniation who underwent contralateral biportal endoscopic surgery. The VAS scores for back and radicular pain were significantly improved compared to preoperative scores. Modified MacNab outcome was good to excellent in 96.3% (26 out of 27 patients). The reduction rate of the facet joint plane was about 4.9% after the contralateral approach indicating a low risk for lumbar stability.

Other experts have documented the biportal endoscopic contralateral sublaminar approach through technical notes, such as Heo et al. [23] and Kim et al. [24] emphasized the advantages associated with this procedure, such as less manipulation of other structures located in the spinal canal (exiting and traversing nerves and dural sac), less bone remodeling, and consequently shorter surgical times. And the expansion of the foraminal area is achieved by removing ventral bony structures with minimal risk of instability, respecting the joint capsule and the ligamentum flavum. This feature is thanks to identification of bone references such as the superior pedicle, IAP, SAP, and intervertebral disc.

The contralateral approach allows access to the lateral and foraminal recess area with minimal bone remodeling compared to ipsilateral techniques in which the facet joint is removed perpendicularly or laminectomies are required. In this approach, the undercutting of the spinous process's base and the contralateral lamina prevents the detachment of the muscles inserted dorsally to these bony structures.

Finally, the excellent visualization of the foramen and the ventral epidural structures cannot be left behind since these are observed from a very different angle than that obtained through a posterior or posterolateral approach. In the biportal endoscopic contralateral sublaminar approach, the surgeon can observe the structures of interest from the front, and through the use of the 30° lens, the depth allows the surgeon to use surgical tools with greater confidence.

Conclusion

In summary, various advantages associated with the biportal endoscopic sublaminar contralateral approach have been observed by different experts, including the preservation of the facet joints, ability to decompress the exiting and traversing nerve roots, less bone work through a direct route to the contralateral side, and excellent visualization of the structures that make up the foramen. However, it is also important to mention that this technique is not infallible and requires experience in biportal endoscopic surgery. Even with the good outcomes reported, more studies with good methodologic quality are needed to confirm the true potential of this method.

References

1. Lee CK, Rauschning W, Glenn W. Lateral lumbar spinal canal stenosis: classification, pathologic anatomy and surgical decompression. Spine (Phila Pa 1976). 1988;13(3):313–20.
2. Jenis LG, An HS. Spine update. Lumbar foraminal stenosis. Spine (Phila Pa 1976). 2000;25(3):389–94.
3. Burton CV, Kirkaldy-Willis WH, Yong-Hing K, Heithoff KB. Causes of failure of surgery on the lumbar spine. Clin Orthop Relat Res. 1981;157:191–9.
4. Porter RW, Hibbert C, Evans C. The natural history of root entrapment syndrome. Spine (Phila Pa 1976). 1984;9(4):418–21.
5. Kunogi J, Hasue M. Diagnosis and operative treatment of intraforaminal and extraforaminal nerve root compression. Spine (Phila Pa 1976). 1991;16(11):1312–20.
6. Stephens MM, Evans JH, O'Brien JP. Lumbar intervertebral foramens. An in vitro study of their shape in relation to intervertebral disc pathology. Spine (Phila Pa 1976). 1991;16(5):525–9.
7. Hasue M, Kunogi J, Konno S, Kikuchi S. Classification by position of dorsal root ganglia in the lumbosacral region. Spine (Phila Pa 1976). 1989;14(11):1261–4.
8. Silav G, Arslan M, Comert A, et al. Relationship of dorsal root ganglion to intervertebral foramen in lumbar region: an anatomical study and review of literature. J Neurosurg Sci. 2016;60(3):339–44.
9. Hasegawa T, An HS, Haughton VM. Imaging anatomy of the lateral lumbar spinal canal. Semin Ultrasound CT MR. 1993;14(6):404–13.
10. Kikuchi S, Sato K, Konno S, Hasue M. Anatomic and radiographic study of dorsal root ganglia. Spine (Phila Pa 1976). 1994;19(1):6–11.
11. Sato K, Kikuchi S. An anatomic study of foraminal nerve root lesions in the lumbar spine. Spine (Phila Pa 1976). 1993;18(15):2246–51.
12. Orita S, Inage K, Eguchi Y, et al. Lumbar foraminal stenosis, the hidden stenosis including at L5/S1. Eur J Orthop Surg Traumatol. 2016;26(7):685–93.
13. Inufusa A, An HS, Lim TH, Hasegawa T, Haughton VM, Nowicki BH. Anatomic changes of the spinal canal and intervertebral foramen associated with flexion-extension movement. Spine (Phila Pa 1976). 1996;21(21):2412–20.
14. Lee CH, Choi M, Ryu DS, et al. Efficacy and safety of full-endoscopic decompression via interlaminar approach for central or lateral recess spinal stenosis of the lumbar spine: a meta-analysis [published correction appears in Spine (Phila Pa 1976). 2019 Feb 15;44(4):E258]. Spine (Phila Pa 1976). 2018;43(24):1756–64.
15. Pairuchvej S, Muljadi JA, Ho JC, Arirachakaran A, Kongtharvonskul J. Full-endoscopic (bi-portal or uni-portal) versus microscopic lumbar decompression laminectomy in patients with spinal stenosis: systematic review and meta-analysis. Eur J Orthop Surg Traumatol. 2020;30(4):595–611.
16. Kashlan ON, Kim HS, Khalsa SSS, et al. Percutaneous endoscopic contralateral lumbar foraminal decompression via an interlaminar approach: 2-dimensional operative video. Oper Neurosurg (Hagerstown). 2020;18(4):E118–9.
17. Kim HS, Patel R, Paudel B, et al. Early outcomes of endoscopic contralateral foraminal and lateral recess decompression via an interlaminar approach in patients with unilateral radiculopathy from unilateral foraminal stenosis. World Neurosurg. 2017;108:763–73.

18. Kim JY, Kim HS, Jeon JB, Lee JH, Park JH, Jang IT. The novel technique of uniportal endoscopic interlaminar contralateral approach for coexisting L5-S1 lateral recess, foraminal, and extraforaminal stenosis and its clinical outcomes. J Clin Med. 2021;10(7):1364.
19. Heo DH, Quillo-Olvera J, Park CK. Can percutaneous biportal endoscopic surgery achieve enough canal decompression for degenerative lumbar stenosis? Prospective case-control study. World Neurosurg. 2018;120:e684–9.
20. Heo DH, Kim JS, Park CW, Quillo-Olvera J, Park CK. Contralateral sublaminar endoscopic approach for removal of lumbar juxtafacet cysts using percutaneous biportal endoscopic surgery: technical report and preliminary results. World Neurosurg. 2019;122:474–9.
21. Akbary K, Kim JS, Park CW, Jun SG, Hwang JH. Biportal endoscopic decompression of exiting and traversing nerve roots through a single interlaminar window using a contralateral approach: technical feasibilities and morphometric changes of the lumbar canal and foramen. World Neurosurg. 2018;117:153–61.
22. Park JH, Jang JW, Park WM, Park CW. Contralateral keyhole biportal endoscopic surgery for ruptured lumbar herniated disc: a technical feasibility and early clinical outcomes. Neurospine. 2020;17(Suppl 1):S110–9.
23. Kim JY, Heo DH. Contralateral sublaminar approach for decompression of the combined lateral recess, foraminal, and extraforaminal lesions using biportal endoscopy: a technical report. Acta Neurochir. 2021;163(10):2783–7.
24. Kim JS, Park CW, Yeung YK, Suen TK, Jun SG, Park JH. Unilateral bi-portal endoscopic decompression via the contralateral approach in asymmetric spinal stenosis: a technical note. Asian Spine J. 2021;15(5):688–700.

Chapter 21
Incidental Dural Tears in Unilateral Biportal Endoscopy

Diego Quillo-Olvera, Javier Quillo-Reséndiz, Alexa Borbolla Ruiz, Michelle Barrera-Arreola, and Javier Quillo-Olvera

Abbreviations

CSF	Cerebrospinal fluid
FL	Flavum ligament
PM	Pseudomeningocele
RF	Radiofrequency
UBE	Unilateral biportal endoscopy
ULBD	Unilateral laminotomy for bilateral decompression

Introduction

The most common complication in spinal surgery due to degenerative diseases is dural tears, occurring in 0.2–20% of cases. Dural tears can cause headaches, meningitis, pseudomeningocele (PM), neurological deterioration, intracranial hemorrhage, postoperative delirium, systemic alterations, and surgical wound infection, all of which prolong hospitalization and increase costs [1, 2].

Unilateral biportal endoscopy (UBE) is a minimally invasive technique based on arthroscopy that uses two portals in a triangled approach to achieve a targeted

D. Quillo-Olvera (✉) · J. Quillo-Reséndiz · M. Barrera-Arreola · J. Quillo-Olvera
The Brain and Spine Care, Minimally Invasive Spine Surgery Group,
Hospital H+ Querétaro, Spine Clinic, Querétaro, México
e-mail: drquilloolvera86@gmail.com; kitnoz@hotmail.com; michelle.barrera@anahuac.mx; neuroqomd@gmail.com

A. B. Ruiz
Anáhuac University School of Medicine, Querétaro, México
e-mail: alexaborbolla@gmail.com

J. Quillo-Olvera et al. (eds.), *Unilateral Biportal Endoscopy of the Spine*,
https://doi.org/10.1007/978-3-031-14736-4_21

surgical goal. The viewing portal is used to introduce the endoscope, through which fluid is continuously irrigated throughout the procedure, which exits through the working portal when the triangular approach is appropriate.

This allows UBE to be called a genuine water-based endoscopic procedure, and at the same time, the continuous irrigation of water and the own endoscopic lens features achieve high-quality real-time imaging of anatomical structures. The working portal, through which the fluid exits, is occupied by any device that facilitates the introduction of standard instruments for spinal surgery [3, 4]. This device is usually customized due to the recent popularity of biportal endoscopy and its limited availability in the market, unlike uniportal endoscopy.

The authors introduce a semi-tubular working sheath of different sizes depending on the depth of the approach in each patient, which facilitates the outflow of fluid, avoiding its stagnation in the created working space, and the introduction of the surgical instruments without damaging the muscles, since they slide into the sheath to be introduced into the surgical field.

Several pathologies can be treated through biportal endoscopic approaches, including cervical, thoracic, and lumbar degenerative processes treated through paramedian, paraspinal approaches, or even recent more lateral modifications of the latter [5–7].

Due to the growing use of the biportal endoscopic technique and its emerging application in various spinal pathologies, it is possible to know the complications related to UBE in more detail. For example, a recent meta-analysis [8] found an overall complication rate of 5%, with dural tears being the most frequent complication followed by epidural hematoma, nerve root injury, insufficient decompression, and postoperative headache.

Based on the current medical literature, this chapter discusses the dural tears in UBE, their consequences, and management options.

Dural Tear in UBE

As already mentioned, the main complication of biportal endoscopic surgery is the dural tear; its prevalence can range from 1.9% to 5.8% [5, 8–12]. The associated factors for its occurrence primarily depend on the technical and case complexity.

Technical factors can include the lack of experience with the technique, blurred visibility due to poor hemostasis, inadequate triangular approach, limitation of the working instrument due to deficient creation of the working space, excessive manipulation of the neural elements, as well as accidents during the procedure; especially during flavectomy, they can cause damage to the dura mater.

Features directly related to the pathological anatomy of a particular case include firm adhesions between the ventral aspect of the flavum ligament (FL) and the dorsum of the dural sac. In addition, hypertrophic meningovertebral ligaments associated with the chronicity of the stenosis, which can be found mainly in the midline attaching the central fold of the dura with the FL or redo surgery, can increase the risk of presenting a dural tear [2, 13, 14].

Other risk factors for dural tears that have been proposed are female gender, advanced age, degenerative spondylolisthesis, and juxtafacet cysts [15].

Some recommendations that may be useful during the biportal endoscopic procedure to reduce the risk of the dural tear are the following:

1. Maintain a clean surgical field at all times through meticulous hemostasis, ensuring a constant hydrostatic pressure (30 mmHg) and confirming the correct outflow through the working portal.
2. The superficial layer of the FL should be removed first with the endoscopic basket scissors. This layer makes it bulky and difficult to remove with the Kerrison punches.
3. If the LF is removed in a piecemeal fashion before each piece is removed with the Kerrison punches, the surgeon should dissect below the LF and above the dural sac with a blunt-tipped angled dissector or nerve hook to ensure that there is no fibrous tissue between the two structures.
4. The angled tip of the Kerrison rongeur should enter as parallel as possible concerning the dural sac to remove the FL. This will prevent biting a fold of the dura.
5. Hydrostatic pressure aids in FL dissection. A water pressure set at 30 mmHg is sufficient, but it is recommended to bring the endoscope closer to the dural sac and FL interface, allowing easy mobilization of epidural fat and identification of adhesions between FL and dural sac.
6. Because the central dural fold is adhered by meningovertebral ligaments to the FL, especially in chronic lumbar stenosis processes, it is recommended to use a fine-tip radiofrequency (RF) probe to cut the ligaments in their most proximal attachment to the FL.
7. It is not recommended to traction the epidural fat in the central dural folding. Instead, the dissection with irrigated saline will allow the fatty tissue to be mobilized, and then the adhesions or meningovertebral ligaments that fix the dural dorsum and the FL can be identified.
8. It is essential to have control of the FL by cardinal exposure of its free edges. Therefore, proper completion of the ipsilateral laminotomy and sublaminar undercutting of the contralateral upper and lower lamina are recommended. Subsequently, it will be possible to visualize the intermediate fold in the FL, located below the base of the previously removed spinous process, which represents the midline. A blunt-tip dissector can separate both sides of the FL and start the flavectomy from medial to lateral. If the lateral free edges of the FL have also been exposed, then en bloc flavectomy may be another option.

Possible Further Events Regarding Dural Tears in UBE

The most feared complication associated with a dural tear missed by the surgeon is cerebrospinal fluid (CSF) leakage. However, there are also other factors that, when present, can increase the risk of presenting a CSF leak, which includes advanced age, obesity, redo surgery, degenerative spondylolisthesis, ossification of the ligamentum flavum, ossification of the posterior longitudinal ligament, limited surgical experience, thrombocytopenia preoperative, chronic use of corticosteroids, inflammatory spondylopathies, and juxtafacet cysts [15–19]. Other diagnoses associated with dural tears are pseudomeningocele, surgical site infection, meningitis, and postoperative problems related to surgical wound closure [20].

Therefore, it is paramount to identify the dural tear and resolve it. In open surgery and microsurgery, it is possible to show a dural tear with CSF outflow when the arachnoid has been transgressed; however, a disadvantage observed in water-based endoscopic techniques (uniportal and biportal) is that continuous fluid irrigation can hide the CSF output, losing sight of the dural tear.

The authors recommend being gentle with the dura and neural tissue, avoiding traction on the neural elements (dural sac, traversing, and exiting nerves). In addition, prevent unnecessary traction of the peridural membrane adhered to the dural sac, avoiding risky maneuvers with the RF probe near the dural sac, maintaining a clean surgical field and adequate hemostasis to allow identification of dural tears.

How to Resolve Dural Tears in UBE?

There is no specific protocol for treating dural tears in UBE. However, various authors [2, 9, 13, 14, 17] have suggested classifying dural tears and making decisions based on their features. In general, if the dural tear is large, the laceration should be repaired directly.

Different options to repair the dural tear in UBE without converting to surgery have been proposed, including analogous dura mater patches, fibrin glue, lining the laceration with hemostatic sponges, fat, and muscle fascia. Direct closure is done with nonabsorbable sutures under endoscopic guidance and with microvascular nontraumatic clips [2, 9, 13, 14, 17]. However, it is suggested that dural tears >1 cm with nerve root herniation or incarceration be directly repaired conventionally to avoid significant short- or long-term sequelae for the patient [2, 17, 21].

In a retrospective analysis, Kim et al. [17] found that 27 (8.2%) patients from 330 who underwent decompression for lumbar spinal stenosis through an interlaminar approach by water-based endoscopy had dural tears. The authors classified them into four types (Table 21.1). The best prognosis was associated with types 1 to 3A and poor for types 3B, 3C, and 4 with a high risk of CSF leak. The surgical tools most associated with the dural damage were Kerrison rongeur, dissectors, endoscopic drilling system, and pituitary forceps in order of relevance.

A collagen-fibrin patch was proposed for the closure of dural tears, in which collagen provides hemostasis while the fibrin creates a sealing barrier with adhesive properties. In addition, nontraumatic microvascular titanium clips can be applied through the working portal in a linear tear for closure. Other treatment options are open surgery with direct repair and duraplasty with fascia lata, muscle, or fat [17].

Table 21.1 Kim et al.'s [17] classification of the type of dura tear in spinal endoscopy

Type	Subtype	Description	Treatment suggested
Type 1 (peripheral): nerve root sleeve tear	A	Dural tear that, regardless of the size, is located in the shoulder of the nerve root sleeve	Accessible for endoscopic dural repair
	B	Dural tear that, regardless of the size, is located in the axilla of the nerve root sleeve	Accessible for endoscopic dural repair
Type 2 (central) dural tear	A	Dural tear size ≤1 cm with normal neural elements	Accessible for endoscopic dural repair
	B	Dural tear size ≤1 cm with neural elements herniated through the tear	Accessible for endoscopic dural repair
	C	Dural tear size ≤1 cm with neural elements incarcerated through the tear	Accessible for endoscopic dural repair enlarging the defect
Type 3: Complex dural tear	A	Dural tear size >1 cm with no entrapment of neural elements. With a stable dural patch adherence on the dural surface	Accessible for endoscopic dural repair
	B	Dural tear size >1 cm with irregular dural laceration OR with an unstable dural patch adherence on the dural surface	Open repair
	C	Incarceration of nerve roots despite endoscopic manipulation regardless of the size of the dural tear	Open repair
Type 4	Unrecognized dural tear		Open repair

Other authors have also proposed the treatment of incidental durotomy in UBE based on different features, including location, size, and regularity of tear margins. Choi et al. [22] recommended that dural tears <4 mm be treated conservatively, with bed rest and observation, and tears >12 mm should be repaired directly, especially those found in the dural sac. Lee et al. [13] suggested microsurgically repairing localized tears in the dural sac and reinforcing the dura mater with a fibrin sealant patch placed through the same endoscopic approach for linear tears in the lateral aspect of the dural sac or the root. Park et al. [23] treated dural tears according to their location and size, suggesting 24-h bed rest and hospital observation for tears <4 mm without surgical intervention, and for durotomies >12 mm, attempt primary closure considering the location and regularity of its margins, using a fibrin sealant patch for lesions with regular margins.

Although it is appreciated as a viable option to repair dural tears through the same endoscopic biportal approach, certain disadvantages can be observed. For example, unlike microsurgery, in biportal endoscopy, one portal is used for the endoscope, and the remaining portal for introducing a surgical tool at once, so that both hands cannot be used to suture the durotomy or perform complex dural reconstructions.

Several attempts to directly repair a dural tear under endoscopic vision to avoid converting surgery have been published [9]. However, microsurgery continues to be the most reliable and safe option to resolve an incidental durotomy. Microsurgery's strengths for the closure of dural tears include the freedom to use instruments with both hands and the assistant support for tissue retracting with a third hand; unlike any water-based endoscopic procedure, it is not possible; the other merit for microsurgery is the relatively short learning curve [24]. Nevertheless, some drawbacks regarding converting the UBE surgery to an open or microsurgical procedure are that muscles and other paraspinal soft tissues can be damaged due to an extensive dissection resulting in postoperative pain, increased risk of instability, increased bleeding, and a more extended hospital stay [9].

Illustrated Cases

Case 1

An 80-year-old male patient diagnosed with lumbar spinal stenosis (LSS) at L4–L5 underwent a left L4–L5 UBE-ULBD approach. During the contralateral flavectomy, a regular linear tear of approximately 4 mm was presented with no evidence of neural elements through the durotomy. A fibrin sealant patch was placed over the dural defect, confirming a stable location of the patch with the endoscope. The patient was left for in-hospital observation for 2 days in bed rest. With no evidence of a CSF leak, he was discharged on the third postoperative day. His evolution was favorable without presenting any complications associated with the dural tear (Fig. 21.1).

Case 2

A 28-year-old female patient who underwent an L5–S1 discectomy with UBE was discharged the day after her surgery without any discomfort. At home, on day 4, the patient presented with swelling in the skin's surgical area, significant headache, and lower back pain. The patient was explored with tubular microsurgery at the same level as past surgery, finding a punctiform dural tear with a CSF leak. The durotomy was treated with a fibrin sealant patch and fibrin glue in addition to antibiotics. The

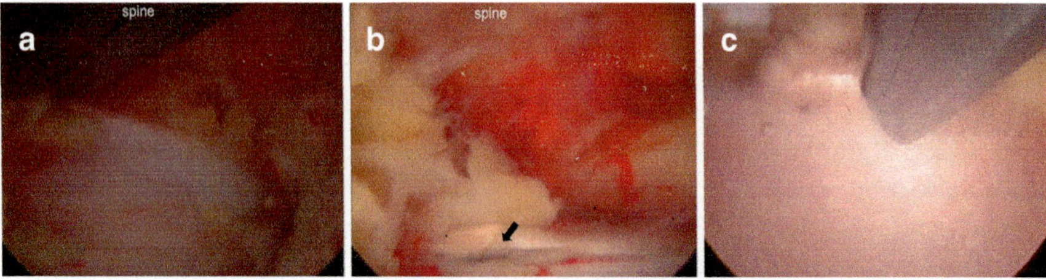

Fig. 21.1 Incidental durotomy of Case 1. (**a**) Contralateral piecemeal flavectomy during a left L4–L5 UBE-ULBD. (**b**) Incidental durotomy (black arrow) located in the lateral surface of the dural sac. (**c**) Fibrin sealant patch placed over the dural defect under endoscopic view

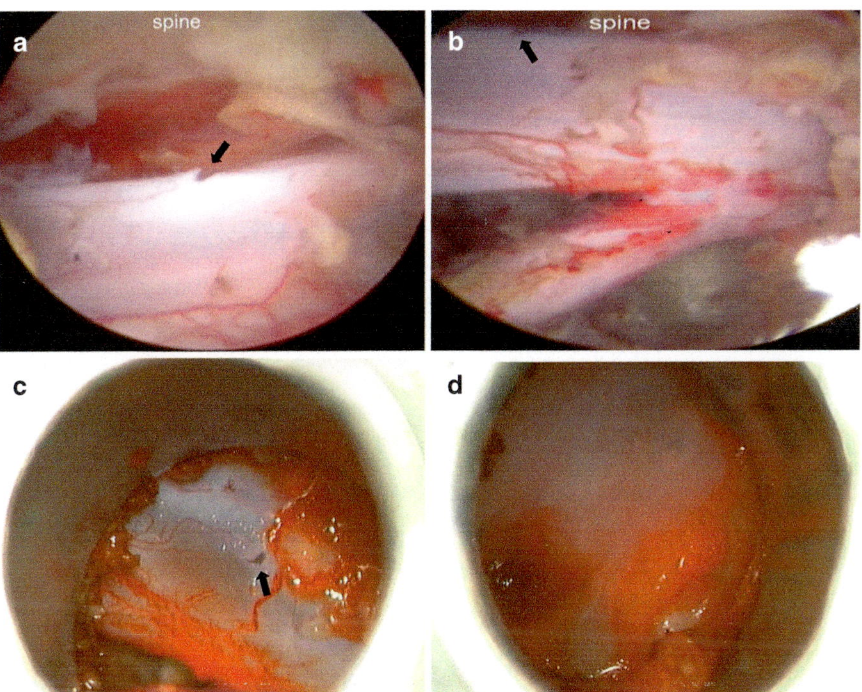

Fig. 21.2 Incidental durotomy of Case 2. (**a**, **b**) Images from a retrospective intraoperative video review found an incidental and inadvertent punctiform dural tear (black arrow) in the central dural fold. (**c**) Intraoperative microscopic view through the tube of dural sac collapsed because of a CSF leak due to a punctiform dural tear (black arrow). (**d**) Fibrin sealant patch and fibrin glue over the dural defect

patient was observed in the hospital for 3 days on bed rest. She was discharged on day 4 with no headache, no back pain, and any discomfort in the surgical area. Her evolution at 12 months was satisfactory, with no sequelae associated with the CSF leak (Fig. 21.2).

Conclusion

Like other spine surgical procedures, UBE is not exempt from complications such as incidental durotomies. Until now, there are no strict protocols to resolve dural tears when they occur during a biportal endoscopic procedure. However, there is evidence on how to decide to deal with this complication, with dural tears in the dorsum of the dural sac, larger than 1 cm, and herniation or incarceration of neural elements being absolute indications to repair the defect directly by open surgery or microsurgery to avoid significant sequelae in the short or long term and affecting the patient quality of life.

References

1. Takenaka S, Makino T, Sakai Y, et al. Dural tear is associated with an increased rate of other perioperative complications in primary lumbar spine surgery for degenerative diseases. Medicine (Baltimore). 2019;98(1):e13970.
2. Kim JE, Choi DJ, Park EJ. Risk factors and options of management for an incidental dural tear in biportal endoscopic spine surgery. Asian Spine J. 2020;14(6):790–800.
3. Eun SS, Eum JH, Lee SH, Sabal LA. Biportal endoscopic lumbar decompression for lumbar disk herniation and spinal canal stenosis: a technical note. J Neurol Surg A Cent Eur Neurosurg. 2017;78(4):390–6.
4. Choi CM, Chung JT, Lee SJ, Choi DJ. How I do it? Biportal endoscopic spinal surgery (BESS) for treatment of lumbar spinal stenosis. Acta Neurochir. 2016;158(3):459–63.
5. Kim JE, Choi DJ, Park EJJ, et al. Biportal endoscopic spinal surgery for lumbar spinal stenosis. Asian Spine J. 2019;13(2):334–42.
6. Heo DH, Eum JH, Jo JY, Chung H. Modified far lateral endoscopic transforaminal lumbar interbody fusion using a biportal endoscopic approach: technical report and preliminary results. Acta Neurochir. 2021;163(4):1205–9.
7. Quillo-Olvera J, Quillo-Reséndiz J, Quillo-Olvera D, Barrera-Arreola M, Kim JS. Ten-step biportal endoscopic transforaminal lumbar interbody fusion under computed tomography-based intraoperative navigation: technical report and preliminary outcomes in Mexico. Oper Neurosurg (Hagerstown). 2020;19(5):608–18.
8. Liang J, Lian L, Liang S, et al. Efficacy and complications of unilateral biportal endoscopic spinal surgery for lumbar spinal stenosis: a meta-analysis and systematic review. World Neurosurg. 2022;159:e91–e102.
9. Hong YH, Kim SK, Suh DW, Lee SC. Novel instruments for percutaneous biportal endoscopic spine surgery for full decompression and dural management: a comparative analysis. Brain Sci. 2020;10(8):516.
10. Lin GX, Huang P, Kotheeranurak V, et al. A systematic review of unilateral biportal endoscopic spinal surgery: preliminary clinical results and complications. World Neurosurg. 2019;125:425–32.
11. Kim JE, Choi DJ. Unilateral biportal endoscopic decompression by 30° endoscopy in lumbar spinal stenosis: technical note and preliminary report. J Orthop. 2018;15(2):366–71.
12. Soliman HM. Irrigation endoscopic decompressive laminotomy. A new endoscopic approach for spinal stenosis decompression. Spine J. 2015;15(10):2282–9.
13. Lee HG, Kang MS, Kim SY, et al. Dural injury in unilateral biportal endoscopic spinal surgery. Global Spine J. 2021;11(6):845–51.
14. Park HJ, Kim SK, Lee SC, Kim W, Han S, Kang SS. Dural tears in percutaneous biportal endoscopic spine surgery: anatomical location and management. World Neurosurg. 2020;136:e578–85.
15. Takahashi Y, Sato T, Hyodo H, et al. Incidental durotomy during lumbar spine surgery: risk factors and anatomic locations: clinical article. J Neurosurg Spine. 2013;18(2):165–9.
16. Murphy ME, Kerezoudis P, Alvi MA, et al. Risk factors for dural tears: a study of elective spine surgery. Neurol Res. 2017;39(2):97–106.
17. Kim HS, Raorane HD, Wu PH, Heo DH, Sharma SB, Jang IT. Incidental durotomy during endoscopic stenosis lumbar decompression: incidence, classification, and proposed management strategies. World Neurosurg. 2020;139:e13–22.
18. Dafford EE, Anderson PA. Comparison of dural repair techniques. Spine J. 2015;15(5):1099–105.
19. Kalevski SK, Peev NA, Haritonov DG. Incidental dural tears in lumbar decompressive surgery: incidence, causes, treatment, results. Asian J Neurosurg. 2010;5(1):54–9.
20. Kang SS, Kim JE, Choi DJ, Park EJ. Pseudomeningocele after biportal endoscopic spine surgery: a case report. J Orthop. 2019;18:1–4.

21. Müller SJ, Burkhardt BW, Oertel JM. Management of dural tears in endoscopic lumbar spinal surgery: a review of the literature. World Neurosurg. 2018;119:494–9.
22. Choi DJ, Jung JT, Lee SJ, Kim YS, Jang HJ, Yoo B. Biportal endoscopic spinal surgery for recurrent lumbar disc herniations. Clin Orthop Surg. 2016;8(3):325–9.
23. Park SM, Park J, Jang HS, et al. Biportal endoscopic versus microscopic lumbar decompressive laminectomy in patients with spinal stenosis: a randomized controlled trial. Spine J. 2020;20(2):156–65.
24. Dhandapani S, Karthigeyan M. "Microendoscopic" versus "pure endoscopic" surgery for spinal intradural mass lesions: a comparative study and review. Spine J. 2018;18(9):1592–602.

Chapter 22
Challenging Cases Treated with UBE: Lumbar Revision Surgery

Javier Quillo-Olvera, Diego Quillo-Olvera, Javier Quillo-Reséndiz, and Michelle Barrera-Arreola

Abbreviations

BESS	Biportal endoscopic spine surgery
IAP	Inferior articular process
LDH	Lumbar disc herniation
LF	Ligamentum flavum
LSS	Lumbar spinal stenosis
MRI	Magnetic resonance imaging
rLDH	Recurrent lumbar disc herniation
SAP	Superior articular process
UBE	Unilateral biportal endoscopy

Introduction

Unsatisfactory results of microsurgical discectomy vary between 5% and 20%, with the recurrence of lumbar disc herniation (rLDH) being the most common cause in 62% of cases [1–5]. The definition proposed by Lee et al. [6] for rLDH is a disc herniation at the same level that appears after a 6-month pain-free interval after the first discectomy [6]. The incidence of rLDH varies between 3% and 18%, and revision surgery is usually necessary for 15–25% [2, 6–10]. The surgical revision consists of a

J. Quillo-Olvera (✉) · D. Quillo-Olvera · J. Quillo-Reséndiz · M. Barrera-Arreola
The Brain and Spine Care, Minimally Invasive Spine Surgery Group,
Hospital H+ Querétaro, Spine Clinic, Querétaro, México
e-mail: neuroqomd@gmail.com; drquilloolvera86@gmail.com; kitnoz@hotmail.com; michelle.barrera@anahuac.mx

J. Quillo-Olvera et al. (eds.), *Unilateral Biportal Endoscopy of the Spine*,
https://doi.org/10.1007/978-3-031-14736-4_22

new microdiscectomy or even lumbar fusion. However, redo surgery can be challenging and associated with incidental durotomy and neural element injury due to peridural scar tissue, in addition to the risk of iatrogenic instability related to a second and more aggressive approach to segmental stabilizing structures [11–14]. Besides, the results of the reoperation may be worse than the results of the initial operation [15].

In a retrospective analysis of 355 patients (2 patients refused to participate in the study and 10 died) consecutively operated for LDH and lumbar spinal stenosis (LSS) with a 10-year follow-up rate of 88.3% (303/343), the authors found a reoperation rate of 22.1% (67/303). Among the leading causes of reoperation were the rLDH, postoperative worsening of spondylolisthesis and instability, insufficient decompression at the level of the laminotomy, and residual foraminal stenosis at the level of the discectomy; 75% of the surgical revisions were at the same level [16].

In this situation, the surgeon should count on surgical options for a safety revision with the least procedure-related collateral effect. Biportal endoscopic spine surgery (BESS), also known as unilateral biportal endoscopy (UBE), is a water-based endoscopic procedure where the surgeon independently uses the surgical instrument from the endoscope because the technique's biportal nature allows the endoscope and the working portal to be introduced through two triangulated channels addressed towards the same pathological target. Visibility is outstanding, thanks to continuous fluid irrigation during the procedure. This feature will allow the surgeon to be more accurate during the revision procedure since it will facilitate the identification of the anatomical structures modified by the first surgery, avoiding a more significant impact on the stabilizing bone structures of the spine and mainly on the neural elements. In addition, one of the characteristics that favor this technique for revision procedures is that the surgeon can use the surgical instruments with greater freedom, allowing to be more delicate and careful with the tissues.

In this chapter, some cases of revision surgery performed by the authors with UBE are presented and discussed, highlighting key points that will serve the reader as important advice.

Indications

1. Revision surgery for recurrent lumbar disc herniation:
   (a) History of a lumbar discectomy procedure
   (b) Recurrent lumbar radiculopathy after at least 6 months of a pain-free period following the first lumbar discectomy
   (c) Recurrent lumbar disc herniation confirmed with MRI at the same level
   (d) Refractory symptoms to conservative measures for at least 4–6 weeks
2. Revision surgery for lumbar re-herniation
3. Revision surgery for lumbar restenosis
4. Revision surgery for lumbar foraminal stenosis

Illustrated Cases

Case 1: Lumbar Re-herniation

A 35-year-old male patient complained of severe radicular pain radiating to both legs, associated with decreased dorsiflexion strength of the left ankle. Preoperative lumbar spine MRI demonstrated a lumbar disc herniation (LDH) with more than 50% spinal canal occupancy at L5–S1 (Fig. 22.1). A microdiscectomy was performed at L5–S1. After that, the patient improved his symptoms and the strength of his left ankle. He was discharged from the hospital on the second postoperative day without incident. However, 5 weeks after surgery, the patient presented with severe sciatic-type pain radiating to the left leg with claudication. A new lumbar spine MRI was performed, revealing a left lateral re-herniation at L5–S1 (Fig. 22.2). The patient underwent surgery for the second time through the UBE technique. During surgery, scar tissue and disc particles adhered to the left S1 nerve root in the left subarticular compartment of L5–S1 were confirmed (Fig. 22.3). A successful neural decompression was achieved after the biportal endoscopic procedure, and the patient was discharged from the hospital on the second day. At the 2-year follow-up, the patient had improved the radicular pain in the left leg entirely and did not report any gait problems, and postoperative MRI showed remodeling of the annulus with ventral epidural scar tissue without compromise to the neural elements. In addition,

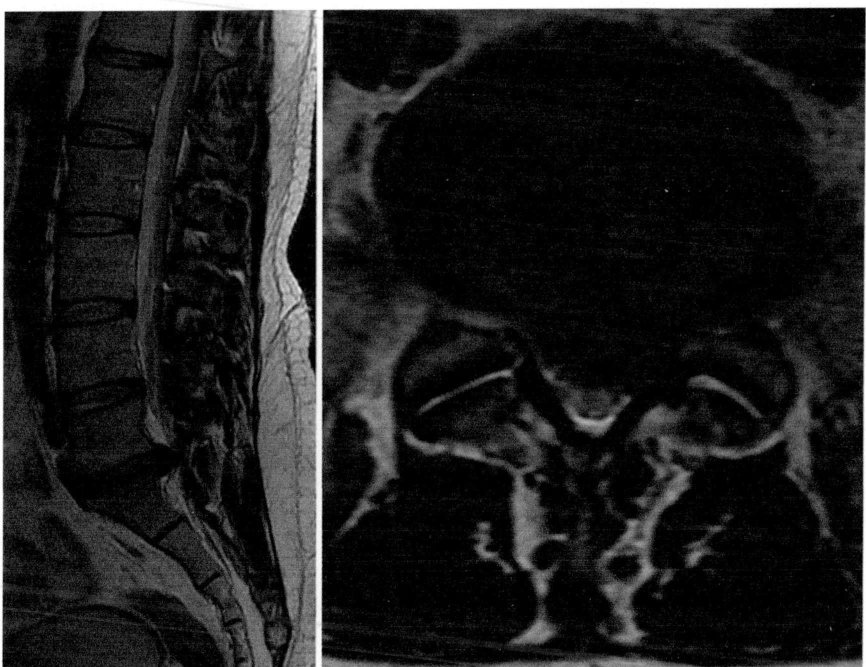

Fig. 22.1 Preoperative lumbar MRI of Case 1. The sagittal and axial views show a massive lumbar disc herniation occupying more than 50% of the spinal canal

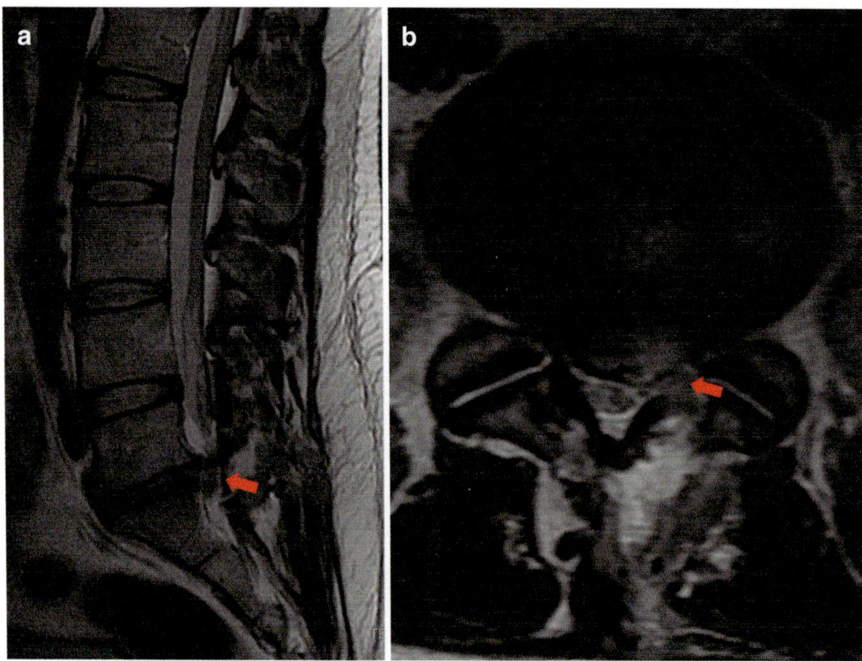

Fig. 22.2 Five-week postoperative lumbar MRI of Case 1. (**a**) The sagittal view shows the postoperative posterior annular defect in L5–S1 and an extruded lumbar disc herniation (red arrow). (**b**) The axial view shows a disc particle in the lateral recess (red arrow)

the left-side facet joint was preserved through the UBE technique and its associated advantages, such as maneuverability of the surgical instruments and excellent visualization quality (Fig. 22.4).

Key Points of Case 1

1. The patient's symptoms must coincide with the radiological findings of the MRI.
2. The triangulation was addressed towards the left L5 lamina to dock both portals over the IAP bone surface (Fig. 22.5).
3. During the endoscopic procedure, the upper lamina and IAP must be identified after dissection of the scar tissue attached. It should be done gently using a curette. Subsequently, we will use various surgical tools such as Kerrison rongeur and a high-speed drill with a diamond tip to complete the laminotomy until the cardinal attachments of ligamentum flavum (LF) are revealed. Later, the flavectomy to release the neural elements should be performed (Fig. 22.6).
4. In summarizing, the most important thing is the identification of the anatomical structures. Use the bone as a safety and orientation landmark. Find a surgical

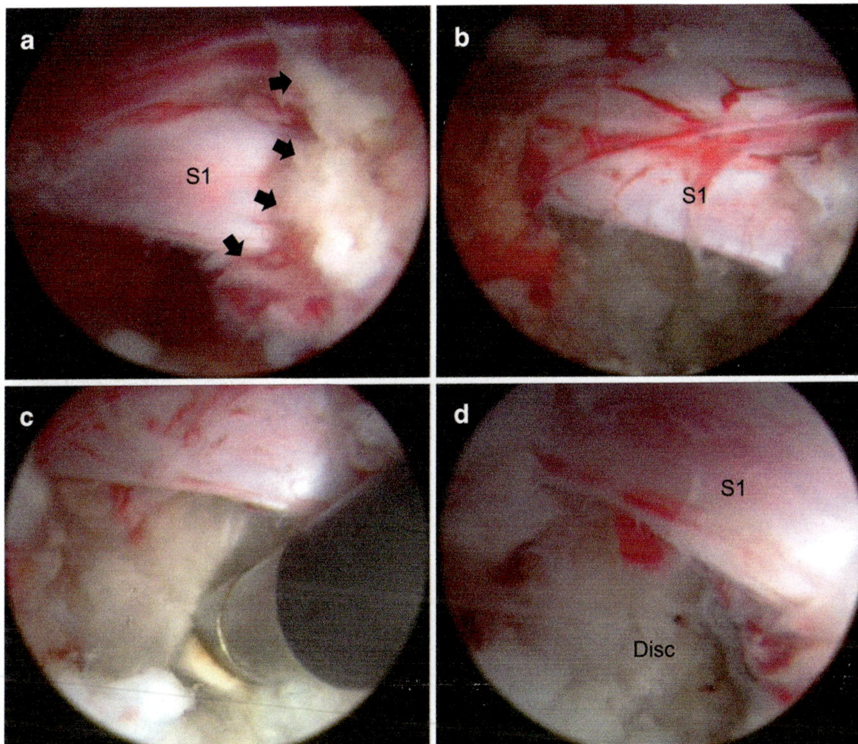

Fig. 22.3 Intraoperative view with the endoscope of Case 1. (**a**) Disc material and scar tissue (black arrows) firmly adhered to the S1 left nerve. (**b**) S1 left nerve decompressed after revision. (**c**) Ablation of the posterior annulus with the radiofrequency probe. (**d**) Final view after left-side neural decompression and cleaning of the epidural space

plane and take advantage of it with a gentle and careful dissection to avoid complications with the dural sac and neural elements. Next, remove the remaining LF and expose the disc by minimally transgressing the lateral recess and facet joints. Finally, perform neural decompression with extreme care.

Case 2: Revision UBE for Lumbar Restenosis

A 62-year-old male patient complained of moderate radicular pain radiating to his left leg associated with paresthesia on the lateral aspect of the calf and dorsum of the left foot for the last 6 months. The patient also presented a 4−/5 paresis in the left-ankle dorsiflexion. He has a history of interspinous device placement 12 years ago at L5–S1. Preoperative MRI of the lumbar spine demonstrated foraminal and subarticular stenosis at L5–S1 on the left side (Fig. 22.7). The patient underwent surgery using a contralateral biportal endoscopic

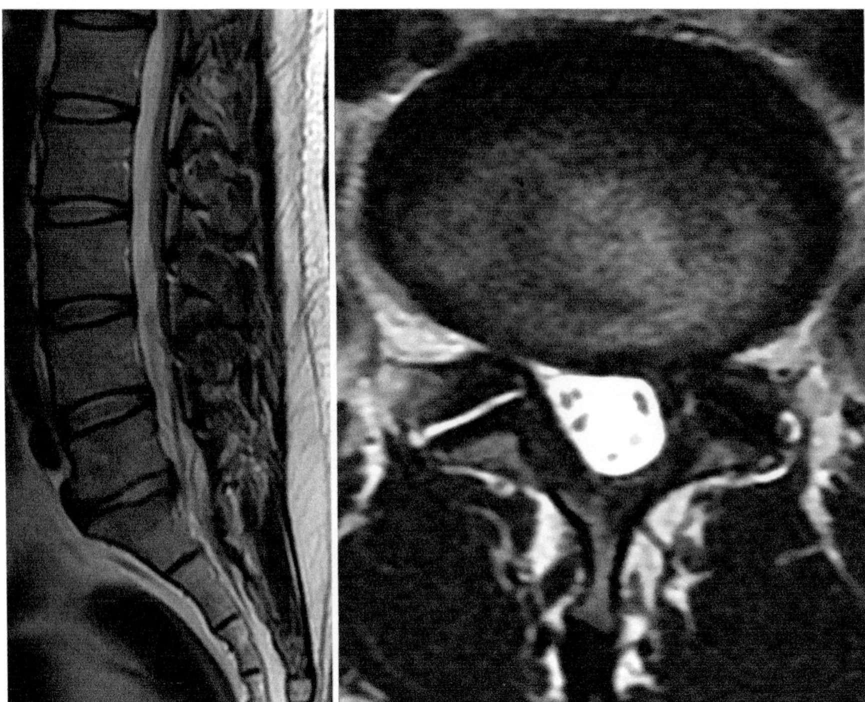

Fig. 22.4 Two-year follow-up postoperative lumbar MRI of Case 1. The neural elements are observed free in the sagittal and axial views

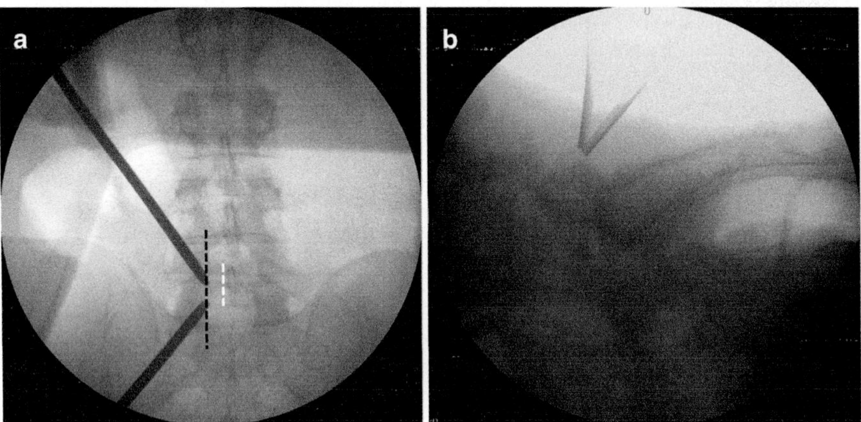

Fig. 22.5 The intraoperative AP and lateral views of the C-arm show the triangulation addressed towards the upper lamina of L5-S1. (**a**) A more lateral trajectory was reached, docking the triangle over the L5 inferior articular process (black dotted line) and not the spinolaminar junction (white dotted line) as usual. (**b**) A lateral view confirms the caudocranial trajectory of the triangle

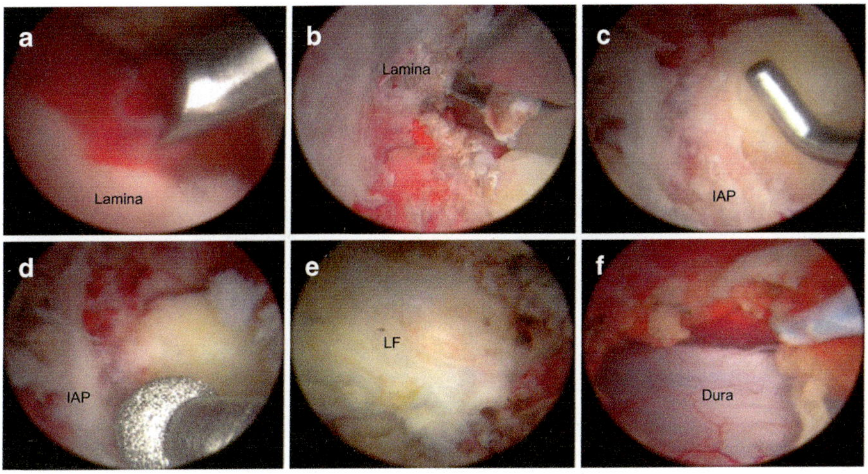

Fig. 22.6 Stepwise technique through the endoscope for a revision due to lumbar re-herniation. (**a**) The upper lamina has been exposed. (**b**) Laminotomy is completed with different surgical tools. (**c**) The cranial attachments of ligamentum flavum (LF) are identified. (**d**) The subarticular area is enlarged with a high-speed drill. (**e**) The LF is exposed before removing it. (**f**) The neural elements are exposed. *IAP* inferior articular process

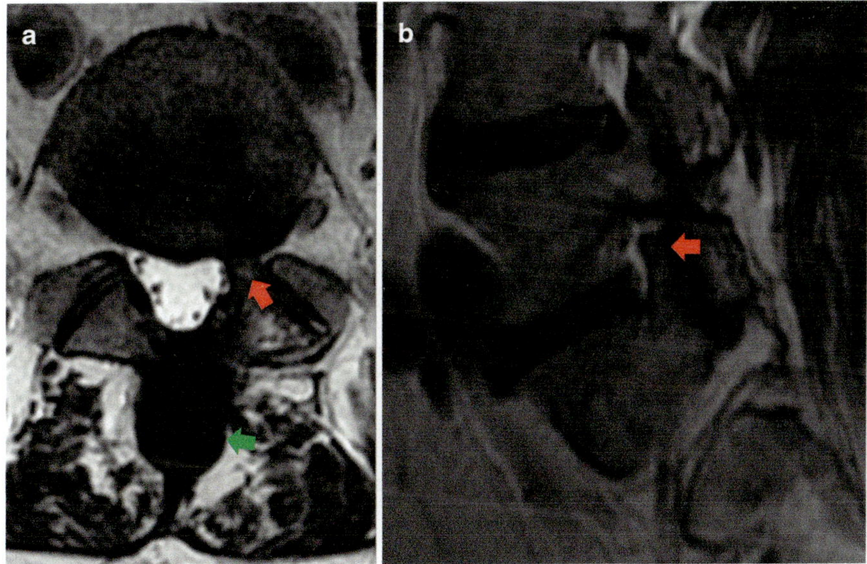

Fig. 22.7 Preoperative lumbar MRI of Case 2. (**a**) The axial view at L5–S1 shows a severe left subarticular stenosis due to a bone excrescence (red arrow). The interspinous device is also observed (green arrow). (**b**) A foraminal stenosis at L5–S1 (red arrow) on the left side is well identified in the sagittal view

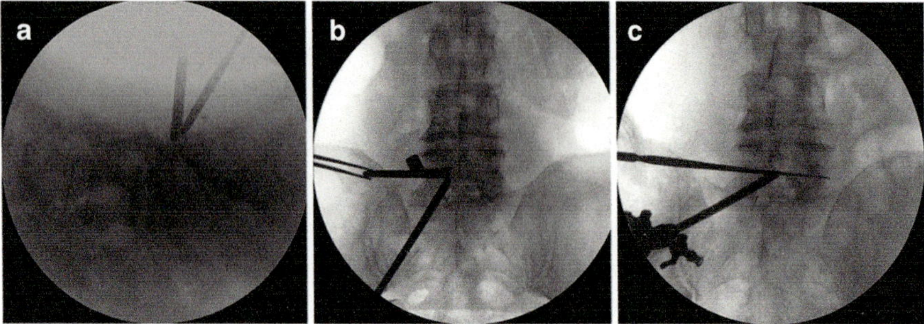

Fig. 22.8 Intraoperative fluoroscopic images of Case 2. (**a**) Lateral view showing the triangulation addressed towards the foramen. (**b**) A paramedian triangular approach docked in the lateral surface and base of the spinous process to enable crossing the midline. (**c**) After decompression of the contralateral subarticular and foraminal spaces. The dissector has been introduced through the foramen and even exits from it

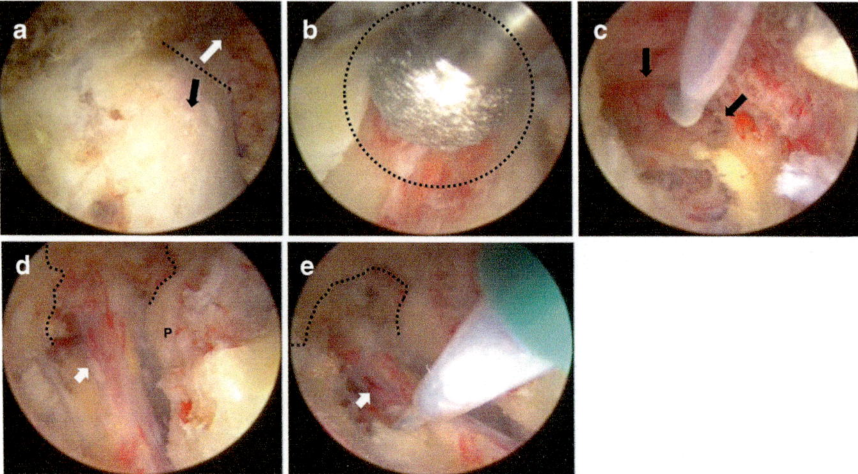

Fig. 22.9 Endoscopic images of Case 2. (**a**) To approach contralaterally in a redo surgery, the spinolaminar junction should be identified (black dotted line). Next, the spinous process (white arrow) and the upper lamina (black arrow) should be identified. (**b**) The spinous process base (black dotted circle) is drilled with a diamond burr. (**c**) The lateral recess and foramen at L5–S1 on the left side are shown (black arrows). (**d**) The left L5 nerve root (white arrow) at L5–S1 has been decompressed, and the foraminal area is represented with the dotted lines. The pedicle (P) can be identified. (**e**) The axillary space can be explored after sufficient contralateral decompression. The white arrow points to the left L5 exiting nerve. The intervertebral foramen has been highlighted with black dotted lines

technique to preserve the facet joint on the left side at L5–S1 (Fig. 22.8). The L5 nerve was decompressed during surgery, and the foraminal area enlarged through the contralateral biportal endoscopic approach (Fig. 22.9). Postoperative lumbar spine MRI demonstrated sufficient decompression in the subarticular

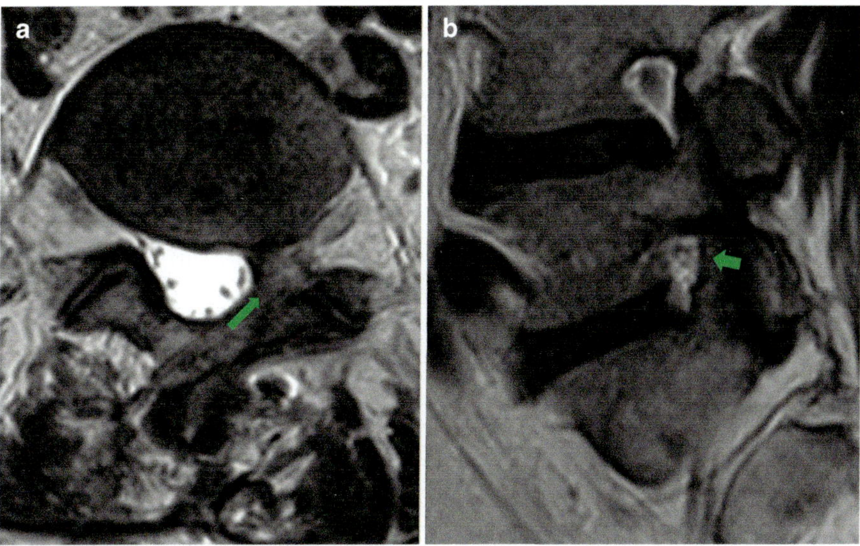

Fig. 22.10 Postoperative lumbar MRI of Case 2. The green arrows point to decompression on (**a**) the subarticular space at L5–S1 on the left side in the axial view and (**b**) the foraminal area in the sagittal view

and foraminal areas. The osteophyte in these locations was removed (Fig. 22.10). The patient's pain in his left leg improved and is still undergoing rehabilitation, improving the strength in the dorsiflexion of the left ankle.

Key Points of Case 2

1. The identification of the spinous process base should be the priority at the beginning of the biportal endoscopic contralateral approach.
2. The biportal endoscopic contralateral approach can have different trajectories, depending on the site of the pathology in the lateral recess or the foramen.
3. Bone removal of the spinous process base is the key to gaining access to the contralateral side.
4. It can be easy to get disoriented on the contralateral side and end up performing a laminotomy. Therefore, the surgeon must identify the inferior articular process (IAP), follow it, and remove it medially. This will allow you to identify the most ventral part of the superior articular process (SAP) and the medial wall of the pedicle. Both are landmarks to find the exiting nerve medially.
5. This approach preserves the contralateral facet joints and the ligamentum flavum. It also avoids dealing with the traversing nerve root and the dural sac, reducing the risk of incidental durotomy, especially in patients previously operated on the same level as Case 2.

Discussion

Biportal endoscopy is an emerging technique that continues to expand its indications. Kang et al. [17] conducted a retrospective study that included 36 patients diagnosed with rLDH. The authors recommend peeling the lamina to have a favorable surgical plane and avoid dealing with the postoperative scar related to the first procedure. The authors compared the results of a group of 20 patients treated with microdiscectomy and 16 patients treated with biportal endoscopy in a setting of rLDH. The authors concluded that biportal endoscopy for rLDH achieved similar results to those obtained through microdiscectomy in revision surgery. However, the biportal technique presented faster pain relief, earlier functional recovery, and better patient satisfaction.

Choy et al. [18] introduced a series of steps for rLDH revision surgery using biportal endoscopy. First, the authors stained the disc with indigo carmine to locate the torn site of the annulus or ruptured disc material under the scar tissue. They also recommended exposing the margin of the lamina and freeing it from the scar, which the authors did from the medial surface of the facet joint to the distal and proximal lamina. Subsequently, they identified the medial edge of the pedicle and performed the adhesiolysis, especially of the scar tissue. This maneuver allowed them access to the epidural space, especially for the traversing nerve root. Finally, the previously stained disc was identified and removed and the procedure concluded by observing the neural element pulsate. The authors highlight the following advantages associated with biportal endoscopy in revision surgery:

- Preservation of the facet joint
- Obtainment of the working space through trimming of the lamina
- Adhesiolysis of the dura without restriction

The range of vision through biportal endoscopy is usually greater than that in uniportal endoscopic procedures due to the floating nature of biportal endoscopic surgery, which translates into the ability to explore with the endoscope the pathology through different perspectives, reducing the traction of neural elements.

Conclusion

Revision surgery to decompress the nerve roots in the lumbar spine is often associated with nerve damage and incidental durotomy due to scar tissue that can disorient the surgeon. For this reason, it is advisable first to identify safety zones that guide the surgeon, such as the bony surfaces of the vertebra. The use of biportal endoscopic surgery for redo surgery has extraordinary advantages such as high-quality visualization, magnification, and lighting. In addition, the technique allows the surgical instrument to be used independently through a different work portal than the endoscope. The surgeon must have the skills and experience to perform revision surgeries using biportal endoscopy.

References

1. Cinotti G, Roysam GS, Eisenstein SM, Postacchini F. Ipsilateral recurrent lumbar disc herniation. A prospective, controlled study. J Bone Joint Surg Br. 1998;80(5):825–32.
2. Cheng J, Wang H, Zheng W, et al. Reoperation after lumbar disc surgery in two hundred and seven patients. Int Orthop. 2013;37(8):1511–7.
3. Aizawa T, Ozawa H, Kusakabe T, et al. Reoperation for recurrent lumbar disc herniation: a study over a 20-year period in a Japanese population. J Orthop Sci. 2012;17(2):107–13.
4. Carragee EJ, Han MY, Suen PW, Kim D. Clinical outcomes after lumbar discectomy for sciatica: the effects of fragment type and annular competence. J Bone Joint Surg Am. 2003;85(1):102–8.
5. Fu TS, Lai PL, Tsai TT, Niu CC, Chen LH, Chen WJ. Long-term results of disc excision for recurrent lumbar disc herniation with or without posterolateral fusion. Spine (Phila Pa 1976). 2005;30(24):2830–4.
6. Lee JK, Amorosa L, Cho SK, Weidenbaum M, Kim Y. Recurrent lumbar disk herniation. J Am Acad Orthop Surg. 2010;18(6):327–37.
7. Shin BJ. Risk factors for recurrent lumbar disc herniations. Asian Spine J. 2014;8(2):211–5.
8. Lebow RL, Adogwa O, Parker SL, Sharma A, Cheng J, McGirt MJ. Asymptomatic same-site recurrent disc herniation after lumbar discectomy: results of a prospective longitudinal study with 2-year serial imaging. Spine (Phila Pa 1976). 2011;36(25):2147–51.
9. Shimia M, Babaei-Ghazani A, Sadat BE, Habibi B, Habibzadeh A. Risk factors of recurrent lumbar disk herniation. Asian J Neurosurg. 2013;8(2):93–6.
10. Suk KS, Lee HM, Moon SH, Kim NH. Recurrent lumbar disc herniation: results of operative management. Spine (Phila Pa 1976). 2001;26(6):672–6.
11. Le H, Sandhu FA, Fessler RG. Clinical outcomes after minimal-access surgery for recurrent lumbar disc herniation. Neurosurg Focus. 2003;15(3):E12.
12. Cinotti G, Gumina S, Giannicola G, Postacchini F. Contralateral recurrent lumbar disc herniation. Results of discectomy compared with those in primary herniation. Spine (Phila Pa 1976). 1999;24(8):800–6.
13. Chen Z, Zhao J, Liu A, Yuan J, Li Z. Surgical treatment of recurrent lumbar disc herniation by transforaminal lumbar interbody fusion. Int Orthop. 2009;33(1):197–201.
14. Waddell G, Kummel EG, Lotto WN, Graham JD, Hall H, McCulloch JA. Failed lumbar disc surgery and repeat surgery following industrial injuries. J Bone Joint Surg Am. 1979;61(2):201–7.
15. Martin BI, Mirza SK, Comstock BA, Gray DT, Kreuter W, Deyo RA. Are lumbar spine reoperation rates falling with greater use of fusion surgery and new surgical technology? Spine (Phila Pa 1976). 2007;32(19):2119–26.
16. Aihara T, Kojima A, Urushibara M, et al. Long-term reoperation rates and causes for reoperations following lumbar microendoscopic discectomy and decompression: 10-year follow-up. J Clin Neurosci. 2022;95:123–8.
17. Kang MS, Hwang JH, Choi DJ, et al. Clinical outcome of biportal endoscopic revisional lumbar discectomy for recurrent lumbar disc herniation. J Orthop Surg Res. 2020;15(1):557.
18. Choi DJ, Jung JT, Lee SJ, Kim YS, Jang HJ, Yoo B. Biportal endoscopic spinal surgery for recurrent lumbar disc herniations. Clin Orthop Surg. 2016;8(3):325–9.

Chapter 23
Unilateral Biportal Endoscopic Transforaminal Lumbar Interbody Fusion: Technique, Variants, and Navigation

Javier Quillo-Olvera, Diego Quillo-Olvera, Javier Quillo-Reséndiz, and Michelle Barrera-Arreola

Abbreviations

ALIF	Anterior lumbar interbody fusion
BESS	Biportal endoscopic spinal surgery
CT	Computed tomography
DLIF	Direct lumbar interbody fusion
EFLIF	Extraforaminal lumbar interbody fusion
ExF	Extraforaminal space
IAP	Inferior articular process
IVS	Intervertebral space
KOL	Key opinion leader
LBP	Lower back pain
LF	Ligamentum flavum
LLIF	Lateral lumbar interbody fusion
LSS	Lumbar spinal stenosis
MISS	Minimally invasive spine surgery
MIS-TLIF	Minimally invasive transforaminal lumbar interbody fusion
MRI	Magnetic resonance imaging
OLIF	Oblique lumbar interbody fusion
PEEK	Polyether ether ketone
PLIF	Posterior lumbar interbody fusion
SAP	Superior articular process
TLIF	Transforaminal lumbar interbody fusion

J. Quillo-Olvera (✉) · D. Quillo-Olvera · J. Quillo-Reséndiz · M. Barrera-Arreola
The Brain and Spine Care, Minimally Invasive Spine Surgery Group,
Hospital H+ Querétaro, Spine Clinic, Querétaro, México
e-mail: neuroqomd@gmail.com; drquilloolvera86@gmail.com; kitnoz@hotmail.com; michelle.barrera@anahuac.mx

J. Quillo-Olvera et al. (eds.), *Unilateral Biportal Endoscopy of the Spine*,
https://doi.org/10.1007/978-3-031-14736-4_23

TP	Transverse process
UBE-TLIF	Unilateral biportal endoscopic transforaminal lumbar interbody fusion
UBE	Unilateral biportal endoscopy
ULBD	Unilateral laminotomy for bilateral decompression
VAS	Visual analog scale

Introduction

Severe degenerative lumbar disease, including intervertebral disc height collapse, facet joint arthritis, and segmental instability, associated with lower back pain (LBP), radiculopathy, or signs of lumbar spinal stenosis (LSS), may require surgical treatment [1, 2]. Transforaminal lumbar interbody fusion (TLIF) is considered a standard technique for posterior lumbar stabilization and fusion. This procedure is associated with a direct decompression of the neural elements involved in degenerative lumbar disease through enlarging the foraminal area; it provides the surgeon with a route to stabilize and fuse the lumbar spine anteriorly and posteriorly by placing an interbody implant filled with different grafts and screwing the spine for cases where it is required [3–5].

Since its introduction by Harms and Jeszenszky [6], the conventional or open TLIF has evolved into a minimally invasive procedure (MIS-TLIF) [7], which is performed through a rigid tubular retractor associated with reduced damage to paraspinal tissues, satisfactory clinical outcomes, and an adequate fusion rate [8–10]. However, the evolution did not end there. TLIF has improved as a technique, mainly due to the benefits generated by technological advances in spine surgery. This innovation has made it possible to potentiate or improve all its attributes, such as planning, identifying anatomical landmarks, boundaries of bone decompression required especially in patients with severe spondylosis, and reducing intraoperative radiation associated with the use of C-arm. The way TLIF has improved in such features was related to intraoperative navigation leading to a more precise and safer surgery for the patient and medical staff [11–16]. In addition, the use of new biological materials and expandable cages has improved the fusion profile, decreased nonunion, and improved the resulting biomechanics of TLIF [17–19].

Recently, the association between full-endoscopic procedures and TLIF has resulted in a transforaminal fusion with high image quality, providing TLIF with more safety, specificity at the site of the pathology, better recognition of the anatomy, and above all, better preparation of the endplates to promote fusion. Not to mention that endoscopy, in addition to its MISS advantages, has benefited TLIF with even lesser damage to the muscles and spinal stabilizing structures, further refining the technique, which has been confirmed by different authors [20–29].

Despite all the advantages that TLIF has acquired when associated with new technologies, one more technique has improved the performance of TLIF. It is called biportal endoscopic spinal surgery (BESS) or unilateral biportal endoscopy

(UBE). This technique has allowed surgeons with experience in microsurgery and uni- or biportal endoscopy to perform more significant decompressions in complex lumbar stenosis and instability cases. In addition, it has recently allowed unilateral biportal endoscopic TLIF (UBE-TLIF) to be associated with intraoperative navigation, thus reducing soft-tissue dissection to find the surgical target and, finally, dislodgment of a larger interbody device [30–32]. In this chapter, the authors describe the UBE-TLIF technique step-by-step, incorporating intraoperative navigation into the technique and placing larger interbody cages in some instances.

Historical Vignettes in Spinal Fusion

The first description of instrumented spinal fusion was made by Dr. Berthold Earnest Hadra in Austin, USA, in 1891 [33], performing a posterior cervical approach and an internal operative spine immobilization by wiring together the spinous process of the sixth and seventh cervical vertebrae. Later, Dr. Chipault, between 1893 and 1895, performed the first five cases of internal fixation for correcting Pott's disease by using Hadra's wiring technique [34]. However, the first descriptions of spinal instability have been found in ancient Indian and Egyptian texts [35–37]. The use of steel rods by Lange in 1908 to stabilize the spine of Pott's disease patients had to be stopped due to the corrosion that steel showed [38]. Hibbs, in 1911, used autologous spinous process bone to create a posterior fixation bridge [39].

Due to the corrosion found by using metal to fuse the vertebral column, Vitallium (an alloy of cobalt, chromium, and molybdenum) was introduced for spine surgery in 1936 by Venable and Stuck. This material was resistant to corrosion and more reliable than other implants used so far [40].

Burns and Capener [41, 42], in 1930, described a spinal approach through the abdominal cavity for an anterior lumbar interbody fusion (ALIF) with autologous bone from the patient's tibia, which was popularized by Lane and Moore later [43].

King [44], during the 1940s, was the first to fix the spine with facet screws to obtain a rigid fixation. However, the short screws used in the facets resulted in a 10% incidence of pseudoarthrosis. Briggs and Milligan [45] were the first to describe the posterior lumbar interbody fusion (PLIF) technique in 1944, and Cloward [46] popularized it in 1953 with some modifications, especially using different bone grafts (autograft and allograft). Harrington introduced his rods for internal spinal fixation in 1962, trying to correct severe scoliosis. This technique spread quickly and was adopted for different uses such as trauma and spondylolisthesis [47, 48].

Nevertheless, the most important concept that Harrington inherited was that the stand-alone spinal instrumentation without fusion is more likely to fail. This allowed the advancement in spinal surgery. Holdsworth related internal fixation problems to a biomechanical concept of spinal instability and, in 1963, reported the two-column model of spinal instability, categorizing subaxial spinal fractures [49].

Roy-Camille [50], in 1970, was the first to describe the use of pedicle screws in combination with a plate, and Steffee, in 1988, suggested combining pedicle screw fixation with interbody fusion to restore load sharing in the anterior column [51–54].

Harms and Rolinger, in 1982, introduced the TLIF technique, which has suffered modifications during the last 30 years [55]. Williams, in 1987, highlighted the potential of polyether ether ketone (PEEK) in spinal fusion; this material is a natural radiolucent polymer with medical applications, reducing a drawback of the titanium: the incompatibility with MRI and CT imaging.

UBE-TLIF Indications and Contraindications

The current indications/contraindications for a UBE-TLIF are the same as conventional TLIF procedure [56].

1. Grade 1 and 2 spondylolisthesis (degenerative or lytic) with mechanical lumbar pain or radicular syndromes
2. Reduced high-grade spondylolisthesis
3. Central canal stenosis with instability
4. Facet joint disease
5. Severe discogenic back pain
6. Lumbar segmental instability
7. Recurrent disc herniation
8. Postlaminectomy instability

Contraindications are the following:

1. Non-reducible high-grade spondylolisthesis
2. Severe osteoporosis
3. Presence of active infection
4. Malignities
5. Traumatic instability
6. Other diseases that prevent surgery

Basic Concepts

Through the biportal endoscopic TLIF, the surgeon will be able to access the IVS to prepare it and dislodge the intersomatic device and bone graft that will allow the lumbar fusion. Endoscopic visualization will allow the surgeon to directly observe the endplate preparation process, ensuring a correct and reliable preparation of a larger surface of the endplates, which is essential to achieving a solid fusion.

In this technique, the goal is identification of the intervertebral disc and make enough space for the discectomy, preparation of the endplates, and placement of the implant and interbody graft, all without affecting the exiting or traversing nerves.

That can be achieved through a lateral foraminotomy, removing the SAP completely to expose the most lateral foraminal and extraforaminal portions of the intervertebral disc. This route is often called the trans-Kambin route, and it has been used successfully by spine surgeons with experience in uniportal endoscopy [57].

However, in cases of multifocal lumbar spinal stenosis with severe spondylosis, it may be necessary to perform a total facetectomy, bilateral laminotomy, or even undercutting of the contralateral facet joint medially. Therefore, the UBE-TLIF can be useful if planned a little more medially, as will be detailed in "UBE-TLIF Surgical Technique" section of this chapter.

There are different maneuvers to achieve the previously mentioned goals. Various authors have systematically described these [20, 30–32, 58]. Kang et al. [58], in an extensive review on the evolution of biportal endoscopic approaches for lumbar transforaminal interbody fusion, reported three methods commonly used by authors from South Korea, the biportal endoscopic posterolateral-TLIF, the biportal endoscopic extraforaminal lumbar interbody fusion (biportal endoscopic-EFLIF), and the modified far-lateral biportal endoscopic TLIF. The difference between them is the location of the entry points for the endoscopic and working portals concerning the index-level pedicles. In addition, the extraforaminal approach and the far-lateral approach may require an extra entry to assist in the placement of the cage. These approaches can be performed through two corridors, the posterolateral and the trans-Kambin (Fig. 23.1). The posterolateral route is more medial than the trans-Kambin [57, 58].

We understand that the principles on which the UBE-TLIF technique is based are the same as those of conventional TLIF:

1. Ipsilateral direct decompression of the neural elements
2. Direct decompression of the central lumbar spinal canal
3. Direct/indirect decompression of the contralateral neural elements

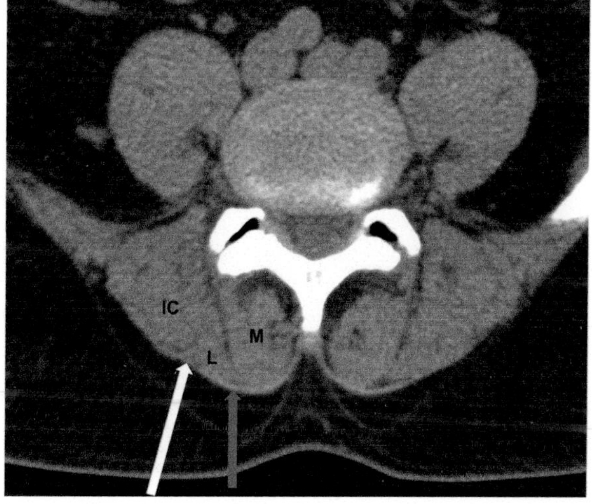

Fig. 23.1 Axial view of lumbar CT at L4–L5 showing the two major routes used in UBE-TLIF. The blue arrow points to the posterolateral approach through the multifidus (M) and longissimus (L) muscles. The white one represents the extraforaminal trajectory, which runs through the longissimus and iliocostalis (IC) muscles

4. Interbody stabilization
5. Segmental lordosis
6. Posterior screw fixation
7. Interbody fusion

Surgical Instruments

The technological requirements of the UBE-TLIF are usually those generally used in any biportal endoscopic procedure, such as a 4 mm outer diameter arthroscope of 0° or 30°. In particular, the authors recommend the use of 30° lenses to have greater depth, especially in contralateral approaches, and to obtain a greater angle of vision by rotating the lens. Continuous saline irrigation can be through a water pressure pump set at 30 mmHg or a gravity-fed system set 1 m above the patient throughout the procedure. In addition, surgical tools such as progressive tubular dilators starting at 5 mm to perform the triangular approach, a standard lumbar spine surgery set, and an underwater drilling system are implemented.

UBE-TLIF Surgical Technique

Step 1: Patient Positioning and Anesthesia

The patient is positioned prone on a radiolucent table on an abdominal support frame or over a specialized spine surgical table. The face and especially the eyes are protected. The knees are flexed to facilitate venous return and prevent thrombosis. Epidural anesthesia is given in cases where one level is treated; however, it is recommended to use general anesthesia in multilevel cases (Fig. 23.2).

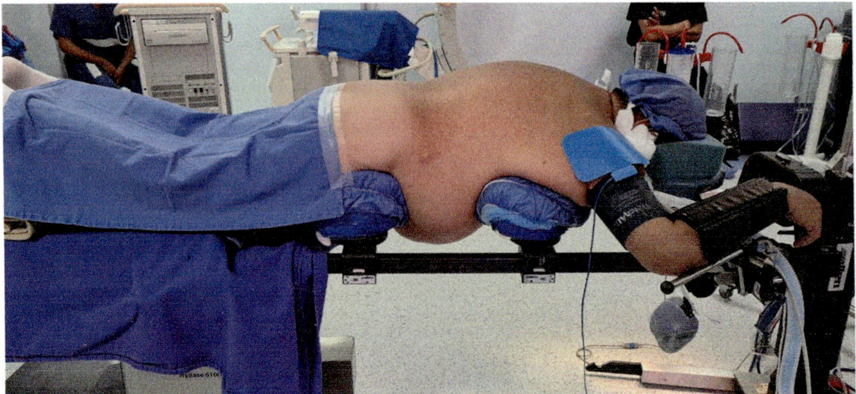

Fig. 23.2 Patient positioning on a specialized spine surgical table for a UBE-TLIF

Step 2: Incision Planning

The approach will be performed on the patient's symptomatic side. Therefore, the planning of skin incisions will depend on the objective of each patient. For this, the authors propose the following preoperative analysis:

1. Is ipsilateral foraminotomy sufficient to reach the intervertebral disc?
2. Is total facetectomy required to decompress the exiting and traversing nerve roots?
3. Is an extended approach to the contralateral side needed in cases of LSS?
4. Is it the ideal case to place a large-sized cage through the far-lateral UBE-TLIF?

Answering these questions will allow the surgeon to define the ideal trajectory (posterolateral or extraforaminal) for each case. Below is the response to that preoperative analysis.

1. *Is ipsilateral foraminotomy sufficient to reach the intervertebral disc?*

   In cases where only the lateral aspect of the facet joint needs to be removed, the SAP can be reached through an extraforaminal route which can be planned 3–4 cm lateral to the index-level pedicles (Fig. 23.3a).
2. *Is total facetectomy required to decompress the exiting and traversing nerve roots?*

   In cases where it is necessary to decompress the exiting and traversing nerve roots, the surgeon must plan an approach that allows him or her to perform a facetectomy that includes the isthmus, inferior articular process (IAP), and SAP. Therefore, the skin incisions should be more medial (posterolateral) than the extraforaminal route. Consequently, we suggest locating the skin incisions 2 cm lateral to the pedicles (Fig. 23.3b).
3. *Is an extended approach to the contralateral side needed in cases of LSS?*

   For patients who require interbody fusion and a unilateral laminotomy with bilateral decompression (ULBD) because of LSS, the ULBD can be planned

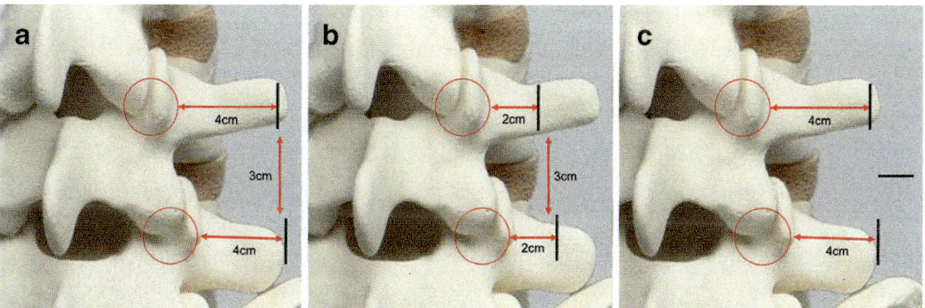

Fig. 23.3 The anatomical model is used to exemplify a right-sided L4–L5 UBE-TLIF. The red circles line the pedicles. The black lines represent the entries for the viewing and working portals. (**a**) Paraspinal extraforaminal approach. (**b**) Paraspinal posterolateral approach. (**c**) Modified far-lateral UBE-TLIF

through a posterolateral approach. After removing the IAP, an experienced surgeon can perform an extended procedure on the contralateral side.

4. *Is it the ideal case to place a large-sized cage through the far-lateral UBE-TLIF?*

   Placing a large OLIF/LLIF cage favors fusion due to its large footprint, enables restoration of segmental lordosis and intervertebral height, and decreases implant subsidence risk. However, care must be taken when attempting to place this type of interbody implant through a route for which they were not intended. The following are exceptions for a modified far-lateral UBE-TLIF:

   (a) A cage of these dimensions can injure the ipsilateral exiting and traversing nerve roots at lumbar levels rostral to L4 (L1–L2, L2–L3, and L3–L4) due to a narrow Kambin corridor.

   (b) The modified far-lateral UBE-TLIF does not replace other lateral techniques such as OLIF or LLIF only for set larger cages in the IVS. Through lumbar posterior approaches, it could be difficult and risky to set cages with similar dimensions of OLIF and LLIF interbody devices in the IVS properly, particularly for beginners.

   (c) Modifying the trajectory of larger interbody devices, like those used in lateral techniques with UBE, could be too risky. In lateral and oblique interbody fusions, the surgeon does not require modifying the cage within the IVS since it is delivered in a determined trajectory (OLIF, LLIF). And precisely, one of the advantages of the lateral techniques (OLIF, LLIF) is avoiding the neural elements' transgression.

   (d) Wide and long cages aim to achieve a larger contact surface between both endplates in order to not only enable fusion and reduce the cage subsidence risk but also allow indirect decompression of the contralateral foramen and the central canal in LSS, which is not reproducible through far-lateral UBE-TLIF.

For these reasons, placement of interbody cages with a considerable length and width through the far-lateral UBE-TLIF does not offer all the advantages for which they were intended, and their use must be at the expert's discretion considering the benefits to be gained on a case-by-case basis.

If a similar lateral and oblique interbody fusion cage is decided to be used through a far-lateral UBE-TLIF, an extra skin incision should be planned at the mid-height of the disc and 5 cm lateral to the pedicles (Fig. 23.3c). The rostrocaudal location of the incisions will depend on both pedicles since the transpedicular screws are usually placed through them. The length between cranial and caudal incisions usually is 3 cm. In the left-sided approach, the surgeon's dominant hand will use the caudal incision for the working portal, and cage placement is easier because the inferior pedicle of the index level is close to the IVS, so the same incision could be used efficiently for delivery of the cage and screwing the spine. However, on the right side, the surgeon's dominant hand uses the cranial incision for the working

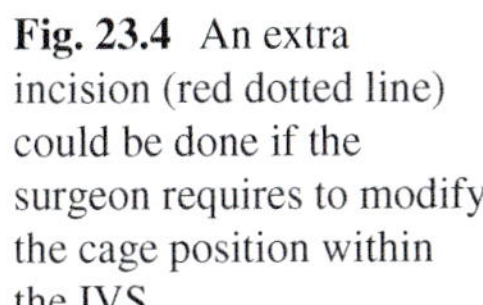

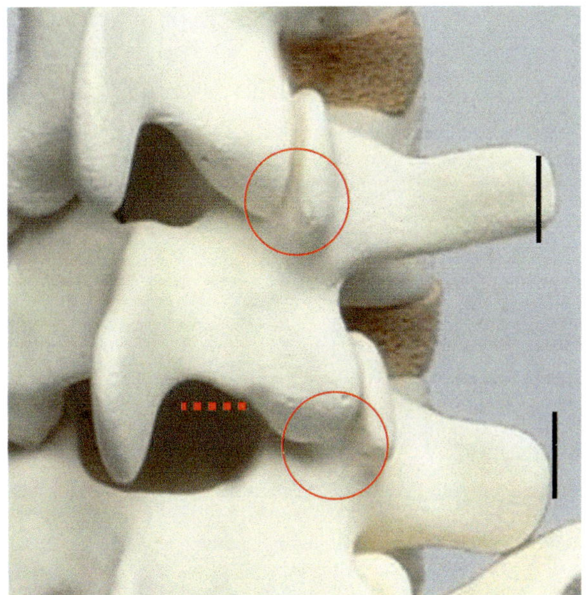

Fig. 23.4 An extra incision (red dotted line) could be done if the surgeon requires to modify the cage position within the IVS

portal, and it does not coincide with the IVS, so the incision should be enlarged to reach the IVS, and the same works for the transpedicular screw or the surgeon could create a third portal similar to the far-lateral UBE-TLIF to introduce the cage on the right side. The surgeon can make an accessory incision in the interlaminar space to manipulate the cage into the IVS and position it as planned (Fig. 23.4).

Step 3: Biportal Paraspinal Approach

The working portal will be created first after appropriately marking the superior and inferior incisions at the index level on the proper side. Then, the initial dilator will be introduced through the wound and directed towards the facet joint. The surgeon should palpate the dorsal aspect of the facet joint with the dilator's tip and slide it towards the transverse process and facet joint junction to finally feel the lateral aspect of the SAP. Subsequently, the following dilators will be introduced progressively until they reach 10 mm of dilation. Finally, the working cannula will be introduced through the initial dilator and left in place to create the next port. The viewing portal will be created similarly, although it will be easier if the dilator inserted through the planned incision is addressed to the working cannula. Finally, the triangular approach should be confirmed by AP and lateral projections of the C-arm (Fig. 23.5).

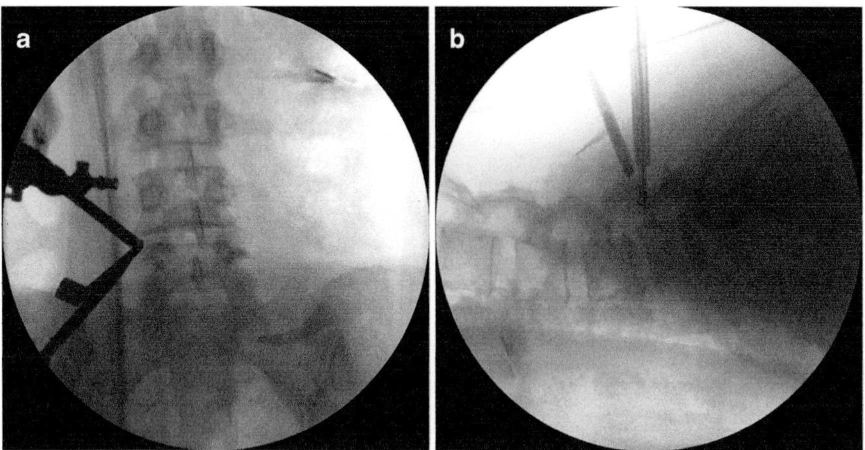

Fig. 23.5 Biportal endoscopic paraspinal approach at L4–L5 on the right side for a UBE-TLIF procedure. (**a**) Both portals are reaching the lateral surface of the facet joint on the AP view of the C-arm. (**b**) The endoscope is slightly out than the RF in the lateral view

Step 4: Neural Decompression

The ipsilateral exiting and traversing nerves, the dural sac, and the contralateral roots can be directly decompressed during UBE-TLIF if the case requires it. That will depend on the bone remodeling that is carried out.

Foraminotomy through SAP resection or total facetectomy will allow decompression of the exiting and traversing nerve roots. An approach extended to the contralateral side through a bilateral laminotomy and medial undercutting of the contralateral facet joint will allow decompression of the neural elements bilaterally.

The SAP can be removed with the high-speed drill, lateral to medial. It is essential to identify its base through the junction with the TP (Fig. 23.6). Specifically, that point gives access to the intervertebral disc. Chisels can be used during foraminotomy to remove the SAP more quickly. Kerrison punches of different sizes and angled tips are helpful when removing the most ventral portion (Fig. 23.7).

The foraminal LF must be preserved while performing the foraminotomy and used as a barrier to avoid damage to the neural elements. After removing the SAP, the ligament can also be removed and the foraminal and extraforaminal space explored.

The surgeon must be careful since the pre-discal space usually contains fat and venous plexuses that will require prior coagulation with the radiofrequency (RF) probe. The disc is exposed and can be identified as a solid white structure. An AP and lateral C-arm projection are obtained to confirm the correct location and trajectory of the approach (Fig. 23.8).

When the patient requires a facetectomy, the SAP and IAP are usually removed. Although the IAP is medial to the SAP, a cleft between both articular processes is

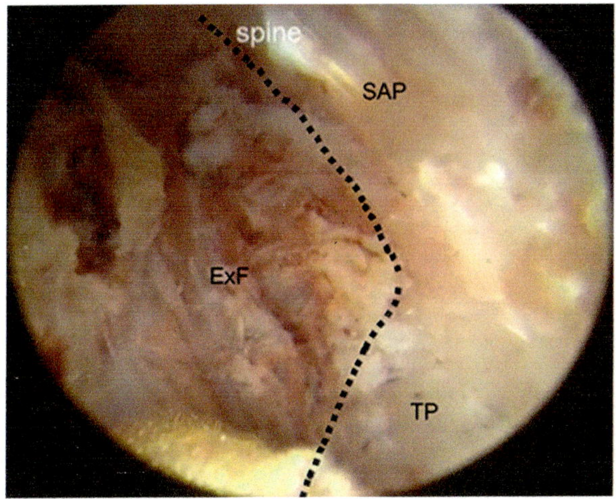

Fig. 23.6 Image obtained with the endoscope during a right L4–L5 UBE-TLIF. The black dotted line shows the SAP and TP junction. The extraforaminal space (ExF) can be identified. *ExF* extraforaminal space, *SAP* superior articular process, *TP* transverse process

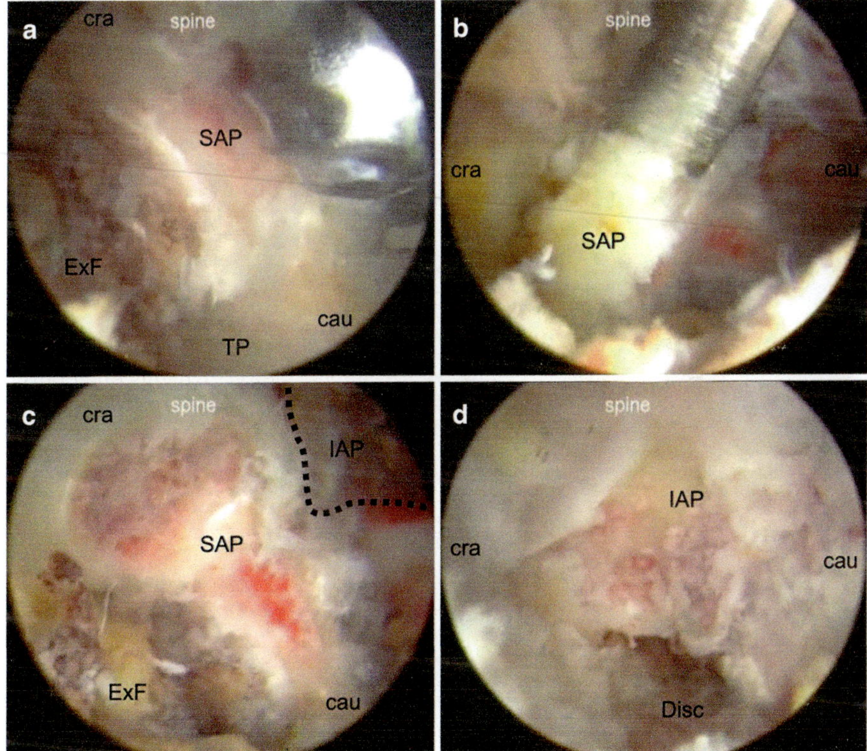

Fig. 23.7 SAP resection during a right L4–L5 UBE-TLIF. (**a**) The high-speed drill is used to remove the dorsal part of the SAP. (**b**) A 6 mm straight chisel is used to remove the apex of the SAP. (**c**) Panoramic view showing the SAP resection process. The IAP can be identified medially and is limited by the black dotted line. (**d**) The SAP was removed entirely, and the IAP and disc were exposed. *Cra* cranial, *Cau* caudal, *SAP* superior articular process, *ExF* extraforaminal space, *TP* transverse process, *IAP* inferior articular process

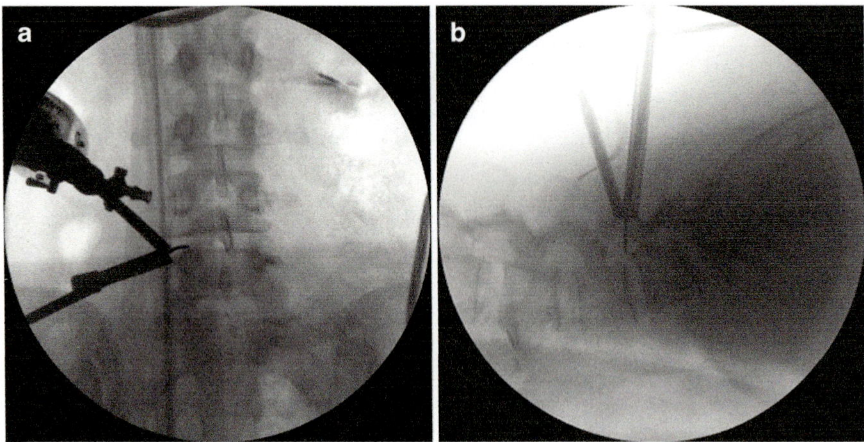

Fig. 23.8 Intraoperative (**a**) AP and (**b**) lateral fluoroscopic projections confirm that the dissector is in the L4–L5 disc through the foraminotomy

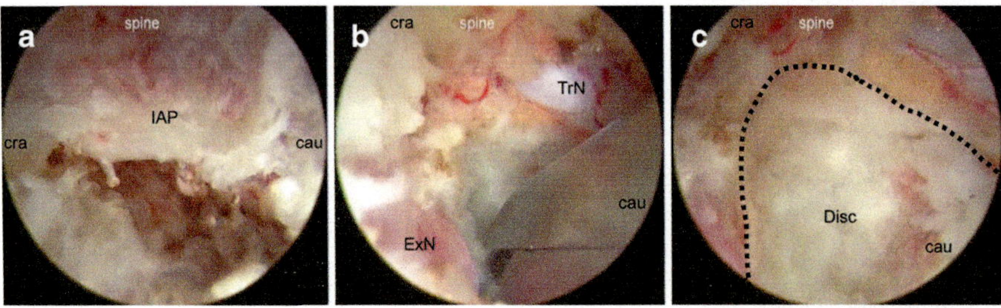

Fig. 23.9 Decompression of the ipsilateral neural elements during a right L4–L5 UBE-TLIF. (**a**) The IAP is exposed. (**b**) Image through the endoscope showing the exiting (ExN) and traversing (TrN) nerve roots after facetectomy. (**c**) The intervertebral disc has been exposed. The area for the discectomy has been delimited with the black dotted line. *Cra* cranial, *Cau* caudal, *IAP* inferior articular process, *ExN* exiting nerve, *TrN* traversing nerve

generally observed during SAP resection. After the flavectomy, the surgeon will identify the exiting and traversing nerves and the intervertebral disc (Fig. 23.9).

If one of the goals of the surgery is also to perform central spinal canal decompression, then the procedure can be conducted as a ULBD. After removing the IAP, the ipsilateral cranial lamina is exposed, and the biportal approach can be advanced medially. The ipsilateral and contralateral sublaminar undercutting can be performed until identified FL attachments. The same process can be applied to the caudal lamina following the SAP base medially.

The surgeon must keep in mind that these direct decompression maneuvers will only be performed if the case requires it, which was previously planned so that the biportal approach may be ideal for specific objectives (Fig. 23.10).

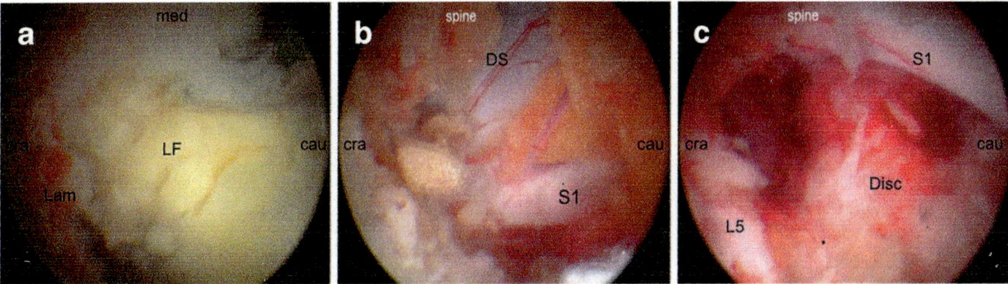

Fig. 23.10 Medial decompression during left L5–S1 UBE-TLIF. (**a**) After the L5–S1 facetectomy, the approach was addressed towards the superior lamina (Lam). As a result, the LF of the spinal canal has been exposed. (**b**) After flavectomy, the dorsal epidural space, dural sac (DS), and traversing nerve S1 are identified. (**c**) Lateral endoscopic image of the same procedure where exiting nerve L5 and traversing S1 are identified, and the disc has been exposed

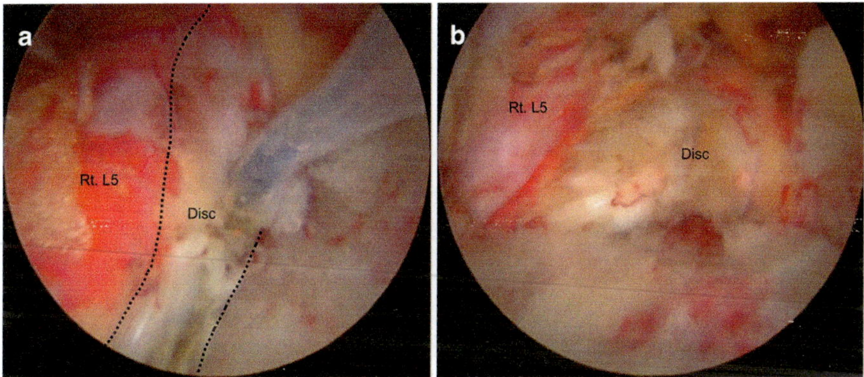

Fig. 23.11 L5–S1 UBE-TLIF on the right side. (**a**) The pre-discal vessels were ablated with the RF. The black dotted lines line the intervertebral disc. In addition, the right L5 exiting nerve is observed cranially (Rt. L5). (**b**) The posterior annulus was exposed (disc), and the L5 exiting nerve (Rt. L5) was identified

Step 5: Biportal Endoscopic Discectomy and Endplate Preparation

The placement of the bone graft, the interbody cage, and the fusion depend on the correct execution of this step. First, the surgeon must identify the intervertebral disc and the nearby neural structures (the exiting and traversing nerves) to avoid injuring them. Next, the posterior annulus should be exposed and the ventral pre-discal epidural vessels and fatty tissue coagulated to obtain a good view of the intervertebral disc (Fig. 23.11). Subsequently, the posterior annulus can be opened with the knife or with the RF to continue with the discectomy, in which pituitary rongeurs are commonly used (Fig. 23.12). During the preparation of the endplates, the surgeon will introduce different instruments (shavers, curettes, and rasps) within the IVS to

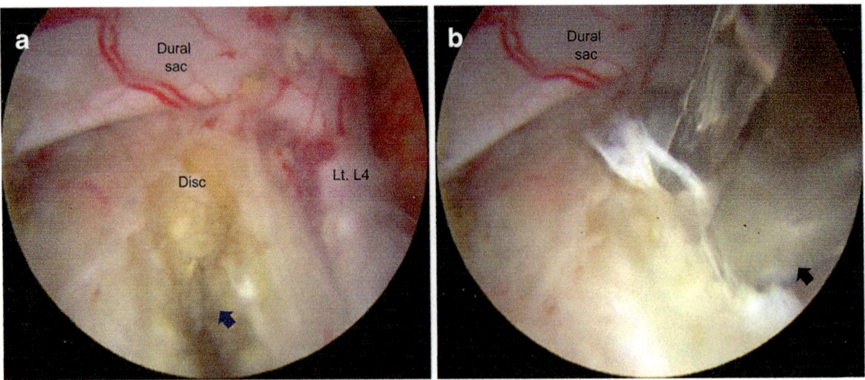

Fig. 23.12 L4–L5 UBE-TLIF on the left side. (**a**) The intervertebral disc (disc) was exposed, and the posterior annulus opened (blue arrow). The neural elements were also identified to avoid damage to them (dural sac and Lt. L4 nerve). (**b**) The pituitary rongeur (black arrow) is used to complete the discectomy under direct visualization with the endoscope

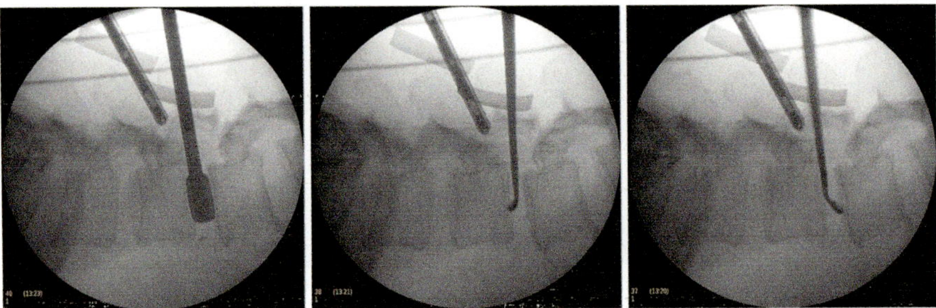

Fig. 23.13 Intraoperative process of endplate preparation during a UBE-TLIF procedure seen on the lateral views of the C-arm

remove the cartilage under direct visualization with the endoscope, avoiding transgression of the endplates due to overpreparation (Fig. 23.13). Finally, the surgeon can observe the final status of the endplates with the endoscope and confirm the correct execution of this step (Fig. 23.14).

Step 6: Graft and Cage Insertion

The IVS is filled with bone graft mixed with any osteoconductive or inductive material through a funnel-shaped delivery device. This instrument is introduced through the working portal under the endoscopic view and confirmed with lateral views of the C-arm (Fig. 23.15). Finally, the TLIF cage (banana- or straight-bullet-nosed tip)

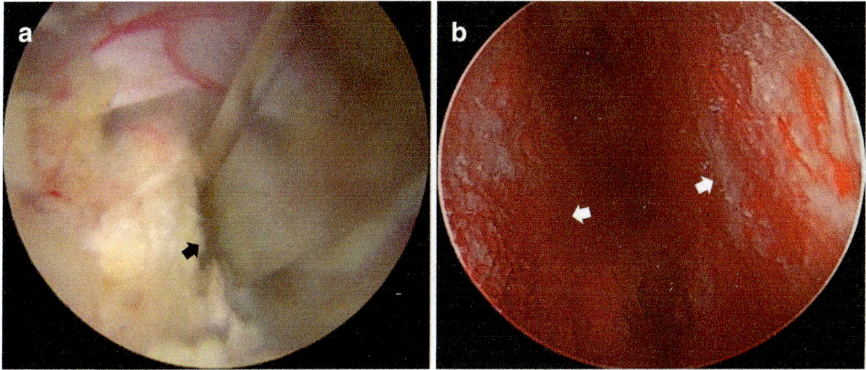

Fig. 23.14 Endplate preparation under direct visualization through the endoscope. (**a**) A shaver is introduced within the intervertebral space (black arrow) to clean up the remaining disc. (**b**) The final state of the endplates (white arrows)

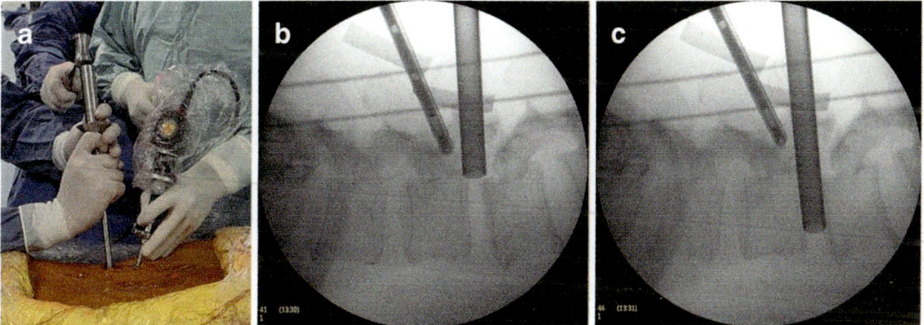

Fig. 23.15 Bone graft delivered within the IVS. (**a**) The funnel-shaped device is placed in the IVS under endoscopic view. (**b**, **c**) The bone graft delivery device is advanced within the IVS and confirmed with the C-arm

filled with the demineralized bone matrix is inserted under direct endoscopic visualization, preventing neural damage. The TLIF cage can be moved inside the IVS if the case requires a different position (Fig. 23.16).

Step 7: Transpedicular Screw Fixation

The incisions on the side where the TLIF was performed can be used to place the pedicle screws. However, on the right side, it is sometimes necessary to increase the incision length used for the working channel (cranial) because it is planned according to the intervertebral space (IVS) and not the superior pedicle. In addition, contralateral transpedicular screws require new incisions, as usual (Fig. 23.17).

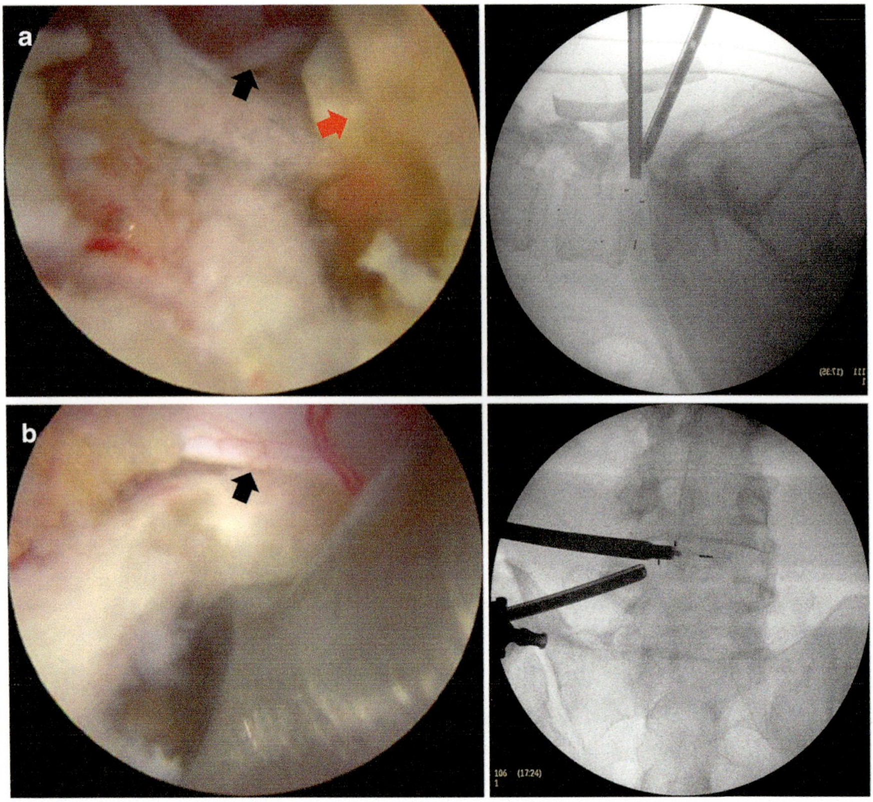

Fig. 23.16 Cage insertion during a UBE-TLIF L4–L5 on the right side. (**a**) The cage (red arrow) is inserted into the IVS under endoscopic visualization to decrease the risk of damage to the neural elements (black arrow). A lateral projection of the C-arm confirms the cage location during its placement. (**b**) The cage was appropriately inserted, and an AP view of the C-arm shows it

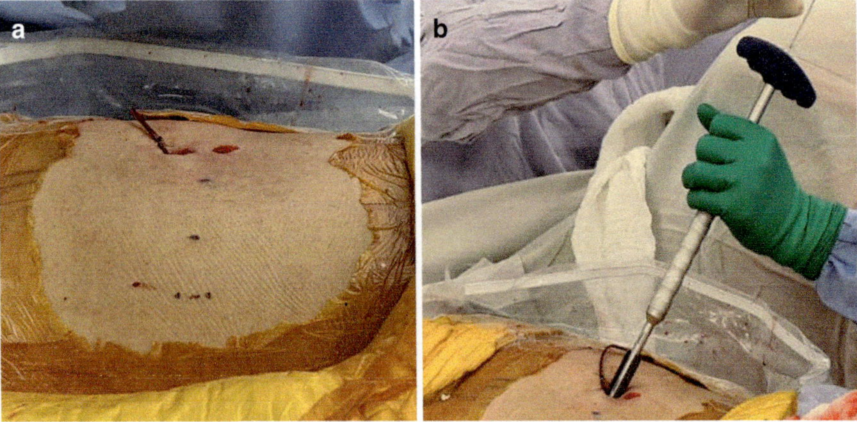

Fig. 23.17 (**a**) The ipsilateral skin incisions can be used for pedicle screws. (**b**) Pedicle screw placement

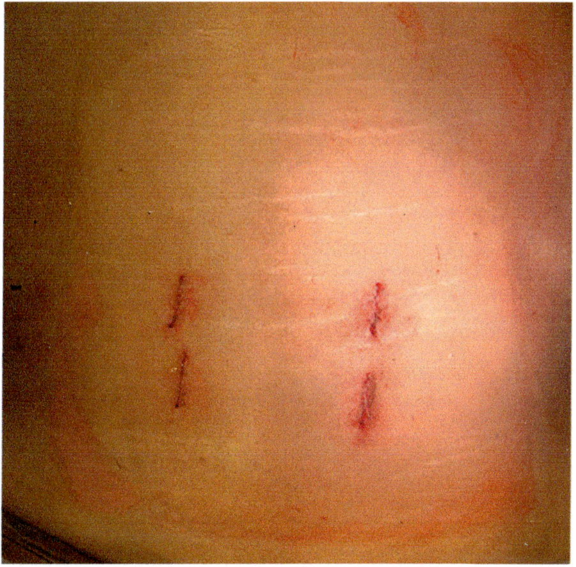

Fig. 23.18 Skin closure after UBE-TLIF in a patient who did not require a drain

Step 8: Wound Closure

The skin incisions are closed with a single suture, and depending on the situation, a drain could be inserted in the caudal, ipsilateral incision to evacuate residual fluid from irrigation or avoid an epidural hematoma (Fig. 23.18).

Modified Far-Lateral UBE-TLIF

This modification to the UBE-TLIF proposed by Heo Dong Hwa and Eum Jin Hwa [31, 59], both KOLs, allows the surgeon to use cages designed for lateral approaches (DLIF, LLIF, OLIF) or larger customized interbody devices in some instances for which the following is required:

1. Have experience with open, microsurgical, and biportal endoscopic TLIF.
2. This technique is recommended at the L4–L5 and L5–S1 levels to avoid damaging any neural element with the sizeable interbody cage.
3. During the procedure, it may be necessary to measure the distance between the lateral edge of the dural sac (traversing nerve root) and the exiting nerve root; this must be greater than 16 mm.

An incision to create a third portal should be located lateral to the working and viewing channels, approximately 5 cm lateral to the index-level pedicles (Fig. 23.3c). This third skin incision will be used to place the cage through the previously prepared IVS. The large interbody cage enters with a more oblique trajectory due to the

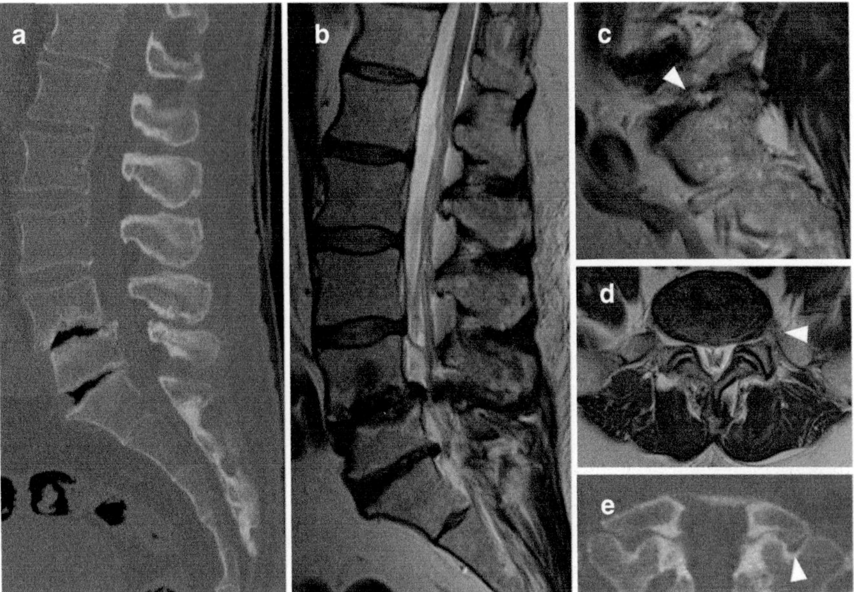

Fig. 23.19 Preoperative images of the Case Example 1. (**a**) Sagittal view of lumbar CT showing a severe degenerative disc disease at L4–L5 and L5–S1, the first one related to the previous spondylodiscitis. (**b**) Central spinal stenosis is noted at L4–L5 and L5–S1 due to severe spondylosis observed at the lumbar MRI on the sagittal view. (**c**) Extraforaminal space at the lateral view of the lumbar MRI showing stenosis at L5–S1 (white arrowhead). (**d**) The same finding (white arrowhead) is observed on the left side at L5–S1 in an axial view of the lumbar MRI. (**e**) The coronal view of the lumbar CT demonstrated extraforaminal stenosis on the left side at L5–S1 (white arrowhead)

lateral nature of the placement process, and with the endoscope, the surgeon confirms that there is no damage to the neural elements.

Subsequently, the cage can be mobilized within the IVS when the case requires it. Finally, the surgeon must confirm adequate hemostasis and if it is necessary to leave an epidural drain before placing the transpedicular screws.

Case 1

A 62-year-old male patient with a history of diabetes mellitus and spondylodiscitis at L4–L5 10 years ago. He complains of severe radicular type pain in his left leg and significant lower back pain. Preoperative lumbar CT showed an ex vacuum phenomenon in the intervertebral spaces of L4–L5 and L5–S1 and changes in the endplates of the intervertebral space L4–L5 associated with previous infection (Fig. 23.19a). Lumbar MRI demonstrated foraminal and extraforaminal stenosis at L5–S1 on the left side associated with radicular type pain in the patient's left leg (Fig. 23.19b–d). The coronal view of the lumbar CT scan confirmed a left L5–S1 extraforaminal stenosis (Fig. 23.19e).

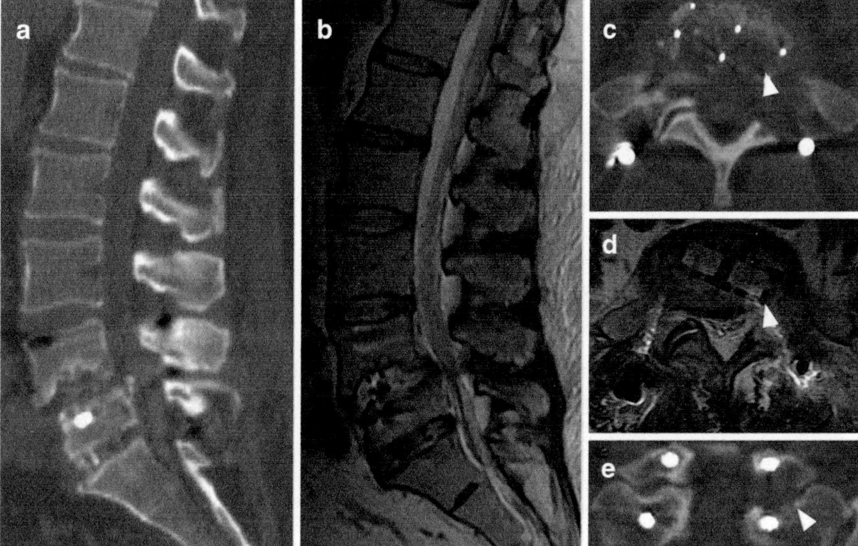

Fig. 23.20 Postoperative images of the Case Example 1. (**a**) The sagittal view of lumbar CT shows restoration of IVS at L4–L5 and L5–S1 with segmental and lumbar lordosis preserved after the UBE-TLIF in both levels. (**b**) The sagittal view of the lumbar MRI showed sufficient decompression on the central spinal canal at L4–L5 and L5–S1. (**c**) Large interbody device (white arrowhead) at L5–S1 on an axial view of lumbar CT. (**d**) The same finding (white arrowhead) on the axial view of lumbar MRI. (**e**) Postoperative imaging of the coronal view of lumbar CT showing the bone remodeling of extraforaminal space at L5–S1 on the left side. The transverse process, SAP, and sacral ala were removed partially to decompress the exiting nerve directly

An extraforaminal paraspinal approach was performed for L4–L5 and L5–S1 to complete the UBE-TLIF of the same levels. At L5–S1, a 10-mm-high, 22-mm-wide, and 45-mm-long with 7 mm of lordosis cage was placed through the far-lateral UBE-TLIF modification. Subsequently, transpedicular fixation was completed at L4–L5–S1 bilaterally. Postoperative lumbar CT demonstrated adequate placement of the interbody cages at L4–L5 and L5–S1 (Fig. 23.20a), and central decompression in the spinal canal at both levels was confirmed on postoperative lumbar MRI (Fig. 23.20b). The large interbody device was seen in a suitable location in the intervertebral space of L5–S1 on postoperative CT and MRI (Fig. 23.20c, d). Also, direct decompression of the extraforaminal space was successfully achieved on the left side (Fig. 23.20e). Preservation of lordosis and restoration of height in both L4–L5 and L5–S1 intervertebral spaces compared to the preoperative state are notable by UBE-TLIF (Fig. 23.21). The patient was discharged the following day with minimal discomfort associated with the procedure and complete resolution of his radicular symptoms and back pain.

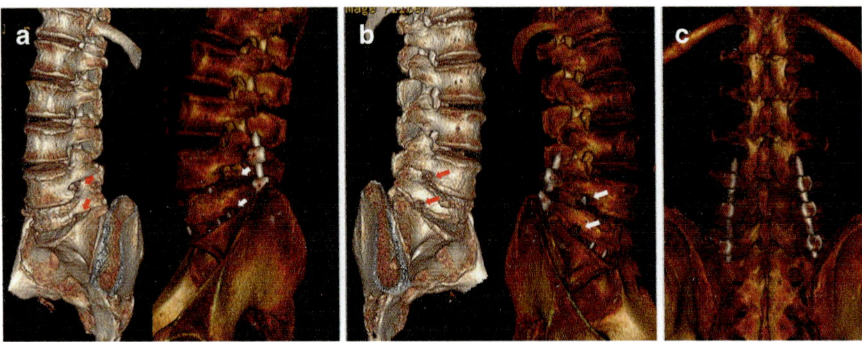

Fig. 23.21 Postoperative 3D lumbar CT reconstruction of Case Example 1. (**a**) Left oblique view of the preoperative (left side) and postoperative (right side) lumbar 3D reconstructions. The red arrows point to the foraminal area at L4–L5 and L5–S1 preoperatively, while the white arrows point to the same foraminal space postoperatively. (**b**) Right oblique view of the preoperative (left side) and postoperative (right side) lumbar 3D reconstructions. The red arrows point to the foraminal area at L4–L5 and L5–S1 preoperatively, while the white arrows point to the same foraminal space after indirect decompression given by the UBE-TLIF in both levels. (**c**) Posterior view of postoperative lumbar 3D reconstruction

UBE-TLIF Under Intraoperative Navigation

Intraoperative navigation in real time is a paradigm in spine surgery. It has been associated with different advantages such as the reduction of operative time, exposure of the patient and the medical staff to radiation-related intraoperative fluoroscopy, and, above all, more accurate surgical procedures, resulting in less procedure-related muscle dissection and trauma as well as more safety for the patient [60].

Its usefulness has not only been confirmed in the precise placement of various devices in the spine, but it is also a handy tool for the surgeon in planning safer trajectories for various procedures such as spinal interbody fusions, direct neural decompressions, and spinal tumor surgery, among others [61, 62].

The merge between endoscopy and navigation might not make much sense pragmatically. One of the advantages of the endoscope is the ability to provide excellent visualization of anatomical structures through continuous fluid irrigation, which allows the surgeon to orient himself or herself by accurately recognizing anatomical structures. However, advanced stages of spondylosis can modify the bone structures that serve as surface landmarks, confusing and disorienting the surgeon and avoiding accomplishing the surgical goals with the endoscope. Another relevant situation is planning the trajectory with which the endoscope will be introduced. This trajectory can be planned with the navigator and make endoscopic surgery more accurate, avoiding unnecessary risks associated with the wrong placement of the endoscopic system.

For this reason, several authors have used 3D real-time image-navigated endoscopy in different circumstances, especially in those that require accuracy and

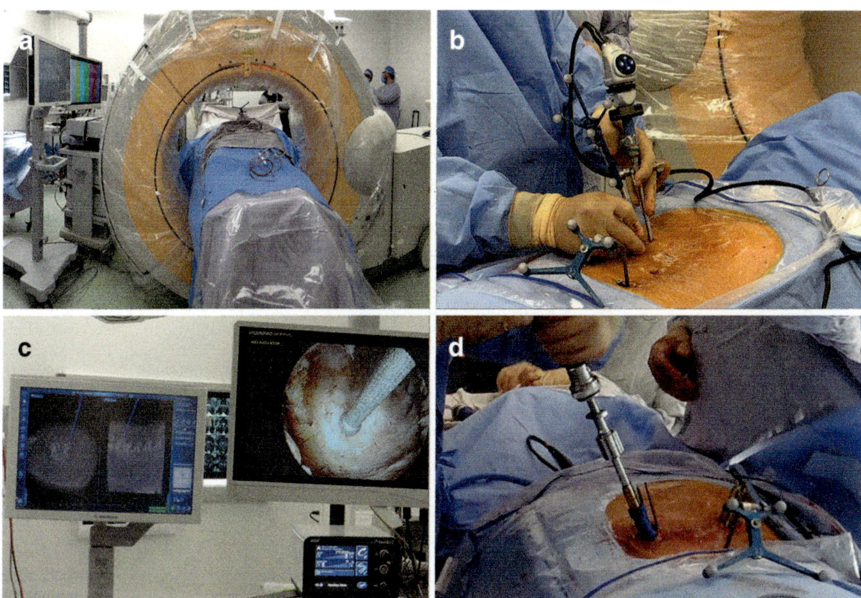

Fig. 23.22 UBE-TLIF under computed tomography-based intraoperative navigation. (**a**) Acquisition of intraoperative tomographic images with the navigation system. (**b**) The surgeon introduces the track to quickly identify the facet joint and observe it with the endoscope. (**c**) Navigation and visualization of the same target, the facet joint. (**d**) Placement of transpedicular screws with navigation to conclude the procedure

recognition of the anatomy due to its complex nature, such as transforaminal and interlaminar decompression of neural structures, and not being the exception in UBE-TLIF [32, 63, 64].

The same authors of this chapter reported the UBE-TLIF technique under intraoperative navigation in 2020 [32]. Using the O-arm system (Medtronic Sofamor Danek, Dublin, Ireland), the biportal endoscopic facetectomy, endplate preparation, and interbody spacer dislodgement were navigated in real time (Fig. 23.22).

This turned out to be of great help, especially in cases with complex anatomical environments, such as:

1. L5–S1 spondylolisthesis with high pelvic incidence.
2. Disorders of the lumbosacral transition in which the surgeon may require extra guidance to identify extraforaminal structures.
3. Severe facet joint spondylosis.
4. Cases in which contralateral decompression of the neural structures is required through the same approach.
5. Severe collapse of the intervertebral disc, making it challenging to identify the entrance to the intervertebral space.
6. Confirm the satisfactory preparation of the intervertebral space or the planned foraminotomy.

In conclusion, the authors noted greater accuracy and safety when performing UBE-TLIF under intraoperative navigation due to the following reasons:

1. The facet joint was quickly located, allowing a correct trajectory to be planned towards the intervertebral space, which also facilitated the placement of the interbody device.
2. Navigating the reference bone structures and later their recognition with the endoscope give the surgeon confidence, allowing a precise dissection and limited surgical field exposure.
3. After facetectomy and decompression of the ipsilateral neural structures, the orientation obtained through navigation to direct decompression towards the contralateral side was simple.
4. An appropriate preparation of the endplates was possible due to high-quality endoscopic imaging working together with the navigation of the intervertebral space in real time. In addition, the transgression of the anterior annulus with the surgical tools and overpreparation of the endplates were also avoided using intraoperative navigation. These steps are usually assessed through images obtained with the fluoroscope. However, real-time navigation during intervertebral space preparation was associated with less exposure to radiation emitted by the fluoroscope.

Short- and medium-term postoperative clinical outcomes of patients who underwent UBE-TLIF under computed tomography-based intraoperative navigation were promising. Adequate direct decompression of the neural elements and a stabilization/fusion process were accomplished, the vast majority of patients considerably improved their preoperative symptoms of leg and back pain, and the null consumption of postoperative opioids was evident.

Illustrated Cases

Case 2

A 56-year-old female patient with a history of full-endoscopic lumbar discectomy at L5–S1 on the right side 5 years ago complained of lower back pain VAS 8/10 and radicular type pain in her right leg VAS 9/10 with 3 months on evolution, without response to conservative treatment. Preoperative lumbar X-ray images demonstrated an unstable grade 2 degenerative spondylolisthesis at L5–S1 (Fig. 23.23a–c). Preoperative lumbar CT showed a decreased height of the intervertebral space and foraminal stenosis on the right side at L5–S1 (Fig. 23.24). Lumbar MRI confirmed significant right-sided foraminal stenosis at L5–S1 without central spinal canal stenosis and agenesis of the left S1 superior articular process (Fig. 23.25). A UBE-TLIF L5–S1 through a right paraspinal approach was performed. The L5 exiting nerve root on the right side was decompressed, and the interbody spacer was

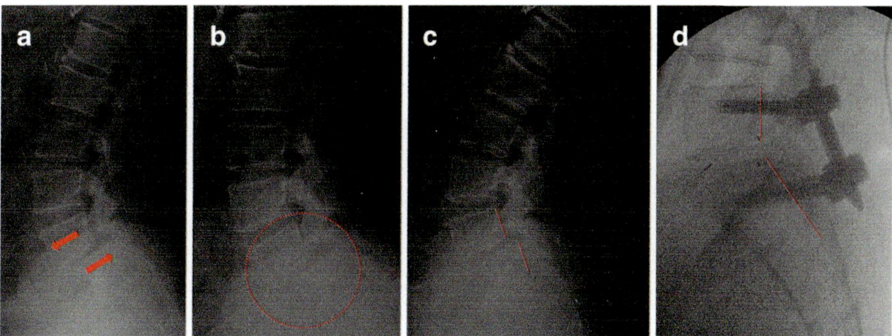

Fig. 23.23 Preoperative lumbar X-ray images of Case 2. (**a**) Neutral lumbar X-ray; the red arrows show a grade 2 L5–S1 spondylolisthesis. (**b**) Lumbar X-ray in flexion; anterior slippage of L5 on S1 and angular instability can be seen within the red dotted circle. (**c**) L5–S1 spondylolisthesis does not reduce with the extension on the lateral X-ray image. (**d**) Postoperative lateral view of L5–S1 after reduction of spondylolisthesis

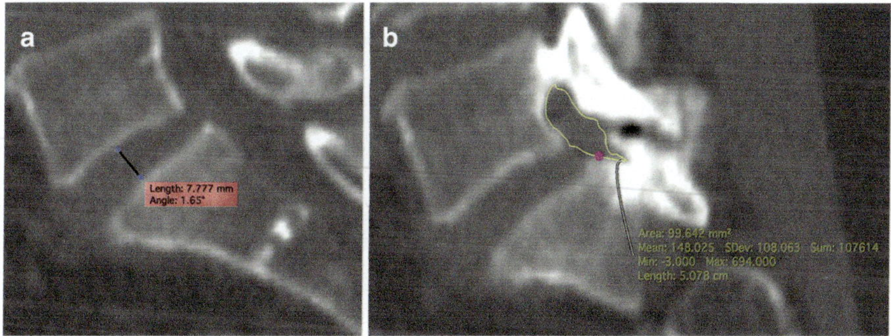

Fig. 23.24 Preoperative measurements in lumbar CT of Case 2. (**a**) Measurement of the intervertebral space. (**b**) Measurement of the foraminal area

placed after the endplates were prepared properly (Fig. 23.26). Spondylolisthesis was reduced, confirmed with the C-arm intraoperatively (Fig. 23.23d). In addition, a postoperative lumbar CT scan showed restitution in the height of the intervertebral space from 7.7 mm preoperatively to 13.6 mm postoperatively, while the foraminal area increased from 99 to 381 mm^2 after foraminotomy, this without affecting the lumbar and segmental lordosis (Fig. 23.27). Postoperative lumbar MRI demonstrated the foraminal decompression achieved by L5–S1 UBE-TLIF (Fig. 23.28). The patient was discharged the following day. The lower back pain decreased substantially from VAS 8/10 to 2/10, while the radicular type pain in the right leg disappeared.

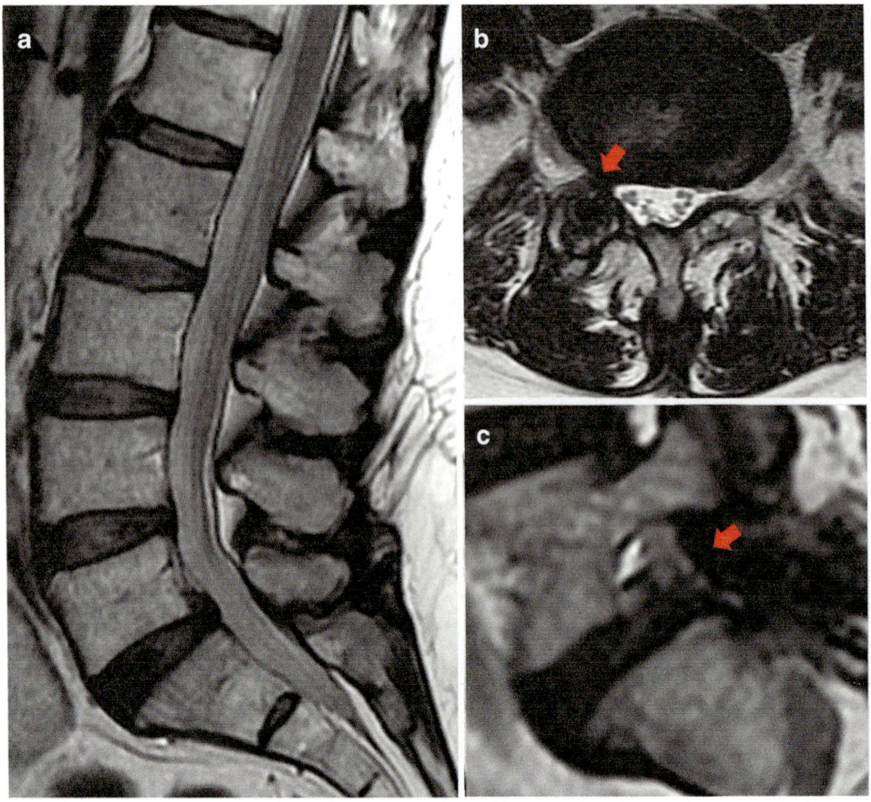

Fig. 23.25 Preoperative lumbar MRI of Case 2. (**a**) Sagittal view. (**b**) Axial view showing foraminal stenosis (red arrow) at L5–S1 on the right side associated with compensatory facet arthrosis due to absence of left facet joint. (**c**) Sagittal view through the right L5–S1 foramen showing severe stenosis (red arrow)

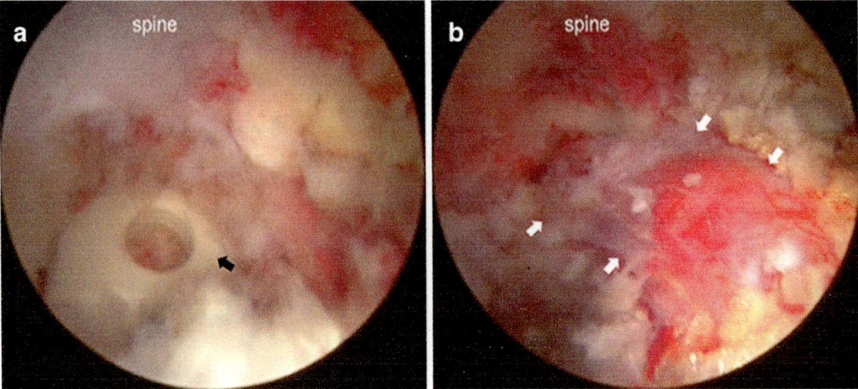

Fig. 23.26 Intraoperative endoscopic images of UBE-TLIF L5–S1 right-side approach of Case 2. (**a**) The black arrow points to the interbody cage in the intervertebral space. (**b**) White arrows point to the L5 exiting nerve free after direct decompression on the right side

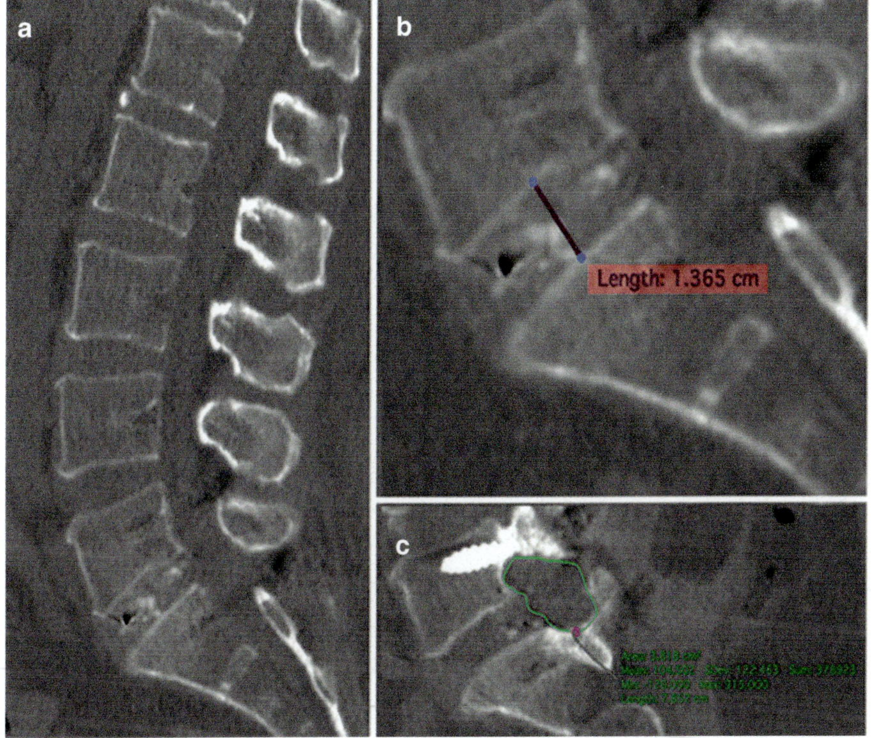

Fig. 23.27 Postoperative lumbar CT scan of Case 2. (**a**) The sagittal view shows proper lumbar and segmental lordosis after UBE-TLIF L5–S1. (**b**) Postoperative intervertebral space height at L5–S1. (**c**) Enlarged foraminal area after biportal endoscopic facet removal

Case 3

A 42-year-old female complains of severe lower back pain, worsening for 2 years. In the last 6 months, the pain has been severe VAS 10/10, limiting lumbosacral movements and requiring potent opioids to control it. In addition, the patient has tried facet and caudal blocks and even two bilateral percutaneous radiofrequency rhizotomy procedures of the medial branch of the dorsal facet ramus at L4, L5, and S1 with transient clinical improvement. Preoperative imaging studies, including X-rays, CT, and MRI of the lumbar spine, demonstrated an unstable grade 2 lytic spondylolisthesis at L5–S1 with a high pelvic incidence (Fig. 23.29a–c). Therefore, an L5–S1 UBE-TLIF with bilateral facetectomies was performed to avoid damaging the neural elements during spondylolisthesis reduction (Fig. 23.30).

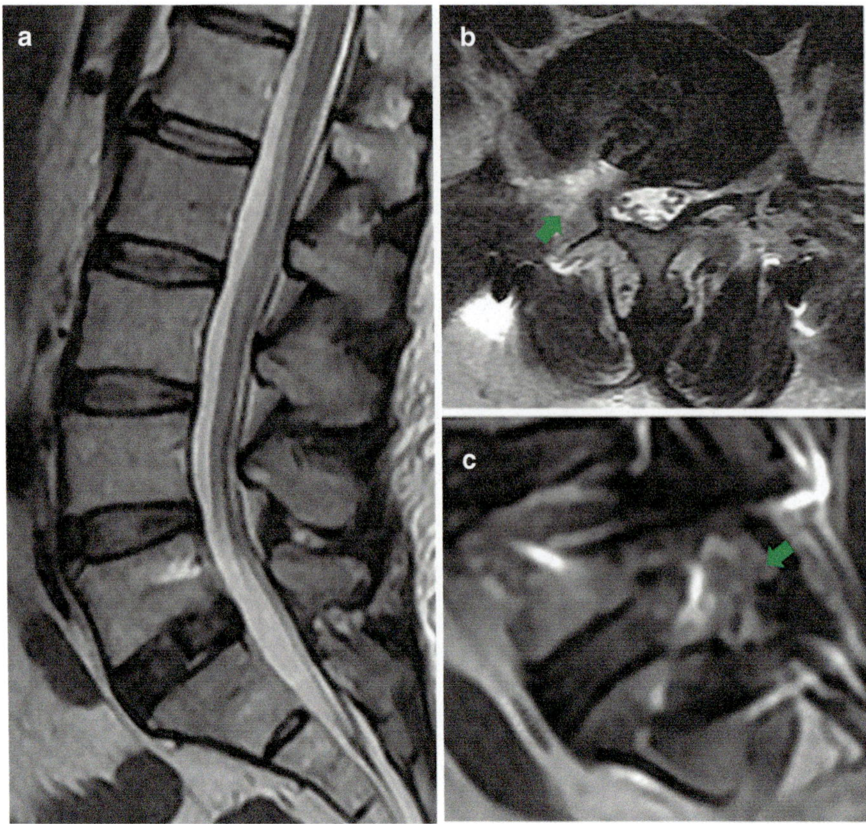

Fig. 23.28 Postoperative lumbar MRI of Case 2. (**a**) Sagittal view. (**b**) The green arrow points to the complete facetectomy at L5–S1 on the right side. (**c**) The enlarged L5–S1 foraminal area (green arrow) after the direct decompression achieved with the UBE-TLIF on the right side

Immediate postoperative imaging studies showed an adequate reduction of the spondylolisthesis and an increase in the height of the intervertebral space of L5–S1 with lumbar lordosis preserved (Fig. 23.29d–f).

The patient was discharged the day after surgery with minimal discomfort associated with the procedure in the surgical area without the need for postoperative opioid consumption. At the 2-year follow-up, the VAS for back pain was 1/10 with a full return to daily activities. In addition, a solid interbody fusion of L5–S1 was observed on the 2-year follow-up lumbar CT (Fig. 23.31).

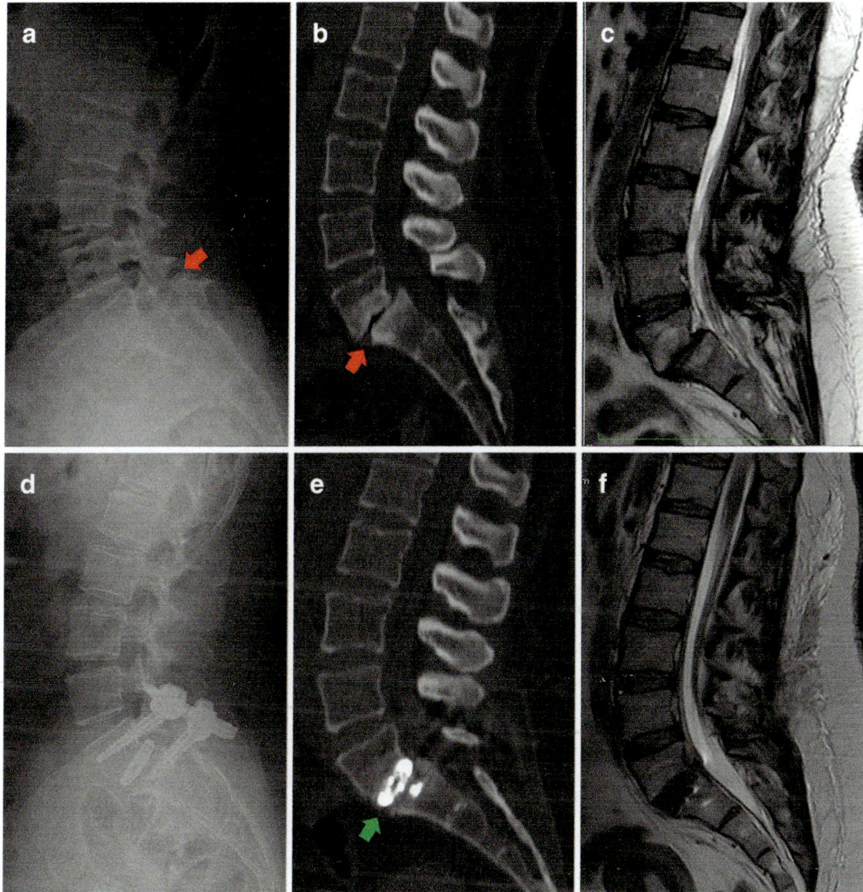

Fig. 23.29 Imaging studies of the lumbar spine of Case 3. (**a**) Preoperative lumbar X-ray on the lateral view; the red arrow points to the unstable spondylolisthesis grade 2 at L5–S1. (**b**) The preoperative lumbar CT scan on the sagittal view shows the slippage of L5 on S1, and a severe disc height collapsed (red arrow). (**c**) Sagittal view of the preoperative lumbar MRI with the same findings at L5–S1. (**d**) Postoperative lumbar X-ray on lateral view showing the interbody cage at L5–S1 and transpedicular screw fixation. (**e**) The postoperative lumbar CT scan on the sagittal view confirmed the spondylolisthesis reduction (green arrow) after UBE-TLIF at L5–S1 with increased intervertebral space height. The lumbar lordosis was not affected. (**f**) The lumbar MRI on the sagittal view showed the same findings with the integrity of the central spinal canal at L5–S1 after the procedure

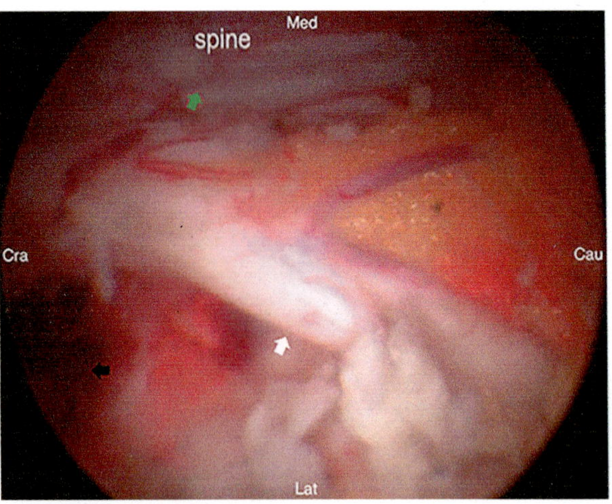

Fig. 23.30 Intraoperative image through the endoscope of Case 3. The black arrow points to the intervertebral space, the white arrow to the S1 root, and the green arrow to the dural sac

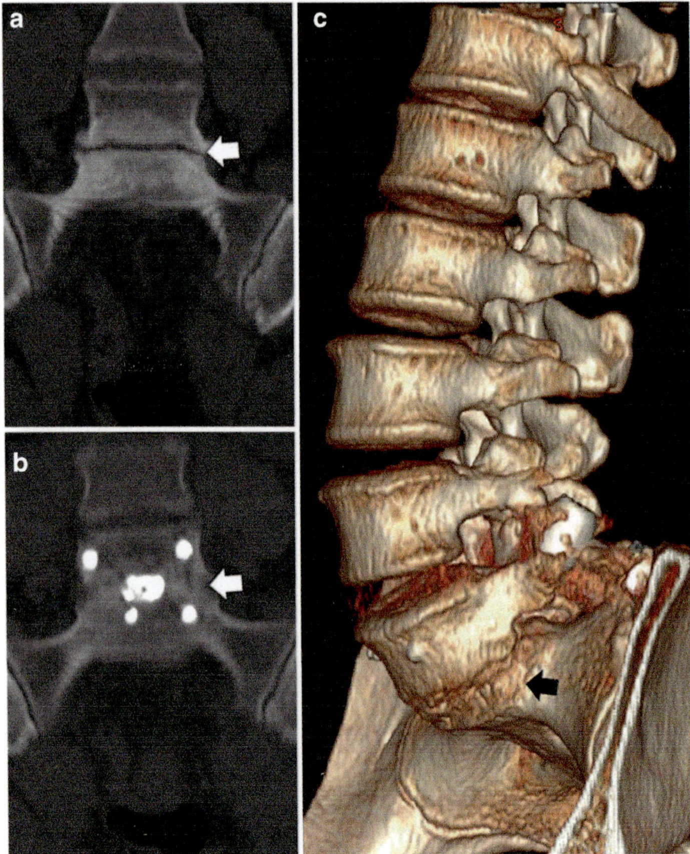

Fig. 23.31 Evaluation of the interbody fusion with the 2-year follow-up lumbar CT of Case 3. (**a**) Coronal view showing the nonfused (white arrow) collapsed disc height at L5–S1. (**b**) Postoperative 2-year follow-up lumbar CT on the coronal view showing solid fusion (white arrow) at L5–S1. (**c**) Lumbar CT 3D reconstruction at 2 years postoperative showing complete interbody fusion (black arrow) at L5–S1 with a solid bone mass

Discussion

Minimally invasive spinal surgical techniques have proven to be effective in reducing damage to paraspinal soft tissues and allowing a faster return to activities of daily living compared to open surgery; other advantages are lower EBL, shorter hospital stays, and lower consumption of analgesics including opioids postoperatively [65].

Several authors have demonstrated the effectiveness of the direct decompression of the neural elements in lumbar degenerative disease through biportal endoscopic surgery [66–69]. In addition, the evolution of minimally invasive techniques in spine surgery has resulted in incorporating the unilateral biportal endoscopic transforaminal lumbar interbody fusion (UBE-TLIF) into the spine surgeon's options as a minimally invasive and highly effective alternative in patients with the same indications for an open or microsurgical TLIF [30].

In the UBE-TLIF, the surgeon can work with both hands through two portals, one to introduce the surgical instruments and the other for the endoscope, with certain independence between the two, which improves performance and comfort during surgery. It is important to note that biportal endoscopy is a water-based technique, so visualization through the endoscope is excellent.

The biportal endoscopic technique is a transmuscular procedure associated with minimal muscle retraction. As it is a technique in which a radiofrequency probe is used to perform hemostasis and not an electrical thermocoagulation, continuous irrigation during the procedure, and minimal exposure to deep soft tissues, the risk of infection at the surgical site is considerably lower compared to other open methods [70, 71]. In addition, the surgical goals that must be achieved through conventional TLIF are also achieved through UBE-TLIF, which include (1) direct decompression, (2) stabilization/fusion, and (3) segmental and lumbar lordosis. However, the side effect associated with the procedure is less in UBE-TLIF than in open TLIF [32].

Some pearls for UBE-TLIF performance include the following:

1. Be clear about the goals of the procedure; this will limit bone work or extend it to achieve the goals set.
2. Identify the particular features of the facet joints, the intervertebral space, and its anatomical relationship with the neural elements. This can be done through preoperative imaging studies.
3. Have extensive experience in paraspinal approaches. Considering the particular goal, if it is only lateral neural decompression, the biportal extraforaminal approach may be sufficient, but if bilateral decompression is required to reach the central or contralateral neural elements, a more medial or posterolateral route may be the option.
4. Avoid over manipulating the neural elements to reduce postoperative sensory disturbances such as paresthesia, dysesthesias, or direct traversing or exiting nerve injury.

5. Make sufficient space to expose the intervertebral disc. This will allow placement of the interbody cage without injuring the traversing or exiting neural elements.
6. Properly prepare the endplates. This step is crucial since overpreparation can damage the endplates and increase the risk of implant subsidence or nonunion, while underpreparation can make interbody implant placement difficult or delay the fusion process.
7. Keep the surgical field clear at all times, which will depend first on a correct triangular approach with a continuous inflow and outflow of saline and appropriate hemostasis with the radiofrequency probe.
8. Apply enough bone graft, autologous and demineralized bone matrix, or even when the case requires other biologics such as morphogenetic protein.
9. Consider the side through which the biportal endoscopic approach will be performed due to particular considerations, especially in right-sided procedures, where the working channel must coincide with the trajectory of the intervertebral space for easier placement of the interbody cage.
10. Consider leaving an epidural drain to avoid the formation of epidural collections such as hematomas.

Conclusion

Over time, encouraging experiences will continue to be added to the medical literature concerning UBE-TLIF, which is associated with acceptable postoperative clinical and radiological outcomes, until now, in the short and medium terms. This procedure appears as one more option for the spine surgeon interested in minimally invasive endoscopic techniques.

References

1. Lan T, Hu SY, Zhang YT, et al. Comparison between posterior lumbar interbody fusion and transforaminal lumbar interbody fusion for the treatment of lumbar degenerative diseases: a systematic review and meta-analysis. World Neurosurg. 2018;112:86–93.
2. Teng I, Han J, Phan K, Mobbs R. A meta-analysis comparing ALIF, PLIF, TLIF and LLIF. J Clin Neurosci. 2017;44:11–7.
3. Rosenberg WS, Mummaneni PV. Transforaminal lumbar interbody fusion: technique, complications, and early results. Neurosurgery. 2001;48(3):569–75.
4. Hee HT, Castro FP Jr, Majd ME, Holt RT, Myers L. Anterior/posterior lumbar fusion versus transforaminal lumbar interbody fusion: analysis of complications and predictive factors. J Spinal Disord. 2001;14(6):533–40.
5. Moskowitz A. Transforaminal lumbar interbody fusion. Orthop Clin North Am. 2002;33(2):359–66.
6. Harms JG, Jeszenszky D. Die posteriore, lumbale, interkorporelle Fusion in unilateraler transforaminaler Technik. Orthop Traumatol. 1998;10(2):90–102.
7. Schwender JD, Holly LT, Rouben DP, Foley KT. Minimally invasive transforaminal lumbar interbody fusion (TLIF): technical feasibility and initial results. J Spinal Disord Tech. 2005;18(Suppl):S1–6.

8. Isaacs RE, Podichetty VK, Santiago P, et al. Minimally invasive microendoscopy-assisted transforaminal lumbar interbody fusion with instrumentation. J Neurosurg Spine. 2005;3(2):98–105.
9. Ozgur BM, Yoo K, Rodriguez G, Taylor WR. Minimally-invasive technique for transforaminal lumbar interbody fusion (TLIF). Eur Spine J. 2005;14(9):887–94.
10. Holly LT, Schwender JD, Rouben DP, Foley KT. Minimally invasive transforaminal lumbar interbody fusion: indications, technique, and complications. Neurosurg Focus. 2006;20(3):E6.
11. Dusad T, Kundnani V, Dutta S, Patel A, Mehta G, Singh M. Comparative prospective study reporting intraoperative parameters, pedicle screw perforation, and radiation exposure in navigation-guided versus non-navigated fluoroscopy-assisted minimal invasive transforaminal lumbar interbody fusion. Asian Spine J. 2018;12(2):309–16.
12. Zhang Y, Xu C, Zhou Y, Huang B. Minimally invasive computer navigation-assisted endoscopic transforaminal interbody fusion with bilateral decompression via a unilateral approach: initial clinical experience at one-year follow-up. World Neurosurg. 2017;106:291–9.
13. Kleck CJ, Johnson C, Akiyama M, Burger EL, Cain CJ, Patel VV. One-step minimally invasive pedicle screw instrumentation using O-arm and stealth navigation. Clin Spine Surg. 2018;31(5):197–202.
14. Liu Z, Jin M, Qiu Y, Yan H, Han X, Zhu Z. The superiority of intraoperative O-arm navigation-assisted surgery in instrumenting extremely small thoracic pedicles of adolescent idiopathic scoliosis: a case-control study. Medicine (Baltimore). 2016;95(18):e3581.
15. Pitteloud N, Gamulin A, Barea C, Damet J, Racloz G, Sans-Merce M. Radiation exposure using the O-arm® surgical imaging system. Eur Spine J. 2017;26(3):651–7.
16. Xiao R, Miller JA, Sabharwal NC, et al. Clinical outcomes following spinal fusion using an intraoperative computed tomographic 3D imaging system. J Neurosurg Spine. 2017;26(5):628–37.
17. Vaishnav AS, Saville P, McAnany S, et al. Retrospective review of immediate restoration of lordosis in single-level minimally invasive transforaminal lumbar interbody fusion: a comparison of static and expandable interbody cages. Oper Neurosurg (Hagerstown). 2020;18(5):518–23.
18. Chang KY, Hsu WK. Spinal biologics in minimally invasive lumbar surgery. Minim Invasive Surg. 2018;2018:5230350.
19. Sayari AJ, Patel DV, Yoo JS, Singh K. Device solutions for a challenging spine surgery: minimally invasive transforaminal lumbar interbody fusion (MIS TLIF). Expert Rev Med Devices. 2019;16(4):299–305.
20. Ahn Y, Youn MS, Heo DH. Endoscopic transforaminal lumbar interbody fusion: a comprehensive review. Expert Rev Med Devices. 2019;16(5):373–80.
21. Zhou Y, Zhang C, Wang J, et al. Endoscopic transforaminal lumbar decompression, interbody fusion and pedicle screw fixation-a report of 42 cases. Chin J Traumatol. 2008;11(4):225–31.
22. Osman SG. Endoscopic transforaminal decompression, interbody fusion, and percutaneous pedicle screw implantation of the lumbar spine: a case series report. Int J Spine Surg. 2012;6:157–66.
23. Jacquot F, Gastambide D. Percutaneous endoscopic transforaminal lumbar interbody fusion: is it worth it? Int Orthop. 2013;37(8):1507–10.
24. Lee SH, Erken HY, Bae J. Percutaneous transforaminal endoscopic lumbar interbody fusion: clinical and radiological results of mean 46-month follow-up. Biomed Res Int. 2017;2017:3731983.
25. He EX, Guo J, Ling QJ, Yin ZX, Wang Y, Li M. Application of a narrow-surface cage in full endoscopic minimally invasive transforaminal lumbar interbody fusion. Int J Surg. 2017;42:83–9.
26. Youn MS, Shin JK, Goh TS, Lee JS. Full endoscopic lumbar interbody fusion (FELIF): technical note. Eur Spine J. 2018;27(8):1949–55.
27. Wu J, Liu H, Ao S, et al. Percutaneous endoscopic lumbar interbody fusion: technical note and preliminary clinical experience with 2-year follow-up. Biomed Res Int. 2018;2018:5806037.
28. Kamson S, Lu D, Sampson PD, Zhang Y. Full-endoscopic lumbar fusion outcomes in patients with minimal deformities: a retrospective study of data collected between 2011 and 2015. Pain Physician. 2019;22(1):75–88.

29. Birkenmaier C, Komp M, Leu HF, Wegener B, Ruetten S. The current state of endoscopic disc surgery: review of controlled studies comparing full-endoscopic procedures for disc herniations to standard procedures. Pain Physician. 2013;16(4):335–44.
30. Kang MS, You KH, Choi JY, Heo DH, Chung HJ, Park HJ. Minimally invasive transforaminal lumbar interbody fusion using the biportal endoscopic techniques versus microscopic tubular technique. Spine J. 2021;21(12):2066–77.
31. Heo DH, Eum JH, Jo JY, Chung H. Modified far lateral endoscopic transforaminal lumbar interbody fusion using a biportal endoscopic approach: technical report and preliminary results. Acta Neurochir. 2021;163(4):1205–9.
32. Quillo-Olvera J, Quillo-Reséndiz J, Quillo-Olvera D, Barrera-Arreola M, Kim JS. Ten-step biportal endoscopic transforaminal lumbar interbody fusion under computed tomography-based intraoperative navigation: technical report and preliminary outcomes in Mexico. Oper Neurosurg (Hagerstown). 2020;19(5):608–18.
33. Hadra BE. Wiring of the vertebrae as a means of immobilization in fractures and Pott's disease. Med Times Reg. 1891;2:1–8.
34. Chipault A. Travaux De Neurologie Chirurgicale; 1986.
35. Kumar K. Spinal deformity and axial traction. Spine (Phila Pa 1976). 1996;21(5):653–5.
36. Hughes JT. The Edwin Smith surgical papyrus: an analysis of the first case reports of spinal cord injuries. Paraplegia. 1988;26(2):71–82.
37. Naderi S, Andalkar N, Benzel EC. History of spine biomechanics: Part I—The pre-Greco-Roman, Greco-Roman, and medieval roots of spine biomechanics. Neurosurgery. 2007;60(2):382–91.
38. Lange F. Support for the spondylitic spine by means of buried steel bars, attached to the vertebrae. Clin Orthop Relat Res. 1986;203:3–6.
39. Hibbs RA. An operation for progressive spinal deformities: a preliminary report of three cases from the service of the orthopaedic hospital. Clin Orthop Relat Res. 2007;460:17–20.
40. Venable CS, Stuck WG. Three years' experience with Vitallium in bone surgery. Ann Surg. 1941;114(2):309–15.
41. Burns BH. An operation for spondylolisthesis. Lancet. 1933;224:1233–9.
42. Capener N. Spondylolisthesis. Br J Surg. 1932;19(75):374–86.
43. Lane JD Jr, Moore ES Jr. Transperitoneal approach to the intervertebral disc in the lumbar area. Ann Surg. 1948;127(3):537–51.
44. King D. Internal fixation for lumbosacral fusion. J Bone Joint Surg Am. 1948;30A(3):560–5.
45. Briggs HH, Milligan PR. Chip fusion of the low back following exploration of the spinal canal. J Bone Jt Surg Am. 1944;26(1):125–30.
46. Cloward RB. The treatment of ruptured lumbar intervertebral discs by vertebral body fusion. I. Indications, operative technique, after care. J Neurosurg. 1953;10(2):154–68.
47. Harrington PR, Dickson JH. Spinal instrumentation in the treatment of severe progressive spondylolisthesis. Clin Orthop Relat Res. 1976;117:157–63.
48. Harrington PR, Tullos HS. Reduction of severe spondylolisthesis in children. South Med J. 1969;62(1):1–7.
49. Holdsworth F. Fractures, dislocations, and fracture-dislocations of the spine. J Bone Joint Surg Am. 1970;52(8):1534–51.
50. Kabins MB, Weinstein JN. The history of vertebral screw and pedicle screw fixation. Iowa Orthop J. 1991;11:127–36.
51. Brantigan JW, Steffee AD, Lewis ML, Quinn LM, Persenaire JM. Lumbar interbody fusion using the Brantigan I/F cage for posterior lumbar interbody fusion and the variable pedicle screw placement system: two-year results from a Food and Drug Administration investigational device exemption clinical trial. Spine (Phila Pa 1976). 2000;25(11):1437–46.
52. Ani N, Keppler L, Biscup RS, Steffee AD. Reduction of high-grade slips (grades III–V) with VSP instrumentation. Report of a series of 41 cases. Spine (Phila Pa 1976). 1991;16(6 Suppl):S302–10.
53. Steffee AD, Sitkowski DJ. Posterior lumbar interbody fusion and plates. Clin Orthop Relat Res. 1988;227:99–102.

54. Steffee AD, Biscup RS, Sitkowski DJ. Segmental spine plates with pedicle screw fixation. A new internal fixation device for disorders of the lumbar and thoracolumbar spine. Clin Orthop Relat Res. 1986;(203):45–53.
55. Harms J, Rolinger H. Die operative Behandlung der Spondylolisthese durch dorsale Aufrichtung und ventrale Verblockung. Z Orthop Ihre Grenzgeb. 1982;120(3):343–7.
56. Uçar BY, Özcan Ç, Polat Ö, Aman T. Transforaminal lumbar interbody fusion for lumbar degenerative disease: patient selection and perspectives. Orthop Res Rev. 2019;11:183–9.
57. Ishihama Y, Morimoto M, Tezuka F, et al. Full-endoscopic trans-Kambin triangle lumbar interbody fusion: surgical technique and nomenclature. J Neurol Surg A Cent Eur Neurosurg. 2021; https://doi.org/10.1055/s-0041-1730970.
58. Kang MS, Heo DH, Kim HB, Chung HT. Biportal endoscopic technique for transforaminal lumbar interbody fusion: review of current research. Int J Spine Surg. 2021;15(Suppl 3):S84–92.
59. Eum JH, Park JH, Song KS, Lee SM, Suh DW, Jo DJ. Endoscopic extreme transforaminal lumbar interbody fusion with large spacers: a technical note and preliminary report. Orthopedics. 2022;2022:1–6.
60. Virk S, Qureshi S. Navigation in minimally invasive spine surgery. J Spine Surg. 2019;5(Suppl 1):S25–30.
61. Sabri SA, York PJ. Preoperative planning for intraoperative navigation guidance. Ann Transl Med. 2021;9(1):87.
62. Stefini R, Peron S, Mandelli J, Bianchini E, Roccucci P. Intraoperative spinal navigation for the removal of intradural tumors: technical notes. Oper Neurosurg (Hagerstown). 2018;15(1):54–9.
63. Oyelese A, Telfeian AE, Gokaslan ZL, et al. Intraoperative computed tomography navigational assistance for transforaminal endoscopic decompression of heterotopic foraminal bone formation after oblique lumbar interbody fusion. World Neurosurg. 2018;115:29–34.
64. Ho TY, Lin CW, Chang CC, et al. Percutaneous endoscopic unilateral laminotomy and bilateral decompression under 3D real-time image-guided navigation for spinal stenosis in degenerative lumbar kyphoscoliosis patients: an innovative preliminary study. BMC Musculoskelet Disord. 2020;21(1):734.
65. Fan S, Hu Z, Zhao F, Zhao X, Huang Y, Fang X. Multifidus muscle changes and clinical effects of one-level posterior lumbar interbody fusion: minimally invasive procedure versus conventional open approach. Eur Spine J. 2010;19(2):316–24.
66. Gao X, Gao L, Chang Z, et al. Case series of unilateral biportal endoscopic-assisted transforaminal lumbar interbody fusion in the treatment of recurrent lumbar disc herniation. Am J Transl Res. 2022;14(4):2383–92.
67. Hua W, Liao Z, Chen C, et al. Clinical outcomes of uniportal and biportal lumbar endoscopic unilateral laminotomy for bilateral decompression in patients with lumbar spinal stenosis: a retrospective pair-matched case-control study. World Neurosurg. 2022;161:e134–45.
68. Heo DH, Lee DC, Park CK. Comparative analysis of three types of minimally invasive decompressive surgery for lumbar central stenosis: biportal endoscopy, uniportal endoscopy, and microsurgery. Neurosurg Focus. 2019;46(5):E9.
69. Park SM, Park J, Jang HS, et al. Biportal endoscopic versus microscopic lumbar decompressive laminectomy in patients with spinal stenosis: a randomized controlled trial. Spine J. 2020;20(2):156–65.
70. Bowers CA, Burns G, Salzman KL, McGill LD, Macdonald JD. Comparison of tissue effects in rabbit muscle of surgical dissection devices. Int J Surg. 2014;12(3):219–23.
71. Heo DH, Son SK, Eum JH, Park CK. Fully endoscopic lumbar interbody fusion using a percutaneous unilateral biportal endoscopic technique: technical note and preliminary clinical results. Neurosurg Focus. 2017;43(2):E8.

Chapter 24
Combination of Uniportal and Biportal Endoscopic Approaches for Tandem Spinal Stenosis

Javier Quillo-Olvera, Diego Quillo-Olvera, Javier Quillo-Reséndiz, and Michelle Barrera-Arreola

Abbreviations

AP	Anteroposterior
CSS	Cervical spinal stenosis
EBL	Estimated blood loss
LSS	Lumbar spinal stenosis
m-JOA	Modified Japanese Orthopaedic Association score
MRI	Magnetic resonance imaging
RF	Radiofrequency
TSS	Tandem spinal stenosis
UBE	Unilateral biportal endoscopy
ULBD	Unilateral laminotomy for bilateral decompression
VAS	Visual analog scale

Introduction

Tandem spinal stenosis (TSS) is defined as the narrowing in the spinal canal diameter that affects two or more noncontiguous regions of the spine, mainly the cervical and lumbar regions simultaneously, and rarely the thoracic region [1–3]. Patients who present with these findings may be asymptomatic. Still, others may have mixed symptoms of myelopathy and radiculopathy of upper and lower extremities, lower

J. Quillo-Olvera (✉) · D. Quillo-Olvera · J. Quillo-Reséndiz · M. Barrera-Arreola
The Brain and Spine Care, Minimally Invasive Spine Surgery Group, Hospital H+ Querétaro, Spine Clinic, Querétaro, México
e-mail: neuroqomd@gmail.com; drquilloolvera86@gmail.com; kitnoz@hotmail.com; michelle.barrera@anahuac.mx

J. Quillo-Olvera et al. (eds.), *Unilateral Biportal Endoscopy of the Spine*, https://doi.org/10.1007/978-3-031-14736-4_24

limb symptoms such as neurogenic claudication, or pain in the neck, lower back, or other spine regions associated with the disease. In addition, gait, bladder, and bowel disorders and simultaneous upper and lower motor neuron syndromes could be present. This clinical presentation can be very confusing for the spine surgeon. Therefore, a high level of suspicion must prevail to give continuity to their prompt attention [1, 4–6].

Nagata et al. [7] investigated the prevalence of spinal stenosis in 931 subjects who underwent whole-spine magnetic resonance imaging (MRI) as part of the Wakayama Spine Study in Japan. The authors excluded patients with prior spinal surgery and under 40 years. They reported a prevalence of image-based cervical spinal stenosis (CSS) of 25%, lumbar spinal stenosis (LSS) of 30%, and TSS of 11%, the latter being more prevalent in congenital spinal stenosis. Among patients with TSS, 10% with CSS and 19% with LSS were symptomatic.

Another study found a close relationship between congenital cervical stenosis and thoracic and LSS in a cohort of 80 patients [8]. Furthermore, a Torg-Pavlov index of 0.78 or less is an independent predictor of TSS, primarily associated with LSS [9].

However, the high variability around the definition of spinal stenosis, inconsistencies in the methodology used to diagnose it, or even asymptomatic cases that are not diagnosed are factors that can bias the true incidence of TSS [10].

One of the most controversial aspects concerning TSS is decision-making for its treatment. Therapeutic measures range from monitoring and alerting about risky postures and activities in asymptomatic patients, painkillers, and physiotherapy in patients with mild symptoms, seeking to control their discomfort. However, some patients could simultaneously have severe myeloradiculopathy and lower limb symptoms, representing a challenging medical context for the spine surgeon. Different circumstances such as age (older or younger than 60 years), physical health status (frail or firm), various comorbidities (diabetes, hypertension, smoking, cancer, liver disease, etc.), and location of the stenosis (contiguous or noncontiguous) will modify the behavior to be followed, including the invasiveness of the proposed treatment.

For this reason, the arguments for first treating the cervical or thoracic over the lumbar spine or vice versa are constant in the literature [10, 11]. In addition, some reports support treating both compression sites in the same or different surgical events [12].

And since there is no evidence of type 1 level of recommendation for the best option for treating TSS, the treatment must be tailored to the symptoms and findings that the patient presents and considering the reasonable judgment, skills, and resources available to the spine surgeon [13].

Due to the above, we decided to carry out a surgical strategy based on water-based endoscopic procedures in patients selected with symptomatic TSS to perform single-stage direct decompression in the cervical and lumbar spine simultaneously. The purpose was to offer an endoscopic ULBD in noncontiguous spinal stenosis through techniques that offered the least associated collateral effect such as intraoperative bleeding, injury to paraspinal elements, and operative time and that allowed a rapid mobilization out of bed, with minor consumption of analgesia [14].

Indications

As mentioned, these patients may present with confusing clinical patterns. Therefore neurological signs related to myelopathy include upper or lower extremity clumsiness, numbness of the upper and/or lower limbs, and gait, bladder, and bowel disturbances. In addition to upper and lower motor neuron signs such as paresis of upper and lower limbs, deep hyperreflexia, Hoffman's sign, clonus, Babinsky, muscular hypotrophy, fasciculations or spasticity, and radicular pain radiated down to the legs raised the suspicion of TSS. Findings in the cervical and lumbar MRI of spinal stenosis related to the described symptoms. Patients with a history of trauma, tumor, cervical and lumbar instability, cervical kyphosis, spinal infection, and other combined injuries were excluded for simultaneous decompressive treatment [15].

Surgical Technique

Step 1: Anesthesia and Positioning

For this procedure, the authors recommend the use of general anesthesia. The eyes are protected to avoid ocular injuries by the position. The face should be supported on a soft surface, allowing the anesthesiologist to control the airway. Subsequently, the patient will be placed prone on an abdominal support frame to reduce the pressure of the epidural venous plexuses and prevent bleeding during the procedure (Fig. 24.1a). Later, the cleaning and drape of the posterior cervical and lumbar regions are done as usual so that the surgical teams can work simultaneously (Fig. 24.1b, c).

Step 2: Operating Room Organization

The cervical and lumbar decompression will be performed simultaneously. Therefore, a couple of expert surgeons in spinal endoscopy will perform cervical and lumbar decompression procedures. One of the advantages of performing a tandem endoscopic spinal decompression is that both uniportal and biportal techniques require minimal personnel assisting the surgeon in the operating theatre since the surgeon performs the procedure by retracting himself or herself when needed through specialized endoscopic instruments [16].

The anesthesiologist will be at the head of the patient. The surgeon in charge of cervical decompression will be lateral to the patient's head and next to him or her, his or her assistant. The fluoroscope will be used as usually in cervical and lumbar spinal procedures. The endoscope and fluoroscope displays will be facing both surgeons. The surgeon who will perform the lumbar biportal endoscopic

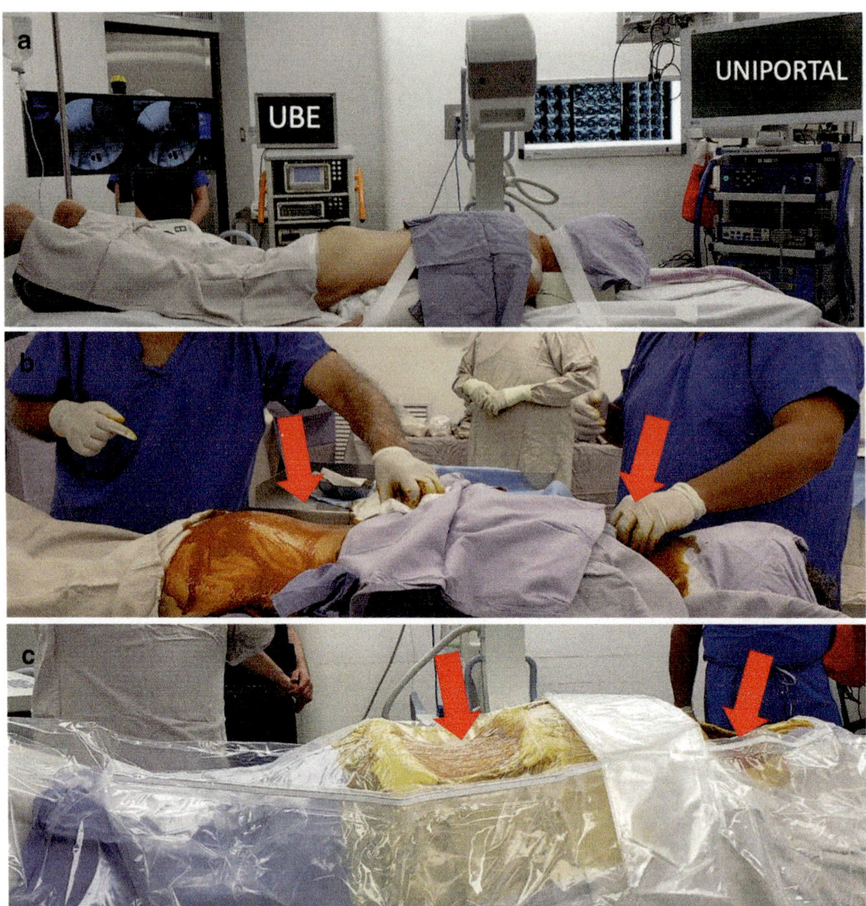

Fig. 24.1 (**a**) Patient in prone. (**b**) The surgical team should clean the cervical and lumbar fields (red arrows). (**c**) Both surgical fields are draped and prepared for simultaneous surgery (red arrows)

decompression will be caudal to the cervical surgeon, and next to the lumbar region, his or her assistant in front of him or her. From this moment on, each surgical team will act independently and simultaneously (Fig. 24.2).

Step 3: Uniportal Endoscopic Cervical ULBD

The cervical uniportal endoscopic approach will be planned as follows. First, the surgeon will require the C-arm to obtain AP and lateral projections. The AP view will define how lateral the approach should be, while the lateral view will determine the rostrocaudal trajectory and confirm the index level.

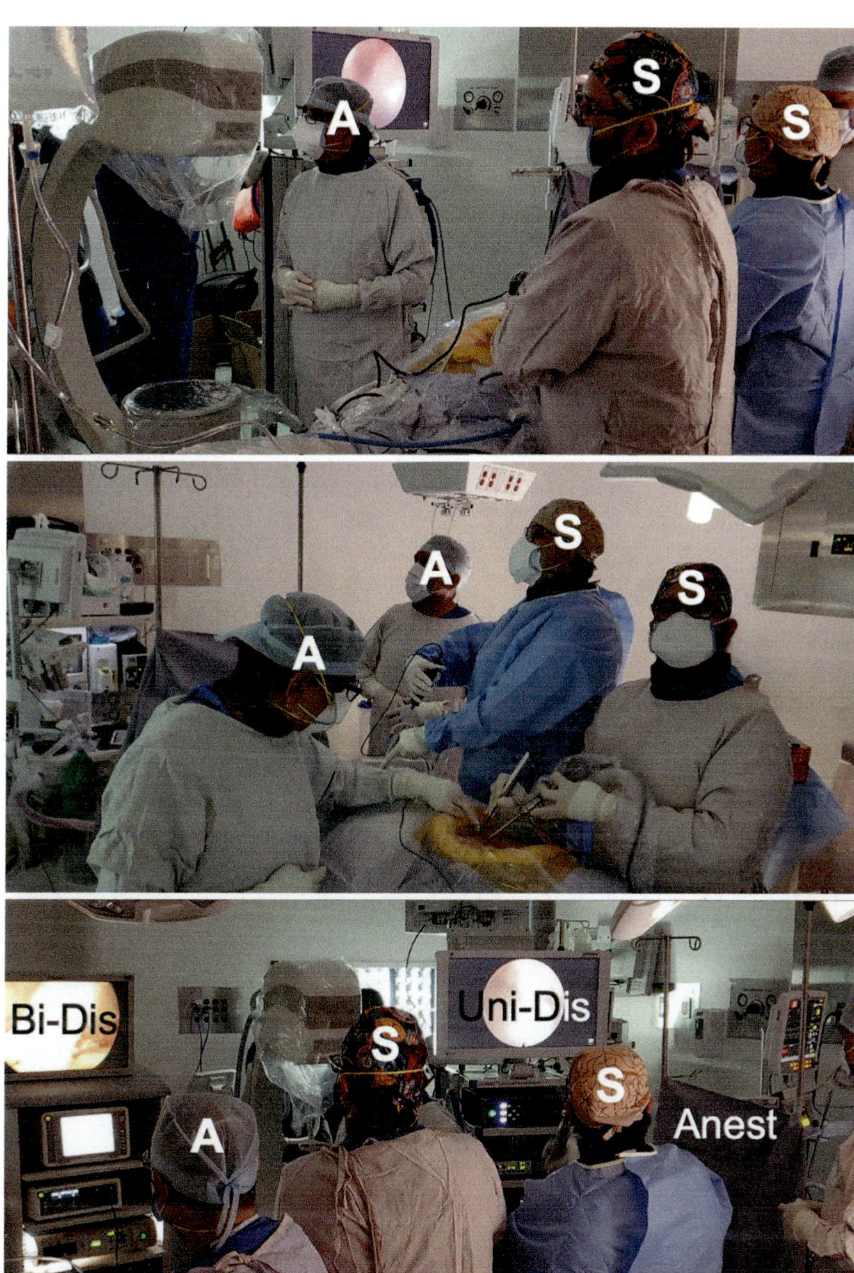

Fig. 24.2 Picture showing different perspectives of OR setup with both surgical teams. *A* assistant, *S* surgeon, *Anest* anesthesiologist, *Bi-Dis* display of biportal procedure, *Uni-Dis* display of uniportal procedure

In the AP view, the surgeon will draw a line medial to the superior and inferior pedicles of the index level (medial interpedicular line). In a true lateral view, the surgeon will draw a line coming from the disc space that passes between the interspinous space of the index level (Fig. 24.3). The intersection of this line with the medial interpedicular line will define the location of the incision.

The surgeon will incise the skin and the superficial cervical aponeurosis through an 8 mm incision. Then, a blunt-tip dilator is advanced through the incision, and the surgeon should feel and palpate the interlaminar space and the V-point with the tip of the dilator. At this point, the surgeon needs to confirm with proper AP and lateral fluoroscopic images the position of the dilator. Finally, the surgeon can introduce the beveled end-tip working cannula. We used a 7.3 mm outer diameter with a 15° angulated lens endoscope (Ilessys Pro, Joimax GmbH, Karlsruhe, Germany).

After introducing the endoscope into the beveled working cannula, the surgeon can remove the soft tissue adjacent to the bone elements using endoscopic pituitary forceps and the RF probe (Endovapor, Joimax GmbH, Karlsruhe, Germany) to identify the V-point.

Subsequently, the surgeon starts with the ipsilateral laminotomy of the upper lamina by using the high-speed endoscopic drill (Shrill, Joimax GmbH, Karlsruhe, Germany) and 3 mm diamond burr until identifying the attachment of the yellow ligament (Fig. 24.4). Next, the same is done in the ipsilateral inferior lamina (Fig. 24.5). Having concluded the ipsilateral bone decompression, the approach is addressed to the spinous process to be undercut starting at the base to get access to the contralateral side. The surgeon should avoid any pressure on the yellow ligament with the instruments or the endoscopic system to prevent a spinal cord injury.

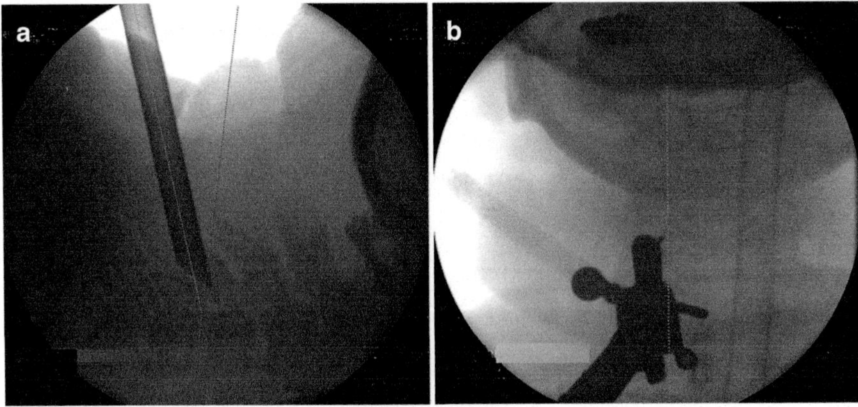

Fig. 24.3 Uniportal endoscopic cervical approach. (**a**) Lateral view of C-arm. The red dotted line represents the disc space, and the blue one passes between the interspinous space. The end-tip beveled working cannula is docked over the V-point. (**b**) The AP view shows the endoscopic system approaching lateral to the mid-interpedicular line (green dotted line)

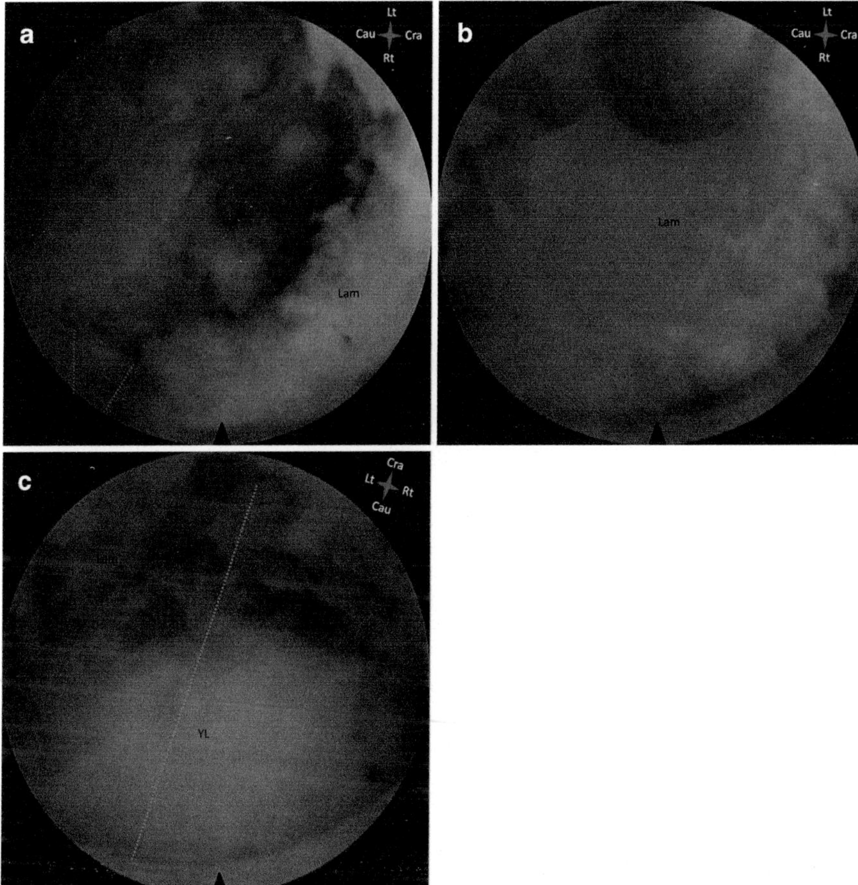

Fig. 24.4 Superior uniportal endoscopic cervical laminotomy. (**a**) The superior lamina is identified; the red dotted lines represent the margins of the V-point. (**b**) Superior laminotomy. (**c**) The cranial attachment of ligamentum flavum is observed after bilateral laminotomy; the green dotted line represents the midline. *Cra* cranial, *Cau* caudal, *Rt* right, *Lt* left, *Lam* lamina, *V* V-point, *YL* yellow ligament

Once the spinous process is undercut sufficiently, the contralateral upper lamina is identified and undercutting is done until the attachment of the yellow ligament appears. After exposing the yellow ligament edges, the surgeon can use the endoscopic nerve hook to detach it with gentle movements avoiding forced retraction to prevent traction on the dural sac. Next, the surgeon will use an especially designed endoscopic Kerrison (Joimax GmbH, Karlsruhe, Germany) rongeur to perform the flavectomy piece by piece or in block, depending on the case, and accomplish the complete direct decompression of the spinal cord, and if the patient requires the exiting nerve also (Fig. 24.6).

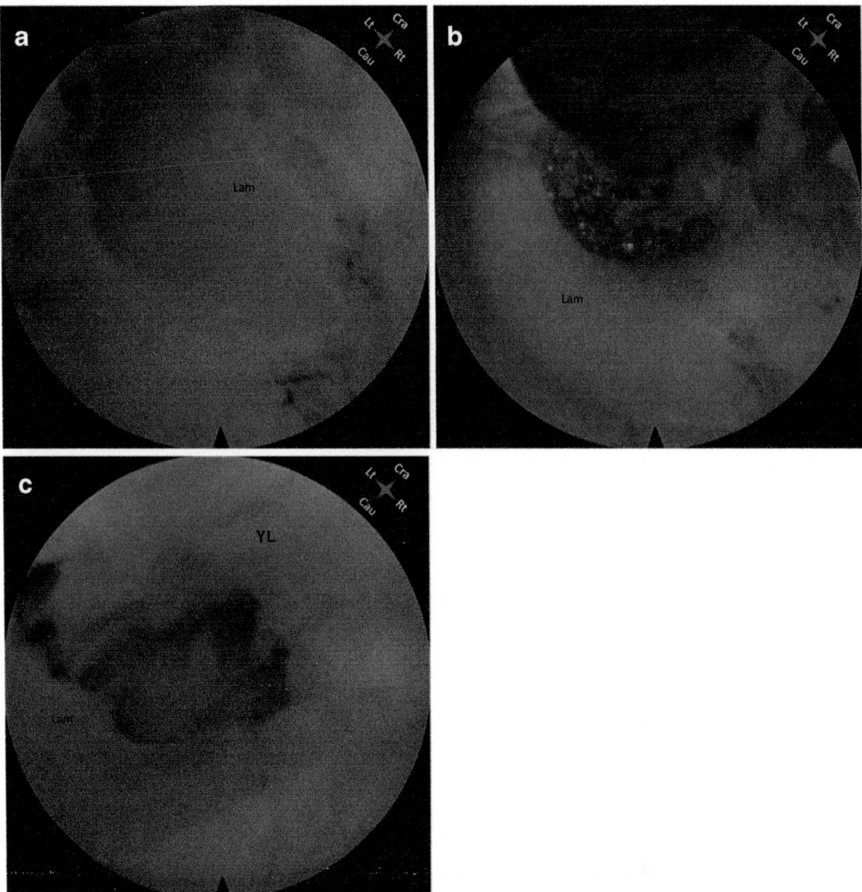

Fig. 24.5 Inferior uniportal endoscopic cervical laminotomy. (**a**) The inferior lamina is identified. (**b**) Inferior laminotomy. (**c**) The caudal attachment of ligamentum flavum is observed. *Cra* cranial, *Cau* caudal, *Rt* right, *Lt* left, *Lam* lamina, *YL* yellow ligament

In cases of multilevel stenosis, the surgeon slids the endoscope to the underlying or adjacent lamina to the index level. Therefore a single skin incision can be used to decompress two or three levels. An epidural drain inserted through the same incision of the approach is recommended. Afterward, the incision is closed with a 3-0 nylon single stitch.

Step 4: Unilateral Biportal Endoscopic Lumbar ULBD

An orthogonal AP view to locate the interlaminar space of the index level is done. It is advisable to plan the incisions as follows: A medial interpedicular line of the index level is drawn in the skin. Then, the midline also. The intervertebral space is

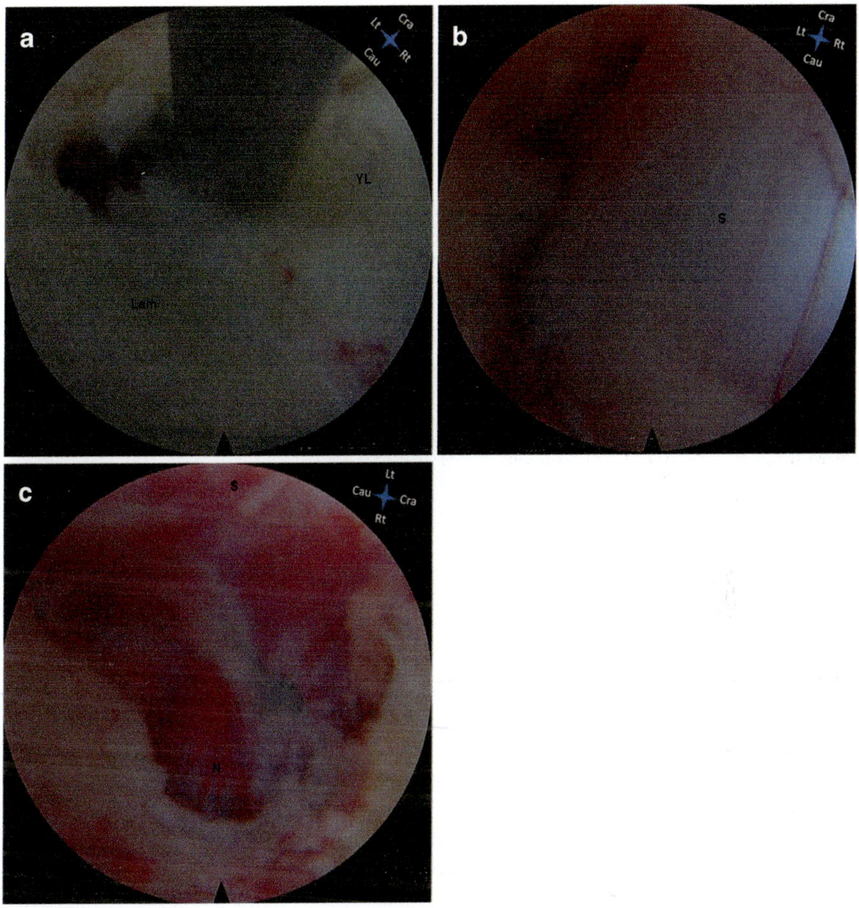

Fig. 24.6 (**a**) Yellow ligament could be removed piece by piece or in block. (**b**, **c**) The dural sac and exiting nerve decompressed. *Cra* cranial, *Cau* caudal, *Rt* right, *Lt* left, *Lam* lamina, *YL* yellow ligament, *S* dural sac, *N* exiting nerve

projected in the skin and drawn. It will allow the surgeon guidance during the approach. The superior and inferior incisions are located slightly lateral to the medial interpedicular line, which generally occurs between 1 and 1.5 cm lateral to the midline and at the level of the superior and inferior pedicles, respectively. Thus, the distance between both incisions usually is around 2.5–3 cm.

Subsequently, a 5–7 mm longitudinal or transverse incision in the skin and thoracolumbar fascia is sufficient in length for inferior and superior incisions. Next, the surgeon introduces a blunt-tip dilator of 6 mm outer diameter through the incision used as a working portal. In the right-side approach, the superior incision is intended for this purpose. On the left side is the contrary.

The dilator is addressed to the upper lamina and the spinous process junction in a craniocaudal and lateromedial trajectory. This trajectory enables the dilator to be inserted, and a working channel is created medially to the multifidus muscle. The surgeon can enlarge the space medial to the multifidus with soft lateral movements with the dilator tip. Finally, the position of the dilator is confirmed in an AP fluoroscopic projection, and the semi-tubular working sheath is advanced along the dilator.

The endoscope trocar will be inserted caudocranially and lateromedially through the inferior incision of the biportal approach. Next, the surgeon must palpate the caudal edge of the upper lamina of the index level with the blunt tip of the trocar and subsequently complete the triangulation of the instruments with both hands, which will be confirmed by fluoroscopy using AP and lateral views. At this point, it is crucial that the surgeon feels the touch between the tip of the trocar and dilator and together palpate the spinolaminar junction. Finally, the surgeon can introduce the endoscope inside the trocar for starting the endoscopic decompression (Fig. 24.7).

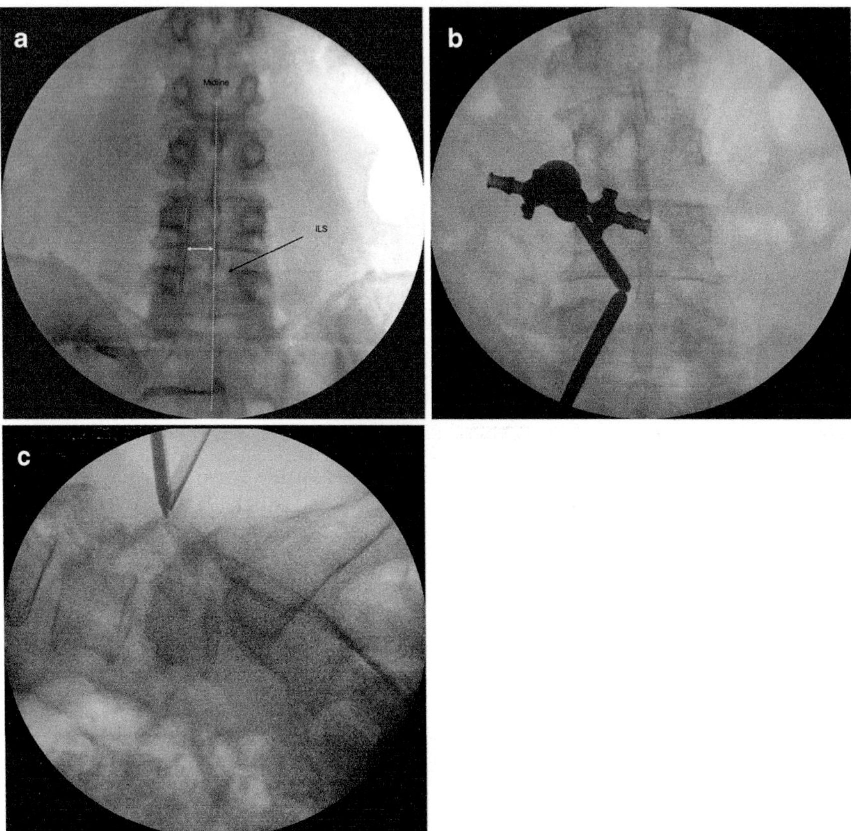

Fig. 24.7 Lumbar paramedian UBE approach. (**a**) An orthogonal AP fluoroscopic view of the lumbar spine. The cranial and caudal incisions were drawn in green and red lines, respectively. The bi-arrow yellow line represents the distance between the midline and the medial interpedicular line (black dotted line). (**b**, **c**) The triangular approach on AP and lateral views of C-arm. *ILS* interlaminar space

Once both ports have been placed and confirmed by fluoroscopy and the saline inflow and outflow are functional, the surgeon can commence the endoscopic procedure. We used a 4 mm outer diameter with a 30° angulated lens endoscope. The first thing is to co-locate the instruments in the surgical field created by the biportal approach. Then, the connective tissue and loose fat located between the lamina and the muscular plane (epiperiosteal space) are removed using pituitary forceps and the RF probe (Smith & Nephew PLC, London, UK) to recognize the spinolaminar junction.

After identifying the bone landmark, the surgeon performs the ipsilateral superior laminotomy using a high-speed drill (NSK Primado 2, Nakanishi Inc., Surgical Division, Kanuma, Japan) with a 3 mm cutting burr until the attachment of the yellow ligament is reached. Bone decompression is performed circumferentially; after the ipsilateral superior laminotomy, the surgeon undercuts the ipsilateral inferior and superior articular processes and the inferior lamina. Bone removal at this area will allow the direct decompression of the ipsilateral subarticular space.

It can be common to deal with bleeding from the bone, having different options to mitigate it. For example, the inflow pressure of the irrigated saline can be increased to reduce bleeding or identify its origin, bone wax, or direct coagulation with the RF probe, and when bleeding is profuse, different brands of hemostatic matrices can be used.

Subsequently, the base of the spinous process is undercut to gain access to the contralateral upper lamina. The approach at this time becomes sublaminar, which means working below the contralateral upper lamina and undercutting its ventral aspect with the drill. This maneuver allows access to the inferior and superior articular process but from a direct view, which will reduce the risk of iatrogenic instability due to over-decompression of the contralateral facet joint.

At this point, the surgeon can detach the yellow ligament using different dissectors and Kerrison rongeur (Aesculap, Tuttlingen, Germany) of various sizes, usually 1, 2, and 3 mm, to remove bone remains. Once circumferential bone decompression has been completed, the yellow ligament is split by the midline and removed piece by piece until the dorsal epidural space is identified. Depending on the chronicity and severity of the compression, there may not be an epidural fat plane.

In this step, the majority of dural tears tend to be present. For this reason, it is highly suggested that when performing the flavectomy, the dorsal epidural space be dissected with the nerve hook since there may be tight meningovertebral ligaments that keep the yellow ligament attached to the dural sac, especially in the sagittal dural fold.

Lateral flavectomy can be performed using curved Kerrison with different tip angles, and the surgeon can rotate the endoscope lens to obtain a broader view of the ipsilateral surgical field using a 30° lens. The flavectomy ends by observing the free and mobile traversing nerves and the dural sac (Fig. 24.8). However, an expert biportal endoscopic surgeon has other specific maneuvers to perform ipsilateral or contralateral foraminotomies that allow him or her to release the exiting nerves if the case so requires (Fig. 24.9).

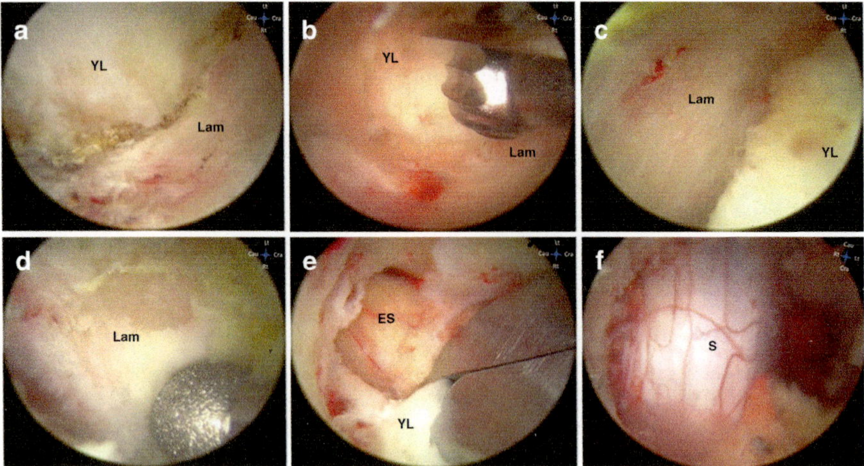

Fig. 24.8 Lumbar UBE-ULBD. (**a**) The superior lamina is identified. (**b**) Ipsilateral and contralateral superior laminotomy. (**c**) The inferior lamina is identified. (**d**) Ipsilateral and contralateral inferior laminotomy. (**e**) Flavectomy. (**f**) Dural sac decompressed. *Cra* cranial, *Cau* caudal, *Rt* right, *Lt* left, *Lam* lamina, *YL* yellow ligament, *Es* epidural space, *S* dural sac

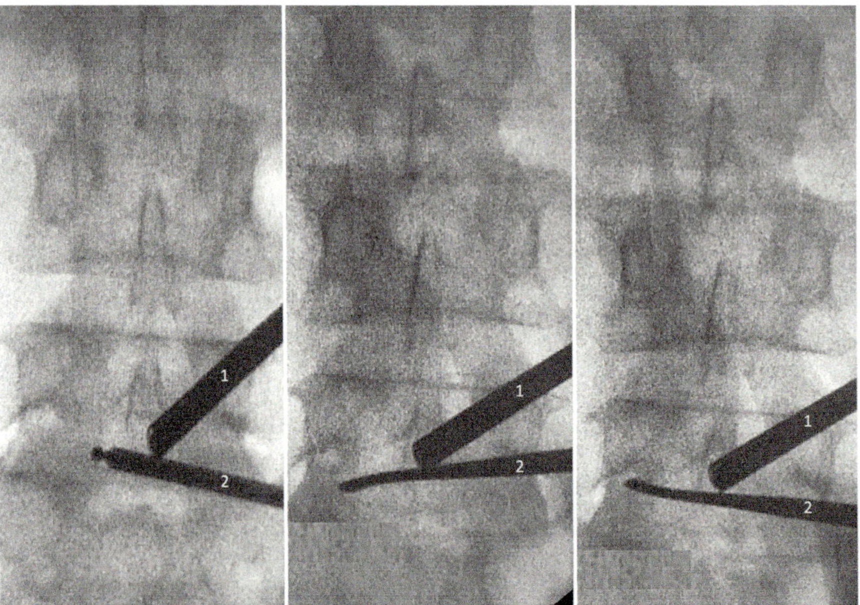

Fig. 24.9 Example of UBE lumbar contralateral medial foraminotomy. (1) Endoscope, (2) surgical instrument

In cases where decompression must be performed at multiple levels, the surgeon decides to use the caudal incision of the decompressed adjacent segment as the working portal for the next level, so he or she only has to make another caudal incision to use as the endoscopic portal.

Finally, a drain in the epidural space is left to evacuate the residual fluid irrigated by the endoscope and reduce the risk of any collection. The incisions are sutured with a 3-0 nylon single stitch, accomplishing the bilateral lumbar decompression.

Illustrated Cases

Case 1

A 78-year-old male presented with a 6-month history of weakness noted while walking. The patient reported numbness of upper and lower limbs, several falls, and trunk instability when sitting last month. In addition, severe electric-shock pain referred in 8/10 on the VAS score radiated down to both legs, which does not improve with any painkiller, including opioids. The patient indicated no back pain. Neurologic examination revealed 4/5 weakness in his limbs bilaterally, throughout hyperreflexia, and bilateral Hoffman and Babinski signs. The preoperative modified Japanese Orthopaedic Association (m-JOA) score was 11/18. The patient also had diabetes mellitus and hypertension. Preoperative cervical MRI revealed cervical spinal stenosis (CSS) at C3–C4, C4–C5, and C5–C6, with a T2-weighted intramedullary increased signal intensity at C3–C4 (Fig. 24.10). In addition, the preoperative lumbar MRI showed central and bilateral subarticular lumbar spinal stenosis (LSS) at L3–L4 and L4–L5 and a fixed grade 1 (Meyerding classification) L4–L5 spondylolisthesis (Fig. 24.11). A single-stage simultaneous uniportal endoscopic cervical ULBD and a lumbar UBE-ULBD were performed approaching through the right side. Operative time was 240 min, the estimated blood loss (EBL) reported was 80 mL, and no postoperative narcotics were required. The patient was discharged the next day with a complete improvement of the pain in the lower extremities. No complications were reported during the procedure. Postoperative MRI of the cervical spine showed adequate bilateral decompression of C3–C4, C4–C5, and C5–C6 with increasing cross-sectional area of the dural sac in the affected levels (Fig. 24.12). Immediately, postoperative lumbar MRI also showed the same findings at the segments with central stenosis (Fig. 24.13). After 12 months, the patient improved to 5/5 in terms of weakness of extremities, and the m-JOA score was 16/18.

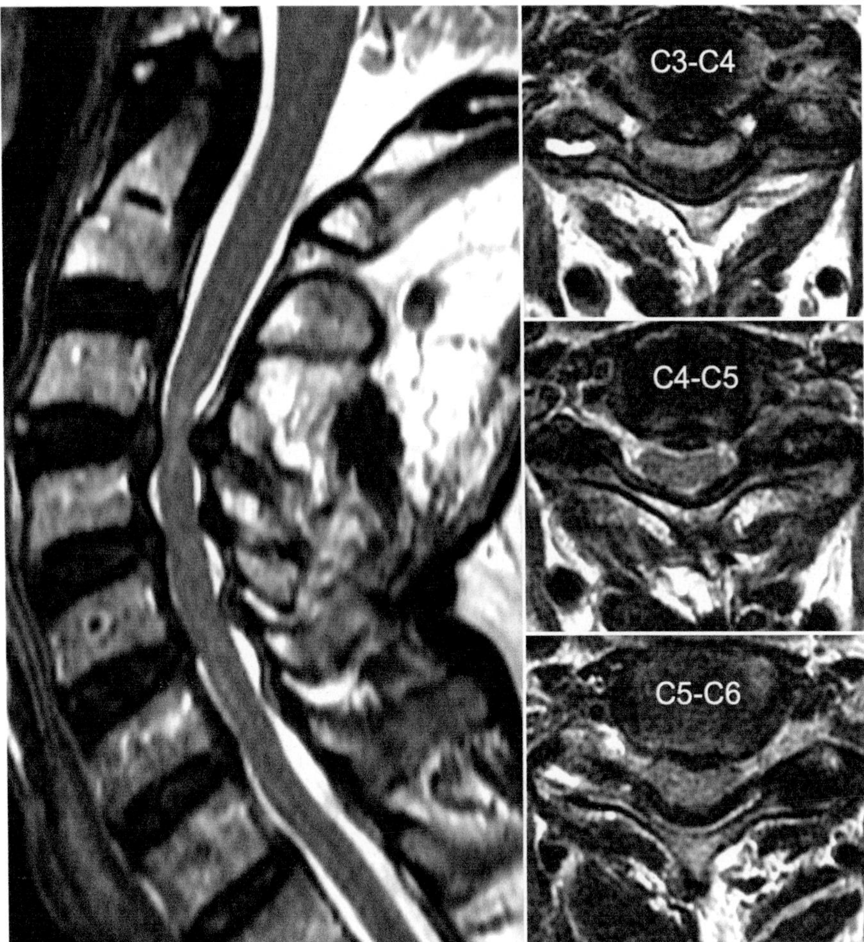

Fig. 24.10 The T2-weighted cervical MRI on sagittal and axial views demonstrated C3–C4, C4–C5, and C5–C6 cervical spinal stenosis

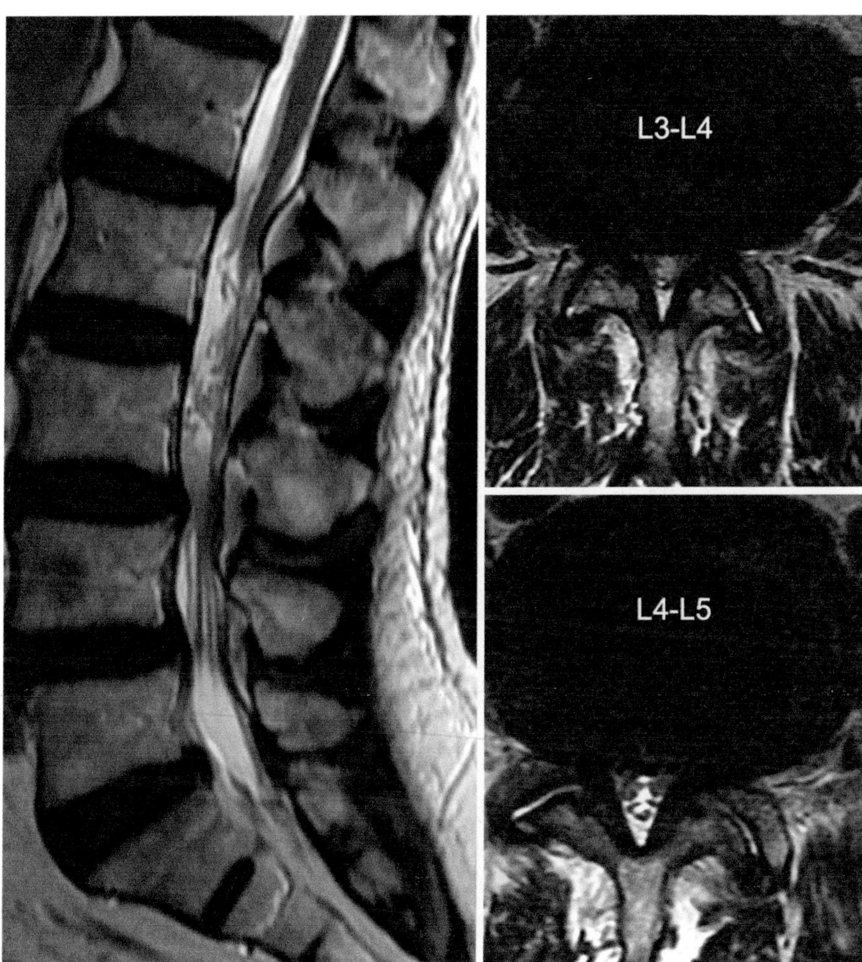

Fig. 24.11 A central and subarticular bilateral lumbar stenosis at L3–L4 and L4–L5 was identified in the T2-weighted lumbar MRI

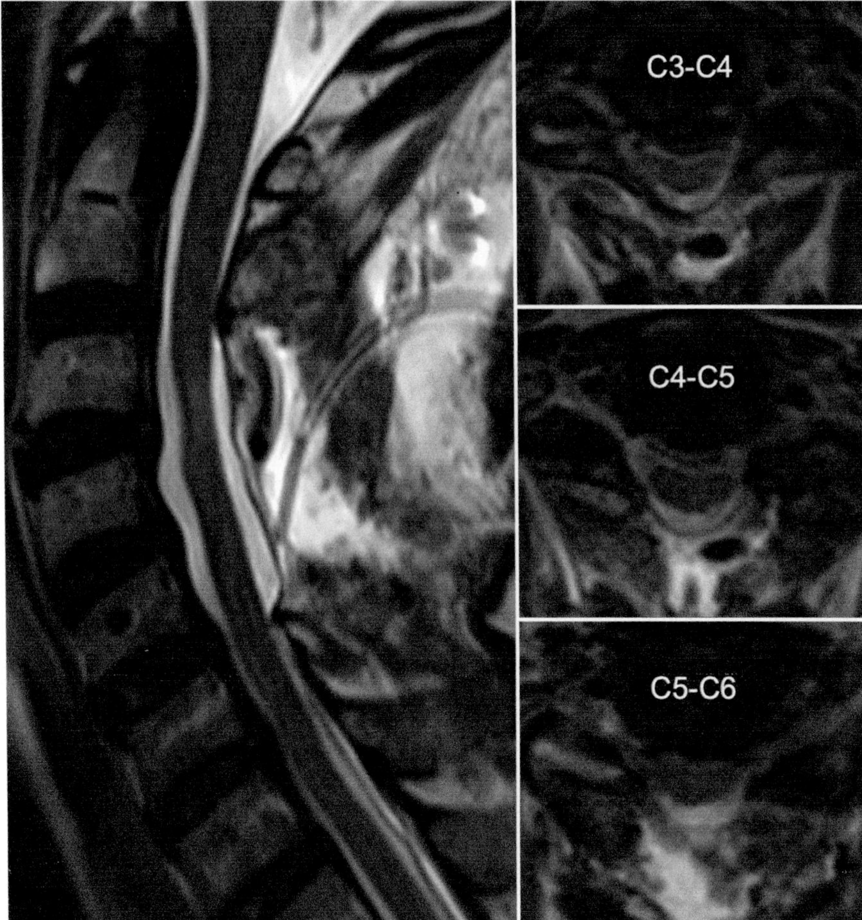

Fig. 24.12 The immediate postoperative cervical MRI showed enough decompression of narrowing levels. Complete bilateral laminotomies were done with the endoscope

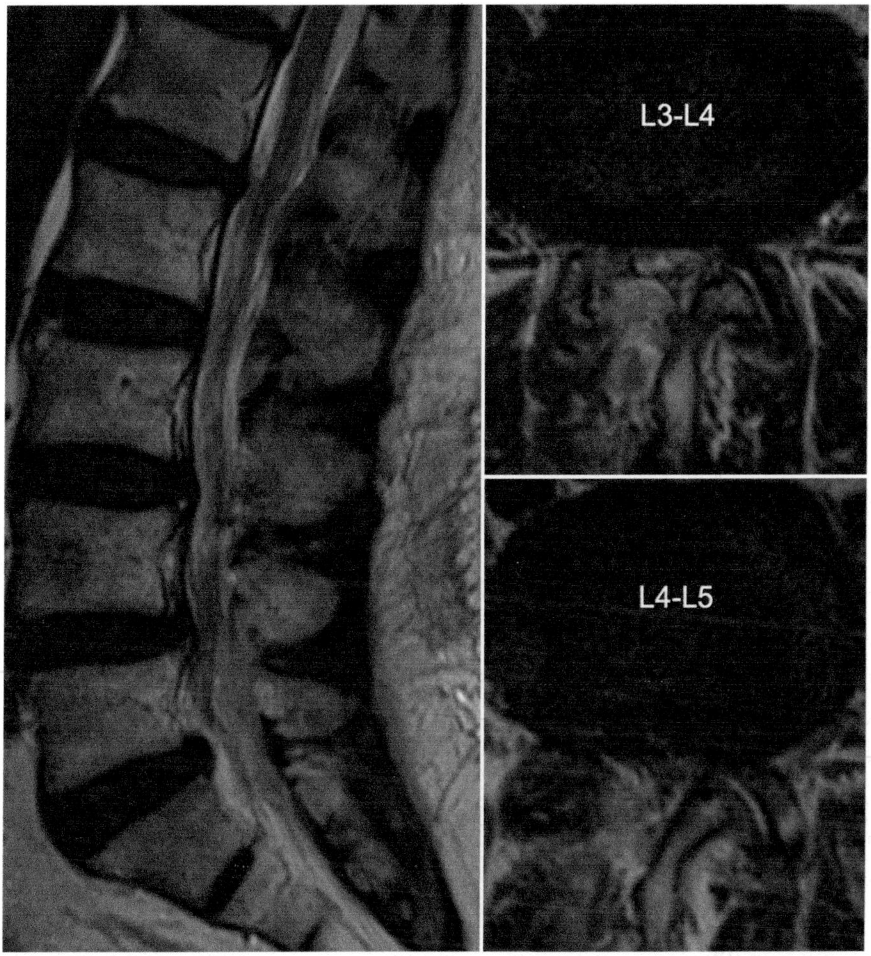

Fig. 24.13 Decompression at L3–L4 and L4–L5 was noted in the immediate postoperative lumbar MRI

Case 2

A 75-year-old male had a considerable medical background: a right femur fracture and knee arthroplasty 6 years ago, diabetes mellitus and hypertension, right bundle-branch block, hypertrophic heart disease with diastolic dysfunction, and mild tricuspid and mitral valve disease. He presented with a 3-month history of spontaneous falls, with a decreased strength in the limbs associated with numbness and severe paresthesia. He reported a significant slowdown in gait. The patient also complained of a painful and spontaneous electric shock-like sensation that lasted a few seconds and radiated from his neck to the entire back when he actively flexed his neck. Neurologic examination revealed −4/5 weakness in his lower limbs, neurogenic claudication, and radicular pain radiated down to both legs VAS 7/10 with mild control obtained with physical therapy and medications. Hoffman sign was present on both sides. No other signs of myelopathy were observed. The preoperative modified Japanese Orthopaedic Association (m-JOA) score was 16/18. Preoperative cervical MRI revealed hypertrophy of ligamentum flavum at C5–C6, which caused mild cervical spinal stenosis (CSS), with no T2-weighted intramedullary increased signal intensity (Fig. 24.14). This finding was associated with the Lhermitte's sign reported by the patient. In addition, the preoperative lumbar MRI showed central lumbar spinal stenosis (LSS) at L2–L3, L3–L4, and L4–L5 (Fig. 24.15). A single-stage

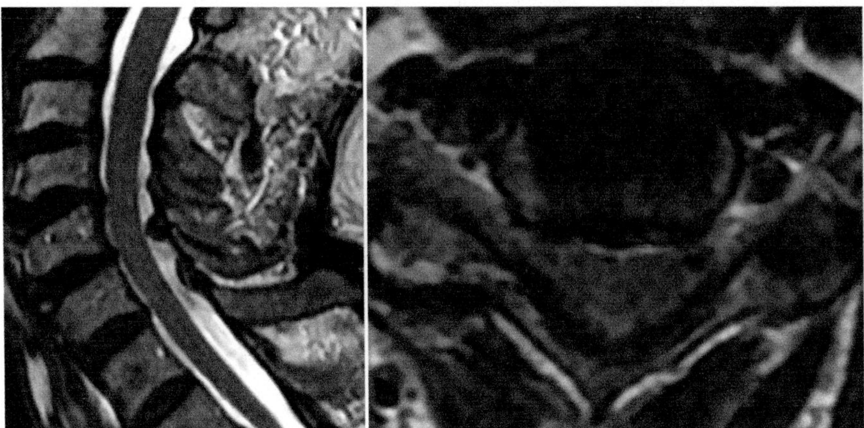

Fig. 24.14 Preoperative T2-weighted cervical MRI on sagittal and axial views. The C5–C6 level denotes hypertrophy of the yellow ligament, causing a narrowing of the spinal canal

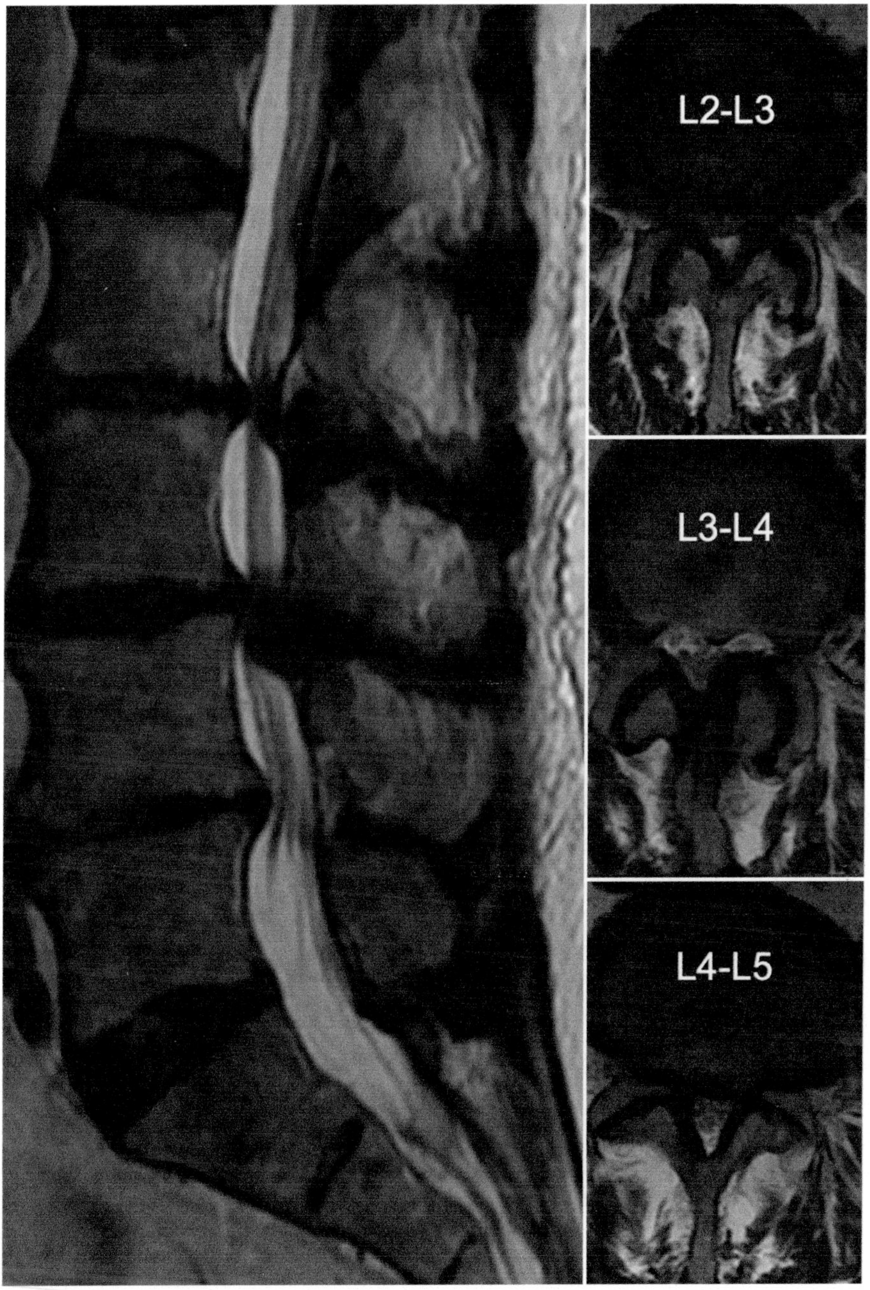

Fig. 24.15 A severe degenerative central spinal stenosis was observed in the preoperative lumbar MRI at L2–L3, L3–L4, and L4–L5

simultaneous uniportal endoscopic cervical ULBD and a lumbar UBE-ULBD were performed approaching through the right side. Operative time was 200 min, the estimated blood loss (EBL) reported was 60 mL, and no postoperative narcotics were required. The patient was discharged the next day with a complete improvement of the Lhermitte's sign and numbness in the lower limbs. No complications were reported during the procedure. Postoperative MRI of the cervical spine showed a complete central decompression of C5–C6 with increasing cross-sectional area of the dural sac in the cervical index level (Fig. 24.16). Immediately, postoperative lumbar MRI also showed the same findings at the segments with central stenosis (Fig. 24.17). After 12 months, the patient did not report a new fall during the walk, and neurogenic claudication disappeared. The 12-month postoperative m-JOA score was 18/18.

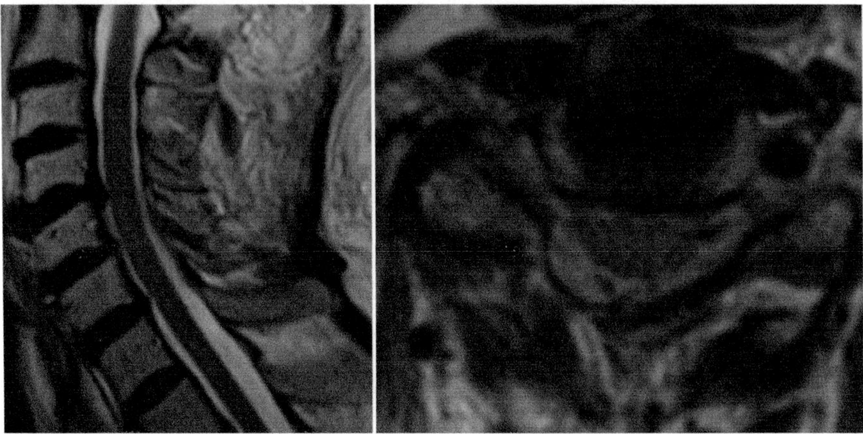

Fig. 24.16 T2-weighted postoperative cervical MRI on sagittal and axial views of C5–C6 with sufficient decompression of the dural sac, observed with expansion

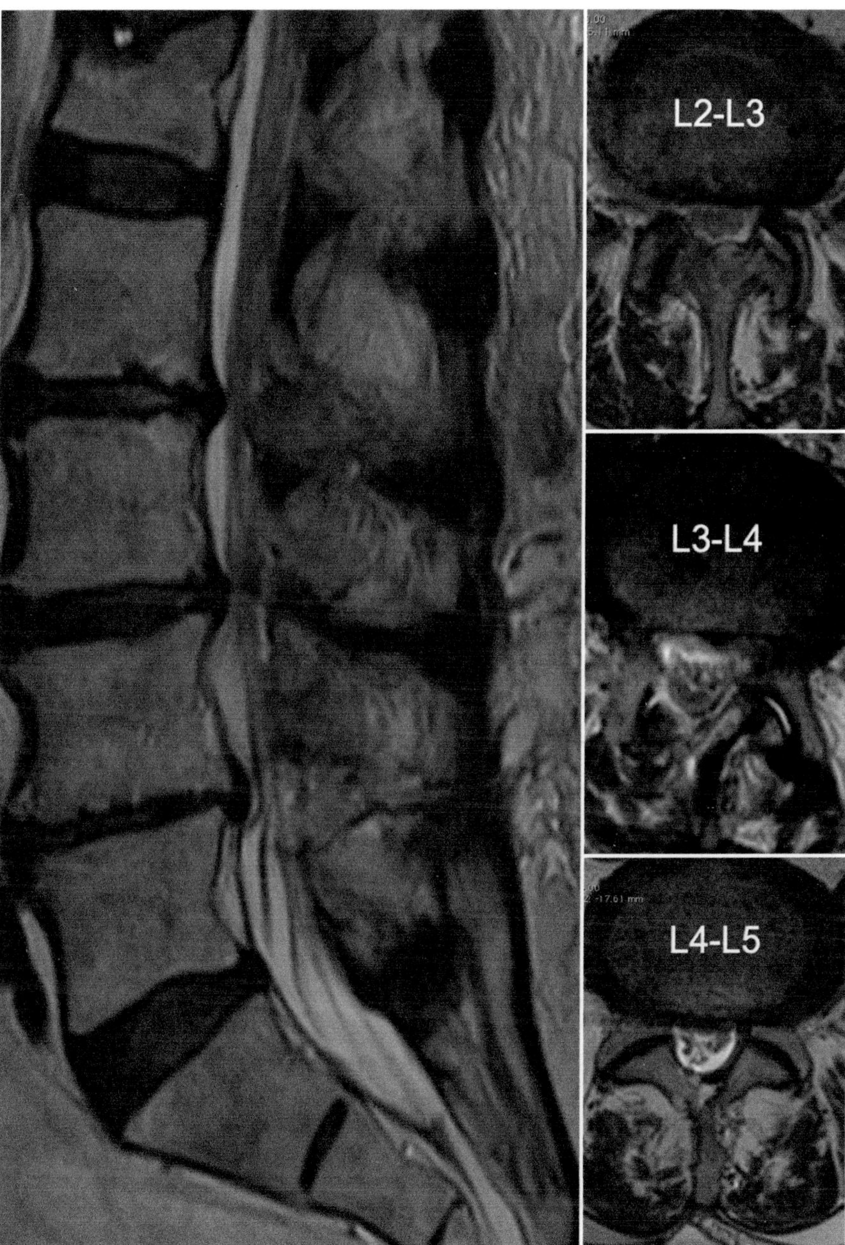

Fig. 24.17 The immediate postoperative lumbar MRI confirmed direct and sufficient decompression at L2–L3, L3–L4, and L4–L5

Discussion

As commented in the introduction, the diagnosis of tandem spinal stenosis can be a challenge for the surgeon because the symptoms derived from two distant compression sites can appear at the same time, or in other cases, one of them can be more significant than the other, which confuses the expert when making decisions regarding the treatment.

The surgeon should determine what compression is the major one clinically. Another critical question is which compression site should be addressed first. If both lesions are seen independently, both will require treatment, which leads us to another question: Should we treat both compression sites simultaneously or in different settings?

We must consider that these patients may present with extravertebral disorders derived from chronic, metabolic, and systemic illnesses. Therefore, we consider that surgical strategy for these patients must be meticulously planned according to each case [17].

We selected patients with symptoms associated with the cervical and lumbar compression generators observed by imaging. The patients should be studied, and the compression sites should be independently analyzed as would usually be done. Later, a posterior approach for direct decompression was considered an appropriate option.

After being sure that a direct decompression procedure on the neural elements could be beneficial and feasible in both cases presented, our second question was which posterior decompression procedure could be ideal in each case. Considering the history of each patient, we opted to choose a procedure with the least possible side effect but highly resolutive for a direct posterior decompression.

For that reason, we choose full-endoscopic spinal procedures. In addition, there is enough literature to support the minimally invasive benefits of spinal endoscopy, such as less aggressiveness to paraspinal soft tissues, less iatrogenic instability, minimal intraoperative bleeding, lower risk of infections and complications associated with the procedure, less hospital stay, and less postoperative opioid consumption. All this allows an earlier return to the activity. In addition, full-endoscopic procedures used for direct decompression of neural elements have been shown to have clinical and radiological outcomes similar to other cervical or lumbar microsurgical techniques for patients with degenerative cervical or lumbar spinal stenosis [18–21].

Therefore, we decided to perform uniportal endoscopic unilateral cervical laminotomy for bilateral decompression (ULBD) because bone remodeling is minor in the cervical spine. In addition, we currently have endoscopic systems with integrated working channels to introduce specially developed surgical tools for bone and soft-tissue removal and hemostasis. We treated the cervical stenosis through this technique in both cases.

Simultaneously, and in the same stage, in the lumbar region, where a significant bone remodeling is planned, and the dissection between the ligamentum flavum and the dural sac requires delicate manipulation to prevent dural tears, we can obtain a benefit in the freedom of the independent handling of the endoscopic lens and surgical instruments. Hence, we opted to use the unilateral biportal endoscopic (UBE) technique for bilateral decompression through the paramedian approach. We treated the lumbar spinal stenosis through this technique in both cases. Combining both techniques achieved simultaneous decompression of distant and symptomatic compression sites. It means that if we perform an isolated decompression of only one site, we would expect to have residual symptoms of another. LaBan and Green reported that after decompression of a clinically predominant site, the other compression site also generates symptoms requiring treatment [22]. That is why we chose to perform simultaneous decompressions in a single stage through two teams of surgeons who are experts in spinal endoscopic techniques.

This strategy made it possible to reduce the incidence of complications associated with other systemic diseases suffered by the patients since other more aggressive procedures would have been less tolerated in simultaneous use, adding morbidity after surgery.

For Case 1, there was no doubt that the patient had cervical spondylotic myelopathy. However, the symptom out of cervical myelopathy was radicular pain radiating to both legs, which was associated with radiological findings of lumbar MRI. For Case 2, the predominant symptoms were related to lumbar spinal stenosis. However, the Lhermitte's sign was associated with stenosis at C5–C6. The surgeon recognized it, and decompression of cervical and lumbar stenosis sites was carried out. In both cases, the patients improved their symptoms significantly after direct decompression.

Limitations

This strategy has drawbacks since not all compressive degenerative pathologies are susceptible to being managed only through a direct posterior decompression, and perhaps the same disease requires a deeper analysis that results in the use of more complex techniques. Therefore, the treatment of tandem stenosis cannot be simultaneous in a single stage.

On the other hand, patients who do not have symptoms derived from both stenosis sites will not require extensive decompression, so that the chosen approach will be tailored on a case-to-case basis.

Another limitation in applying this strategy is that it requires both surgeons' significant experience in full-endoscopic spine procedures, and a detailed organization within the operating room to both endoscopic techniques (cervical and lumbar) is carried out without setbacks.

The strategy also requires an adequate anesthetic team that evaluates risks and benefits between the different anesthetic modalities to be used in this type of patient in whom the surgical time is expected to be prolonged, in a single position.

How to Avoid Complications

1. A detailed planning includes the surgical procedure and the operating room setup, including the location of surgical assistants for each operative team, which will offer ergonomics and avoid accidents or contamination of the surgical equipment that lead to an increase in the risk of infections.
2. Intraoperative neuromonitoring (IONM) is helpful in patients with spondylotic cervical myelopathy in whom direct decompression has been planned; its use can prevent iatrogenic lesions.
3. During cervical endoscopic ULBD, a meticulous decompression is meaningful, starting with circumferential bone decompression continuing with careful dissection of the dorsal epidural space, including the space between the ligamentum flavum and the dural sac, which will prevent dural tears.
4. It is also important to avoid traction and excessive manipulation of the dural sac as much as possible since the spinal cord is highly susceptive to these circumstances.
5. Hemostasis with the RF probe must be accurate but of low intensity to avoid thermal injuries that would be catastrophic at the cervical level.
6. It is advisable to use a dorsal epidural drain after cervical decompression during the next 24 h if the surgeon appreciated a procedure with a bleeding tendency. It will prevent a residual epidural hematoma.
7. It is essential to locate the spinolaminar junction at the lumbar level. It gives guidance to the surgeon to continue with lumbar UBE-ULBD.
8. Care must be taken when performing lumbar flavectomy, especially in the midline, since we can find firm adhesions between the flavum and the dural sac through hypertrophic meningovertebral ligaments.
9. Lumbar epidural drainage is recommended, especially in cases of multilevel lumbar decompression through the UBE technique.
10. When decompressing both lateral recesses, we must avoid excessive bone remodeling on the medial aspect of the facet joints to avoid iatrogenic instability.

Conclusion

Although tandem spinal stenosis is not a frequent pathology, its treatment remains controversial and depends on each surgeon's experience. The short- and medium-term clinical outcomes of the patients who underwent the strategy reported in this chapter to treat cervical and lumbar stenosis simultaneously and in a single stage were encouraging. However, a meticulous and precise selection of the ideal patient in which this type of minimally invasive techniques are sufficient to achieve adequate direct decompression of the neural elements is required.

References

1. Baker JF. Evaluation and treatment of tandem spinal stenosis. J Am Acad Orthop Surg. 2020;28:229–39.
2. Hu PP, Yu M, Liu XG, Liu ZJ, Jiang L. Surgeries for patients with tandem spinal stenosis in cervical and thoracic spine: combined or staged surgeries? World Neurosurg. 2017;107:115–23.
3. Schaffer JC, Raudenbush BL, Molinari C, Molinari RW. Symptomatic triple-region spinal stenosis treated with simultaneous surgery: case report and review of the literature. Global Spine J. 2015;5:513–21.
4. Overley SC, Kim JS, Gogel BA, Merrill RK, Hecht AC. Tandem spinal stenosis: a systematic review. JBJS Rev. 2017;5:e2.
5. Dagi TF, Tarkington MA, Leech JJ. Tandem lumbar and cervical spinal stenosis. Natural history, prognostic indices, and results after surgical decompression. J Neurosurg. 1987;66:842–9.
6. Alvin MD, Alentado VJ, Lubelski D, Benzel EC, Mroz TE. Cervical spine surgery for tandem spinal stenosis: the impact on low back pain. Clin Neurol Neurosurg. 2018;166:50–3.
7. Nagata K, Yoshimura N, Hashizume H, Ishimoto Y, Muraki S, Yamada H, et al. The prevalence of tandem spinal stenosis and its characteristics in a population-based MRI study: The Wakayama Spine Study. Eur Spine J. 2017;26:2529–35.
8. Miyazaki M, Kodera R, Yoshiiwa T, Kawano M, Kaku N, Tsumura H. Prevalence and distribution of thoracic and lumbar compressive lesions in cervical spondylotic myelopathy. Asian Spine J. 2015;9:218–24.
9. Iizuka H, Takahashi K, Tanaka S, Kawamura K, Okano Y, Oda H. Predictive factors of cervical spondylotic myelopathy in patients with lumbar spinal stenosis. Arch Orthop Trauma Surg. 2012;132:607–11.
10. Pennington Z, Alentado VJ, Lubelski D, Alvin MD, Levin JM, Benzel EC, et al. Quality of life changes after lumbar decompression in patients with tandem spinal stenosis. Clin Neurol Neurosurg. 2019;184:105455.
11. Luo CA, Kaliya-Perumal AK, Lu ML, Chen LH, Chen WJ, Niu CC. Staged surgery for tandem cervical and lumbar spinal stenosis: which should be treated first? Eur Spine J. 2019;28:61–8.
12. Cao J, Gao X, Yang Y, Lei T, Shen Y, Wang L, et al. Simultaneous or staged operation for tandem spinal stenosis: surgical strategy and efficacy comparison. J Orthop Surg Res. 2021;16:214.
13. Naderi S, Mertol T. Simultaneous cervical and lumbar surgery for combined symptomatic cervical and lumbar spinal stenoses. J Spinal Disord Tech. 2002;15:229–32.
14. Song Q, Zhu B, Zhao W, Liang C, Hai B, Liu X. Full-endoscopic lumbar decompression versus open decompression and fusion surgery for the lumbar spinal stenosis: a 3-year follow-up study. J Pain Res. 2021;14:1331–8.
15. Minamide A, Yoshida M, Nakagawa Y, Okada M, Takami M, Iwasaki H, et al. Long-term clinical outcomes of microendoscopic laminotomy for cervical spondylotic myelopathy: a 5-year follow-up study compared with conventional laminoplasty. Clin Spine Surg. 2021; https://doi.org/10.1097/BSD.0000000000001200.
16. Kim HS, Wu PH, Jang IT. Rationale of endoscopic spine surgery: a new paradigm shift in spine surgery from patient's benefits to public interest in this new era of pandemic. J Minim Invasive Spine Surg Tech. 2021;6:S77–80.
17. Jannelli G, Baticam NS, Tizi K, Truffert A, Lascano AM, Tessitore E. Symptomatic tandem spinal stenosis: a clinical, diagnostic, and surgical challenge. Neurosurg Rev. 2020;43:1289–95.
18. Pairuchvej S, Muljadi JA, Ho JC, Arirachakaran A, Kongtharvonskul J. Full-endoscopic (bi-portal or uni-portal) versus microscopic lumbar decompression laminectomy in patients with spinal stenosis: systematic review and meta-analysis. Eur J Orthop Surg Traumatol. 2020;30:595–611.
19. Park SM, Park J, Jang HS, Heo YW, Han H, Kim HJ, et al. Biportal endoscopic versus microscopic lumbar decompressive laminectomy in patients with spinal stenosis: a randomized controlled trial. Spine J. 2020;20:156–65.

20. Ahn Y. The current state of cervical endoscopic spine surgery: an updated literature review and technical considerations. Expert Rev Med Devices. 2020;17:1285–92.
21. Tang S, Mok TN, He Q, Li L, Lai X, Sin TH, et al. Comparison of clinical and radiological outcomes of full-endoscopic versus microscopic lumbar decompression laminectomy for the treatment of lumbar spinal stenosis: a systematic review and meta-analysis. Ann Palliat Med. 2021; https://doi.org/10.21037/apm-21-198.
22. LaBan MM, Green ML. Concurrent (tandem) cervical and lumbar spinal stenosis: a 10-yr review of 54 hospitalized patients. Am J Phys Med Rehabil. 2004;83:187–90.

Part V
Cervical

Chapter 25
Unilateral Biportal Endoscopic Posterior Cervical Foraminotomy and Discectomy

Javier Quillo-Olvera, Diego Quillo-Olvera, Javier Quillo-Reséndiz, and Michelle Barrera-Arreola

Abbreviations

ACDF	Anterior cervical discectomy and fusion
CT	Computed tomography
MRI	Magnetic resonance imaging
PCF	Posterior cervical foraminotomy
PECF	Posterior endoscopic cervical foraminotomy
RF	Radiofrequency
RLN	Recurrent laryngeal nerve
UBE-PCF	Unilateral biportal endoscopic posterior cervical foraminotomy
VAS	Visual analog scale

Introduction

Unilateral biportal endoscopic posterior cervical foraminotomy (UBE-PCF) was reported in 2016 [1]. This technique depends on the correct triangulation of two ports, one used to introduce the endoscope and the second for surgical instruments commonly used in microsurgical procedures of the cervical spine. Through the

Supplementary Information The online version contains supplementary material available at [https://doi.org/10.1007/978-3-031-14736-4_25].

J. Quillo-Olvera (✉) · D. Quillo-Olvera · J. Quillo-Reséndiz · M. Barrera-Arreola
The Brain and Spine Care, Minimally Invasive Spine Surgery Group,
Hospital H+ Querétaro, Spine Clinic, Querétaro, México
e-mail: neuroqomd@gmail.com; drquilloolvera86@gmail.com; kitnoz@hotmail.com; michelle.barrera@anahuac.mx

J. Quillo-Olvera et al. (eds.), *Unilateral Biportal Endoscopy of the Spine*,
https://doi.org/10.1007/978-3-031-14736-4_25

continuous flow of saline, the visualization of the anatomy is clear, precise, and similar to that observed in microsurgery.

Full-endoscopic PCF has also been reported [2]. One of the most critical differences between uniportal and biportal endoscopic PCF is that in the biportal technique, the surgeon can freely and more comfortably mobilize the surgical instrument introduced through the working channel, allowing more confidence in the exploration of the cervical epidural space. This is vital, mainly due to the neural elements dealt with.

This procedure is highly selective and targeted. The goal of UBE-PCF is the direct decompression of the neural elements at the foramen. From this perspective, UBE-PCF can be an option for lateral herniated discs or spondylotic cervical radiculopathy and an alternative to anterior cervical approaches in which discectomy and fusion (ACDF) or arthroplasty takes place for similar cases. However, UBE-PCF has specific indications that give it a very defined value without displacing the other procedures mentioned.

Indications

The success of this technique depends on the proper choice of the patient and an adequate decompression of neural elements involved in the pathology [3]. In addition, UBE-PCF should be addressed only to the lateral space of the cervical canal to avoid manipulation of the spinal cord (Fig. 25.1). Other endoscopic biportal techniques to treat cervical spinal stenosis will be reviewed in another chapter.

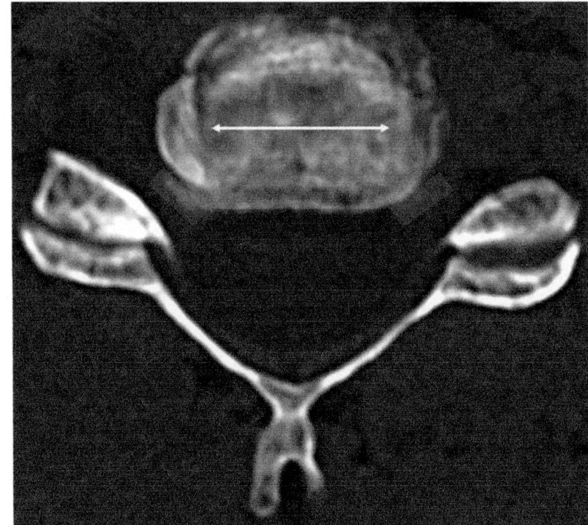

Fig. 25.1 Axial view of C5–C6 with right-sided foraminal stenosis. The white bi-arrow represents the space between the uncinate processes reserved for anterior cervical approaches. The red bar shows the epidural space unsuitable for UBE-PCF and the green ones the optimal lateral area for foraminotomy

The following are the indications of UBE-PCF:

1. Foraminal cervical disc herniations located lateral to the edge of the spinal cord in imaging studies
2. Symptomatic unilateral radiculopathy caused by spondylotic foraminal stenosis
3. Incomplete anterior decompression resulting in persistent or recurrent radiculopathy after ACDF or arthroplasty
4. Failure of conservative treatment for at least 4–8 weeks

A relative contraindication for this procedure is a history of cervical surgery through a posterior approach at the same level since it could be challenging. The UBE-PCF is not recommended for bilateral compressive radiculopathy that comes from the same level, central disc protrusion, calcified herniated discs, cervical spondylotic myelopathy, axial neck pain as the primary symptom, lateral mass hypoplasia, or any degree of cervical instability or deformity since other techniques are more appropriate for these situations.

Surgical Instruments

A 0° or 30° arthroscopic lens can be used for this technique. However, the authors find it helpful to use the 30° endoscopic angulated lens to reach a more extended visualization of anatomy by rotating the endoscope (Fig. 25.2). Besides, common surgery tools used in microsurgical spinal procedures are fitting, such as different water-based drill systems, curette, nerve hooks, dissectors, dilators, Kerrison punches, and pituitary forceps, except for a semi-tubular customized working sheath (Fig. 25.3).

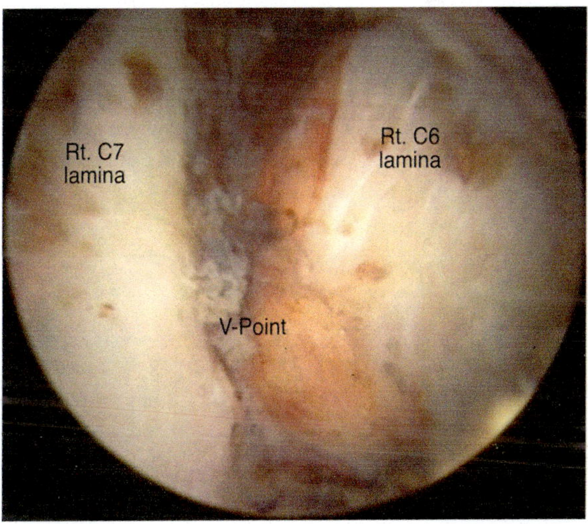

Fig. 25.2 The initial view of bone landmarks through a 30° endoscope during a UBE-PCF

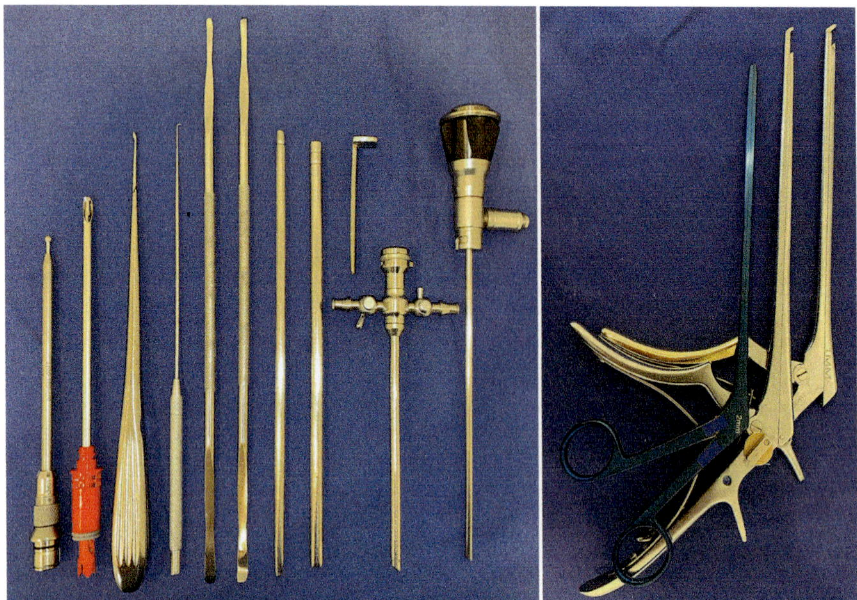

Fig. 25.3 Surgical instruments used during a UBE-PCF

Surgical Technique

Step 1: Patient Positioning and Anesthesia

The patient is placed prone in a reverse Trendelenburg position on an abdominal support frame to decrease abdominal pressure. All bony prominences in contact with the surgical table are protected to avoid prolonged direct contact and postoperative pain. In addition, special attention should be put on the face to be covered after controlling the airway, which the anesthesiology team must constantly be monitoring. It will prevent facial edema, pressure sores, and even major eye complications from direct pressure. The reverse Trendelenburg position is ideal for improving venous return and preventing venous epidural bleeding. The shoulders must be pulled gently to avoid traction injuries of the cervical plexus. The use of general anesthesia is recommended for this procedure. After that, the patient can be draped sterilely (Fig. 25.4).

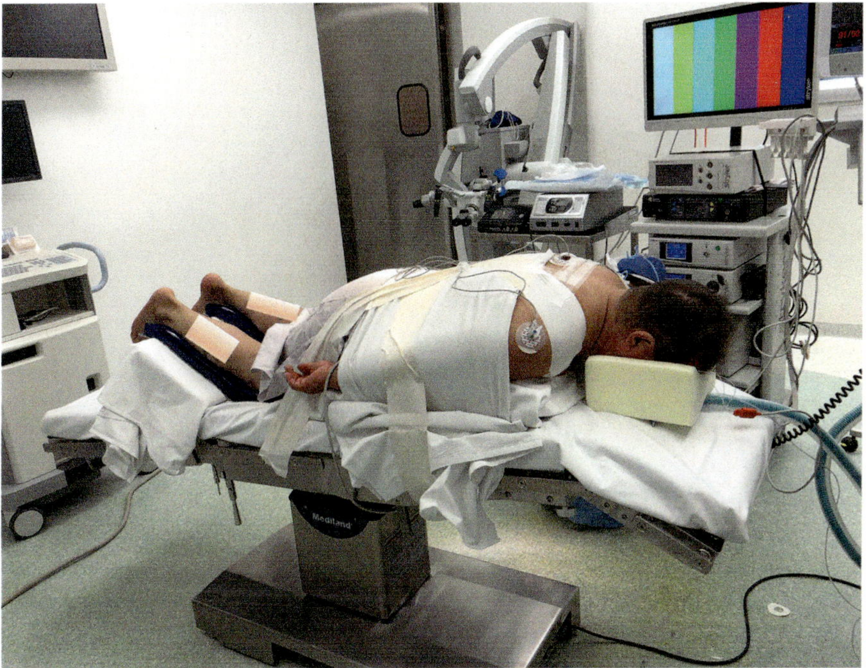

Fig. 25.4 Reverse Trendelenburg position for UBE-PCF

Step 2: Location of Entry Points

The cranial incision will be used for the working portal in a right-sided approach, while the caudal incision is for the endoscope. In the left-sided approach, it will be the opposite. The general stepwise technique to locate the entries for both ports is the following: under intraoperative use of the fluoroscope, the AP view will serve to identify the facet joints. First, a medial interarticular line will be drawn in the skin. Then, the incisions will be planned slightly lateral to this line. Later, in the lateral projection, the index level will be identified. The lower endplate will serve as a reference to plan the cranial incision. The caudal entry will be located from 2 to 3 cm inferior. The bone landmark is the intersection of both laminae, also known as the V-point. Then the surgeon will introduce the endoscope and the surgical tools depending on the side where he or she is working (Fig. 25.5).

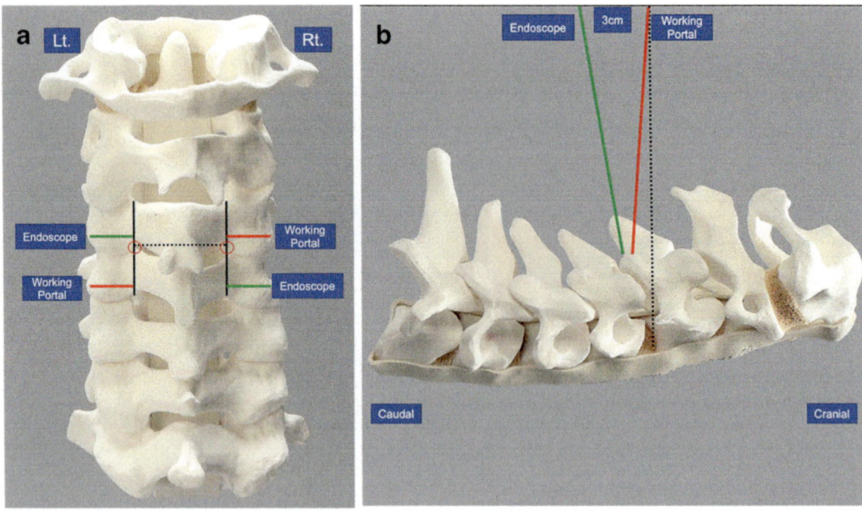

Fig. 25.5 (**a**) Anteroposterior view of the cervical spine. The black lines represent the interarticular line. The black dotted line illustrates the index level's inferior endplate. The red circles are the V-point on both sides. (**b**) Lateral view of the cervical spine. The base of the triangular approach is of 3 cm length

Step 3: Triangular Approach

Two skin incisions of 7 mm in length, transverses or longitudinal, are made. It is recommended to incise the fascia to allow adequate inflow and outflow of the saline during the procedure and prevent fluid stagnation in the tissues. Subsequently, a 6 mm dilator is introduced through both incisions. The surgeon should perform a triangular approach by palpating the lower edge of the superior lamina and the V-point with the dilator tip. After addressing both initial dilators towards the same bone landmark, a dilation is done progressively by introducing 7 and 8 mm dilators on each one. Finally, both ports can be used as planned (Fig. 25.6).

Step 4: Foraminotomy

Once the V-point and the distal part of the superior and inferior laminae are identified, bone removal can begin. For this purpose, a water-based drill system with a 3 mm diamond burr tip is used to prevent damage to neural elements. Foraminotomy is also performed with Kerrison punches of different sizes.

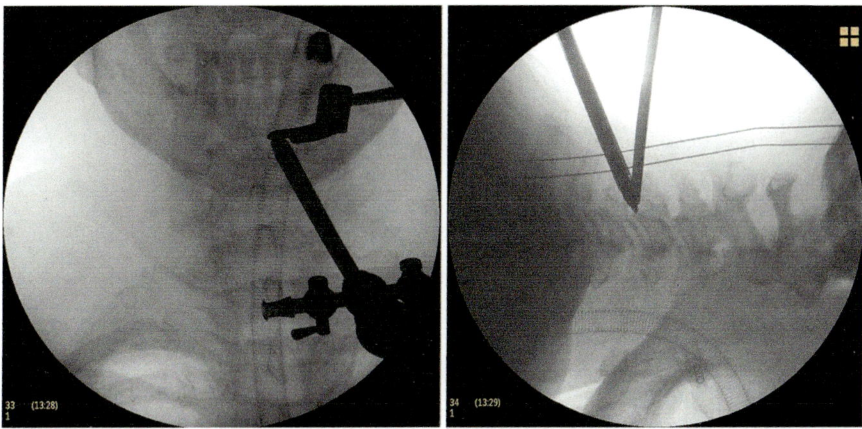

Fig. 25.6 Right paramedian posterior cervical unilateral biportal endoscopic approach. The endoscope has been placed caudal and the working channel cranial

The medial aspect of superior and inferior articular processes is removed to enlarge the V-point. The underlying structure is the yellow ligament and below the peridural fat and vessels.

The radiofrequency (RF) probe is used for hemostasis with low intensity, especially while drilling the cancellous bone of the facet joint and pedicle or for perineural tissue and epidural vessels associated with profuse bleeding. In addition, sometimes inferior medial pediculectomy is performed to reach the intervertebral space. Finally, the perineural membrane or adhesive bands should be removed to visualize the exiting nerve (Fig. 25.7).

Step 5: Discectomy

After the foraminotomy and identifying the exiting nerve root, a medial pediculectomy of the inferior pedicle allows access to the axillary space where the intervertebral disc can be reached. Also, this maneuver decreases the dural sac's retraction, avoiding manipulation of the spinal cord.

Next, a dissector or nerve hook helps to dissect the protrusion. Then, the surgeon can open the annulus or release the extrusion with the RF probe or other blunt-tip instruments to remove the herniated disc. Subsequently, the fragment is removed using pituitary forceps until the exiting nerve and the axillary space are observed free.

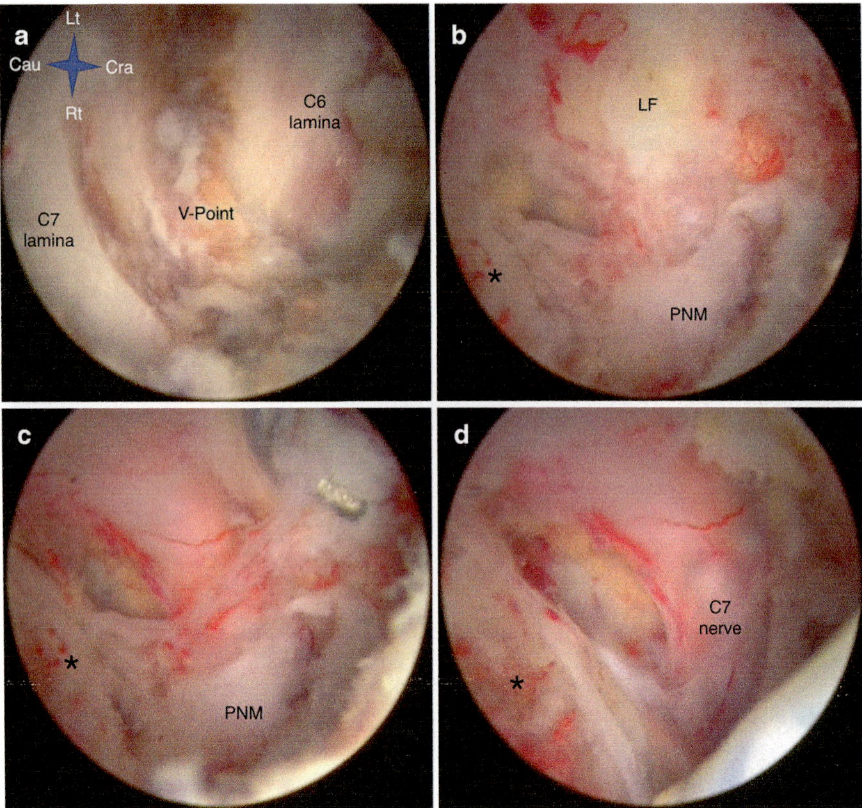

Fig. 25.7 Right C6–C7 UBE-PCF. (**a**) V-point enlarged. (**b**) Foraminotomy with medial pediculectomy (asterisk). (**c**) Tight perineural membrane (PNM). (**d**) Right C7 exiting nerve decompressed. *LF* ligamentum flavum, *Cra* cranial, *Cau* caudal

In the case of upward disc migration, or a shoulder particle location, the medial pediculectomy should be performed in the superior pedicle of the index level. Careful exploration of the epidural space is advised to avoid excessive bleeding from peridiscal vessels. In addition, meticulous hemostasis is recommended to prevent postoperative epidural hematomas, which would have significant implications for the patient. Finally, after observing the nerve free without restrictions for mobilizing it, a drain can be left in the dorsal epidural space and the skin incisions closed (Fig. 25.8).

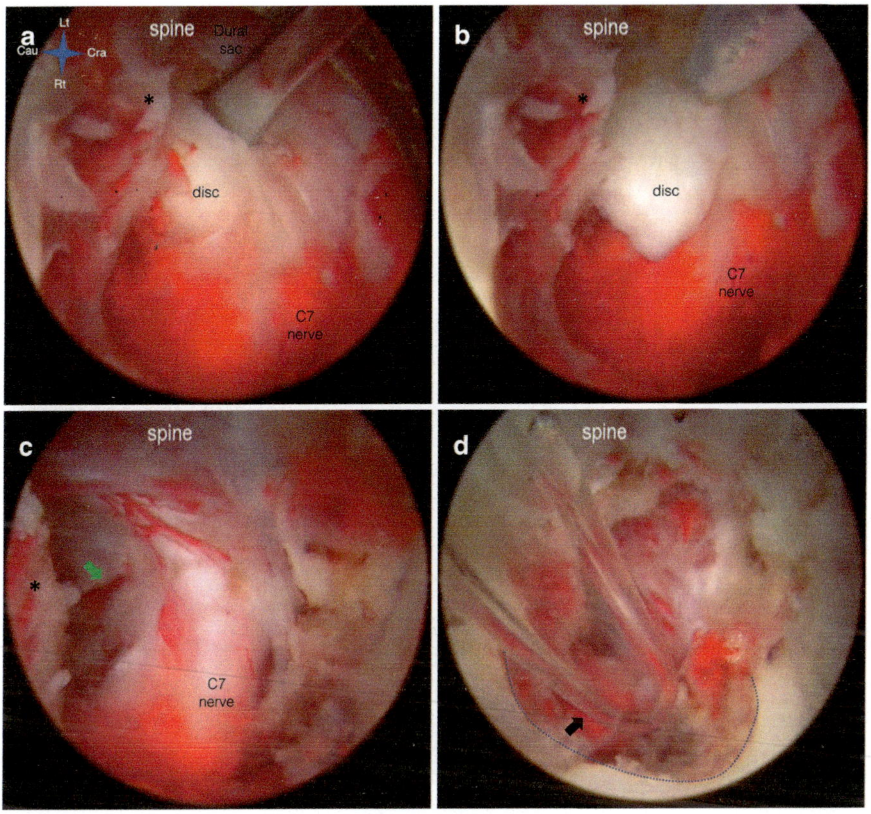

Fig. 25.8 Right C6–C7 PCF and discectomy through UBE. (**a**) C6–C7 posterior cervical foraminotomy (PCF) with medial pediculectomy (asterisk) of C7 has been performed to expose the disc located in the axilla. (**b**) Subannular exploration with a 90° hook-tip RF probe resulted in the disc fragment release. (**c**) The green arrow points to the axillary area free from disc particles, and the right C7 exiting nerve is decompressed. (**d**) The black arrow shows the drain left in the space made by the foraminotomy lined by the blue dotted line. *Cra* cranial, *Cau* caudal

Illustrated Cases

Case 1

A 65-year-old male patient with severe electrical pain in the left arm without cervical axial pain. The pain starts in the left shoulder and runs down the anterolateral aspect of the arm to the thumb. Pain is associated with significant paresthesia on the palmar aspect of the left thumb and index finger.

Neurological examination revealed decreased strength for the following movements: arm abduction, elbow flexion, and wrist extension, all on the left side. In addition, the bicipital and stylorradial reflexes decreased on the left compared to those on the right side. After trying conservative treatment for 6 weeks, the pain got worse (VAS 8/10), decreasing the strength to 4−/5.

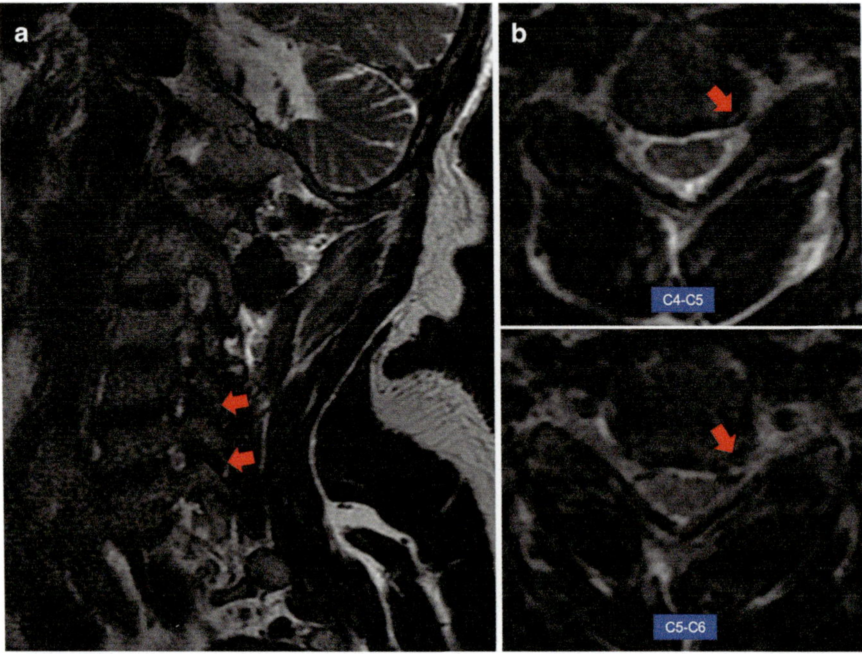

Fig. 25.9 Case 1 preoperative cervical MRI. (**a**) The sagittal view showed a decrease in the foraminal area at C4–C5 and C5–C6 on the left side (red arrows). (**b**) Sagittal views of C4–C5 and C5–C6 on MRI showing left foraminal stenosis (red arrows) at both levels

Cervical X-rays showed moderate spondylosis at low levels of the subaxial spine. Cervical MRI demonstrated foraminal stenosis at C4–C5 and C5–C6 on the left side, coinciding with the C5 and C6 radiculopathy reported by the patient (Fig. 25.9). After explaining the different surgical options, a UBE-PCF for the left C4–C5 and C5–C6 levels was chosen.

The procedure was uneventful, and the patient was discharged from the hospital 1 day after, improving the radicular pain in his left arm (VAS 0/10). The sensitivity disturbances in the thumb and index finger disappeared. An immediate postoperative cervical CT scan revealed sufficient foraminal decompression at C4–C5 and C5–C6 levels (Fig. 25.10). In addition, the patient showed progressive improvement in the strength of limited movements seen preoperatively during subsequent visits, recovering his motor deficit in month three postoperatively.

Case 2

A 45-year-old woman complained of severe (VAS 8/10) shock electric-type pain from the mid-scapular space radiated down her right arm of 7 weeks on evolution. Pain does not improve with opioid use. The neurological examination showed a decrease of the strength 4−/5 in the triceps muscle, wrist flexion, and extension of the fingers on the right side. In addition, the right triceps reflex was abolished.

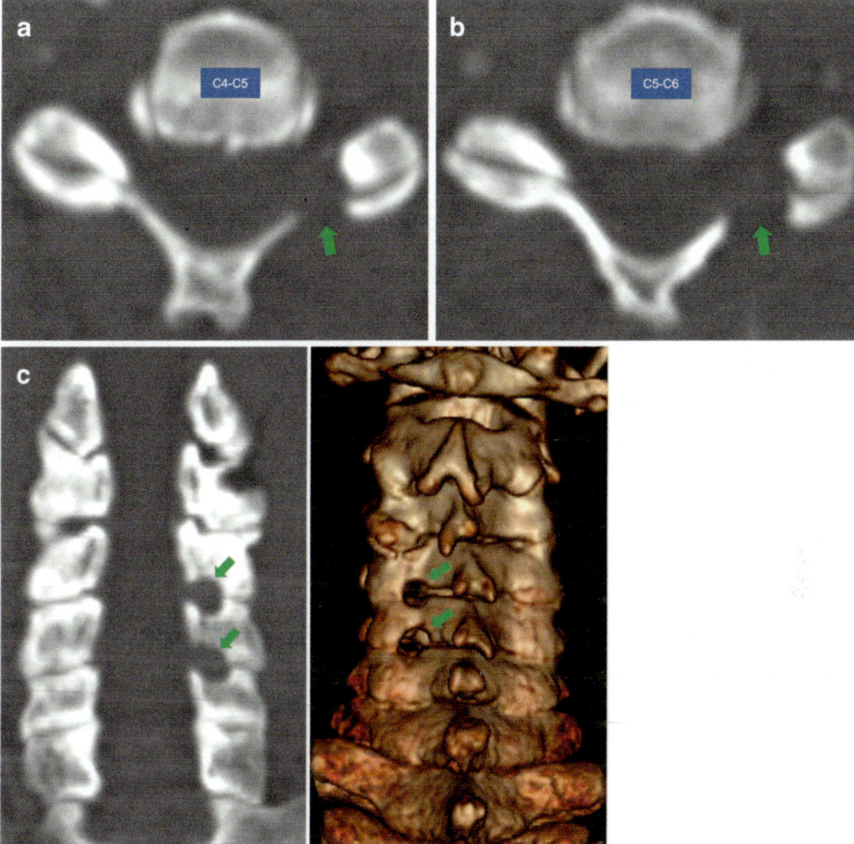

Fig. 25.10 Immediate postoperative cervical CT scan of Case 1. (**a**) Axial view demonstrating the left foraminotomy at C4–C5 and (**b**) C5–C6. (**c**) The coronal view of the same study (left) and the 3D CT reconstruction (right) show preservation of more than 50% of the facet joint at both levels. Green arrows point to foraminal decompression

No instability was noted in the cervical X-rays, and the patient did not report neck pain. Preoperative cervical MRI showed a right centrolateral disc herniation at C6–C7 in contact with the dural sac and compressing the C7 nerve root (Fig. 25.11).

A right-sided UBE-PCF plus discectomy at C6–C7 was offered, among other surgical possibilities. A small laminoforaminotomy and a medial pediculectomy of the right C7 pedicle were performed to avoid traction of the neural elements. As a result, the herniated disc was found in the axillary space of the C7 exiting nerve of the right side, and it was removed without any incident (Video 25.1).

After surgery, the patient was discharged with minimal analgesia and general measures. The pain in the right arm decreased to VAS 1/10 immediately after surgery. In the 1-month postoperative follow-up, the patient no longer reported pain,

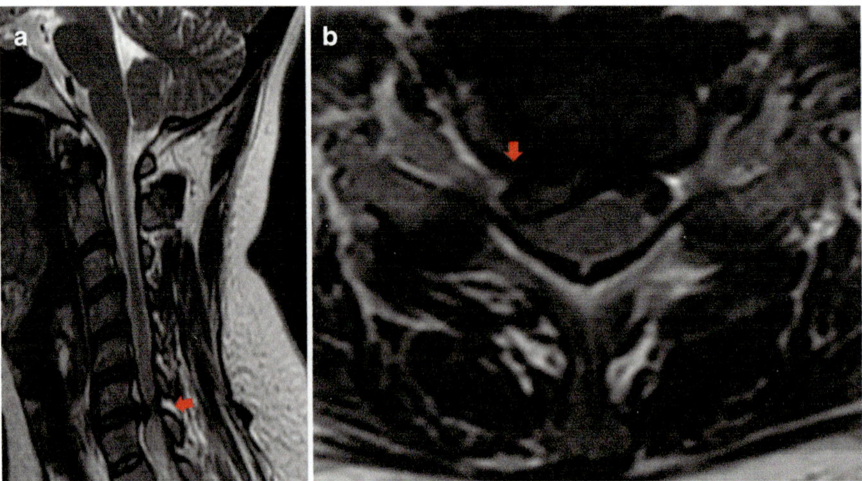

Fig. 25.11 Case 2 preoperative cervical MRI. (**a**) An extruded disc particle at C6–C7 is shown in the sagittal view (red arrow). (**b**) The axial view demonstrates exiting nerve root compression (red arrow) because the disc herniated at C6–C7 on the right side

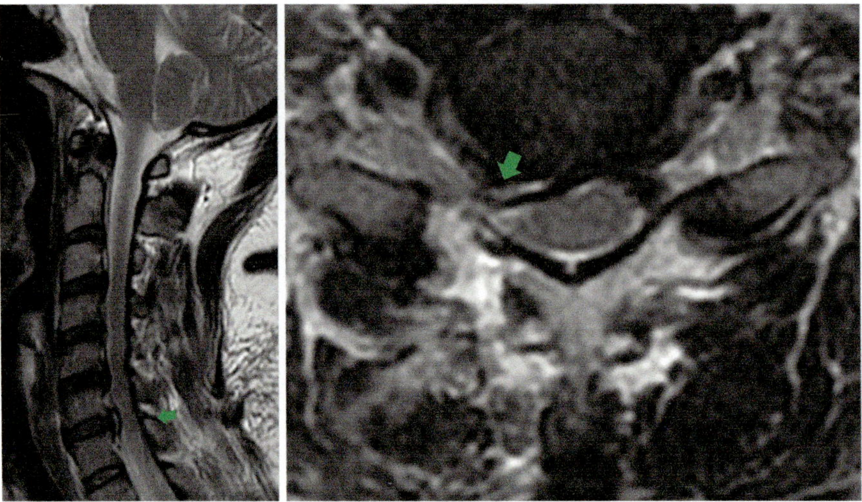

Fig. 25.12 Postoperative MRI of the cervical spine from Case 2. Complete disc removal and enough decompression through the UBE-PCF were achieved

and the triceps muscle weakness with the other movement limitations improved. No adverse events related to the procedure were reported.

Immediate postoperative MRI and CT scan of the cervical spine demonstrated successful decompression of the C7 nerve root and complete fragmentectomy of the herniated disc on the right side (Figs. 25.12 and 25.13).

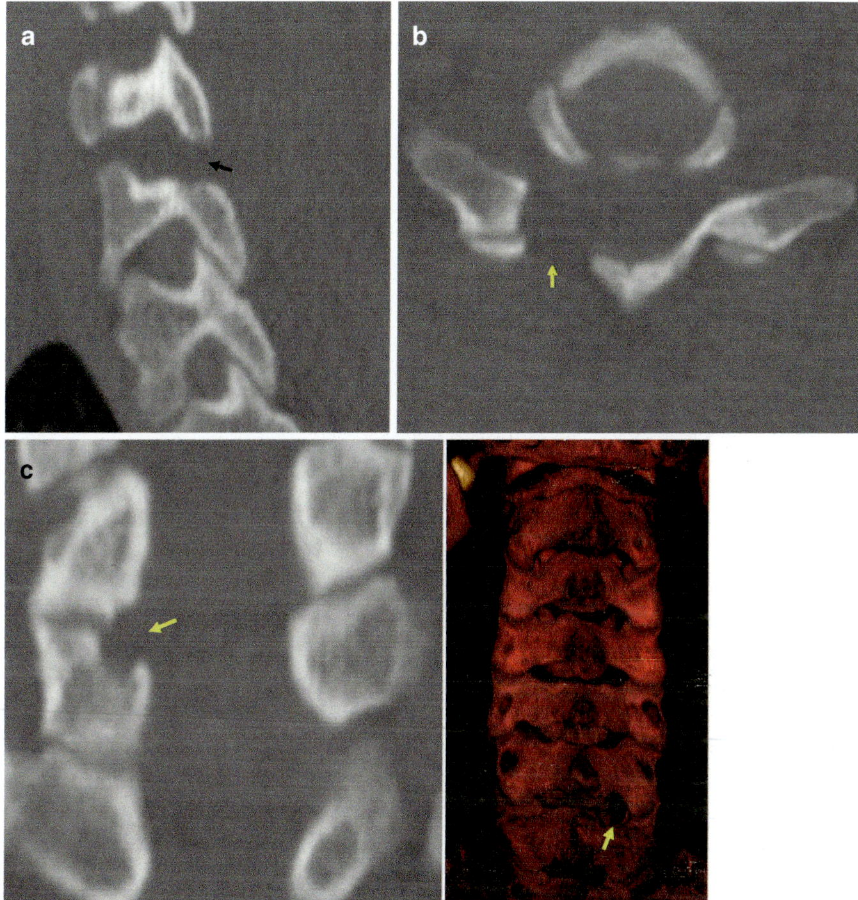

Fig. 25.13 Case 2 postoperative cervical CT scan. (**a**) Foraminotomy (black arrow) at C6–C7 in a midsagittal view is shown. (**b**) Enough bone decompression with the facet joint preserved on the right side at C6–C7 (yellow arrow). (**c**) A minor bone defect (yellow arrows) at C6–C7 on the right side is noted in the coronal view (left) and 3D-reconstructed CT scan

Discussion

Posterior cervical foraminotomy (PCF) is an accurate alternative for treating unilateral radicular symptoms caused by lateral disc herniation or spondylosis in the intervertebral foramen that affect the exiting nerve [4].

Other options such as anterior cervical approaches are widely accepted for treating bilateral radiculopathy. However, there are some complications such as dysphagia, postoperative hematoma, unilateral recurrent laryngeal nerve (RLN) palsy, cerebrospinal fluid leakage, accidental esophageal perforation, worsening of preexisting radicular symptoms, temporary unilateral Horner syndrome, implant failure, superficial surgical wound infection, adjacent segment disease, pseudoarthrosis, and other graft-related problems reported in anterior cervical discectomy and fusion (ACDF) [5].

This chapter describes a different technique for performing PCF called unilateral biportal endoscopy (UBE) in detail. Unlike full-endoscopic posterior cervical foraminotomy (PECF), in which the working instruments are introduced through the endoscope, in biportal endoscopy, the surgeon can use the surgical tool independently of the arthroscope in a similar way to the microsurgical procedure. This feature lets the surgeon use the instruments with a certain degree of freedom.

With the emergence of minimally invasive spinal surgery, the surgeon seeks, in addition to effectiveness against the pathology, a lesser impact on the patient related to the chosen technique—water-based endoscopic procedures, including uni- and biportal, offer decrease in the procedure-related collateral effect, leading to a better short-term clinical outcome [6–8].

Ruetten et al. [2, 9] introduced PECF and reported encouraging results associated with preserving the intervertebral disc and movement in the treated segment. However, a factor to consider when adopting this technique is the high cost of a full-endoscopic uniportal suit. Therefore, accessing these highly specialized technologies may be limited in countries with low or medium income.

Also, learning these techniques can be difficult due to multiple variables such as the location of training centers far from the workplace of surgeons with interest in endoscopy, a steep and challenging learning curve, and the difficulty of acquiring early skills since few academic programs worldwide consider spinal endoscopy as part of their training for neurosurgeons or orthopedists.

However, the evolution of spinal surgery has made it possible to implement endoscopic visualization technologies used by other specialties and adapt them to treat spinal pathologies. For example, arthroscopic surgery for various joint problems is commonly used by orthopedic surgeons.

Park et al. [1], in 2017, introduced the unilateral biportal endoscopic posterior cervical foraminotomy (UBE-PCF). The authors reported favorable outcomes in 13 patients who underwent this technique. Among the most significant procedure-related advantages were a relatively short hospital stay and an acceptable profile of complications. Furthermore, promising clinical and radiological results confirmed the technique's effectiveness.

In addition to achieving excellent visualization with the arthroscopic lens and freedom with the working instrument in the surgical field, the surgeon precisely finds two situations familiar through the UBE-PCF technique: the first is that the surgical tools are those that are commonly used in microsurgical procedures. Second, the anatomy visualized with the endoscope is similar to that seen through the microscope because UBE-PCF is a posterior cervical technique.

As already mentioned, UBE requires, like uniportal endoscopic surgery, the continuous irrigation of fluid to obtain a clear visualization of the surgical field. However, in the cervical region, care must be taken regarding irrigation pressure, especially in the epidural space. The recommendation is to maintain a pressure of

30 mmHg or less, preventing the fluid from being stagnant in the paravertebral tissue by maintaining a continuous inflow and outflow achieved through a successful triangular approach [10–12].

A general concern associated with a PCF procedure is the excessive facet joint removal and the risk of iatrogenic instability. Therefore, the surgeon should plan the procedure to evaluate the complete dimensions of the facet joints, the V-point location, and the neural elements within the cervical spinal canal and foramen. Recently, an anatomical imaging-based study measured the distance between the lateral edge of the dural sac and the V-point bilaterally on MRI and 3D-reconstructed CT scan in 80 patients. The authors concluded that sometimes more bone removal is required for decreasing the risk of neural damage, especially at C5–C6 and C6–C7 in elderly patients since the dural sac edge is located more laterally [13]. Accurate identification of bone landmarks with the arthroscope allows having the complete visuospatial perception of the joint. This is feasible because the arthroscopic lens is handled independently of the working channel and freely mobilized. The 0° lenses offer a panoramic view, while the 30° arthroscope can be rotated for a more extended view. As a recommendation, it is suggested to preserve at least 50% of the facet joint to avoid procedure-related segmental instability [14–15].

Regarding the muscle injury that leads to postoperative neck pain, the UBE-PCF can be similar to uniportal endoscopic surgery, with the difference that in this technique, an independent port is added.

After creating the endoscopic and working ports, a space overlying the bone elements is enlarged by dissection with the two dilators, which will make it easier to co-locate the surgical tool with the endoscope. This space is located below the deep muscular plane and is filled with fat and connective tissue. This epiperiosteal space is maintained during surgery with continuous saline irrigation; therefore, there is no need to detach the multifidus muscle since the UBE-PCF is placed medially and below it when the technique is performed correctly.

Another general procedure-related concern is controlling bleeding during a PCF. However, in the biportal endoscopic technique, we have different maneuvers such as using a bipolar radiofrequency probe to locate and stop specific bleeding sources, using hemostatic materials through the working channel if necessary, or a transient increase of the continuous flow pressure to achieve correct hemostasis.

A factor that positively influences the results of a UBE-PCF is the experience obtained through microsurgical procedures; since the method by which a PCF is performed does not matter, the same surgical principles of microsurgery are applied in biportal endoscopy. Thus, an additional recommendation is to be familiar with microsurgery and then unilateral biportal endoscopy.

The following complications can be seen during a UBE-PCF: access-related pain, nerve injury, spinal cord injury, intraoperative bleeding, postoperative epidural hematoma, dural injury, postoperative neurological deficit, neurological deterioration associated with high-pressure irrigation, infection, surgical-induced segmental instability, and persistent symptoms [16–18].

Tips and Pearls

- Proper patient selection ensures good postoperative outcomes.
- Experience with microsurgical spine procedures before biportal endoscopy is a key for shortening the learning curve.
- Appropriate triangular approach consists of (a) creating both ports, (b) dissection and enlarging the epiperiosteal space above the bone landmarks, (c) orienting by palpating with the dilators the bone landmarks, (d) co-locating the surgical instrument with the endoscope in the surgical field, and (e) confirming the inflow and outflow of the saline.
- Identify the V-point for starting with the drilling.
- Preserve as much as possible the ligamentum flavum until bone decompression ends. It is a barrier that protects the neural elements.
- Be meticulous with hemostasia. The radiofrequency probe, Gelfoam sponge, bone wax, hemostatics, and irrigation pressure increase are available options for treating surgical bleeding.
- After foraminotomy, the disc can be hindered by the medial aspect of the pedicle. Therefore, a medial pediculectomy can be done to achieve disc herniation.
- Avoid any neural tissue retraction during your approach.
- Try to preserve at least 50% of the facet joint with your approach.
- UBE-PCF is a targeted technique. Try to disturb as little as possible around anatomy.
- A drain on the dorsal epidural space could be left after the procedure to prevent fluid collection, especially a postoperative hematoma.

Conclusion

The UBE-PCF is a feasible and minimally invasive method to decompress the exiting nerve root within the cervical intervertebral foramen. The clear visualization of the anatomy and the ability to use surgical instruments with some freedom in the surgical field are features that differentiate it from microsurgery and the uniportal endoscopic technique. This technique can be highly effective in selected cases. However, spine surgeons' experience with biportal endoscopic surgery and being prepared for adverse scenarios such as bleeding or disorientation in the surgical field should be considered to prevent complications.

References

1. Park JH, Jun SG, Jung JT, Lee SJ. Posterior percutaneous endoscopic cervical foraminotomy and diskectomy with unilateral biportal endoscopy. Orthopedics. 2017;40(5):e779–83.
2. Quillo-Olvera J, Lin GX, Kim JS. Percutaneous endoscopic cervical discectomy: a technical review. Ann Transl Med. 2018;6(6):100.
3. Ahn Y. Percutaneous endoscopic cervical discectomy using working channel endoscopes. Expert Rev Med Devices. 2016;13(6):601–10.
4. van Geest S, Kuijper B, Oterdoom M, et al. CASINO: surgical or nonsurgical treatment for cervical radiculopathy, a randomised controlled trial. BMC Musculoskelet Disord. 2014;15:129.
5. Fountas KN, Kapsalaki EZ, Nikolakakos LG, et al. Anterior cervical discectomy and fusion associated complications. Spine (Phila Pa 1976). 2007;32(21):2310–7.
6. Fessler RG, Khoo LT. Minimally invasive cervical microendoscopic foraminotomy: an initial clinical experience. Neurosurgery. 2002;51(5 Suppl):S37–45.
7. Kim KT, Kim YB. Comparison between open procedure and tubular retractor assisted procedure for cervical radiculopathy: results of a randomized controlled study. J Korean Med Sci. 2009;24(4):649–53.
8. Winder MJ, Thomas KC. Minimally invasive versus open approach for cervical laminoforaminotomy. Can J Neurol Sci. 2011;38:262–7.
9. Ruetten S, Komp M, Merk H, Godolias G. A new full-endoscopic technique for cervical posterior foraminotomy in the treatment of lateral disc herniations using 6.9-mm endoscopes: prospective 2-year results of 87 patients. Minim Invasive Neurosurg. 2007;50(4):219–26.
10. Kang T, Park SY, Lee SH, Park JH, Suh SW. Assessing changes in cervical epidural pressure during biportal endoscopic lumbar discectomy. J Neurosurg Spine. 2020;2020:1–7.
11. Kang MS, Park HJ, Hwang JH, Kim JE, Choi DJ, Chung HJ. Safety evaluation of biportal endoscopic lumbar discectomy: assessment of cervical epidural pressure during surgery. Spine (Phila Pa 1976). 2020;45(20):E1349–56.
12. Hong YH, Kim SK, Hwang J, et al. Water dynamics in unilateral biportal endoscopic spine surgery and its related factors: an in vivo proportional regression and proficiency-matched study. World Neurosurg. 2021;149:e836–43.
13. Kim JY, Kim DH, Lee YJ, et al. Anatomical importance between neural structure and bony landmark: clinical importance for posterior endoscopic cervical foraminotomy. Neurospine. 2021;18(1):139–46.
14. Adamson TE. Microendoscopic posterior cervical laminoforaminotomy for unilateral radiculopathy: results of a new technique in 100 cases. J Neurosurg. 2001;95(1 Suppl):51–7.
15. Jagannathan J, Sherman JH, Szabo T, et al. The posterior cervical foraminotomy in the treatment of cervical disc/osteophyte disease: a single-surgeon experience with a minimum of 5 years' clinical and radiographic follow-up. J Neurosurg Spine. 2009;10:347–56.
16. Yang JS, Chu L, Chen L, Chen F, Ke ZY, Deng ZL. Anterior or posterior approach of full-endoscopic cervical discectomy for cervical intervertebral disc herniation? A comparative cohort study. Spine (Phila Pa 1976). 2014;39(21):1743–50.
17. Komp M, Oezdemir S, Hahn P, Ruetten S. Full-endoscopic posterior foraminotomy surgery for cervical disc herniations. Vollendoskopische dorsale Foraminotomie zur Operation des zervikalen Bandscheibenvorfalls. Oper Orthop Traumatol. 2018;30(1):13–24.
18. Joh JY, Choi G, Kong BJ, Park HS, Lee SH, Chang SH. Comparative study of neck pain in relation to increase of cervical epidural pressure during percutaneous endoscopic lumbar discectomy. Spine (Phila Pa 1976). 2009;34(19):2033–8.

Chapter 26
Unilateral Biportal Endoscopic Posterior Inclinatory Cervical Foraminotomy

Javier Quillo-Olvera, Diego Quillo-Olvera, Javier Quillo-Reséndiz, and Michelle Barrera-Arreola

Abbreviations

ACDF	Anterior cervical discectomy and fusion
Cau	Caudal
Cra	Cranial
CT	Computed tomography
IAP	Inferior articular process
LF	Ligamentum flavum
Lt	Left
Med	Medial
MRI	Magnetic resonance imaging
NDI	Neck Disability Index
NSAID	Nonsteroidal anti-inflammatory drug
PCF	Posterior cervical foraminotomy
PCIF	Posterior cervical inclinatory foraminotomy
RF	Radiofrequency
Rt	Right
SAP	Superior articular process
UBE	Unilateral biportal endoscopy

Supplementary Information The online version contains supplementary material available at [https://doi.org/10.1007/978-3-031-14736-4_26].

J. Quillo-Olvera (✉) · D. Quillo-Olvera · J. Quillo-Reséndiz · M. Barrera-Arreola
The Brain and Spine Care, Minimally Invasive Spine Surgery Group,
Hospital H+ Querétaro, Spine Clinic, Querétaro, México
e-mail: neuroqomd@gmail.com; drquilloolvera86@gmail.com; kitnoz@hotmail.com; michelle.barrera@anahuac.mx

J. Quillo-Olvera et al. (eds.), *Unilateral Biportal Endoscopy of the Spine*,
https://doi.org/10.1007/978-3-031-14736-4_26

UBE-PCIF Unilateral biportal endoscopic posterior cervical inclinatory foraminotomy
VAS Visual analog scale

Introduction

It is estimated that the overall incidence of cervical radiculopathy is 83.2 per 100,000 people annually, with a higher incidence in men (107.3/100,000) than in women (63.5/100,000), mainly between the fourth and fifth decades of life [1, 2].

This pathology is caused by compression of one or multiple cervical nerve roots due to a herniated disc or cervical spondylosis that affects the intervertebral foramen. Patients with this condition usually present pain in the upper extremities associated with sensory disturbances and strength deficit that correlate with the nerves involved [3].

The diagnosis of cervical radiculopathy is based on the patient's symptoms, physical findings on neurological examination, and imaging studies such as X-rays, MRI, and CT scan of the cervical spine. Different authors have reported the main symptoms with which patients with this disease debut. These include pain in the arm (93.4–100%), neck pain (52%), sensitivity disorders (68–70%), and objective weakness (35.7–65%) [4–8].

Therapeutic options usually include conservative management because approximately 75–90% of patients will evolve favorably between 4 and 8 weeks after starting symptoms [1, 9–11]. The most commonly used conservative options are nonsteroidal anti-inflammatory drugs (NSAIDs), epidural steroid injections, and various physical therapy techniques. However, in patients who do not present a favorable evolution despite multiple conservative management attempts, surgical options include anterior cervical discectomy and fusion (ACDF), cervical arthroplasty, and posterior cervical foraminotomy (PCF).

Since 1940, PCF has been utilized to decompress the nerve root involved in foraminal disease directly [12]. Over time, this procedure has evolved, and recently with the emergence of minimally invasive techniques for spinal surgery, PCF has been performed through tubular accesses and uniportal and biportal endoscopy [4, 13–16].

The surgeon has adapted the PCF procedure to innovative techniques to reduce the biomechanical and functional impact on the patient. However, some concerns related to this procedure have been reported in the literature, such as the progression of the adjacent segment followed by PCF [17, 18], cervical kyphosis, iatrogenic instability especially in patients older than 60 years with <10° of lordosis preoperatively, and history of posterior cervical surgery [7].

Postoperative degeneration of the segment after a PCF seems to be related to the integrity of the facet joint. A study showed that segmental hypermobility could result from the resection of more than 50% of the facet joint. Therefore, the more the joint is preserved after a PCF, the lower the risk of biomechanical issues related

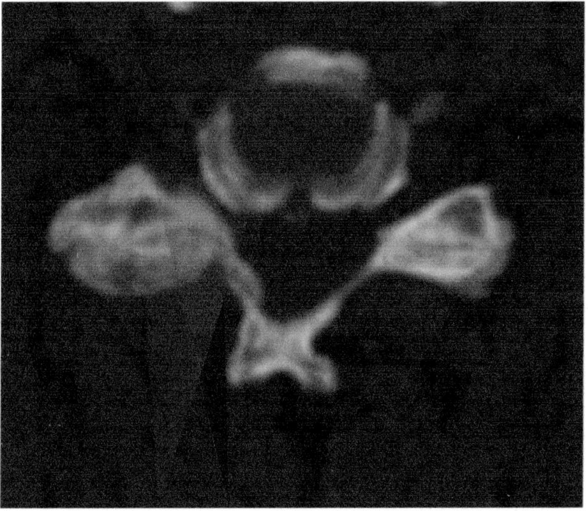

Fig. 26.1 Axial view of the cervical CT scan. The red triangle represents the PCIF, while the green one the ipsilateral posterior paramedian approach

to the procedure [19]. A PCF procedure can also be associated with persistent neck pain, mainly due to muscle stripping. It could be related to chronic neck pain [20]. However, despite the above, the rate of complications of PCF reported is 1.5–3.3%, within which infections, radiculitis, dural tears, and injury to neural elements have also been announced [5, 21, 22].

Chang et al. [23] in 2010 described the inclinatory technique for PCF, arguing that a cervical foraminotomy performed in an oblique, mediolateral trajectory preserves more of the facet joint. The posterior cervical inclinatory foraminotomy (PCIF) was recently implemented through unilateral biportal endoscopy (UBE) by Song et al. [24]. With the PCIF, the V-point is reached in a mediolateral and inclinatory form different from the posterior paramedian approach, which addresses it dorsally. Therefore, performing a tunnel-shaped foraminotomy to follow the pathway of the exiting nerve root is feasible (Fig. 26.1). This chapter describes in detail the UBE-PCIF technique.

Indications

The indications for the UBE-PCIF are the same as for any PCF:

1. Lateral soft disc herniation affecting the exiting nerve root
2. Persistent symptomatic unilateral radiculopathy caused by spondylotic foraminal stenosis
3. Incomplete anterior decompression resulting in persistent or recurrent radiculopathy after ACDF or arthroplasty
4. Failure of conservative treatment for at least 4–8 weeks

The feasibility of performing UBE-PCIF at multiple levels is based on the reported outcomes by different authors in one- or two-level PCF for patients with unilateral symptoms. Others have even performed PCF for three-level disease with encouraging results [4, 5, 8, 18]. In UBE, the surgeon can slide the endoscope and the working tool to reach the cranial or caudal level with the same approach. This technique requires comprehensive experience with microsurgery, particularly cervical and endoscopic (uni- or biportal) procedures.

Contraindications for performing this procedure are previous posterior cervical surgery or revision surgery. However, it is usually a relative contraindication since the feasibility of performing revision UBE-PCIF is challenging for the surgeon. Also, there are other absolute contraindications for this procedure such as bilateral compressive radiculopathy that comes from the same level, central disc protrusion, calcified herniated discs, cervical spondylotic myelopathy, axial neck pain as the primary symptom, lateral mass hypoplasia, or any degree of cervical instability or deformity since other techniques are more appropriate for these situations.

Surgical Instruments

Even though the reported UBE-PCIF technique [24] mentions using a 0° arthroscopic lens, the authors consider advantages in using lenses with other angles. For example, the 0° lens can be particularly effective in a panoramic view of the surgical field. However, with UBE-PCIF, the surgeon can make a tunnel-shaped approach because the ventral aspect of the facet joint is undercutting in an inclinatory angled trajectory. For this reason, the 30° arthroscopic lens helps to perform the bone tunnel under the facet joint. Other surgical tools are standard instruments commonly used for cervical microsurgical procedures: curettes, nerve hook, dissectors, dilators, Kerrison punches, and pituitary forceps.

It is important to use a specialized drilling system to work in water. The authors use a semi-tubular customized working sheet for the work portal that facilitates the introduction of tools in the surgical field, minimizing damage to the muscle and allowing continuous flow of the saline.

Surgical Technique

In general, biportal endoscopic surgery can be systematized in established steps to avoid incidents and facilitate the surgeon's performance. The first stage of a biportal endoscopic procedure is as follows:

1. Meticulous preoperative planning to perform the triangular approach with the dilators.
2. The correct location of entries in the skin to address a particular target should always be kept in mind. Water-based endoscopic surgery (uniportal and biportal) is a targeted set of procedures. Hence, lesser damage to paraspinal tissues could be achieved.

3. A successful triangulation addressed to the target.
4. Palpation of the bone landmark with dilators to guide the surgeon. It will be confirmed by intraoperative fluoroscopy.
5. Creating an underlying space to the bone surface will allow to observe the anatomy clearly and contribute to a correct flow of irrigated solution during the procedure.
6. Confirm the correct inflow and outflow of the saline.

The second stage of the biportal endoscopic procedure is the execution of the surgery to achieve the planned goals under endoscopic view, which will be explained below.

Step 1: Patient Positioning and Anesthesia

The patient is placed in a reverse Trendelenburg prone position on an abdominal frame to decrease abdominal pressure, and facilitate the venous return, thus indirectly reducing intraoperative bleeding (Fig. 26.2). The same considerations regarding the position for a PCF should be followed (Chap. 25 in "Step 1: Patient Positioning and Anesthesia"). The recommended anesthesia for this procedure is general.

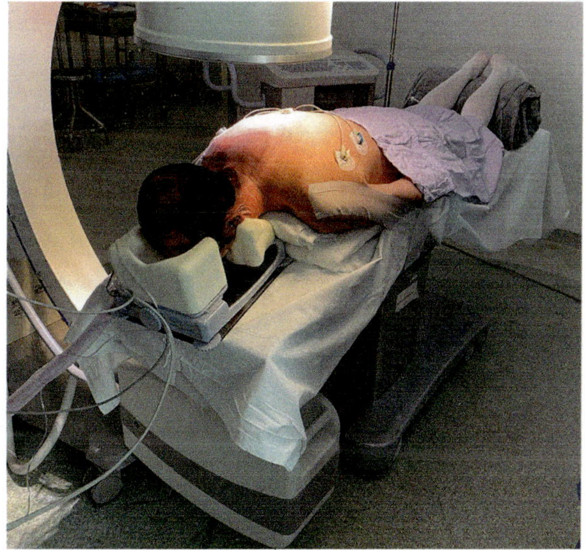

Fig. 26.2 Patient positioning for a UBE-PCIF

Step 2: Location of Entry Points

The surgeon should be on the opposite side of the foraminotomy. First, a line that passes lateral to the spinous processes is drawn to have an initial reference of the approach. This reference is confirmed by palpation. The following line references the V-point; the surgeon should mark a line medial to the facet joints. Both lines are confirmed in an AP view of the C-arm. Next, the surgeon will draw a line that passes through the intervertebral disc in the lateral view. Therefore, the incisions will be 1.5 cm cranial and 1.5 cm caudal to this line, meaning that there will be a 3 cm distance between the two incisions so that the endoscope and the work tool are not obstructed.

Similar to a contralateral approach, the right-handed surgeon will use the cranial incision to create the endoscopic portal and the caudal incision for the working portal to address a pathology on the right side. However, the surgeon will place on the right side for a left-sided pathology, and the ports' arrangement will be the opposite (Fig. 26.3).

Step 3: Triangular Approach

Two transverse or longitudinal 7 mm skin incisions are made in the previously located entries. The fascia should be cut to introduce the dilator and enable a correct inflow and outflow of solution during surgery. Subsequently, a pair of 6 mm dilators

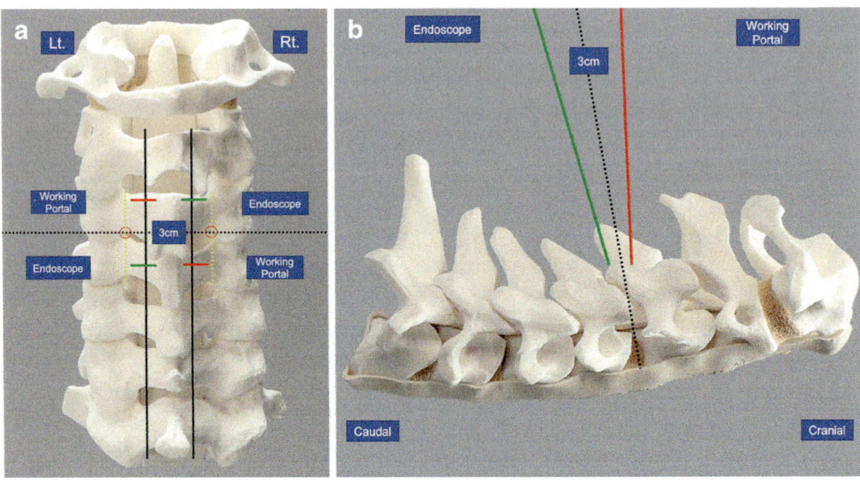

Fig. 26.3 Planning to locate the incisions in a UBE-PCIF. (**a**) AP view of anatomical model showing the references followed during a UBE-PCIF. The black lines pass slightly lateral to the cervical spinous processes. The yellow dotted lines are medial to the facet joints. The black dotted line represents the disc space. The red circles are located at the V-point on each side. The cranial incision (green line) is for the endoscope on the right side, and the caudal incision (red line) is for the working canal. On the left side, it is the opposite. (**b**) Lateral view of the same anatomical model showing the references for planning a UBE-PCIF

are introduced into the incisions with a mediolateral inclinatory trajectory. This is the key step for performing a correct inclinatory approach since only 10°–15° of angulation is enough to reach the V-point. However, if the angle of the approach is greater, there is a risk of addressing the dilator to other vital cervical structures (Fig. 26.4). Then, the surgeon must palpate the following bone references with both dilators: the lower edge of the superior lamina, the superior border of the inferior lamina, and the confluence of both or the V-point of the index level (Video 26.1). Both ports can be used after creating the space above the bone landmarks and dilating both channels by the progressive introduction of 7 and 8 mm dilators (Fig. 26.5).

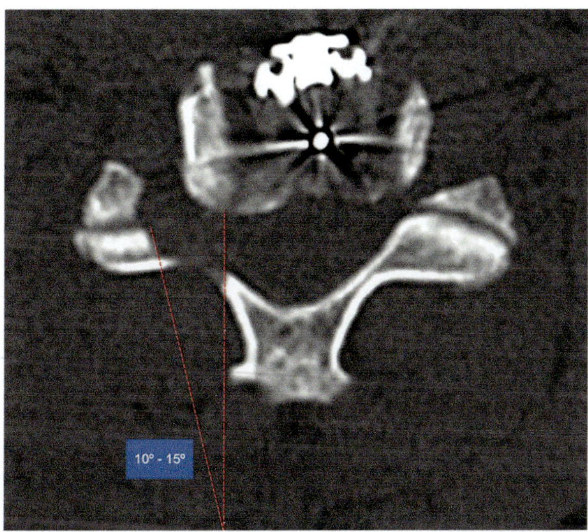

Fig. 26.4 Trajectory angle of a right biportal endoscopic inclinatory foraminotomy at C4–C5

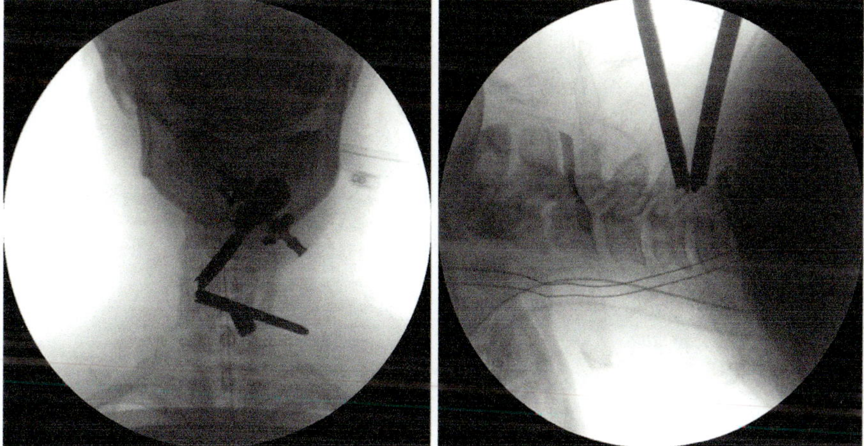

Fig. 26.5 Biportal endoscopic approach for a right posterior cervical inclinatory foraminotomy at C5–C6. Note that the endoscopic portal is cranial, and the working portal is caudal

Step 4: UBE-Posterior Cervical Inclinatory Foraminotomy

After inserting the endoscope, the first thing to confirm is an appropriate inflow and outflow of saline. Then, co-location of both ports in the surgical field is necessary to start with the endoscopic procedure. Next, the surgeon must coagulate with the radiofrequency (RF) probe the soft tissue over the bone surfaces to achieve a more detailed visualization and identify the landmarks. Afterward, the foraminotomy begins drilling of the bone references. It is recommended to use a 3 mm diamond burr tip to avoid any injury to the neural elements. The surgeon should drill out the superior edge of the inferior lamina, the V-point, and the inferior border of the upper lamina.

The surgeon must identify the superior articular process (SAP) by drilling the bone elements. Below this structure, there may or may not be ligamentum flavum (LF) covering the distal part of the exiting nerve root. The bone drill must follow the trajectory of the nerve root. Within the foramen, venous plexuses surrounding the nerve root are found, and hemostasis must be meticulous without damaging the nerve to allow clear visualization of the surgical field. Finally, visualization and free mobilization of the nerve root are the endpoints of the decompression. A nerve hook can be introduced above the nerve into the foramen to feel the free space (Fig. 26.6). After having confirmed adequate decompression, an epidural drain can be left to reduce the risk of collections such as hematomas, and the incisions are closed (Fig. 26.7).

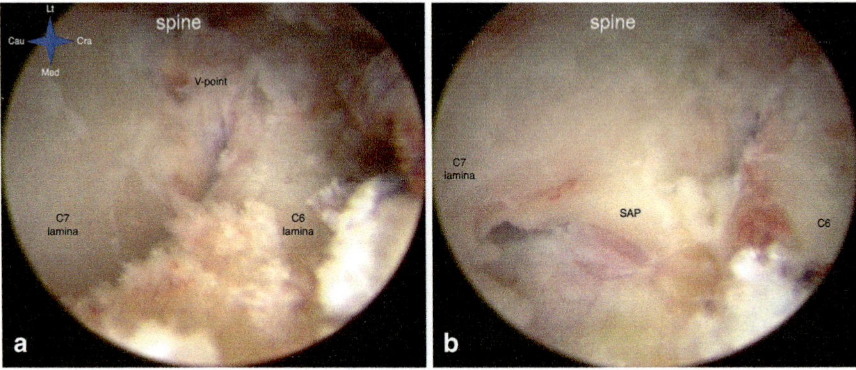

Fig. 26.6 Endoscopic biportal approach for a left posterior cervical inclinatory foraminotomy at C6–C7. (**a**) The bone landmarks have been exposed. Observe the mediolateral perspective obtained with the 30° endoscope of the V-point. (**b**) Both lamina's distal part has been drilled out, and the SAP was exposed. (**c**) C7 exiting nerve root has been decompressed. (**d**) Panoramic view confirming the tunnel-shaped foraminotomy through an inclinatory approach in left C6–C7. *Cra* cranial, *Cau* caudal, *Lt* left, *Med* medial, *SAP* superior articular process, *IAP* inferior articular process, *LF* ligamentum flavum

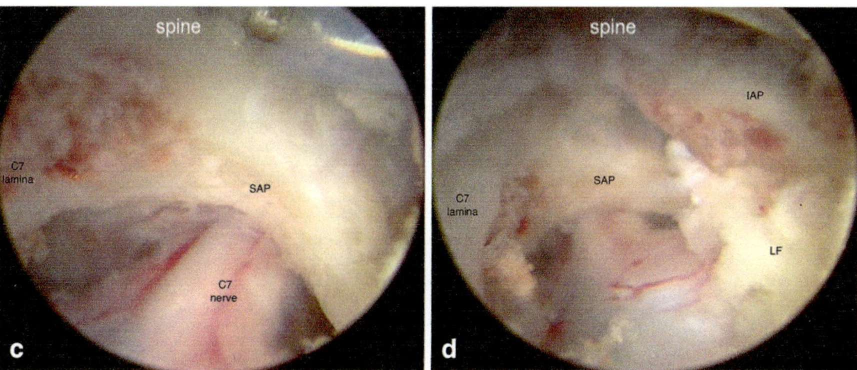

Fig. 26.6 (continued)

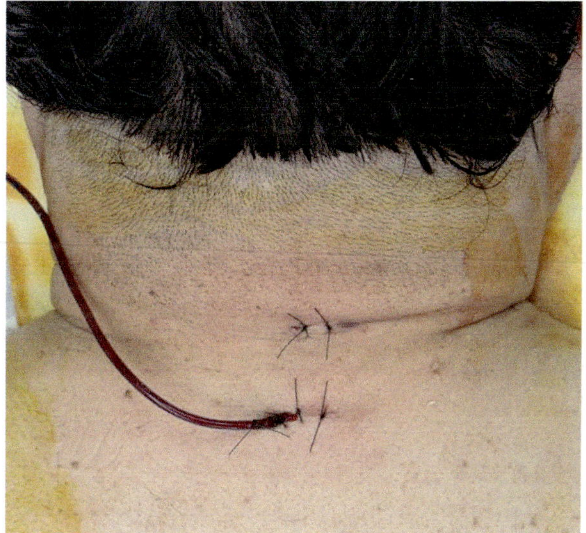

Fig. 26.7 Skin incisions closed and drainage

Illustrated Cases

Case 1

A 62-year-old male with radicular pain in the right arm (VAS 8/10) and neck pain (VAS 6/10) was treated with 4 months on evolution. The pain radiated from the interscapular region and ran down his upper extremity's lateral aspect, reaching the hand. The patient complained of paresthesia in the right hand's first three fingers, and the pain did not improve with potent opioids.

The neurological examination showed a weakness in the biceps and triceps of the right arm (4−/5) and the extension and flexion of the right wrist (4−/5). In addition, the right triceps reflex was abolished at the time of examination.

Preoperative X-ray images of the cervical spine demonstrated a collapse in the height of the C6–C7 disc space (Fig. 26.8). The axial views of the CT scan showed severe right foraminal stenosis at C5–C6 caused by facet hypertrophy and bilateral

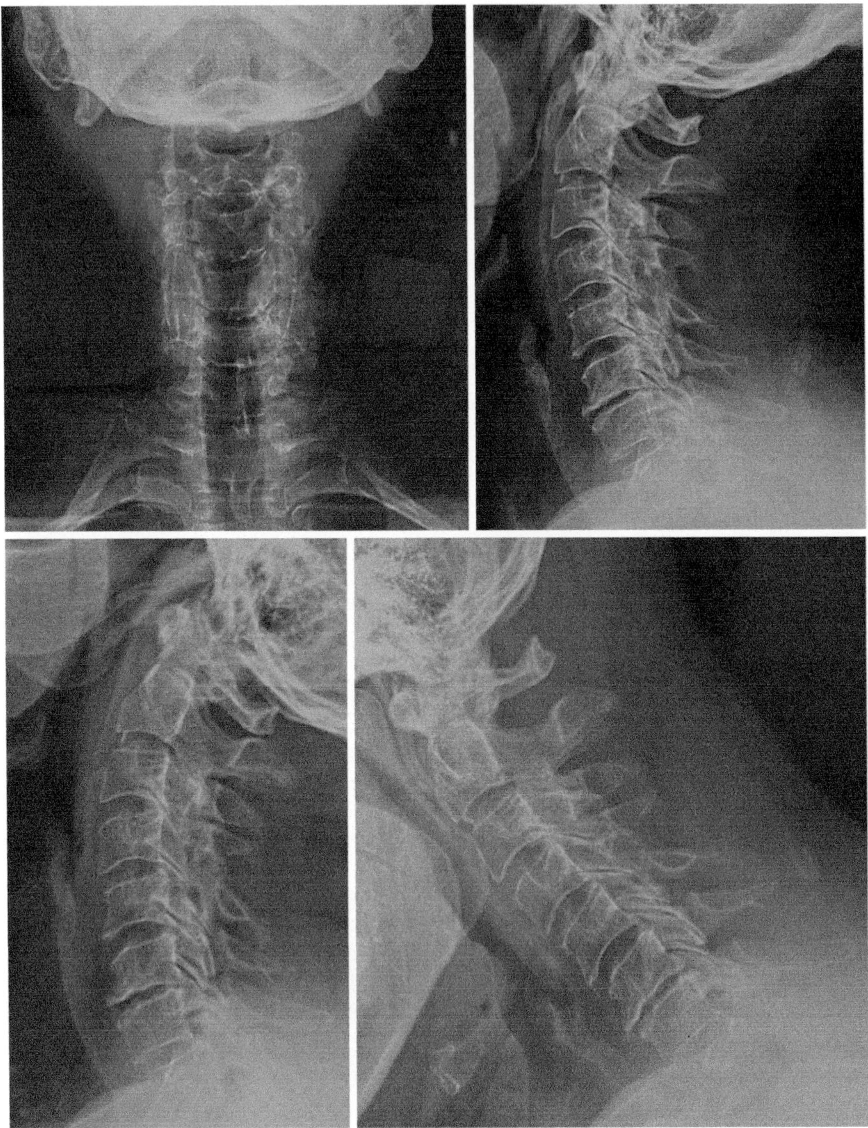

Fig. 26.8 Case 1 preoperative X-rays of the cervical spine. A degenerative disc disease with disc collapse is observed in C6–C7

right foraminal stenosis in C6–C7 predominantly on the right side, related to uncinate hypertrophy (Fig. 26.9). Cervical MRI confirmed the findings observed in CT scan (Fig. 26.10).

The diagnosis was symptomatic compressive C6 and C7 right-sided radiculopathy and axial neck pain, and a UBE-PCIF at C5–C6 and C6–C7 on the right side was offered. A long trajectory of the right C7 nerve root compressed by the severe spondylosis of the uncinate process and bilateral foraminal stenosis due to the significant collapse of the disc space was noted in the CT scan at the C6–C7. Therefore, it was decided to combine this level with an ACDF to avoid recurrent symptoms.

No complications were reported during the procedure. The inclinatory foraminotomies were performed in C5–C6 and C6–C7 on the right side and later the ACDF in C6–C7 during the same surgical time. A severe compression in the right C6 and C7 exiting nerves due to spondylosis was noted during the decompression. The firm periradicular membrane was detached from both nerves (Video 26.2).

The patient was discharged 1 day after surgery with encouraging outcomes. His right arm and neck pain improved immediately after the procedure to VAS 1/10, and the drain was removed 16 h later. No postoperative opioids were required.

At the 15-day follow-up visit, the patient improved the right biceps, triceps, and wrist strength to 4+/5, and a complete recovery was observed until the 3-month follow-up.

Postoperative studies demonstrated the restoration of intervertebral height at C6–C7 and adequate placement of the intersomatic implant (Fig. 26.11). In addition, sufficient decompression was observed in the postoperative MRI and CT scan imaging studies at C5–C6 and C6–C7 (Fig. 26.12).

Case 2

A 54-year-old female with severe electric shock-like pain in the left arm VAS 9/10 with 6 weeks on evolution underwent surgery. The pain was resistant to multiple

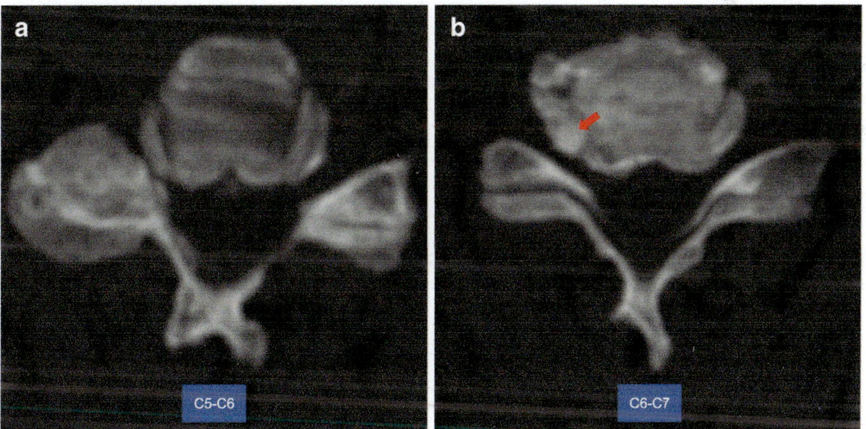

Fig. 26.9 Axial views of the CT scan from Case 1. (**a**) C5–C6. (**b**) C6–C7, the red arrow points to the right uncinate hypertrophy at that level

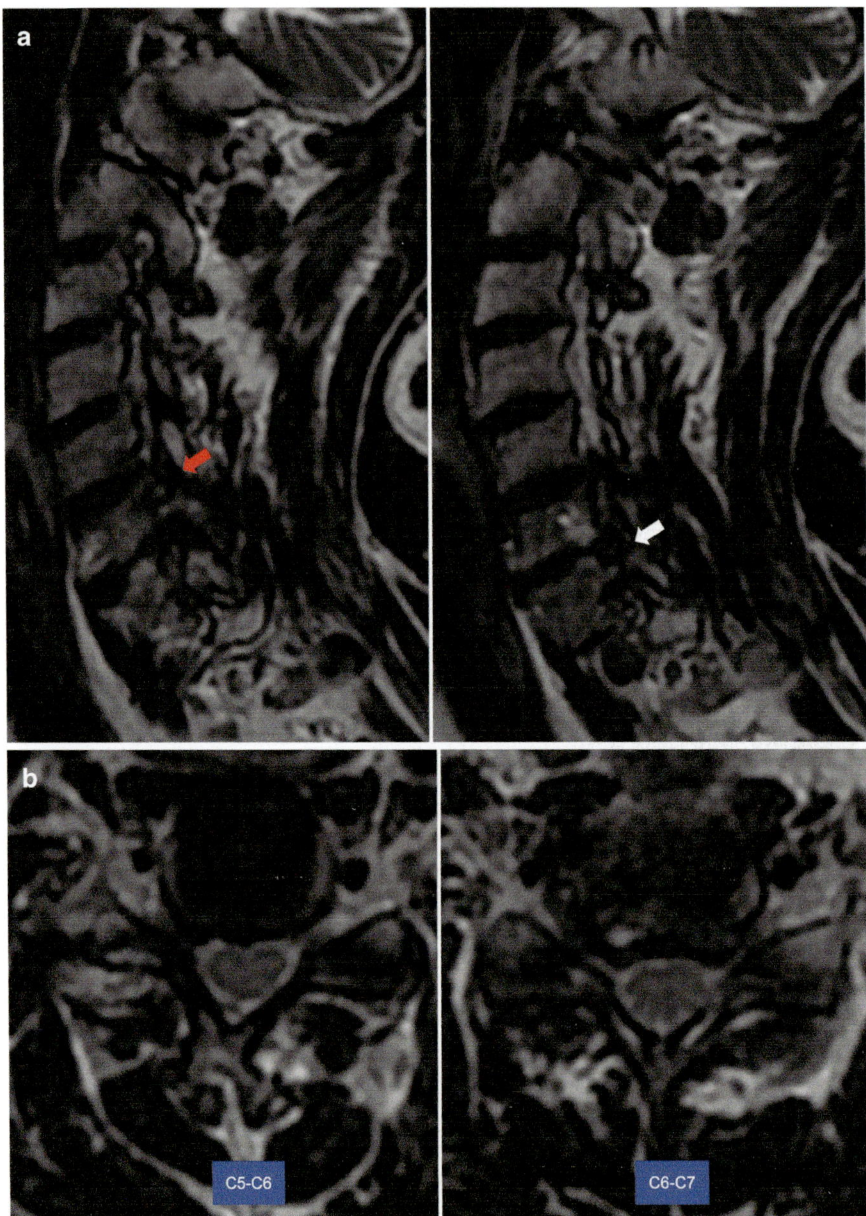

Fig. 26.10 Case 1 preoperative cervical MRI. (**a**) The oblique sagittal views on the right side showed foraminal stenosis at C5–C6 (red arrow) and C6–C7 (white arrow). (**b**) Axial views of the MRI of both levels

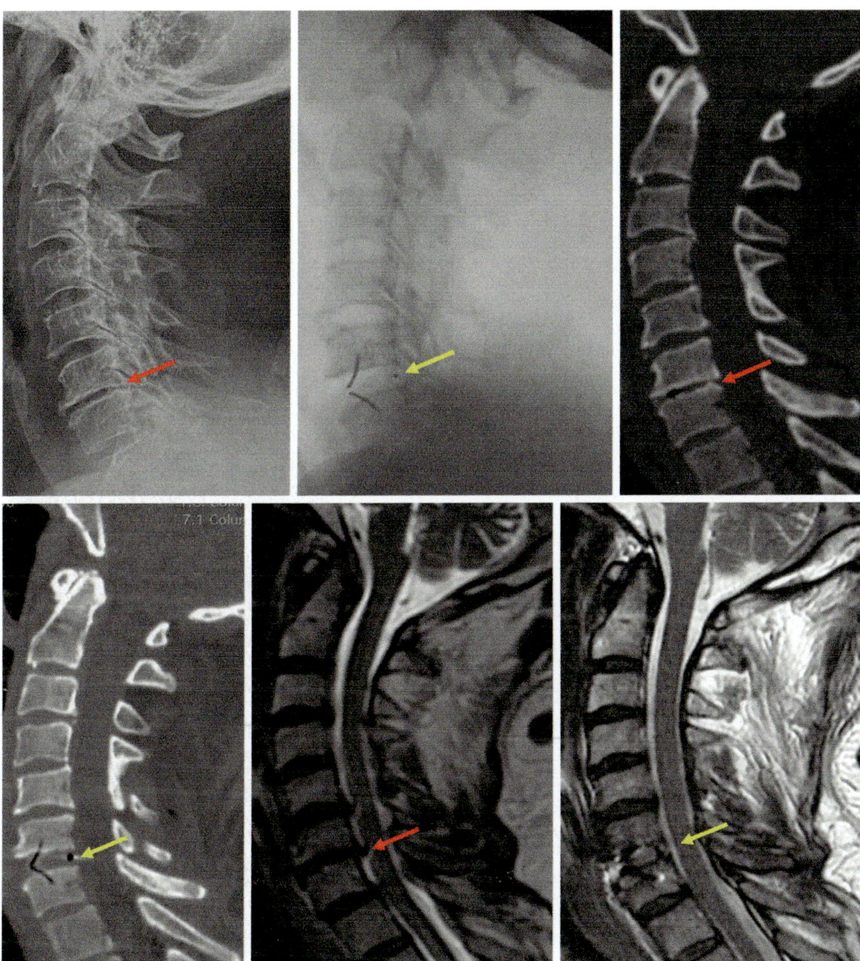

Fig. 26.11 Lateral and sagittal views of cervical X-rays, CT scan, and MRI of Case 1 comparing the preoperative (red arrow) and postoperative (yellow arrow) C6–C7 status

conservative measures, including NSAIDs, opioids, and physical therapy. Her pain started in the upper interscapular region and radiated down the lateral aspect of the shoulder and arm until the first three fingers of the left hand. The patient also complained of numbness in the palmar aspect of the first three fingers from her left hand. The neurological examination demonstrated decreased elbow extension strength (4−/5) and flexion and extension of the wrist (4+/5) of the left upper limb. Preoperative cervical MRI demonstrated foraminal stenosis at the C5–C6 and C6–C7 levels (Fig. 26.13).

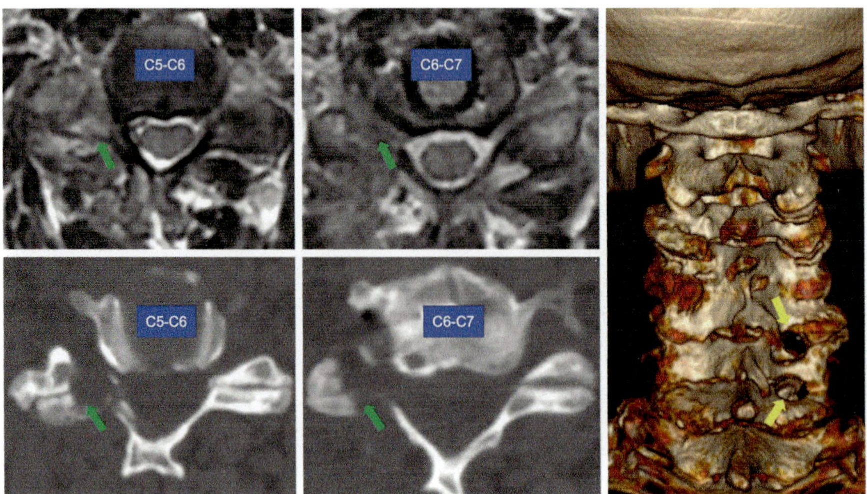

Fig. 26.12 Postoperative cervical MRI (upper panel) and CT scan (lower panel) axial views of Case 1. The green arrow points to the postoperative bone defect left by the UBE-PCIF procedure. The 3D CT scan shows the foraminotomies at C5–C6 and C6–C7 on the right side (yellow arrow)

Among the treatment options suggested to the patient, posterior cervical foraminotomies with a biportal endoscopic inclinatory technique at C5–C6 and C6–C7 on the left side were chosen. The C6–C7 inclinatory foraminotomy was the first one. Only tight bands were found when exploring the epidural space in the C7 axilla, and they were coagulated with the nerve hook-type bipolar radiofrequency.

Subsequently, the C5–C6 level was reached using the sliding technique. The foraminotomy was performed by first removing the upper edge of the C6 lamina until visualizing the SAP, which was partially removed. Next, the C6 nerve root was identified and freed from epidural adhesions. It was also possible to confirm a disc protrusion ventral to the nerve root and approached axillary (Video 26.3).

No incidents were reported during the procedure. The pain and numbness in the upper extremity improved markedly after the surgery (VAS 0/10). In addition, the weakness in the left wrist improved 2 weeks after the procedure, and the left triceps muscle strength deficit fully recovered in the postoperative month.

Postoperative imaging studies (MRI and CT scan) of the cervical spine demonstrated adequate decompression with the foraminotomies performed at C5–C6 and C6–C7 on the left side (Fig. 26.14).

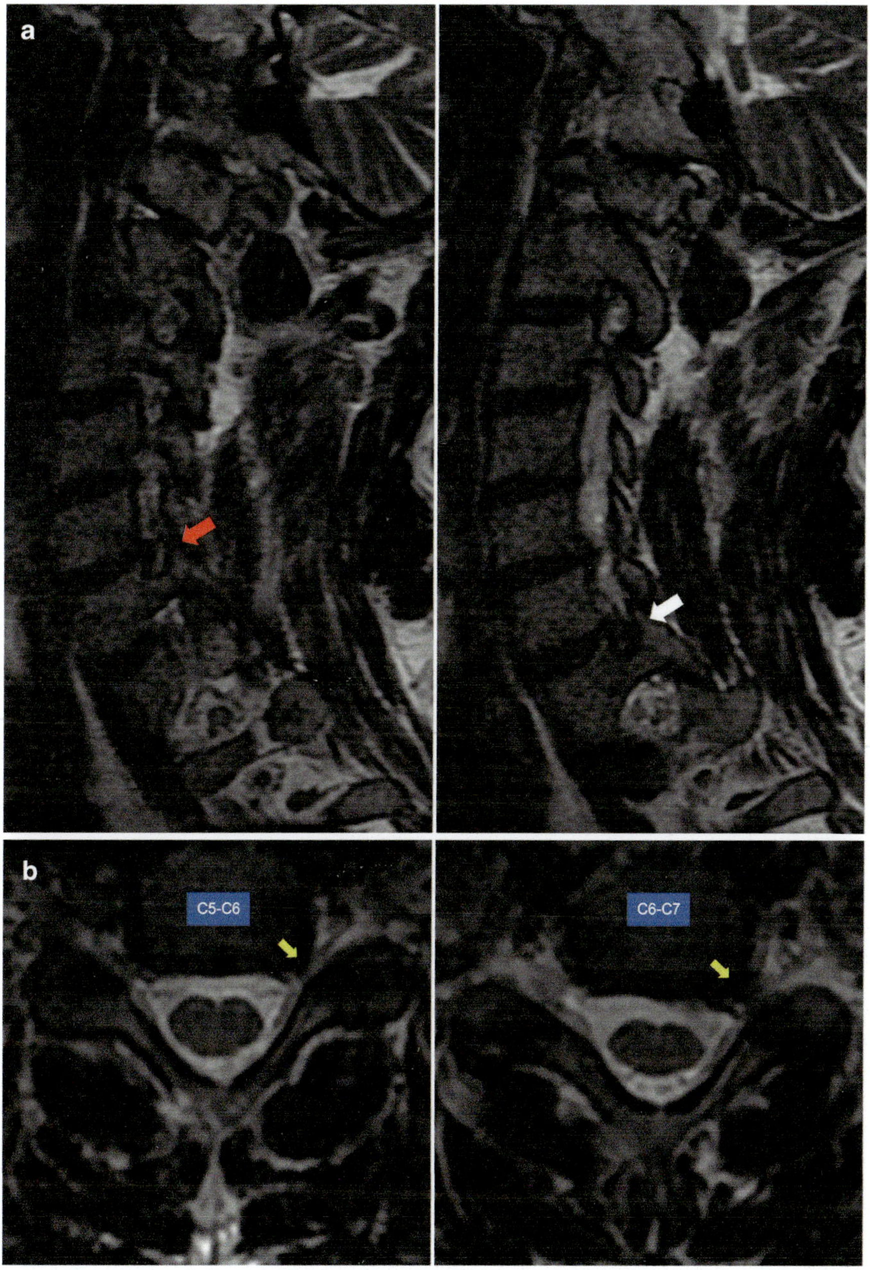

Fig. 26.13 Case 2 preoperative cervical MRI. (**a**) Left oblique sagittal views showing foraminal stenosis at C5–C6 (red arrow) and C6–C7 (white arrow). (**b**) Both levels (C5–C6 and C6–C7) with foraminal stenosis are associated with a lateral disc protrusion (yellow arrows)

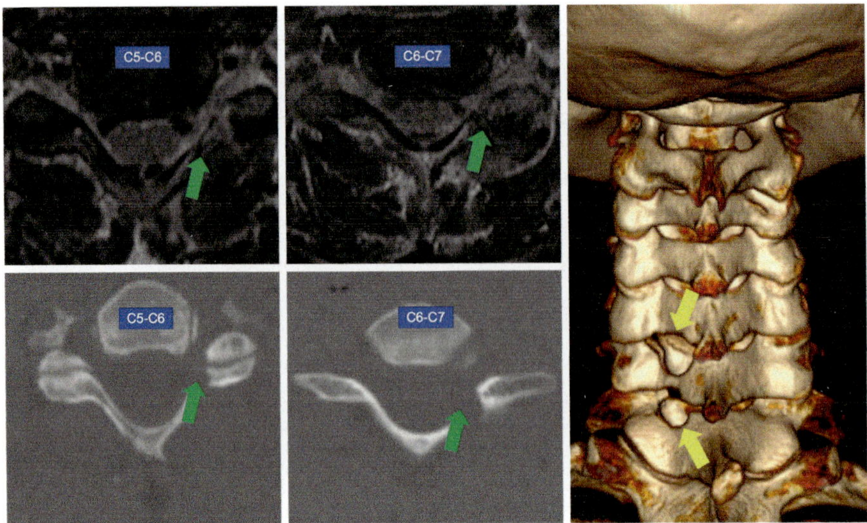

Fig. 26.14 Postoperative axial views of cervical MRI (upper panel) and CT scan (lower panel) from Case 2. The green arrow points to the postoperative bone defect left by the UBE-PCIF procedure on the left side. The 3D CT scan shows the foraminotomies at C5–C6 and C6–C7 on the left side (yellow arrow)

Discussion

Anterior cervical approaches for treating compressive radiculopathy have shown encouraging results over time. However, procedure-related morbidity for fusion or arthroplasty ranges from 13.2% to 19.3% [25, 26]. Different treatment options such as PCF have been used to treat highly selected patients to reduce collateral effects on the patient. Recently, more minimally invasive techniques have modified the PCF's performance for this purpose [2, 4].

Complications associated with uniportal endoscopic cervical foraminotomy are similar to those reported using any other technique. The following complications have been reported: access-related neck pain, injury or irritation of spinal nerves and spinal cord, intraoperative bleeding or postoperative epidural bleeding, dural damage, headache, seizures or postoperative neurological deficit caused by the increased pressure of continuous irrigation system, infections, impaired wound healing, surgical induced instability, and persistent symptoms [27, 28].

The reported effectiveness in patients who underwent PCF for cervical radiculopathy is 70–97% [3]. The clinical outcomes of the cases presented in this chapter are similar to those published in different series. For example, Skovrlj et al. [18] reported results from a series of 70 patients who underwent PCF and were followed for 32.1 months. The authors found a decrease in pain immediately after surgery, which was analyzed with scales such as the neck disability index (NDI) and the visual analog scale (VAS) for neck and arm pain; the improvement was also sustained during the follow-up time. Ruetten et al. [4] reported effectiveness with uniportal endoscopic PCF of 89% in 89 patients followed for 2 years.

PCF performed through a biportal endoscopic approach with an oblique or inclinatory angled trajectory is a relatively new adaptation introduced by Song et al. [24] in 2020. The authors treated 7 patients (3 men and 4 women) with a mean age of 59 ± 12.1 years, and 11 cervical levels, of which 3 underwent a discectomy through the same approach, and in 8 only exiting nerve decompression was performed. The patients were followed for 6.42 ± 2.99 months. The mean time of hospitalization was 5.71 ± 3.86 days. At the end of the follow-up, the authors did not observe any sagittal disbalance, instability, or disc height collapse regarding the UBE-PCIF. Radiculopathy symptoms improved from 7.71 ± 0.75 to 0.85 ± 0.69 in the postoperative VAS score and from 60.85 ± 26.85 to 10.57 ± 5.74 postoperatively in the NDI score.

These results remain similar to those reported in other PCF series and the cases illustrated in this chapter. Among their complications, they registered a durotomy treated with Gelfoam and a fibrin sealing patch without cerebrospinal fluid leakage.

The procedure-related advantages noted with the UBE-PCIF are the following:

1. The preservation of the facet joint is considerable since the mediolateral inclinatory (oblique) trajectory allows a more specific tunnel-shaped approach that follows the pathway of the exiting nerve root. For this purpose, an undercut of the ventral aspect of the facet joint is needed and not unroof the facet joint.
2. The transmuscular approach is more medial than the paraspinal, which means it crosses fewer muscles due to its sagittal and inclinatory nature compared with other more lateral procedures. As a result, it can provide a minimum postoperative neck pain.
3. This approach allows decompressing longer exiting nerve root length when necessary, preserving the dorsal part of the facet joint because the facet joint is not reached perpendicular but oblique.
4. The axillary area of the nerve root is easily accessible through this approach because the surgeon drills out the junction of the lamina and the SAP, which reaches directly starting the surgery.
5. The advantages associated with the biportal endoscopic technique include the visualization obtained through the endoscope and the clean surgical field due to continuous irrigation during the whole procedure and using the freer working instrument.

The technique's disadvantages lie in its complexity, especially when there is no experience in other biportal endoscopic procedures. In addition, decompression of the more distal part of the exiting nerve requires skills through the endoscope and surgical instruments to prevent a nerve root injury. Therefore, this technique can be complex for young surgeons starting their learning curve.

Tips and Pearls

- Correct triangulation with a mediolateral inclinatory trajectory is very important for the correct execution of the UBE-PCIF technique.
- The surgeon should not exaggerate the angle of the inclinatory trajectory as it may lose its orientation or injure vital cervical structures.

- The authors suggest that the first dilator be introduced to create the working portal with the ideal angulation concerning the case. Subsequently, the second dilator to create the endoscopic portal will only address the first one.
- It is highly recommended to perform an adequate epiperiosteal dissection to create sufficient space. This will lead to an easier and faster co-location of both portals in the surgical field.
- This approach can quickly access the axillary space by removing the medial part of the index level's laminofacet junction. Therefore, this landmark can guide the surgeon and facilitate the recognition of SAP.
- Due to the inclinatory trajectory of the approach, the surgeon can immediately locate the exit nerve root. Therefore, care must be taken during the drill out of the bone elements since there may be no ligamentum flavum protecting the exiting nerve. Only a thin periradicular membrane can be found over the nerve.
- The use of microsurgical curettes and angled-tip chisels can facilitate the removal of the most distal part of the SAP.
- It is necessary to have a bipolar radiofrequency with a blunt and fine tip to coagulate the periradicular venous plexuses since other broad-tip RF probes could damage the nerve.
- An anatomical based planning is essential for any case. For example, large and bifid spinous processes could obstruct the inclinatory trajectory. Furthermore, this UBE-PCIF is not recommended for central decompression of the cervical spinal canal.
- Leaving a drain at the end of the procedure can prevent epidural collections in the foraminotomy or the cervical spinal canal.

Conclusion

Posterior cervical inclinatory foraminotomy through the biportal endoscopic technique (UBE-PCIF) may be an option for patients with unilateral radiculopathy caused by stenosis of the foramen. The advantages of this approach are preserving more of the facet joint, especially in cases where it is required to decompress long tracts of the exiting nerve root. Other advantages regarding using the biportal endoscopic technique are the clear visualization of the anatomical structures through the endoscope and the continuous irrigation of saline during the procedure. However, this technique requires a steeper learning curve, so great experience with other biportal endoscopy procedures is advised.

References

1. Radhakrishnan K, Litchy WJ, O'Fallon WM, Kurland LT. Epidemiology of cervical radiculopathy. A population-based study from Rochester, Minnesota, 1976 through 1990. Brain. 1994;117(Pt 2):325–35.

2. Fessler RG, Khoo LT. Minimally invasive cervical microendoscopic foraminotomy: an initial clinical experience. Neurosurgery. 2002;51(5 Suppl):S37–45.
3. Dodwad SJ, Dodwad SN, Prasarn ML, Savage JW, Patel AA, Hsu WK. Posterior cervical foraminotomy: indications, technique, and outcomes. Clin Spine Surg. 2016;29(5):177–85.
4. Ruetten S, Komp M, Merk H, Godolias G. Full-endoscopic cervical posterior foraminotomy for the operation of lateral disc herniations using 5.9-mm endoscopes: a prospective, randomized, controlled study. Spine (Phila Pa 1976). 2008;33(9):940–8.
5. Church EW, Halpern CH, Faught RW, et al. Cervical laminoforaminotomy for radiculopathy: symptomatic and functional outcomes in a large cohort with long-term follow-up. Surg Neurol Int. 2014;5(Suppl 15):S536–43.
6. Zeidman SM, Ducker TB. Posterior cervical laminoforaminotomy for radiculopathy: review of 172 cases. Neurosurgery. 1993;33(3):356–62.
7. Jagannathan J, Sherman JH, Szabo T, Shaffrey CI, Jane JA. The posterior cervical foraminotomy in the treatment of cervical disc/osteophyte disease: a single-surgeon experience with a minimum of 5 years' clinical and radiographic follow-up. J Neurosurg Spine. 2009;10(4):347–56.
8. Grieve JP, Kitchen ND, Moore AJ, Marsh HT. Results of posterior cervical foraminotomy for treatment of cervical spondylitic radiculopathy. Br J Neurosurg. 2000;14(1):40–3.
9. Rhee JM, Yoon T, Riew KD. Cervical radiculopathy. J Am Acad Orthop Surg. 2007;15(8):486–94. https://doi.org/10.5435/00124635-200708000-00005.
10. Woods BI, Hilibrand AS. Cervical radiculopathy: epidemiology, etiology, diagnosis, and treatment. J Spinal Disord Tech. 2015;28(5):E251–9.
11. Alentado VJ, Lubelski D, Steinmetz MP, Benzel EC, Mroz TE. Optimal duration of conservative management prior to surgery for cervical and lumbar radiculopathy: a literature review. Global Spine J. 2014;4(4):279–86.
12. Scoville WB. Recent developments in the diagnosis and treatment of cervical ruptured intervertebral discs. Proc Am Fed Clin Res. 1945;2:23.
13. Tumialán LM, Ponton RP, Gluf WM. Management of unilateral cervical radiculopathy in the military: the cost effectiveness of posterior cervical foraminotomy compared with anterior cervical discectomy and fusion. Neurosurg Focus. 2010;28(5):E17.
14. Adamson TE. The impact of minimally invasive cervical spine surgery. Invited submission from the Joint Section Meeting on Disorders of the Spine and Peripheral Nerves, March 2004. J Neurosurg Spine. 2004;1(1):43–6.
15. Hilton DL Jr. Minimally invasive tubular access for posterior cervical foraminotomy with three-dimensional microscopic visualization and localization with anterior/posterior imaging. Spine J. 2007;7(2):154–8.
16. Park JH, Jun SG, Jung JT, Lee SJ. Posterior percutaneous endoscopic cervical foraminotomy and diskectomy with unilateral biportal endoscopy. Orthopedics. 2017;40(5):e779–83.
17. Clarke MJ, Ecker RD, Krauss WE, McClelland RL, Dekutoski MB. Same-segment and adjacent-segment disease following posterior cervical foraminotomy. J Neurosurg Spine. 2007;6(1):5–9.
18. Skovrlj B, Gologorsky Y, Haque R, Fessler RG, Qureshi SA. Complications, outcomes, and need for fusion after minimally invasive posterior cervical foraminotomy and microdiscectomy. Spine J. 2014;14(10):2405–11.
19. Zdeblick TA, Zou D, Warden KE, McCabe R, Kunz D, Vanderby R. Cervical stability after foraminotomy. A biomechanical in vitro analysis. J Bone Joint Surg Am. 1992;74(1):22–7.
20. Caridi JM, Pumberger M, Hughes AP. Cervical radiculopathy: a review. HSS J. 2011;7(3):265–72.
21. Henderson CM, Hennessy RG, Shuey HM Jr, Shackelford EG. Posterior-lateral foraminotomy as an exclusive operative technique for cervical radiculopathy: a review of 846 consecutively operated cases. Neurosurgery. 1983;13(5):504–12.
22. Kumar GR, Maurice-Williams RS, Bradford R. Cervical foraminotomy: an effective treatment for cervical spondylotic radiculopathy. Br J Neurosurg. 1998;12(6):563–8.

23. Chang JC, Park HK, Choi SK. Posterior cervical inclinatory foraminotomy for spondylotic radiculopathy preliminary. J Korean Neurosurg Soc. 2011;49(5):308–13.
24. Song KS, Lee CW. The biportal endoscopic posterior cervical inclinatory foraminotomy for cervical radiculopathy: technical report and preliminary results. Neurospine. 2020;17(Suppl 1):S145–53.
25. Bertalanffy H, Eggert HR. Complications of anterior cervical discectomy without fusion in 450 consecutive patients. Acta Neurochir. 1989;99(1–2):41–50.
26. Tasiou A, Giannis T, Brotis AG, et al. Anterior cervical spine surgery-associated complications in a retrospective case-control study. J Spine Surg. 2017;3(3):444–59.
27. Yang JS, Chu L, Chen L, Chen F, Ke ZY, Deng ZL. Anterior or posterior approach of full-endoscopic cervical discectomy for cervical intervertebral disc herniation? A comparative cohort study. Spine (Phila Pa 1976). 2014;39(21):1743–50.
28. Komp M, Oezdemir S, Hahn P, Ruetten S. Full-endoscopic posterior foraminotomy surgery for cervical disc herniations. Vollendoskopische dorsale Foraminotomie zur Operation des zervikalen Bandscheibenvorfalls. Oper Orthop Traumatol. 2018;30(1):13–24.

Chapter 27
Biportal Endoscopic Posterior Decompression for Degenerative Cervical Myelopathy

Wei Zhang, Cheng Wei, and Javier Quillo-Olvera

Abbreviations

ACCF	Anterior cervical corpectomy and fusion
ACDF	Anterior cervical discectomy and fusion
AP	Anteroposterior
BESS	Biportal endoscopic spine surgery
CT	Computed tomography
DCM	Degenerative cervical myelopathy
FJ	Facet joint
FL	Flavum ligament
IAP	Inferior articular process
ILS	Interlaminar space
Lt	Left
MISS	Minimally invasive spine surgery
mJOA	Modified Japanese Orthopedic Association

Supplementary Information The online version contains supplementary material available at [https://doi.org/10.1007/978-3-031-14736-4_27].

W. Zhang
Department of Orthopaedics, Hangzhou Traditional Chinese Medicine Hospital Affiliated to Zhejiang Chinese Medical University, Hangzhou, China
e-mail: volcano8060@163.com

C. Wei
Department of Orthopaedics, Hangzhou Ding Qiao Hospital, Hangzhou, China
e-mail: 837283441@qq.com

J. Quillo-Olvera (✉)
The Brain and Spine Care, Minimally Invasive Spine Surgery Group, Hospital H+ Querétaro, Spine Clinic, Querétaro, México
e-mail: neuroqomd@gmail.com

J. Quillo-Olvera et al. (eds.), *Unilateral Biportal Endoscopy of the Spine*,
https://doi.org/10.1007/978-3-031-14736-4_27

MRI	Magnetic resonance imaging
MVL	Meningovertebral ligament
OPLL	Ossification of posterior longitudinal ligament
RF	Radiofrequency
Rt	Right
SAP	Superior articular process
SP	Spinous process
UBE	Unilateral biportal endoscopy
ULBD	Unilateral laminotomy for bilateral decompression

Introduction

Progressive spinal cord compression associated with age-related degenerative changes that may include facet arthropathy, spondylosis, and disc degeneration; subluxation of the vertebral bodies; and hypertrophy, ossification, or calcification of the supporting ligaments, which can narrow the cervical spinal canal, is commonly referred to as degenerative cervical myelopathy (DCM) [1, 2].

Repeated static and dynamic injury to the spinal cord in a setting of DCM causes vascular changes, specific inflammation, alterations in the brain-spinal cord barrier, and apoptosis, causing demyelination, neuronal death, and astrogliosis [3, 4].

DCM incidence and prevalence in North America are estimated to be 41 and 605 per million, respectively. Although this may not be accurate throughout the world, the degenerative spinal disease is becoming more constant concerning increasing age in the world population [5, 6]. Therefore, DCM diagnosis should include detailed patient history, a complete neurological exam, X-rays, CT, and MRI studies.

Surgical strategies to decompress the spinal cord in DCM may be limited, especially in aging patients with multiple comorbidities and a high risk of complications. Anterior cervical discectomy and fusion (ACDF) may not be an appropriate option in patients who have previously undergone anterior approach of the neck, when the compression vector is predominantly dorsal, or in patients in whom failure of the fusion process is anticipated due to their comorbidities, in addition to the well-known associated postoperative dysphagia, especially in multilevel and octogenarians [7–10]. Laminoplasty and laminectomy have been associated with damage to the posterior cervical soft tissues, including muscles and ligaments, persistent axial pain, restriction of neck movements, loss of cervical lordosis, restenosis, and even kyphotic deformity [8, 11–13].

Due to the above, multiple techniques to decompress the spinal cord in the cervical region in patients with DCM have been postulated [14–18] to preserve the paraspinal muscles, posterior elements such as the lamina, spinous process, supra- and interspinous ligaments, and facet joints.

Among minimally invasive spine surgery (MISS) techniques, biportal endoscopic surgery stands out for many reasons. Multiple authors have confirmed its effectiveness in decompressing lumbar neural elements [19–25]. Furthermore, the versatility with which the surgical procedure is carried out is remarkable when compared to uniportal endoscopy; the maneuverability of the two ports, one for the endoscope and the other for the working tools, used independently, and the ability to use surgical instruments similar to those used in microsurgery make biportal endoscopic surgery (BESS) a feasible option to perform spinal cord decompression in patients with DCM. This chapter describes the biportal endoscopic technique for posterior cervical decompression.

Indications and Contraindications

Patients with cervical spinal cord compression due to degenerative causes should be allocated in different populations regarding the severity of the myelopathy [26]. Therefore, they can be classified as follows:

1. Mild myelopathy: defined as a modified Japanese Orthopedic Association (mJOA) score of 15–17
2. Moderate myelopathy: mJOA = 12–14
3. Severe myelopathy: mJOA = 11
4. Nonmyelopathic patients with evidence of cord compression

Fehlings et al. [27] developed the following recommendations based on a study for guideline development:

1. For patients with severe DCM (mJOA = 0–11), the recommendation is surgical treatment.
2. For patients with moderate DCM (mJOA = 12–14), surgical treatment is recommended.
3. For patients with mild DCM (mJOA = 15–17), the recommendation is to offer early surgical treatment before progressing to a more severe state. If conservative treatment is provided, the patient should be offered close monitoring and education about the possible progressive evolution of symptoms derived from spinal cord compression. If there is neurological deterioration during follow-up, surgical treatment should be advised.
4. For nonmyelopathic patients with evidence of spinal cord compression on imaging but no signs or symptoms of radiculopathy: The recommendation is not surgical but to advise the patient on what decision to make in the face of the possibility of neurological deterioration and closely monitor its evolution.
5. For nonmyelopathic patients with evidence of spinal cord compression on imaging and signs and symptoms of radiculopathy: These patients should be informed that there is a high possibility of developing cervical myelopathy. Therefore, surgery is recommended, but if conservative treatment is chosen, close surveillance and alerts should be given to possible early signs and symptoms of myelopathy for recognition and prompt surgical treatment.

Knowing which patients must undergo surgery for DCM, the chosen method will depend on the pathological characteristics of the compression and the patient. Senile patients with a history of significant comorbidities may not tolerate or present complications associated with orthodox decompression methods such as laminectomies, multilevel ACDF, ACCF, and posterior cervical fixation. MISS for posterior cervical decompression may be an option, of which BESS would be well indicated. Mainly patients with a posterior compression vector such as hypertrophy of the flavum ligament (FL), myeloradiculopathy due to central or foraminal cervical spondylosis, or stenosis associated with ossification of the posterior longitudinal ligament (OPLL), and multilevel stenosis not more than three levels.

However, it is not recommended to perform BESS for DCM associated with instability; OPLL involving more than 50% of the canal, congenital stenosis, and soft and central cervical disc herniation; and other causes of cervical stenosis such as trauma, infections, tumors, and deformity, since these warrant another therapeutic protocol.

Surgical Technique

Step 1: Patient Positioning and Anesthesia

The patient is placed in a reverse Trendelenburg prone position on an abdominal frame to decrease abdominal pressure, and facilitate the venous return, thus indirectly reducing intraoperative bleeding (Fig. 27.1). The recommended anesthesia for this procedure is general.

Step 2: Planning for Entry Points

A horizontal line is drawn through the intervertebral space at the index level. Then, a longitudinal line tangential to the medial border of the lateral masses (Son's line) or even at the midpoint of the lateral masses (Zhang's line) will determine how lateral the approach should be. Subsequently, the incisions will be located 1–1.5 cm above and below the intervertebral space of the index level (Fig. 27.2). If a multilevel decompression is required, the caudal incision will be used as the cranial for the lower segment, and the caudal will be located 1–1.5 cm below the next intervertebral level.

Step 3: Posterior Cervical Biportal Approach

The surgeon will make a pair of 7 mm incisions in the skin and fascia. The incisions can be made transverse or longitudinal. It is advised that the fascia be incised appropriately to allow the continuous flow of saline during the procedure. The working

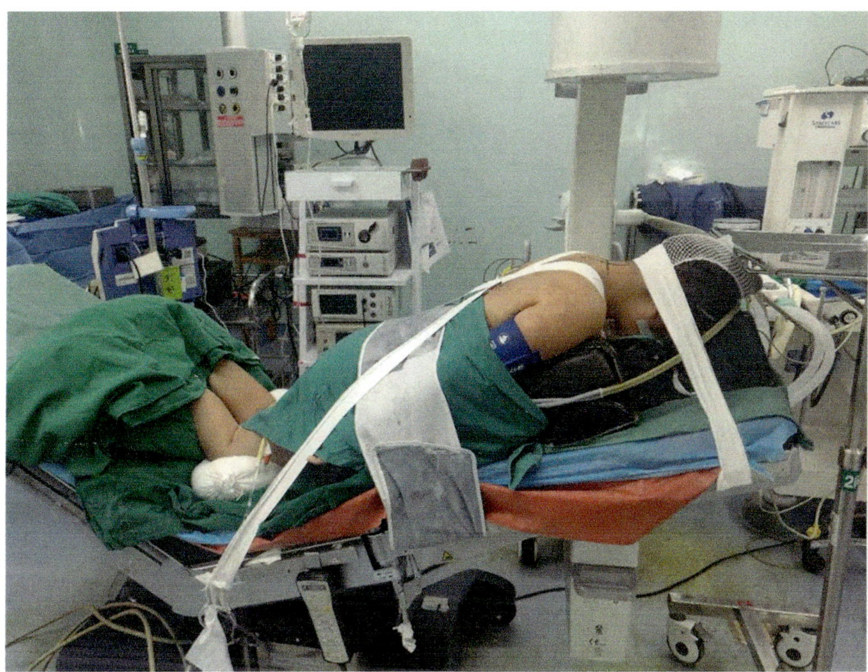

Fig. 27.1 Reverse Trendelenburg prone position for posterior cervical unilateral biportal endoscopy (UBE) decompression

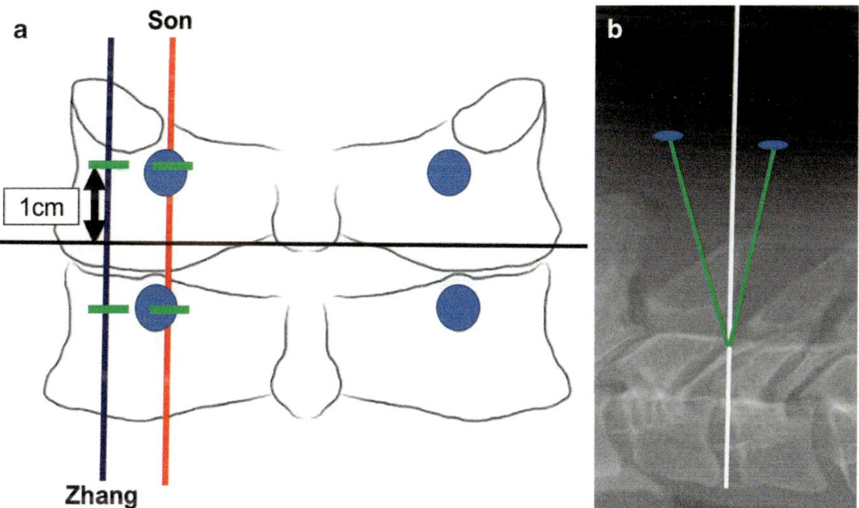

Fig. 27.2 Planning the incisions for a posterior cervical biportal endoscopic decompression. (**a**) Anatomical design showing a cervical level in AP view. Son's line passes medial to the lateral masses, while Zhang's line passes through the midpoint of the facet joints. The incisions will be located 1–1.5 cm above and below the intervertebral space intersecting one of these two lines. (**b**) Lateral view of a cervical X-ray. The disc space is intersected by the white line. The green lines represent the biportal triangular approach, and the blue circles both incisions

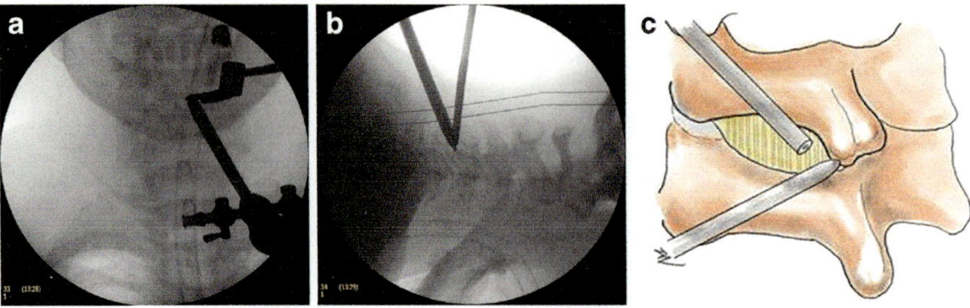

Fig. 27.3 Triangular approach. (**a**) C-arm AP view showing both portals on the right side. Both portals are addressed towards the spinolaminar junction, and the working cannula is in the cranial incision and the endoscopic trocar in the caudal. (**b**) The same triangular approach in the lateral view. (**c**) Drawing exemplifying the biportal approach with the two instruments meeting in the spinolaminar junction

portal will be created first. It must be remembered that the surgeon will be ipsilateral to the approach side, and in right-sided procedures, with a right-handed surgeon, the cranial incision will be used for the working portal and the caudal incision for the endoscopic. On the left side, this will be the opposite. A 5 mm dilator will be used to initiate the triangular approach. This dilator will be inserted through the incision used as a working portal and addressed towards the spinolaminar junction. Upon palpation, the surgeon will dissect the ipsilateral superior lamina bone surface and feel its inferior border at the index level. Subsequently, dilators with a larger diameter will be introduced sequentially until reaching the 7 mm outer diameter. Finally, the working cannula will be inserted. This process will be confirmed by intraoperative fluoroscopy in AP and lateral projections. The same process will be carried out with the viewing portal (Fig. 27.3).

Step 4: Creating the Working Space

When inserting the endoscope, it is essential to confirm the correct flow of the irrigated saline. First, the fluid must exit through the working portal. Subsequently, the surgeon must identify the surgical tool with the endoscope, called the co-location of both instruments. For beginners, it could be time consuming.

The authors recommend simplifying the instrument's location with the endoscope by correctly approaching the spine through the biportal technique. If both ports are crossed, the endoscope will not be able to visualize the surgical instrument, and if either of the two portals is located outside the surgical field, they will not be able to be met at the same point. Therefore, during the biportal triangular approach, the surgeon must create each port independently. Next, he or she must address the dilator used to create each port to a common point, the spinolaminar junction. Subsequently, both portals must coincide in that bone landmark before introducing the endoscope. Finally, the surgeon must feel that both dilators introduced through the incisions coincide, palpate the same anatomical reference, and confirm it with C-arm images.

The working space will be created by removing or coagulating the soft tissue adjacent to the bony elements to identify them (Fig. 27.4). The surgeon must observe with the endoscope both laminae (upper and lower) of the index level, the interlaminar space, the V-point (confluence of both laminae), and the ipsilateral facet joint (Fig. 27.5; Video 27.1).

Step 5: Over-the-Top Circumferential Bone Removal

This step consists of performing decompression in both circumferential and over-the-top fashion. The surgeon will use the high-speed drilling system with a 3 mm diamond burr tip to reduce the neural elements' risk of transgressing. In addition, he

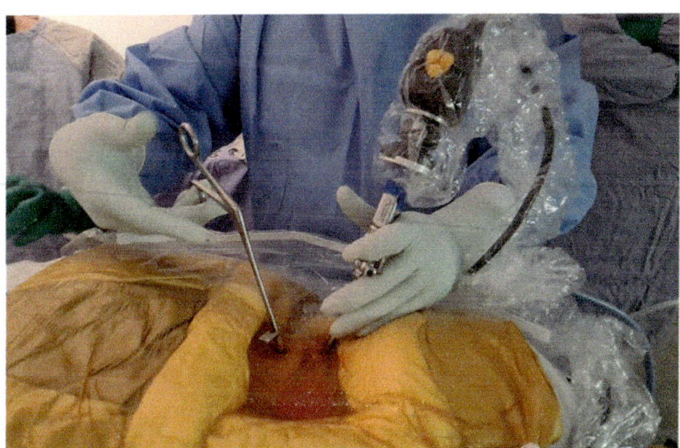

Fig. 27.4 The working space is created with the RF probe or pituitary forceps; moreover, the surgeon should confirm the proper inflow and outflow through both portals

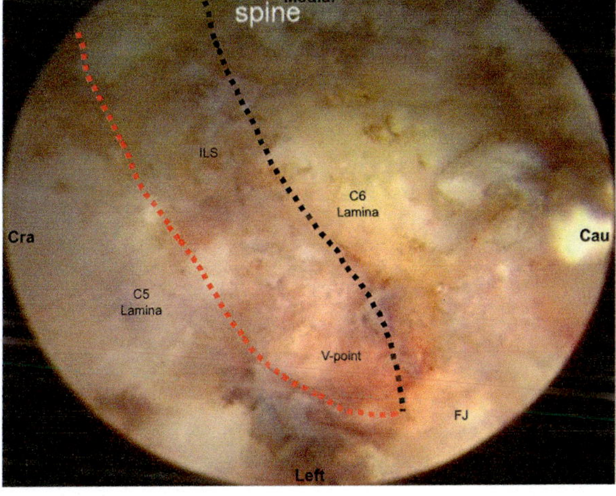

Fig. 27.5 Posterior cervical unilateral biportal endoscopic (UBE) decompression of C5–C6 on the left side. After creating the working space, the bone references can be identified. The red dotted line limits the inferior border of C5 lamina, and the black dotted line edges the upper margin of C6 lamina; both confluence in the V-point. *Cra* crania, *Cau* caudal, *ILS* interlaminar space, *FJ* facet joint

or she will use the ligamentum flavum as a protective barrier for the dural sac. Bone decompression consists of circumferentially performing a superior and inferior laminotomy until identifying the craniocaudal attachments of the flavum ligament (FL). The same will happen with the ipsilateral and contralateral undercutting of both facet joints (FJs). It can be removed when finding the lateral portion of the FL on both sides. Unilateral laminotomy with bilateral decompression (ULBD) is achieved when the surgeon removes the spinous process's base to address the contralateral side, similar to a lumbar ULBD. However, unlike other MISS techniques, in BESS, there is no need to turn to the surgical table since the endoscope allows the visualization of contralateral structures if we angle its trajectory, and the 30° lens will enable us to achieve a more lateral and deep view, which in these cases is very useful. The surgeon must always keep in mind that he or she is working in the cervical region. For this reason, he or she must avoid any excessive manipulation in the central canal nor apply pressure with any instrument. Bone decompression can be completed using Kerrison punches of different sizes (Fig. 27.6; Video 27.2).

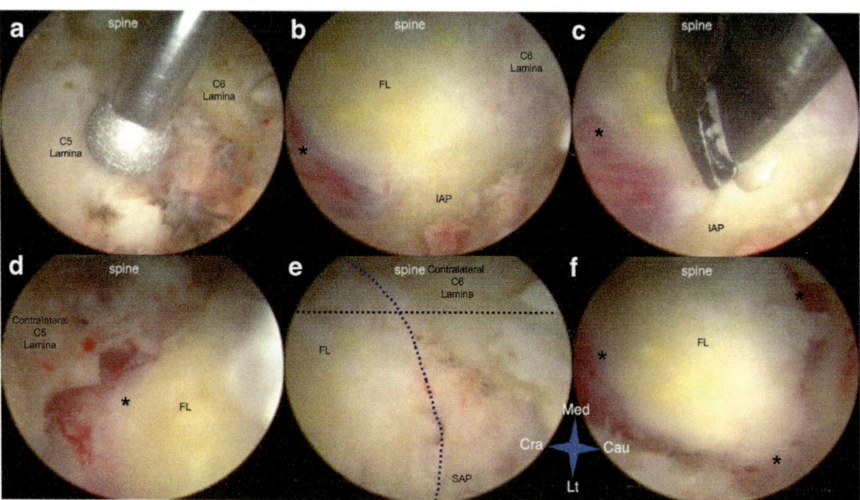

Fig. 27.6 Bone removal during a left-sided C5–C6 posterior cervical UBE decompression. (**a**) The circumferential bone removal starts with the ipsilateral superior laminotomy. (**b**) The endpoint of the bone removal is when the FL attachments (asterisk) are identified. (**c**) The undercutting of IAP and SAP first in the ipsilateral side and after in the contralateral. (**d**) Contralateral superior laminotomy. (**e**) Contralateral inferior laminotomy. (**f**) Complete FL detached. *Cra* cranial, *Cau* caudal, *Med* medial, *Lt* left, *FL* flavum ligament, *IAP* inferior articular process, *SAP* superior articular process, (asterisk) attachments of FL

Step 6: Flavectomy and Neural Decompression

After circumferential bone decompression and exposing the attachments of the FL, it will be removed. The flavectomy can be en bloc or also piecemeal (Fig. 27.7). A crucial consideration in this step is to meticulously remove its ventral aspect from the dural sac due to possible adhesions or meningovertebral ligaments that can firmly fix it to the dorsal part of the dural sac, elevating the risk of a dural injury (Fig. 27.8). After flavectomy, the dural sac must be inspected, and dural pulsation and exhaustive hemostasis are confirmed; finally, epidural drainage can be left, and the incisions are closed to conclude the procedure (Video 27.3).

Fig. 27.7 En bloc flavectomy after C5–C6 UBE-ULBD

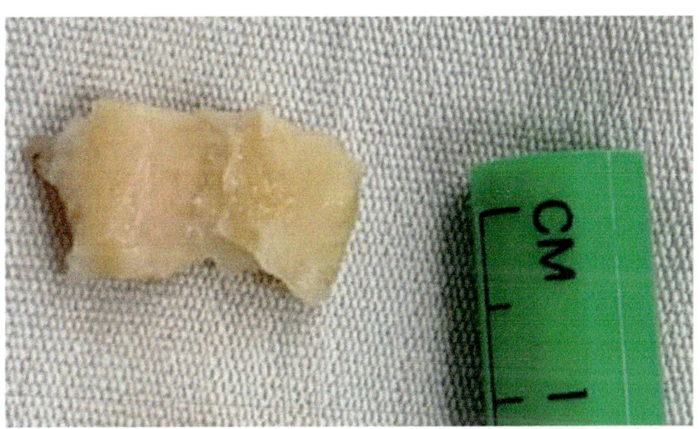

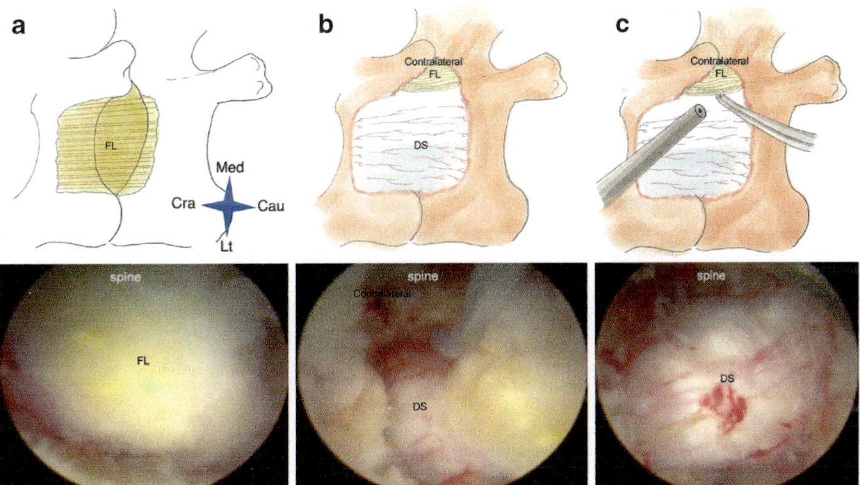

Fig. 27.8 Blocks composed of draws (upper) and endoscopic intraoperative images (lower) showing the flavectomy and direct decompression of the dural sac in a left-sided C5–C6 UBE-ULBD. (**a**) The free edges of the FL have been exposed cardinally. (**b**) The flavectomy is extended to the contralateral side. (**c**) The dural sac at C5–C6 has been decompressed bilaterally

Illustrated Case

Case 1

An 88-year-old male in whom his family noted difficulty moving his arms and legs with 4 weeks of evolution. The patient cannot stand or walk and has numbness in the limbs with anesthesia in both hands. He also has hypertension, has suffered two heart attacks, and is receiving antiplatelet therapy. Neurological examination revealed quadriparesis of 3/5, exacerbated tendon reflexes, and bilateral Babinski's sign. The patient had an increased range of motion at C4–C5 observed on lateral flexion and extension X-ray films (Fig. 27.9). Preoperative cervical MRI showed a multilevel cervical spinal stenosis at C2–C3, C3–C4, and C3–C5, with compression of the spinal cord predominantly at C3–C4 and C4–C5 due to hypertrophy of the ligamentum flavum, as well as hyperintensity in T2-weighted image at C4–C5 (Fig. 27.10). He was diagnosed with severe DCM (mJOA = 8) and underwent surgery using a posterior cervical UBE-ULBD C2–C3, C3–C4, and C4–C5 and subsequently an ACDF C4–C5 in a second stage. The radiological outcomes were satisfactory. The postoperative cervical MRI showed an adequate spinal cord decompression (Fig. 27.11). At the 6-month follow-up, the patient improved his mJOA score to 12, returning to walking with assistance and improving limb numbness.

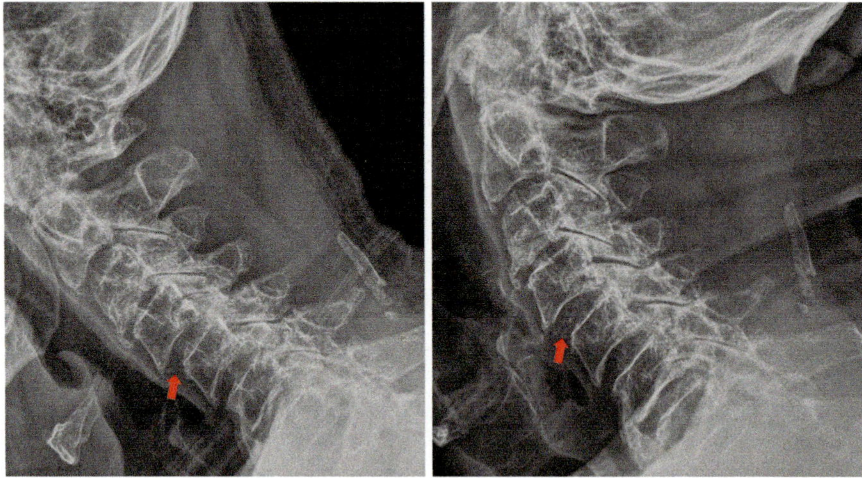

Fig. 27.9 Preoperative cervical X-ray on lateral flexion and extension films of Case 1. The red arrow points to C4–C5 instability

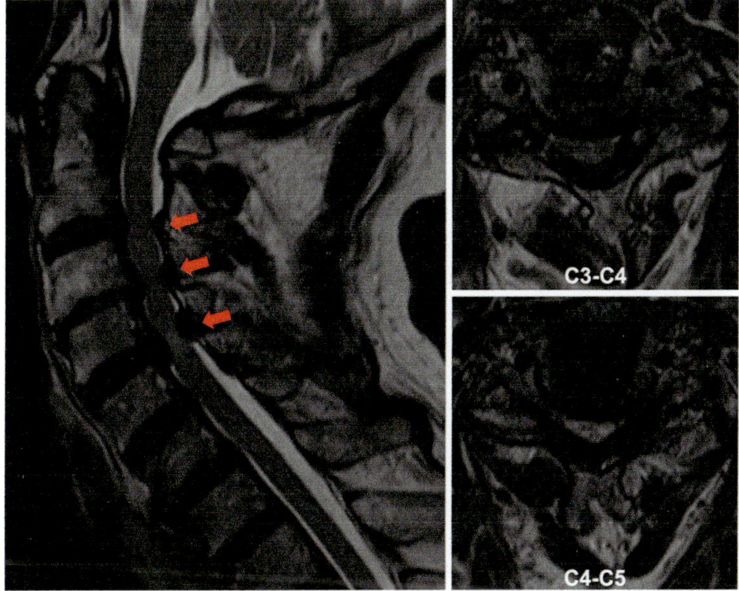

Fig. 27.10 Preoperative cervical MRI of Case 1. The red arrows point to C2–C3, C3–C4, and C4–C5 spinal cord compression on the sagittal view. The axial views at C3–C4 and C4–C5 show severe central stenosis due to FL hypertrophy

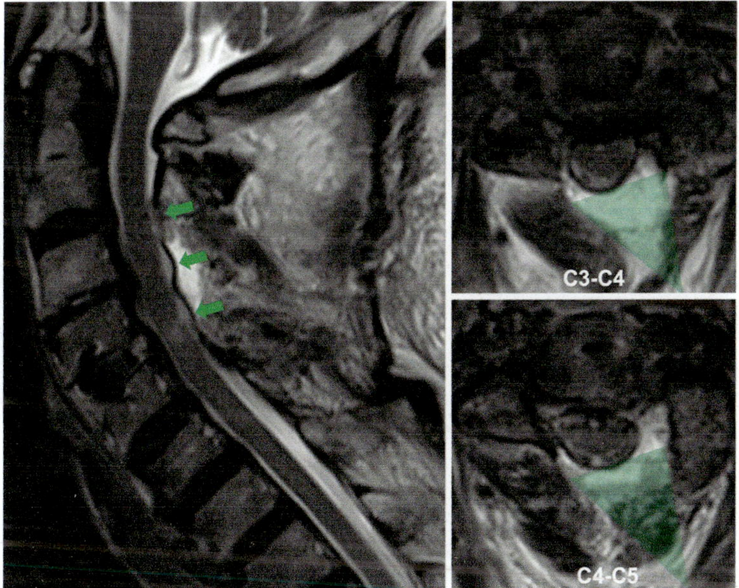

Fig. 27.11 The postoperative cervical MRI of Case 1 shows a C4–C5 intersomatic stabilization through an ACDF procedure in the sagittal view. Also, sufficient spinal cord decompression can be observed at C2–C3, C3–C4, and C4–C5 achieved by a posterior cervical multilevel UBE-ULBD. In addition, the axial views at C3–C4 and C4–C5 demonstrated expansion of the dural sac after the surgery

Discussion

Direct decompression of the spinal cord through biportal endoscopic surgery is a minimally invasive option associated with preserving the extensor muscles of the neck, facet joints, inter- and supraspinous ligaments, and other paraspinal muscles, as occurs with tubular microsurgery and other minimally invasive techniques [28].

These advantages finally make it possible to preserve the segment's motion and avoid the impact that a more aggressive surgery would have on the health of a patient with DCM who is elderly and has other morbidities.

According to a 2017 study [27], the incidence of complications in patients treated surgically for DCM is low and includes cervical axial pain (5.6%), laryngeal nerve injury/dysphagia (2.2%), instrumentation/graft complication (2.0%), C5 radiculopathy or palsy (1.9%), pseudoarthrosis (1.8%), infection (2.1%), adjacent segment disease (1.5%), dural tear/cerebrospinal fluid leak (1.4%), worsening of myelopathy (1.3%), hematoma (0.9%), new radiculopathy/palsy (not C5) (0.9%), neurologic deterioration (0.9%), delayed wound healing (0.8%), dysphonia (0.7%), postoperative deformity (0.5%), bed sores (0.8%), death (0.3%), stroke/transient ischemia attack (0.3%), esophageal injury (0.0%), cardiopulmonary events (3.3%), fracture (2.1%), and reoperation/revision surgery (1.4%). Despite its low incidence, it is still worrying that an elderly patient suffers a complication related to the surgical procedure due to the random clinical course that can follow after the adverse event.

Minimally invasive unilateral laminotomy with bilateral decompression (ULBD) is not new [9, 17]. However, what is new is performing it through biportal endoscopic surgery (BESS), due to the multiple technical advantages observed in its execution, for example:

In spinal cord decompression of the cervical spine, precision and adequate maneuverability of the surgical instruments are required to avoid excessive manipulation of the dural sac, traction of the neural elements, and pressure on them that lead to irreparable neurological damage.

Although this is related to the skills of each surgeon, the technique plays an important role. For example, in uniportal endoscopic surgery, the surgeon must learn to control the surgical instrument, the working cannula, and the endoscopic system all at the same time. The loss of control of any device that integrates the uniportal endoscopic technique would be catastrophic. In this technique, the surgeon controls the endoscopic system and the working cannula with the nondominant hand and the surgical instrument with the dominant hand. However, long-sized surgical tools compared with standard microsurgical instruments are used in most uniportal spinal endoscopic systems, which could be problematic for use through the integrated-lens working channel. That is usually tough for surgeons without training in full endoscopy, so cervical procedures are not recommended until a high level of experience is reached [18].

In biportal endoscopic surgery, the surgeon has the freedom to move his or her surgical instrument without restrictions and independently of the endoscopic lens. In addition, using the endoscopic lens with greater freedom and from different inclination angles provides safety and confidence during the procedure. However, this advantage does not replace the need to have a comprehensive experience in posterior cervical approaches through open surgery, microsurgery, tubular surgery, and later uni- or biportal endoscopy.

Another critical issue related to water-based endoscopic procedures (uniportal and biportal) is the water pressure entering the epidural space during the operation. Continuous fluid irrigation enables clear, high-quality visualization of anatomical structures, allowing precise endoscopic surgery.

However, the hydrostatic pressure of the irrigated fluid can be associated with epidural hypertension with large-scale neurological effects, which is why the surgeon must set the initial water pressure between 20 and 30 mmHg in his or her posterior cervical UBE procedure [29]. Avoid increasing pressure during the procedure. And always before continuing with the biportal endoscopic procedure, the surgeon must confirm the inflow and outflow of the saline through the cannula located in the working portal and avoid in any way that the irrigated saline stagnates the soft tissues [30]. Another recommendation is to avoid performing the flavectomy until bone decompression has been completed.

Another recommendation for the surgeon is to leave an epidural drain at the end of the biportal endoscopic procedure to avoid collections, such as hematomas. However, adequate hemostasis should always be the priority throughout the surgery. It can be achieved using the bipolar RF probe with a minimum intensity to avoid a thermal injury of the spinal cord. Also, bone wax in the bleeding derived from the laminotomy or the medial undercutting of the FJ can be used, and there are also several hemostatic matrices on the market as a suitable option in cases of layer bleeding.

After decompression, the dural sac should be explored before removing the endoscope from the surgical field to recognize inadvertent dural tears leading to cerebrospinal fluid leakage. In the case of identifying a punctiform dural tear, it is possible to choose to seal it with an analogous patch of dura mater and fibrin glue. If the tear is larger, direct closure should be considered on a case-by-case basis.

Conclusion

Posterior cervical decompression through UBE-ULBD is a novel and feasible option to treat cervical spinal cord compression in patients with DCM in selected cases. Its advantages are those observed in other minimally invasive cervical procedures, such as preserving cervical stabilizing structures and a minor collateral effect in elderly patients with other morbidities. In addition, posterior cervical UBE-ULBD is associated with excellent visualization and greater freedom with the working instrument introduced into the surgical field independently of the endoscope. However, there is little evidence confirming superior results of the posterior cervical UBE-ULBD versus other minimally invasive options. Therefore, its use is at the surgeon's discretion experienced in biportal endoscopic surgery.

References

1. Tetreault L, Goldstein CL, Arnold P, et al. Degenerative cervical myelopathy: a spectrum of related disorders affecting the aging spine. Neurosurgery. 2015;77(Suppl 4):S51–67.
2. Yamaguchi S, Mitsuhara T, Abiko M, Takeda M, Kurisu K. Epidemiology and overview of the clinical spectrum of degenerative cervical myelopathy. Neurosurg Clin N Am. 2018;29(1):1–12.
3. Akter F, Kotter M. Pathobiology of degenerative cervical myelopathy. Neurosurg Clin N Am. 2018;29(1):13–9.
4. Kalsi-Ryan S, Karadimas SK, Fehlings MG. Cervical spondylotic myelopathy: the clinical phenomenon and the current pathobiology of an increasingly prevalent and devastating disorder. Neuroscientist. 2013;19(4):409–21.
5. Nouri A, Tetreault L, Singh A, Karadimas SK, Fehlings MG. Degenerative cervical myelopathy: epidemiology, genetics, and pathogenesis. Spine (Phila Pa 1976). 2015;40(12):E675–93.
6. Fehlings MG, Tetreault L, Nater A, et al. The aging of the global population: the changing epidemiology of disease and spinal disorders. Neurosurgery. 2015;77(Suppl 4):S1–5.
7. Kim J, Heo DH, Lee DC, Chung HT. Biportal endoscopic unilateral laminotomy with bilateral decompression for the treatment of cervical spondylotic myelopathy. Acta Neurochir. 2021;163(9):2537–43.
8. Zhu C, Cheng W, Wang D, Pan H, Zhang W. A helpful third portal for unilateral biportal endoscopic decompression in patients with cervical spondylotic myelopathy: a technical note. World Neurosurg. 2022;161:75–81.
9. Minamide A, Yoshida M, Nakagawa Y, et al. Long-term clinical outcomes of microendoscopic laminotomy for cervical spondylotic myelopathy: a 5-year follow-up study compared with conventional laminoplasty. Clin Spine Surg. 2021;34(10):383–90.
10. Puvanesarajah V, Jain A, Shimer AL, Singla A, Shen F, Hassanzadeh H. Complications and mortality following one to two-level anterior cervical fusion for cervical spondylosis in patients above 80 years of age. Spine (Phila Pa 1976). 2017;42(9):E509–14.
11. Hosono N, Yonenobu K, Ono K. Neck and shoulder pain after laminoplasty. A noticeable complication. Spine (Phila Pa 1976). 1996;21(17):1969–73.
12. Hosono N, Sakaura H, Mukai Y, Fujii R, Yoshikawa H. C3–6 laminoplasty takes over C3–7 laminoplasty with significantly lower incidence of axial neck pain. Eur Spine J. 2006;15(9):1375–9.
13. Kawaguchi Y, Matsui H, Ishihara H, Gejo R, Yoshino O. Axial symptoms after en bloc cervical laminoplasty. J Spinal Disord. 1999;12(5):392–5.
14. Liu J, Ebraheim NA, Sanford CG Jr, et al. Preservation of the spinous process-ligament-muscle complex to prevent kyphotic deformity following laminoplasty. Spine J. 2007;7(2):159–64.
15. Shiraishi T, Fukuda K, Yato Y, Nakamura M, Ikegami T. Results of skip laminectomy-minimum 2-year follow-up study compared with open-door laminoplasty. Spine (Phila Pa 1976). 2003;28(24):2667–72.
16. Adamson TE. Microendoscopic posterior cervical laminoforaminotomy for unilateral radiculopathy: results of a new technique in 100 cases. J Neurosurg. 2001;95(1 Suppl):51–7.
17. Minamide A, Yoshida M, Yamada H, et al. Clinical outcomes of microendoscopic decompression surgery for cervical myelopathy. Eur Spine J. 2010;19(3):487–93.
18. Carr DA, Abecassis IJ, Hofstetter CP. Full endoscopic unilateral laminotomy for bilateral decompression of the cervical spine: surgical technique and early experience. J Spine Surg. 2020;6(2):447–56.
19. Hua W, Chen C, Feng X, et al. Clinical outcomes of uniportal and biportal lumbar endoscopic unilateral laminotomy for bilateral decompression in patients with lumbar spinal stenosis: a retrospective pair-matched case-control study. World Neurosurg. 2022;161:e134–45.
20. Pao JL. A review of unilateral biportal endoscopic decompression for degenerative lumbar canal stenosis. Int J Spine Surg. 2021;15(Suppl 3):S65–71.
21. Liang J, Lian L, Liang S, et al. Efficacy and complications of unilateral biportal endoscopic spinal surgery for lumbar spinal stenosis: a meta-analysis and systematic review. World Neurosurg. 2022;159:e91–e102.

22. Kim JY, Heo DH. Contralateral sublaminar approach for decompression of the combined lateral recess, foraminal, and extraforaminal lesions using biportal endoscopy: a technical report. Acta Neurochir. 2021;163(10):2783–7.
23. Kim JS, Park CW, Yeung YK, Suen TK, Jun SG, Park JH. Unilateral bi-portal endoscopic decompression via the contralateral approach in asymmetric spinal stenosis: a technical note. Asian Spine J. 2021;15(5):688–700.
24. Heo DH, Lee DC, Park CK. Comparative analysis of three types of minimally invasive decompressive surgery for lumbar central stenosis: biportal endoscopy, uniportal endoscopy, and microsurgery. Neurosurg Focus. 2019;46(5):E9.
25. Heo DH, Quillo-Olvera J, Park CK. Can percutaneous biportal endoscopic surgery achieve enough canal decompression for degenerative lumbar stenosis? Prospective case-control study. World Neurosurg. 2018;120:e684–9.
26. Tetreault L, Kopjar B, Nouri A, et al. The modified Japanese Orthopaedic Association scale: establishing criteria for mild, moderate and severe impairment in patients with degenerative cervical myelopathy. Eur Spine J. 2017;26(1):78–84.
27. Fehlings MG, Tetreault LA, Riew KD, et al. A clinical practice guideline for the management of patients with degenerative cervical myelopathy: recommendations for patients with mild, moderate, and severe disease and nonmyelopathic patients with evidence of cord compression. Global Spine J. 2017;7(3 Suppl):70S–83S.
28. Hernandez RN, Wipplinger C, Navarro-Ramirez R, et al. Ten-step minimally invasive cervical decompression via unilateral tubular laminotomy: technical note and early clinical experience. Oper Neurosurg (Hagerstown). 2020;18(3):284–94.
29. Hong YH, Kim SK, Hwang J, et al. Water dynamics in unilateral biportal endoscopic spine surgery and its related factors: an in vivo proportional regression and proficiency-matched study. World Neurosurg. 2021;149:e836–43.
30. Kang MS, Park HJ, Hwang JH, Kim JE, Choi DJ, Chung HJ. Safety evaluation of biportal endoscopic lumbar discectomy: assessment of cervical epidural pressure during surgery. Spine (Phila Pa 1976). 2020;45(20):E1349–56.

Part VI
Special Considerations

Chapter 28
Biportal Endoscopic Posterior Decompression of Thoracic Spinal Stenosis Due to Ossification of Ligamentum Flavum

Wei Zhang, Yipeng Chen, and Javier Quillo-Olvera

Abbreviations

AP	Anteroposterior
Cau	Caudal
Cra	Cranial
CSF	Cerebrospinal fluid
CT	Computed tomography
EP	Evoked potentials
IAP	Inferior articular process
IONM	Intraoperative neuromonitoring
JOA	Japanese Orthopedic Association score for myelopathy
LF	Ligamentum flavum
MRI	Magnetic resonance imaging
OLF	Ossification of ligamentum flavum
OPLL	Ossification of posterior longitudinal ligament
RF	Radiofrequency
SAP	Superior articular process
UBE	Unilateral biportal endoscopy
ULBD	Unilateral laminotomy for bilateral decompression

W. Zhang (✉) · Y. Chen
Department of Orthopaedics, Hangzhou Traditional Chinese Medicine Hospital Affiliated to Zhejiang Chinese Medical University, Hangzhou, China
e-mail: volcano8060@163.com; chen-yi-peng@163.com

J. Quillo-Olvera
The Brain and Spine Care, Minimally Invasive Spine Surgery Group, Hospital H+ Querétaro, Spine Clinic, Querétaro, México
e-mail: neuroqomd@gmail.com

J. Quillo-Olvera et al. (eds.), *Unilateral Biportal Endoscopy of the Spine*,
https://doi.org/10.1007/978-3-031-14736-4_28

Introduction

Ossification of the ligamentum flavum (OLF) in the thoracic region is a rare cause of myelopathy. Thoracic OLF may be due to two factors, one systemic and the other local. The first is associated with heredity, abnormal metabolism of carbohydrates, calcium, abnormal secretion of gender hormone, and its degeneration. Local factors include mechanical stress on the ligament entheses. In addition, the hypertrophic and ossified ligamentum flavum narrows the thoracic spinal canal, compressing the spinal cord and triggering neurological symptoms [1, 2].

This pathology is usually common in East Asian countries, including Japan, China, and Korea. However, it has also been reported in different parts of the world, including West countries [3–5].

Various studies have analyzed the incidence of OLF, especially in Japan. Kawaguchi et al. [6] investigated the entire spine of 178 patients with CT scans. They reported that 64.6% of patients with ossification of the posterior longitudinal ligament (OPLL) in the cervical region also had thoracic OLF. Sato et al. [7] analyzed 265 patients who underwent surgery for thoracic myelopathy, showing that OLF was the generator of compression in 52%, OLF combined with OPLL was responsible in 9% of patients, and 65% of OLF was located at T10–T11 and T11–T12. Moon et al. [8] reported a prevalence of thoracic OLF of 16.9%, with T10–T11 being the most affected in 2134 Korean individuals.

Regarding the clinical presentation of thoracic OLF, patients with increased deep tendon reflexes predominantly in both legs compared to those in the arms and flaccid paralysis of the lower extremities with muscle atrophy and weakness should have a high suspicion for thoracic OLF, and imaging studies to study thoracic and lumbar spine should be recommended [2].

Surgical treatment to decompress the spinal cord of the thoracic spine in patients with OLF is urged due to the progression of neurological deterioration due to spinal cord compression, especially in patients with a spastic gait, associated muscle weakness in the lower extremities, and bladder and bowel disorders [2]. Surgical methods include open-door-type laminectomy, en bloc laminectomy, fenestration, and hemilaminectomy [9–14]. This chapter describes the unilateral biportal endoscopy (UBE) technique to resolve thoracic spinal cord compression by OLF.

Relevant Anatomy and Pathological Findings

The thoracic lamina is usually broad, sloping, and longer than the cervical vertebrae. The thoracic spinous process is long and thin with a caudal course. The facet joints are oriented in the coronal plane, with the inferior facet of the superior vertebra overlapping the superior facet of the inferior vertebra. At the thoracolumbar junction, the orientation of the facet joints becomes more sagittal.

The ligamentum flavum (LF) in the thoracic spine has two portions on each side, medially the interlaminar and laterally the capsular portion. The LF is attached to the cephalad lamina's ventral side and the caudal lamina's dorsal side. The LF extends to the intervertebral foramen area but only covers the upper half of the foramen [11].

The thoracic level most affected by OLF is T10–T11 because it receives maximum tensile strength [7, 8, 14]. Thoracic OLF originates in the capsular portion of the LF and extends to its interlaminar part. Ossification then enlarges anteriorly toward the spinal canal, sometimes forming a nodular or tuberous mass in the midline [15].

OLF gradually extends from the dorsal to the ventral surface of the LF, and at some point, during the disease, the dural sac may ossify and even blend with the LF. Therefore, recognizing this phenomenon before surgery is of utmost importance to avoid complications such as dural tears or cerebrospinal fluid (CSF) leak.

Muthukumar [16] retrospectively reviewed imaging studies, including CT and MRI of 20 patients with thoracic OLF treated surgically to determine the dural sac's ossification patterns. Of the 20 patients with OLF, 8 had intraoperative evidence of dural ossification, including dural lacerations. Of the 8 patients with this finding, radiological evidence of dural involvement was found in 7. The author described two radiological signs: a "tram-track sign" consisting of a hyperdense bone excrescence on CT with a central hypodensity. The other was called the "comma sign," characterized by uniform ossification of the dura around one-half of the circumference of the dura. The same signs could be observed on MRI. Miyakoshi et al. [17] reported that 62% of patients with OLF had dural "adhesions." Li et al. [18] found that one of seven patients had dural ossification in their case series. Another series report even up to 40% incidence in dural ossification and OLF [19].

The CT-based thoracic OLF classification on axial images divides the ossification into five types as follows [20]:

1. Lateral type: The OLF is located only at the capsular portion and is detected in the lateral parts of the spinal canal.
2. Extended type: The ossification is only on the surface of LF but extends to the interlaminar portion of the ligament.
3. Enlarged type: The OLF protrudes into the canal without midline fusion of both interlaminar parts of LF.
4. Fused type: Both interlaminar parts ossified are fused in the midline, but a groove is still observed.
5. Tuberous type: A tuberous or nodular ossification protrudes into the spinal canal.

And on sagittal images ossification of the ligamentum flavum (OLF) is round and beak-shaped in anatomical pathology [11, 21].

Indications for Biportal Endoscopic Decompression of Thoracic Spinal Stenosis

1. Ossification of thoracic ligamentum flavum
2. Thoracic hypertrophied LF (interlaminar and capsular portion)
3. Soft and lateral thoracic disc herniation causing lateral stenosis
4. Neurological deterioration according to the imaging finding

Contraindications include infection, kyphotic deformity, severe spinal cord compression that requires a different approach to prevent neurological damage, tumor, and multilevel stenosis. The biportal endoscopic decompression is only for decompressing the spinal cord; however, if a different technique is required to stabilize or fuse the thoracic spine, it should be performed independently. A minimally invasive technique for thoracic OLF with a complex pattern of dural adhesions or ossification is not recommended because of the high need for dural reconstruction techniques that can be difficult to perform through UBE [22, 23].

Surgical Technique

It is recommended to mark the thoracic index level preoperatively to prevent wrong-level spine surgery. The patient is positioned prone on a radiolucent Jackson table with an abdominal support frame, and the procedure will be performed under general anesthesia. Intraoperative neuromonitoring (IONM) with evoked potentials (EP) is recommended (somatosensory and motor). Under an AP view of the C-arm, the index level is identified and confirmed with the preoperative mark.

Translaminar thoracic spinal decompression with biportal endoscopy requires proper placement of the ports for the endoscope and the working channel. First, the surgeon must identify the medial margin of the index-level pedicles and the superior edge of the index-level transverse process. Then, the incisions can be planned 1.5 cm above and below an imaginary line tangential to the superior border of the spinous process and at the medial margin of both pedicles (Fig. 28.1).

It should be remembered that if it is approached from the right side, and the surgeon is right-handed, the superior incision is used for the working portal, and the inferior one for the endoscopic portal, being the opposite on the left side.

After marking the entry points, it is suggested to create the working portal first and then the viewing one. First, a 6–8 mm transverse or longitudinal incision will be made in the skin and fascia. Afterward, a 6 mm tubular dilator will be inserted toward the spinolaminar junction. Then, progressive dilators are introduced through the first one sequentially. The same process will be carried out to create the viewing portal. The surgeon should feel the palpation between both tubular dilators and palpate the spinolaminar junction with both.

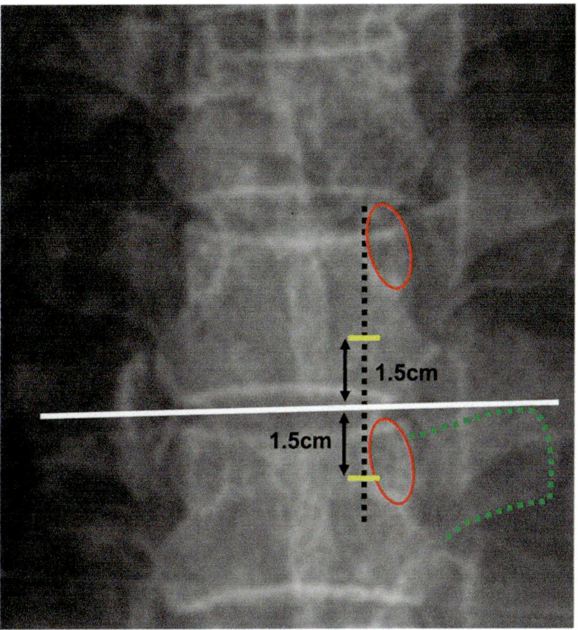

Fig. 28.1 Intraoperative fluoroscopic based landmarks for planning the two portals of UBE posterior thoracic decompression. A mid-pedicular line (black dotted line) passing tangentially to the medial margin of the pedicles (red circles) should be identified. A line (white line) passing tangentially to the upper edge of the transverse process (green dotted line) is also marked. Finally, two incisions (yellow lines), one 1.5 cm above and the other 1.5 cm below the white line over the mid-pedicular line, are planned

The endoscope will be introduced in the viewing portal and the surgical instruments through the working portal. The correct inflow and outflow of the irrigated fluid will be verified. If an automatic irrigation pump is used, a 30 mmHg is set. Next, the working space must be created. Under endoscopic view, the radiofrequency (RF) probe will be used to clean the soft tissue on the surface of the lamina, which will reveal the junction of the lamina with the LF medially (Fig. 28.2).

The high-speed drill's 3 mm diamond head is used to thin the ipsilateral lamina and the OLF. First, the surgeon must identify the medial portion of the inferior articular process (IAP) and lower edge of the superior lamina, then the upper edge of the inferior lamina, and the interlaminar part of LF. Next, bone removal is performed with the high-speed drill circumferentially until it reaches the inferior vertebra's superior articular process (SAP), and a partial medial facetectomy is completed. In addition, the 1 or 2 mm 130° angled-tip Kerrison rongeur can enlarge the laminectomy, avoiding touching the dura (Fig. 28.3).

The surgeon can also use the drill to remove thick portions of the lamina or LF, leaving a thin layer adhered to the dural sac. Later, this layer can be removed with a fine microdissector avoiding retraction of the dura or leaving it floating, reducing the risk of a dural tear (Fig. 28.4).

The operation field of the contralateral side is larger than that on the ipsilateral side. In addition, the small nerve detacher effectively separates the adhesion between the contralateral ossified ligament and the dura. Therefore, it is best to deal with contralateral ossification using a bur with a protective sheath. The biportal

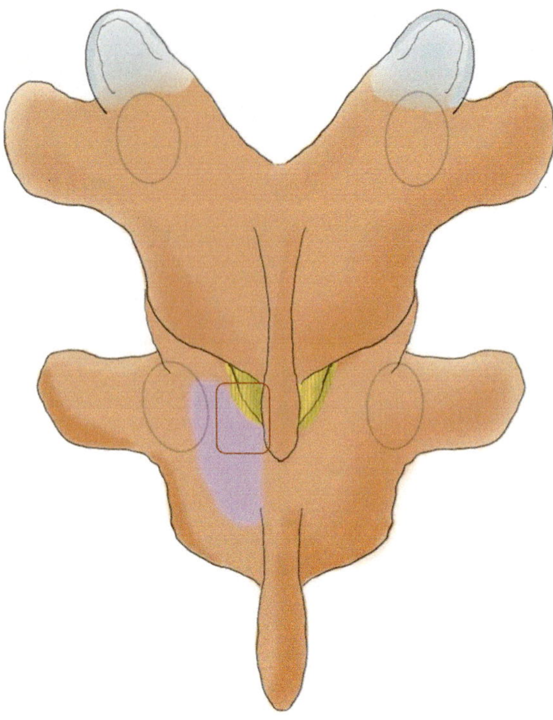

Fig. 28.2 The procedure can begin when the bone landmarks that conform to a small interlaminar window (red rectangle) have been identified

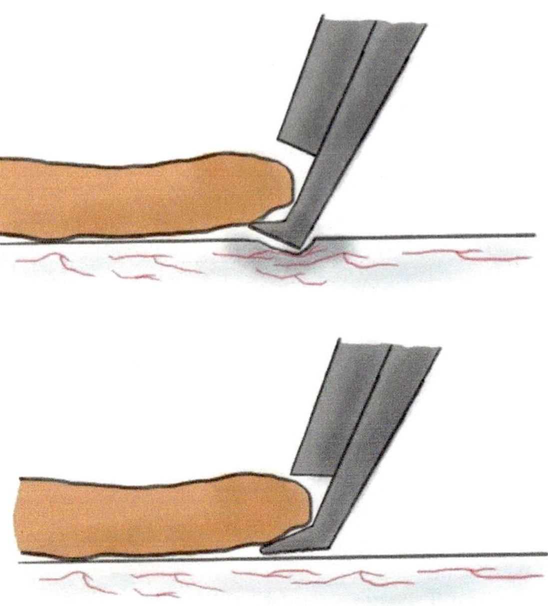

Fig. 28.3 The use of a 130° thin-blade Kerrison rongeur avoids touching the dural sac

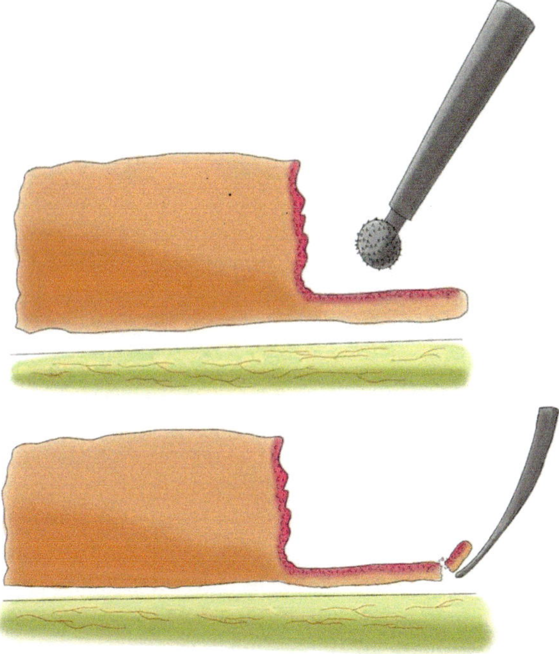

Fig. 28.4 The surgeon can drill the lamina leaving a thin layer, and then a microdetacher to lift the bone fragments completes the decompression

endoscopic thoracic decompression allows the proper identification of all boundaries of the OLF after circumferential bone removal. After the decompression is complete, a drainage tube is placed, and the incision is sutured.

Postoperative Measures

Prophylactic antibiotics are routinely used after surgery. Depending on the drainage, the drainage tube is generally removed after 24–48 h if there is no CSF leakage. It is usually removed after 5–7 days if CSF leakage occurs.

Surgical Procedure Essentials

Biportal endoscopic surgery is a targeted technique, so the translaminar approach is always suggested instead of the interlaminar in the thoracic region. The thoracic OLF usually occurs in the capsular portion of the LF and extends to its interlaminar part. For this reason, the translaminar approach has the advantage of directly addressing the medial edge of the facet joint and the inferior lamina. The other reason is that it allows direct circumferential decompression to find the limits of the

LF. Anatomically, the thoracic interlaminar space is reduced compared to the lumbar (Fig. 28.5).

Kang et al. [24] reported the biportal endoscopic technique for posterior thoracic decompression. The authors make helpful recommendations to avoid serious complications, for example, identifying all OLF limits during decompression. Also, leave only a thin layer in contact with the dura to remove it last and confirm by endoscopic visualization the pulsation of the dural sac after decompression.

The precise point to start bone removal is very important. Since the thoracic lamina is very wide, the surgeon must identify the point where the external layer of ligamentum flavum reaches the inferior lamina to precisely start bone drilling there. This medial and caudal point to the inferior lamina can be observed as anatomically different from the yellow color of the LF, with it being pink. This transition can be recognized through the endoscope and used as a starting landmark for bone work (Fig. 28.6).

Preoperative planning is crucial since thoracic OLF may require only ipsilateral OLF decompression or be a thoracic ULBD procedure. Preoperative imaging studies, including thoracic CT scan and MRI, will allow us to determine if there is dural ossification and, based on intraoperative findings, decide whether the OLF can be removed entirely or left floating to avoid CSF leakage. If it is determined to float the OLF or ossification of the dura mater, then adequate pulsation of the dural sac should be confirmed after cardinal detachment of the OLF.

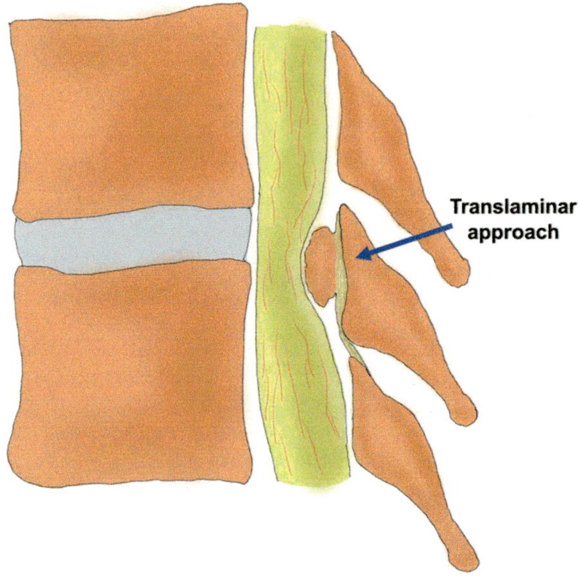

Fig. 28.5 The translaminar route in the thoracic spine

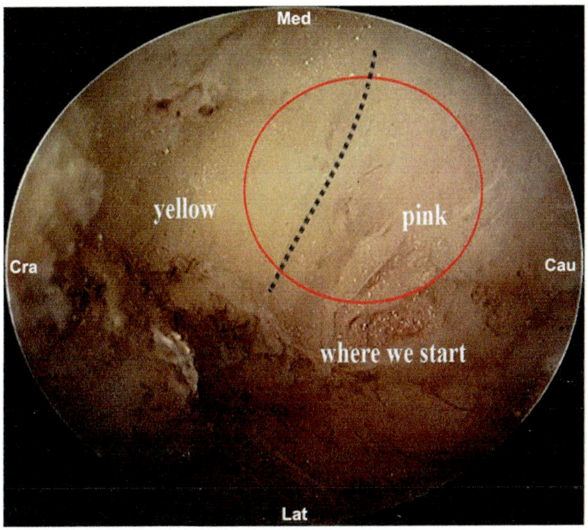

Fig. 28.6 The yellow and pink color transition due to a small thoracic interlaminar space can be identified with the endoscope for starting the bone drilling

Finally, any hematoma or epidural collection should be prevented due to the risk of compression and ischemia of the thoracic spinal cord leading to neurological deterioration. Various hemostatic matrices on the market can be used if basic maneuvers such as RF, bone wax, or hemostatic sponges are not enough. It is also recommended to leave a drain at the end to evacuate the remaining fluid irrigated by the endoscopic system or residual epidural blood.

Illustrated Case

Case 1

A 55-year-old female presented with paraparesis 3/5 and bowel and bladder disturbances since 3 weeks on evolution. Neurological examination revealed an inability to walk, exalted tendon reflexes in the lower extremities, and bilateral Babinski's sign. In addition, preoperative imaging studies demonstrated spinal cord compression at T1–T2 due to OLF on the left side (Fig. 28.7). Therefore, a right-sided contralateral UBE approach for posterior thoracic decompression was planned and successfully performed on the patient. During surgery, it was possible to identify the SAP and, consequently, the lateral margins of the LF. Subsequently, a flavectomy and adequate hemostasis were performed (Fig. 28.8). Postoperative images confirmed sufficient decompression of the spinal cord (Fig. 28.9).

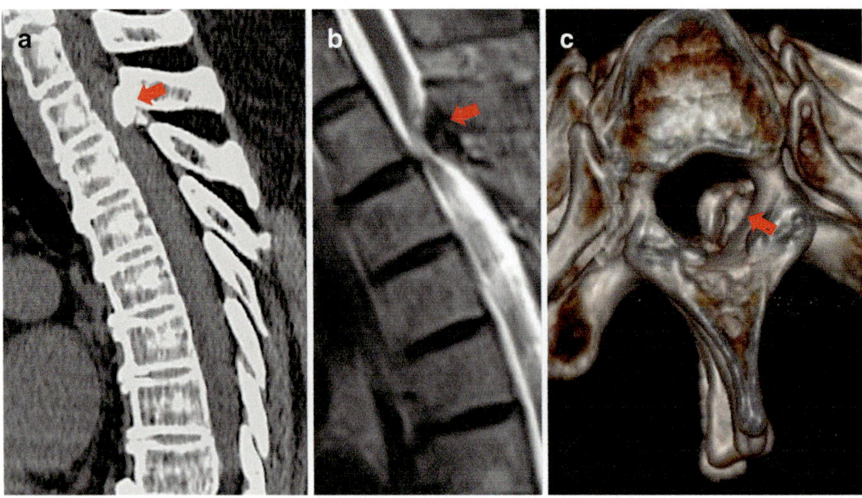

Fig. 28.7 Preoperative images of Case 1. (**a**) The sagittal view of the thoracic CT scan shows an OLF at T1–T2 (red arrow). (**b**) A severe spinal cord compression was observed in the sagittal view of the MRI (red arrow). (**c**) An axial view of the 3D CT reconstructed demonstrated an OLF on the right side (red arrow)

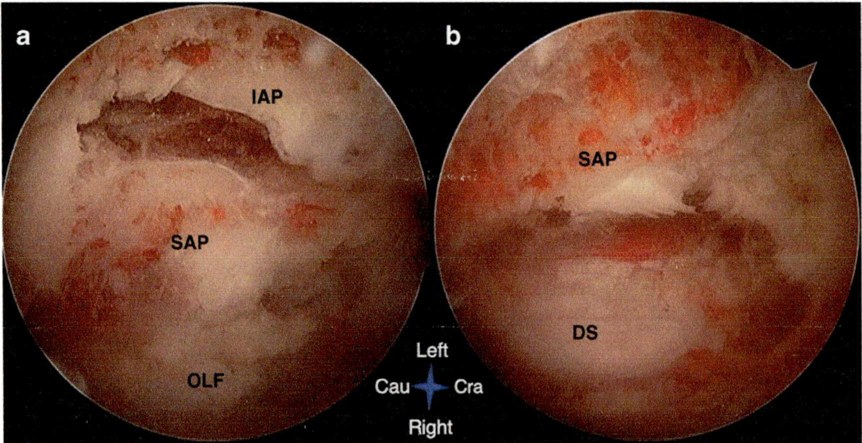

Fig. 28.8 Intraoperative images through the endoscope of Case 1. (**a**) After contralateral laminotomy, the IAP and SAP on the left side and the lateral attachment of OLF were identified. (**b**) The dural sac decompressed after OLF removal. (**c**) Proper hemostasis of the central spinal canal using a sponge (white arrow). (**d**) A drainage (blue arrow) is placed on the epidural space. *Cra* cranial, *Cau* caudal, *IAP* inferior articular process, *SAP* superior articular process, *DS* dural sac, *OLF* ossification of ligamentum flavum

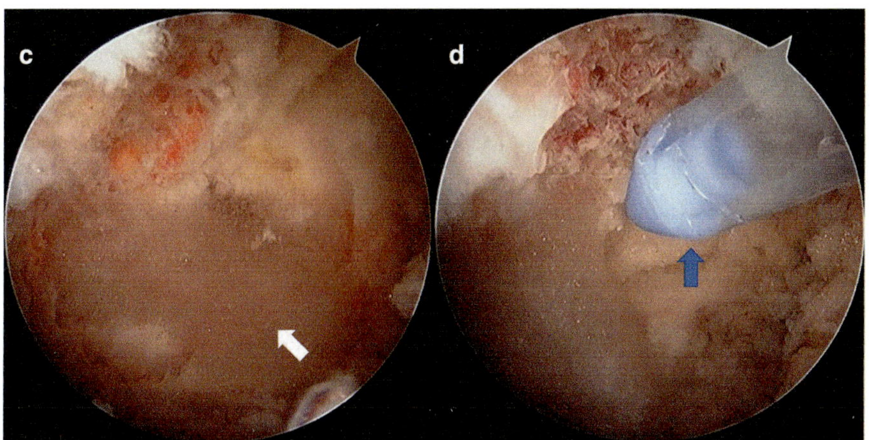

Fig. 28.8 (continued)

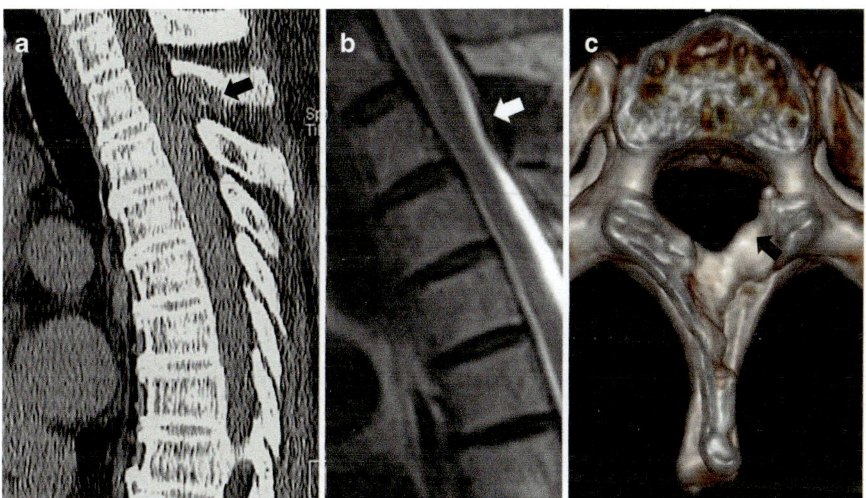

Fig. 28.9 Postoperative images of Case 1. Total removal of OLF is observed in (**a**) thoracic CT scan (black arrow), (**b**) MRI (white arrow), and (**c**) axial view of 3D CT reconstructed (black arrow)

Discussion

It is essential to mention that despite achieving adequate decompression of the spinal cord through any technique, including UBE, the clinical results may not be consistent since these will depend on other factors such as the time since the onset of symptoms and the treatment in addition to the severity of the neurological deterioration measured through the JOA score and which may be irreversible. Nevertheless, the rate of improvement in functional status after surgery is around 40–54% according to different series of posterior thoracic decompression [11, 17, 25, 26].

The reported complication rate also depends on the series studied; however, a recent meta-analysis [27] reported a rate of around 35%. Among the most frequent complications associated with posterior thoracic decompression, dural tears are the most frequent with 18.4%, and CSF leak associated with dural tears was the second most frequent complication with an incidence of 12.1% [27]. Because of this, techniques that provide more excellent clearness in the visualization of anatomical structures may result in minor anatomical transgression when attempting to remove the OLF. In this case, despite having the concept of detaching the OLF and leaving it floating [28], the UBE technique allows high-quality visualization of the OLF and its attachments to the bone structures, allowing a decision to be made based on intraoperative findings whether to leave or not floating to the OLF to decrease the risk of a dural tear and CSF leak.

Another complication observed when decompressing the thoracic spinal cord in patients with OLF is early neurological deterioration, with an incidence of 5.7% [27]. It can be caused by epidural hematomas [26], excessive manipulation of the dural sac, and consequently injury to the thoracic spinal cord [29]. We found another advantage for UBE here since the surgeon can work with both hands. One is used to handle the endoscope, and the other uses the surgical instruments freely in the working field. Therefore, accuracy is achieved with UBE compared to other minimally invasive and endoscopic techniques decreasing the excessive manipulation of neural structures. It should be noted that UBE for posterior thoracic decompression requires expertise obtained with other spinal surgery techniques. Hemostasis achieved through biportal endoscopy is adequate. Although there are different options to perform it correctly, the fluid irrigated through the endoscope during the procedure allows a clean surgical field and accurately determines where particular bleeding comes from. The RF probe and other options such as bone wax, sponges, and various hemostatic matrices can also be used.

Finally, one of the risks when performing posterior thoracic decompression due to OLF is iatrogenic instability resulting from excessive bone removal. The considerable damage of facet joints during thoracic decompression can cause progressive kyphotic deformity and associated neurological deterioration, in addition to OLF in adjacent levels close to the deformity [13, 14, 30]. Because biportal endoscopy is a targeted and specific technique, this risk may be reduced since the surgeon can visualize bone elements such as the IAP and SAP and only remove them medially until the OLF attachment is observed. Therefore, decompression is usually more selective through UBE, avoiding excessive bone remodeling and, in turn, reducing the need for fusion.

Infections have been reported in posterior thoracic decompressions, up to 3.5–5.8% [27, 31], associated with hemostasis or drainage failure and triggering a hematoma with the risk of infection. However, since biportal endoscopy relies on continuous fluid irrigation, the risk of infection associated with UBE is unlikely.

Conclusion

OLF-related thoracic myelopathy is rare compared to other degenerative diseases of the thoracic spine; however, its clinical and functional impact on the patients is usually considerable. Decompressive surgical treatment remains the most recommended option when the patient shows neurological deterioration. Biportal endoscopy is a promising and emerging minimally invasive option that can reduce the complication profile associated with other thoracic spinal cord decompression techniques with acceptable radiological outcomes, even similar to more aggressive methods. More scientific evidence is needed, with adequate methodology, to determine the role of biportal endoscopy in thoracic OLF.

References

1. Li M, Wang Z, Du J, Luo Z, Wang Z. Thoracic myelopathy caused by ossification of the ligamentum flavum: a retrospective study in Chinese patients. J Spinal Disord Tech. 2013;26(1):E35–40.
2. Hirabayashi S. Ossification of the ligamentum flavum. Spine Surg Relat Res. 2017;1(4):158–63.
3. Inamasu J, Guiot BH. A review of factors predictive of surgical outcome for ossification of the ligamentum flavum of the thoracic spine. J Neurosurg Spine. 2006;5(2):133–9.
4. Shiokawa K, Hanakita J, Suwa H, Saiki M, Oda M, Kajiwara M. Clinical analysis and prognostic study of ossified ligamentum flavum of the thoracic spine. J Neurosurg. 2001;94(2 Suppl):221–6.
5. Jayakumar PN, Devi BI, Bhat DI, Das BS. Thoracic cord compression due to ossified hypertrophied ligamentum flavum. Neurol India. 2002;50(3):286–9.
6. Kawaguchi Y, Nakano M, Yasuda T, et al. Characteristics of ossification of the spinal ligament; incidence of ossification of the ligamentum flavum in patients with cervical ossification of the posterior longitudinal ligament - analysis of the whole spine using multidetector CT. J Orthop Sci. 2016;21(4):439–45.
7. Sato T, Aizawa T. Current status of thoracic myelopathy. Sekitsui Sekizui (Spine & Spinal Cord). 2009;22(2):136–41. Japanese
8. Moon BJ, Kuh SU, Kim S, Kim KS, Cho YE, Chin DK. Prevalence, distribution, and significance of incidental thoracic ossification of the ligamentum flavum in Korean patients with back or leg pain: MR-based cross sectional study. J Korean Neurosurg Soc. 2015;58(2):112–8.
9. Zhong ZM, Wu Q, Meng TT, et al. Clinical outcomes after decompressive laminectomy for symptomatic ossification of ligamentum flavum at the thoracic spine. J Clin Neurosci. 2016;28:77–81.
10. Ando K, Imagama S, Ito Z, et al. Predictive factors for a poor surgical outcome with thoracic ossification of the ligamentum flavum by multivariate analysis: a multicenter study. Spine (Phila Pa 1976). 2013;38(12):E748–54.
11. Aizawa T, Sato T, Sasaki H, Kusakabe T, Morozumi N, Kokubun S. Thoracic myelopathy caused by ossification of the ligamentum flavum: clinical features and surgical results in the Japanese population. J Neurosurg Spine. 2006;5(6):514–9.
12. Ahn DK, Lee S, Moon SH, Boo KH, Chang BK, Lee JI. Ossification of the ligamentum flavum. Asian Spine J. 2014;8(1):89–96.
13. Nishiura I, Isozumi T, Nishihara K, Handa H, Koyama T. Surgical approach to ossification of the thoracic yellow ligament. Surg Neurol. 1999;51(4):368–72.

14. Okada K, Oka S, Tohge K, Ono K, Yonenobu K, Hosoya T. Thoracic myelopathy caused by ossification of the ligamentum flavum. Clinicopathologic study and surgical treatment. Spine (Phila Pa 1976). 1991;16(3):280–7.
15. Kubota T, Kawano H, Yamashima T, Ikeda K, Hayashi M, Yamamoto S. Ultrastructural study of calcification process in the ligamentum flavum of the cervical spine. Spine (Phila Pa 1976). 1987;12(4):317–23.
16. Muthukumar N. Dural ossification in ossification of the ligamentum flavum: a preliminary report. Spine (Phila Pa 1976). 2009;34(24):2654–61.
17. Miyakoshi N, Shimada Y, Suzuki T, et al. Factors related to long-term outcome after decompressive surgery for ossification of the ligamentum flavum of the thoracic spine. J Neurosurg. 2003;99(3 Suppl):251–6.
18. Li F, Chen Q, Xu K. Surgical treatment of 40 patients with thoracic ossification of the ligamentum flavum. J Neurosurg Spine. 2006;4(3):191–7.
19. Jaffan I, Abu-Serieh B, Duprez T, Cosnard G, Raftopoulos C. Unusual CT/MR features of putative ligamentum flavum ossification in a North African woman. Br J Radiol. 2006;79(944):e67–70.
20. Sato T, Tanaka Y, Aizawa T, et al. Surgical treatment for ossification of ligamentum flavum in the thoracic spine and its complications [in Japanese]. Spine Spinal Cord. 1998;11:505–10.
21. Kuh SU, Kim YS, Cho YE, et al. Contributing factors affecting the prognosis surgical outcome for thoracic OLF. Eur Spine J. 2006;15(4):485–91.
22. An B, Li XC, Zhou CP, et al. Percutaneous full endoscopic posterior decompression of thoracic myelopathy caused by ossification of the ligamentum flavum. Eur Spine J. 2019;28(3):492–501.
23. Baba S, Oshima Y, Iwahori T, Takano Y, Inanami H, Koga H. Microendoscopic posterior decompression for the treatment of thoracic myelopathy caused by ossification of the ligamentum flavum: a technical report. Eur Spine J. 2016;25(6):1912–9.
24. Kang MS, Chung HJ, You KH, Park HJ. How I do it: biportal endoscopic thoracic decompression for ossification of the ligamentum flavum. Acta Neurochir. 2022;164(1):43–7.
25. He S, Hussain N, Li S, Hou T. Clinical and prognostic analysis of ossified ligamentum flavum in a Chinese population. J Neurosurg Spine. 2005;3(5):348–54.
26. Chen XQ, Yang HL, Wang GL, et al. Surgery for thoracic myelopathy caused by ossification of the ligamentum flavum. J Clin Neurosci. 2009;16(10):1316–20.
27. Osman NS, Cheung ZB, Hussain AK, et al. Outcomes and complications following laminectomy alone for thoracic myelopathy due to ossified ligamentum flavum: a systematic review and meta-analysis. Spine (Phila Pa 1976). 2018;43(14):E842–8.
28. Wang W, Kong L, Zhao H, et al. Thoracic ossification of ligamentum flavum caused by skeletal fluorosis. Eur Spine J. 2007;16(8):1119–28.
29. Liao CC, Chen TY, Jung SM, Chen LR. Surgical experience with symptomatic thoracic ossification of the ligamentum flavum. J Neurosurg Spine. 2005;2(1):34–9.
30. Wang T, Yin C, Wang D, Li S, Chen X. Surgical technique for decompression of severe thoracic myelopathy due to tuberous ossification of ligamentum flavum. Clin Spine Surg. 2017;30(1):E7–E12.
31. Li Z, Ren D, Zhao Y, et al. Clinical characteristics and surgical outcome of thoracic myelopathy caused by ossification of the ligamentum flavum: a retrospective analysis of 85 cases. Spinal Cord. 2016;54(3):188–96.

Chapter 29
Biportal Endoscopic Lumbar Facet Joint Denervation for Symptomatic Facet Joint Syndrome

Diego Quillo-Olvera, Javier Quillo-Reséndiz, Daniella Andrea Ponce de León Camargo, Michelle Barrera-Arreola, and Javier Quillo-Olvera

Abbreviations

BESS	Biportal endoscopic surgery
CLBP	Chronic low back pain
CT	Computed tomography
DMB	Dorsal medial branch
FJ	Facet joint
IAP	Inferior articular process
LBP	Low back pain
MRI	Magnetic resonance imaging
NSAIDs	Nonsteroidal anti-inflammatory drugs
OR	Operative room
RF	Radiofrequency
SAP	Superior articular process
TNF-α	Tumor necrosis factor-alpha
TP	Transverse process
UBE	Unilateral biportal endoscopy

D. Quillo-Olvera (✉) · J. Quillo-Reséndiz · M. Barrera-Arreola · J. Quillo-Olvera
The Brain and Spine Care, Minimally Invasive Spine Surgery Group,
Hospital H+ Querétaro, Spine Clinic, Querétaro, México
e-mail: drquilloolvera86@gmail.com; kitnoz@hotmail.com; michelle.barrera@anahuac.mx; neuroqomd@gmail.com

D. A. P. de León Camargo
Anáhuac University School of Medicine, Querétaro, México
e-mail: daniellaponcedeleon@gmail.com

J. Quillo-Olvera et al. (eds.), *Unilateral Biportal Endoscopy of the Spine*,
https://doi.org/10.1007/978-3-031-14736-4_29

Introduction

Chronic low back pain (CLBP) has a prevalence of 4.2–20.3% in the general population, and degeneration and inflammation of the facet joint (FJ) are frequent causes that account for at least 20–40% of cases [1]. Articular facets are authentic synovial joints; they have 1–1.5 mL contained synovial fluid within the intra-articular space surrounded by a synovial membrane, a hyaline cartilage surface, and a 1 mm thick fibrous capsule made up of collagen fibers in a transverse arrangement. The innervation is provided by the dorsal medial branch (DMB), which originates from the posterior main branch and contains neurons capable of providing nociceptive and proprioceptive information on the facet [2]. The morphology of each FJ shows an inferior articular process (IAP) emerging from the upper vertebrae and a superior articular process (SAP) ascending from the lower vertebrae; the lamina joins the articular processes on both sides.

The shape and orientation of the FJs determine the role played by each joint to protect the spine against excessive movement or force. In other words, the FJ works to hold, stabilize, and prevent the spine from an injury by allowing a specific limited range of motion for safety in all planes [2, 3]. This chapter discusses basic concepts of lumbar FJs, the low back pain (LBP) generated by these joint structures, and their treatment through radiofrequency (RF) denervation with the biportal endoscopic technique or UBE.

Facetogenic Pain

FJ pain has been related to different injury mechanisms, including capsular stretch, entrapment of synovial villi between articular surfaces, nerve impingement due to osteophytes, and release of inflammatory substances [4–8]. Various inflammatory mediators, including prostaglandins, cytokines (1B- and 6-interleukins), and tumor necrosis factor (TNF-α), have been found in FJ's inflamed cartilage and synovial tissue, and these have been related to the inflammatory response in lumbar degenerative disease [2].

Revel et al. [9], in 1998, proposed seven clinical parameters associated with a positive response to FJ anesthesia. Parameters include age greater than 65 years, pain not exacerbated by coughing, pain not worsened by hyperextension, pain not worsened by forward flexion, pain not worsened when rising from forward flexion, pain not worsened by extension-rotation, and pain well relieved by recumbency. The authors concluded that the presence of at least 5–7 criteria could discriminate 100% of those who would respond and 66% of those who would not react to FJ anesthesia. Therefore, diagnostic facet block remains the best tool available to identify lumbar facet pain, although it is associated with a high rate of false positives between 27% and 41% [10]. However, false-negative results can also be related to anatomical variants in facet innervation, inadvertent venous uptake during the procedure, or technique failure [11]. This is relevant since a decrease in LBP of 50% or more after a diagnostic facet block can predict the results of DMB radiofrequency ablation [2].

Clinically, facetogenic pain can affect the entire back. At the cervical level, pain occurs in the neck and can radiate to the head and shoulders. At the thoracic level, pain with neuralgic characteristics may present in the paraspinal and mid-back region, and chest pain may also be present. Finally, pain radiates to the buttocks and the lower extremities' proximal areas in the lumbar region. In 1927, Putti suggested that local and degenerative inflammation of the facets could generate radiculopathy due to irritation of the nerve roots [12–14].

Deterioration of lumbar FJs seems to be a significant contributor to LBP. X-rays provide minimal information about the degree of facet degeneration, whereas computed tomography (CT) and magnetic resonance imaging (MRI) provide more specific information. Pathria et al. [15], in 1987, introduced an MRI-based classification of FJ degeneration as follows: Grade 0: normal width of 2–4 mm; Grade 1: slight narrowing and irregularity facet; Grade 2: moderate narrowing and irregularity facet plus sclerosis and osteophyte formation; Grade 3: severe narrowing with loss of joint space, sclerosis, and mild osteophyte formation; and Grade 4: severe subarticular erosion, osteophytes, or subchondral cyst.

Several options for treating lumbar FJ pain including conservative treatment, intra-articular injections, facet joint nerve blocks, and radiofrequency ablation under different modalities are available [10, 16, 17]. In the early 1970s, Rees [18] introduced percutaneous denervation for discogenic back pain with a success rate of 99%, and Shealy [19, 20] described the currently used technique based on the intraoperative fluoroscopy. However, the percutaneous approach to denervate FJs may not accurately identify the DMB; therefore, it is associated with unsatisfactory long-term results. Some studies have theorized that pain relief is temporary and lasts for less than 12 months [21–24].

The treatment of facetogenic pain involves a multimodal approach that consists of conservative treatment with nonsteroidal anti-inflammatory drugs (NSAIDs) and depression and anxiety management [2]. Short-term pain relief is provided by periarticular or intra-articular infiltration with local steroids and anesthetics, but long-term benefits are not guaranteed [25, 26].

The evolution of the percutaneous needle technique for FJ denervation gave rise to endoscopic denervation using RF. The latter has the advantage of directly visualizing the DMB, allowing complete and broader denervation of the FJ with better long-term outcomes [27–30].

However, there are limitations in accessing uniportal endoscopy for facet joint denervation. These include the high costs of various highly specialized uniportal endoscopic devices for facet denervation, various health policies regulating access to medical supplies in different countries, steeper learning curve, and difficulty for learning spinal endoscopy.

Given this situation, biportal endoscopic surgery (BESS) has been expanding its indications, and since it is a true water-based endoscopic technique, the visualization of the structures is usually similar to that obtained through uniportal endoscopy.

That means it may be feasible to triangulate both ports of the biportal technique to reach the junction of the transverse process and the facet joints in the lumbar spine and thus perform an RF facet joint denervation under direct visualization. The biportal endoscopic approach has proven to be more accessible for the spine surgeon, more versatile in the maneuverability of the endoscope and the working instrument (the RF probe), and much less expensive than uniportal endoscopy.

Indications

It is advised that the patient has a history of CLBP and that at least two diagnostic facet blocks have been positive with nondurable results, thus confirming facet-induced LBP. This procedure is not recommended in patients with other apparent causes of LBP (instability, trauma, infection, discogenic, tumor). In addition, it is advised to have a history of failure of conservative medical treatment with medications and physical therapy for at least 3 months.

Surgical Technique

Under conscious sedation, the patient is placed in the prone position under an abdominal support frame, and the surgical area at the lumbar region is appropriately draped. Then, AP and lateral views will be obtained with the C-arm.

First, the junction between the transverse process and SAP (TP-SAP) is identified in the AP view of the lumbar spine at the index level. Subsequently, the 6–7 mm skin incisions will be located 2–3 cm lateral to the TP-SAP junction and 1.5 cm above and below it (Fig. 29.1).

In a right-sided approach, a right-hand surgeon will use the cranial incision to introduce the RF probe and the caudal incision for the endoscope. On the left side, this will be the opposite. Also, in cases where RF ablation of the DMB is required at multiple levels, the caudal incision will be used as the cranial incision for the next level.

For biportal endoscopic facet denervation, a set of 5 and 6 mm progressive tubular dilators, a 30° arthroscopic lens, RF probe with a 90° angled tip, working cannula, and a tissue dissector are required, in addition to a 2 mm pituitary forceps and a 2 mm Kerrison rongeur. The skin of both incisions will be infiltrated with a local anesthetic. The surgeon will be ipsilateral to the side of the approach (Fig. 29.2).

The surgeon will first create the working channel by inserting the 6 mm dilator through the incision used for this purpose (on the right side, the cranial, and on the left the caudal). The trajectory of the dilator will be lateral-to-medial and cranial-to-caudal on the right side. The latter will be the opposite on the left. The goal is to palpate the junction between the transverse process and the SAP. Subsequently, the customized semi-tubular working cannula will be introduced through the 6 mm

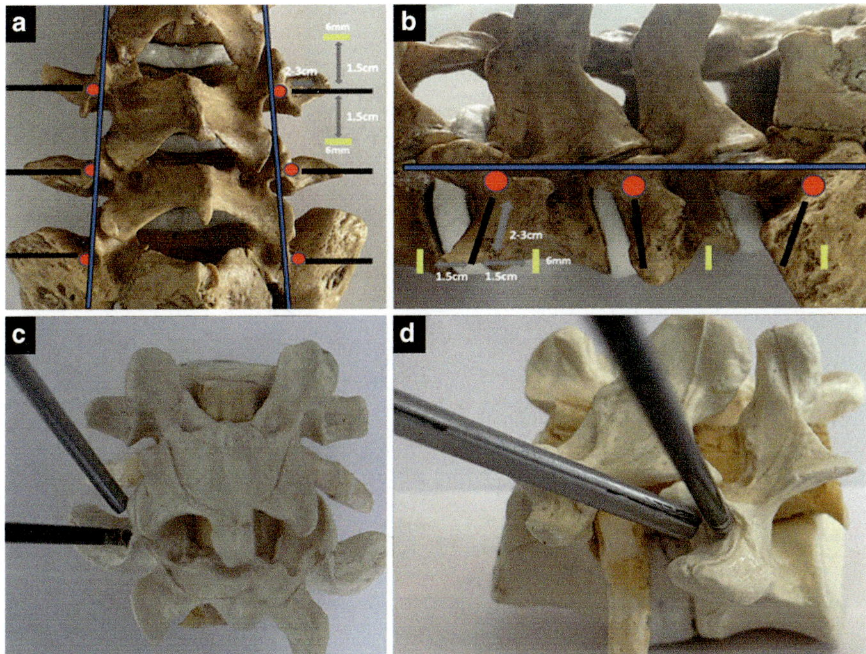

Fig. 29.1 Biportal endoscopic approach to the lumbar TP-SAP junction for facet DMB ablation. (**a**) The TP-SAP junction is identified (red dot) on a lumbar anatomical model on AP view, and the skin incisions are planned according to that point. (**b**) Lateral oblique view of the TP-SAP junction in a lumbar anatomical model. (**c**) Representation of an endoscopic biportal approach for FJ lumbar denervation in an anatomical model on an AP view. (**d**) Same representation as (**c**) with an oblique lateral view. *TP* transverse process, *SAP* superior articular process, *DMB* dorsal medial branch

dilator, and the endoscope's trocar will continue to be introduced towards the same TP-SAP junction so that both ports coincide at the same point. These maneuvers should be confirmed with the C-arm in AP view (Fig. 29.3).

Once the endoscope is introduced in the surgical field, 25 or 30 mmHg is sufficient pressure set for the fluid irrigated during the procedure. Subsequently, the surgeon must confirm the exit of the fluid through the working portal. After that, the working instrument will be located in the surgical field with the endoscope over the TP-SAP junction. Next, the surgeon needs to identify the landmarks to avoid transgressing the intertransverse space, which can cause fluid to leak into the retroperitoneum or violate the foramen in its ventral part with the consequent injury to the exiting nerve root.

Having identified the transverse process (TP) and the SAP, the RF is used under endoscopic visualization to clean the soft tissue adjacent to the bony elements (or create the working space). The surgeon will then visualize the dorsal facet branches and ablate them without mishap (Fig. 29.4).

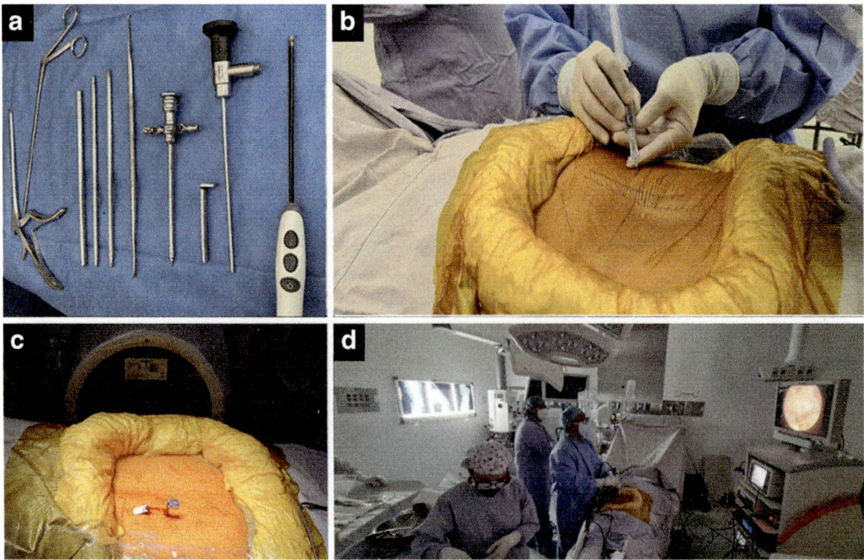

Fig. 29.2 Intraoperative images during a biportal endoscopic lumbar FJ denervation procedure. (**a**) Surgical tools. (**b**) Local anesthesia infiltrated before the surgery. (**c**) After creating both portals, the semi-tubular customized working cannulas were docked under C-arm on the TP-SAP junction. (**d**) OR setup. *OR* operative room, *TP* transverse process, *SAP* superior articular process, *DMB* dorsal medial branch

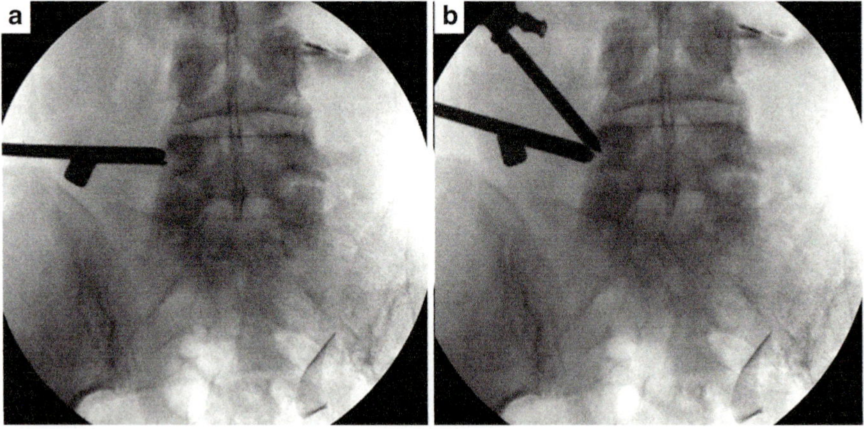

Fig. 29.3 An intraoperative fluoroscopic sequence of a biportal endoscopic approach for lumbar FJ denervation on the left side. (**a**) The working portal is addressed to the TP-SAP junction. (**b**) The triangular approach is completed with the endoscopic trocar addressed to the same point as the first dilator. *TP* transverse process, *SAP* superior articular process, *FJ* facet joint

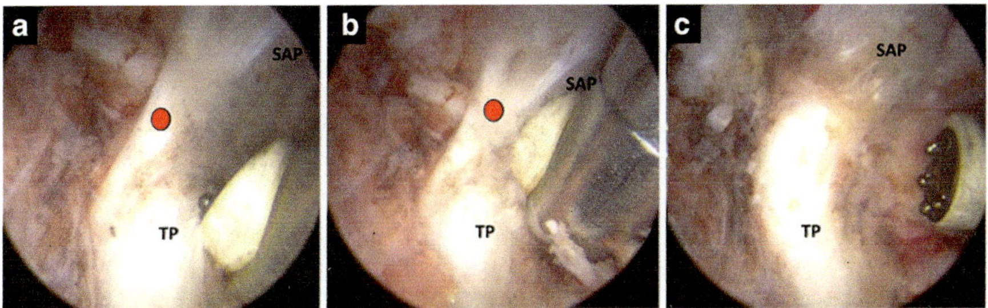

Fig. 29.4 Biportal endoscopic denervation, intraoperative view. (**a**) The DMB (red circle) is identified in the junction of the transverse process (TP) and SAP junction. (**b**) The ablation of the DMB is performed with the RF probe. (**c**) Denervation is confirmed with the endoscope. *DBM* dorsal medial branch, *TP* transverse process, *SAP* superior articular process

Finally, the biportal endoscopic system will be removed not before confirming perfect hemostasis. Then, the skin incisions will be closed with a single stitch, and the procedure will be finished. In this case, no drainage will be left because the procedure is quick, and the surgical assistant will confirm that the same amount of solution irrigated is the same as that collected.

Perioperative Care

The patient will receive appropriate antibiotics 1 h before the procedure. It is suggested to speak with the patient to inform the possible procedure-expected outcomes and how the surgery will be driven under conscious sedation to reduce the procedure-related stress. After surgery, the patient will remain under observation for 6 h and be treated with minimal analgesia, for example, paracetamol IV 1 g, single dose, to assess the postoperative pain threshold and make decisions about the care with which he or she will be discharged. The patient may be discharged in acceptable physical condition, walking and moving his or her back without restrictions, and instructions will be given for the use of mild-acting NSAIDs for 5–7 days and mild activity until next visit on postoperative day 10.

Discussion

Endoscopic denervation of the DMB is part of the evolution of percutaneous techniques. The main benefit of this technique is the ability to directly observe the landmarks such as joint capsule fibers and nervous branches, enabling the performance of extensive denervation. In addition, by implementing this technique, ablation can be more precise.

It has been reported that the patients who most benefit from endoscopic denervation are those under 60 years. This may occur due to central sensitization in older patients with chronic pain. Also, those treated with neurolysis of the DMB at 1–2 joint levels have better improvement in the LBP than those treated on 3 or more levels [1].

BESS dorsal branch ablation meets the same neurolysis objectives as percutaneous RF and uniportal endoscopic rhizotomy. In addition, the correct triangulation of both portals addressed to the TP-SAP junction makes it possible to identify the bone landmarks and DMB accurately.

In addition, the advantages associated with the biportal endoscopic technique include its low cost, the ability to use the RF probe without restriction in the surgical field since it is not introduced through the endoscopic lens, and an easier learning curve compared with uniportal endoscopy, which makes this procedure attractive. On the other hand, it is evident that the triangular approach for creating both ports takes slightly longer than the uniportal endoscopy and that the biportal technique also requires some experience and adaptation on the part of the surgeon. Still, these are not important limitations to reproducing the technique in selected cases with greater safety and effectiveness since the endoscopic view through the biportal procedure has a wide range to observe the TP, the SAP, and the whole FJ, thanks to the fact that the endoscope also has a range of freedom independent of the working portal.

Conclusion

Endoscopic techniques can be considered helpful for lumbar DMB denervation, including BESS. Biportal endoscopic technique is associated with lower costs and a shorter learning curve than uniportal endoscopy. In addition, surgical targets are reached through both ports percutaneously with slim 5–6 mm dilators avoiding excessive damage to the paraspinal muscles and giving the biportal endoscopic technique its characteristic of minimal invasiveness. However, studies with large samples and appropriate methodology are needed to determine the long-term pros and cons of biportal endoscopic facet joint denervation.

References

1. Meloncelli S, Germani G, Urti I, et al. Endoscopic radiofrequency facet joint treatment in patients with low back pain: technique and long-term results. A prospective cohort study. Ther Adv Musculoskelet Dis. 2020;12:1759720X20958979.
2. Cohen SP, Raja SN. Pathogenesis, diagnosis, and treatment of lumbar zygapophysial (facet) joint pain. Anesthesiology. 2007;106(3):591–614.
3. Xue Y, Ding T, Wang D, et al. Endoscopic rhizotomy for chronic lumbar zygapophysial joint pain. J Orthop Surg Res. 2020;15(1):4.

4. Tessitore E, Molliqaj G, Schatlo B, Schaller K. Clinical evaluation and surgical decision making for patients with lumbar discogenic pain and facet syndrome. Eur J Radiol. 2015;84(5):765–70.
5. Igarashi A, Kikuchi S, Konno S, Olmarker K. Inflammatory cytokines released from the facet joint tissue in degenerative lumbar spinal disorders. Spine (Phila Pa 1976). 2004;29(19):2091–5.
6. Gellhorn AC, Katz JN, Suri P. Osteoarthritis of the spine: the facet joints. Nat Rev Rheumatol. 2013;9(4):216–24.
7. Kim JS, Kroin JS, Buvanendran A, et al. Characterization of a new animal model for evaluation and treatment of back pain due to lumbar facet joint osteoarthritis. Arthritis Rheum. 2011;63(10):2966–73.
8. Schulte TL, Filler TJ, Struwe P, Liem D, Bullmann V. Intra-articular meniscoid folds in thoracic zygapophysial joints. Spine (Phila Pa 1976). 2010;35(6):E191–7.
9. Revel M, Poiraudeau S, Auleley GR, et al. Capacity of the clinical picture to characterize low back pain relieved by facet joint anesthesia. Proposed criteria to identify patients with painful facet joints. Spine (Phila Pa 1976). 1998;23(18):1972–7.
10. Boswell MV, Manchikanti L, Kaye AD, et al. A best-evidence systematic appraisal of the diagnostic accuracy and utility of facet (zygapophysial) joint injections in chronic spinal pain. Pain Physician. 2015;18(4):E497–533.
11. Kaplan M, Dreyfuss P, Halbrook B, Bogduk N. The ability of lumbar medial branch blocks to anesthetize the zygapophysial joint. A physiologic challenge. Spine (Phila Pa 1976). 1998;23(17):1847–52.
12. Boswell MV, Colson JD, Sehgal N, Dunbar EE, Epter R. A systematic review of therapeutic facet joint interventions in chronic spinal pain. Pain Physician. 2007;10(1):229–53.
13. Cohen SP, Huang JH, Brummett C. Facet joint pain—advances in patient selection and treatment. Nat Rev Rheumatol. 2013;9(2):101–16.
14. Putti V. New concepts in the pathogenesis of sciatica pain. Lancet. 1927;2:53–60.
15. Pathria M, Sartoris DJ, Resnick D. Osteoarthritis of the facet joints: accuracy of oblique radiographic assessment. Radiology. 1987;164(1):227–30.
16. Datta S, Lee M, Falco FJ, Bryce DA, Hayek SM. Systematic assessment of diagnostic accuracy and therapeutic utility of lumbar facet joint interventions. Pain Physician. 2009;12(2):437–60.
17. Manchikanti L, Kaye AD, Boswell MV, et al. A systematic review and best evidence synthesis of the effectiveness of therapeutic facet joint interventions in managing chronic spinal pain. Pain Physician. 2015;18(4):E535–82.
18. Rees WE. Multiple bilateral subcutaneous rhizolysis of segmental nerves in the treatment of the intervertebral disc syndrome. Ann Gen Pract. 1971;26:126–7.
19. Shealy CN. Percutaneous radiofrequency denervation of spinal facets. Treatment for chronic back pain and sciatica. J Neurosurg. 1975;43(4):448–51.
20. Shealy CN. Facet denervation in the management of back and sciatic pain. Clin Orthop Relat Res. 1976;115:157–64.
21. Cohen SP, Bhaskar A, Bhatia A, et al. Consensus practice guidelines on interventions for lumbar facet joint pain from a multispecialty, international working group. Reg Anesth Pain Med. 2020;45(6):424–67.
22. Kim MH, Kim SW, Ju CI, Chae KH, Kim DM. Effectiveness of repeated radiofrequency neurotomy for facet joint syndrome after microscopic discectomy. Korean J Spine. 2014;11(4):232–4.
23. Leclaire R, Fortin L, Lambert R, Bergeron YM, Rossignol M. Radiofrequency facet joint denervation in the treatment of low back pain: a placebo-controlled clinical trial to assess efficacy. Spine (Phila Pa 1976). 2001;26(13):1411–7.
24. van Wijk RM, Geurts JW, Wynne HJ, et al. Radiofrequency denervation of lumbar facet joints in the treatment of chronic low back pain: a randomized, double-blind, sham lesion-controlled trial [published correction appears in Clin J Pain. 2005 Sep–Oct;21(5):462]. Clin J Pain. 2005;21(4):335–44.
25. Manchikanti L, Singh V, Falco FJ, Cash KA, Pampati V. Evaluation of lumbar facet joint nerve blocks in managing chronic low back pain: a randomized, double-blind, controlled trial with a 2-year follow-up. Int J Med Sci. 2010;7(3):124–35.

26. Wu T, Zhao WH, Dong Y, Song HX, Li JH. Effectiveness of ultrasound-guided versus fluoroscopy or computed tomography scanning guidance in lumbar facet joint injections in adults with facet joint syndrome: a meta-analysis of controlled trials. Arch Phys Med Rehabil. 2016;97(9):1558–63.
27. Li ZZ, Hou SX, Shang WL, Song KR, Wu WW. Evaluation of endoscopic dorsal ramus rhizotomy in managing facetogenic chronic low back pain. Clin Neurol Neurosurg. 2014;126:11–7.
28. Jeong SY, Kim JS, Choi WS, Hur JW, Ryu KS. The effectiveness of endoscopic radiofrequency denervation of medial branch for treatment of chronic low back pain [published correction appears in J Korean Neurosurg Soc. 2014 Nov;56(5):454]. J Korean Neurosurg Soc. 2014;56(4):338–43.
29. Yeung A, Gore S. Endoscopically guided foraminal and dorsal rhizotomy for chronic axial back pain based on cadaver and endoscopically visualized anatomic study. Int J Spine Surg. 2014;8:23.
30. Divizia M, Germani G, Urti I, Imani F, Varrassi G, Meloncelli S. Endoscopic neuromodulation of suprascapular nerve in chronic shoulder pain: a case report. Anesth Pain Med. 2020;10(2):e103624.

Chapter 30
The Role of Unilateral Biportal Endoscopy in Thoracolumbar Burst Fractures

Javier Quillo-Olvera, Diego Quillo-Olvera, Javier Quillo-Reséndiz, and Michelle Barrera-Arreola

Abbreviations

CT	Computed tomography
EBL	Estimated blood loss
ICU	Intensive care unit
LBP	Lower back pain
MRI	Magnetic resonance imaging
NSAIDs	Nonsteroidal anti-inflammatory drugs
SCI	Spinal cord injury
UBE	Unilateral biportal endoscopy
VAS	Visual analog scale

Introduction

AO Spine has classified thoracolumbar spinal trauma in the AO Spine Thoracolumbar Spine Injury Classification to group injuries into different types and improve the reliability of their diagnosis, also facilitating communication between experts and

Supplementary Information The online version contains supplementary material available at [https://doi.org/10.1007/978-3-031-14736-4_30].

J. Quillo-Olvera (✉) · D. Quillo-Olvera · J. Quillo-Reséndiz · M. Barrera-Arreola
The Brain and Spine Care, Minimally Invasive Spine Surgery Group,
Hospital H+ Querétaro, Spine Clinic, Querétaro, México
e-mail: neuroqomd@gmail.com; drquilloolvera86@gmail.com; kitnoz@hotmail.com; michelle.barrera@anahuac.mx

J. Quillo-Olvera et al. (eds.), *Unilateral Biportal Endoscopy of the Spine*,
https://doi.org/10.1007/978-3-031-14736-4_30

improving the comparison of clinical results, allowing greater homogeneity in the therapeutic decisions made based on this classification [1, 2].

Despite having this classification, the decision of whether to treat thoracolumbar vertebral fractures surgically, especially burst fractures with neurological deterioration, remains controversial. Even the surgical intervention time in patients with a neurological deficit is based on clinical results extrapolated chiefly from studies on spinal cord injury [3]. Therefore, it is essential to comment which patients with thoracolumbar fractures can benefit from surgical treatment.

According to the AO Spine Thoracolumbar Spine Injury Classification, type A, with subtypes A0, A1, and A2 without neurological deterioration (N0), or a partial and transient neurological deficit (N1), generally would not require surgical treatment. However, the case should be reassessed when neurological impairment progresses (N2: radicular, N3: incomplete, and N4: complete) because an added inadvertent lesion may go unnoticed.

Treatment of subtypes A3 and A4 or burst fractures remains debatable. Some authors recommend surgical treatment for patients even without neurological deficit (N0) but with:

- Segmental kyphosis of 20°–35°
- The collapse of >50% vertebral body height
- >50% involvement of the canal due to retropulsed fragment

Others prefer to offer conservative treatment to patients with minimal neurological impairment (N0, N1, or Frankel D) without the characteristics mentioned above. However, conservative management requires prolonged immobilization, and the results reported in patients with a neurological deficit are not very encouraging [4–11].

Thoracolumbar burst fractures can be associated with instability, ligament injury, facet joint dislocation, diastasis of the spinous process, and subluxation. These features make it necessary to reclassify these lesions, and therefore surgical treatment must be offered [12, 13].

In the case of B1 type (Chance) fractures without neurological deterioration (N0) or minimal (N1), and only with a bone component, without displacement and no kyphosis, conservative treatment is accepted as an option. But, in cases where instability, kyphosis, severe pain, inability to walk, deformity, or neurological deterioration are anticipated, or radiological or clinical modifiers (M1 and M2) suggest progressive deterioration, surgical treatment may be offered. Lastly, surgical treatment is recommended for the remaining types of fractures (B2, B3, and C) due to their high probability of causing progressive neurological deterioration or deformity [12, 13].

To preserve the neurological function in a setting of thoracolumbar fracture is a priority. Biportal endoscopic decompression could be an option, especially in burst fractures with bone fragments encroaching the spinal canal. There are advantages associated with biportal endoscopic surgery that can be particularly useful, especially in patients with trauma and some other comorbidity who find it difficult to tolerate a "second hit" through early surgery; therefore, a technique that allows decompression of the nervous system with minimal physiological stress has the possibility of being better tolerated.

Biportal endoscopic surgery has a particular purpose: to allow the spine surgeon to perform direct decompression of the nervous system, with the least possible side effects. In turn, the surgeon can rely on other techniques to achieve the goals required in each singular case, such as stabilization, fixation, and fusion. The authors then discuss the role of the UBE technique in thoracolumbar burst fractures.

Indications

These are the indications recommended to perform a UBE decompression in a setting of thoracolumbar burst fracture:

1. Sufficient experience with the paramedian UBE approach.
2. Technological resources to employ the UBE technique.
3. A medical staff familiar with the UBE technique.
4. Diagnosed thoracolumbar burst fracture categorized as A3 or A4 by the AO Spine Thoracolumbar Spine Injury Classification.
5. Single level injured.
6. Progressive or established (more than 6 and before 24 h) neurological deterioration (N2, N3, N4) based on the AO Spine Thoracolumbar Spine Injury Classification, associated with a specific compromise of the neural elements (spinal cord, cauda equina, or specific nerve root) observed in imaging studies (retropulsed bone fragment within the spinal canal, >50% of stenosis regarding that, etc.).
7. Hemodynamically stable patient, with conditions to be operated on.
8. Be prepared to use other techniques to accomplish specific goals on a case-by-case basis.
9. Not having any of the above would contraindicate the biportal endoscopic decompression procedure.

Surgical Instruments

The technical requirements to perform a biportal endoscopic procedure include a complete laminectomy set containing dissectors, root retractor, nerve hook, pituitary forceps, and Kerrison rongeur of different sizes. In addition, it is necessary to have a drilling system that can be used in water, specialized radiofrequency probes for endoscopy, and 0° or 30° endoscopic lenses. The 0° endoscope will allow us a panoramic view, while in the 30° endoscope, a more lateral view is reached (Fig. 30.1).

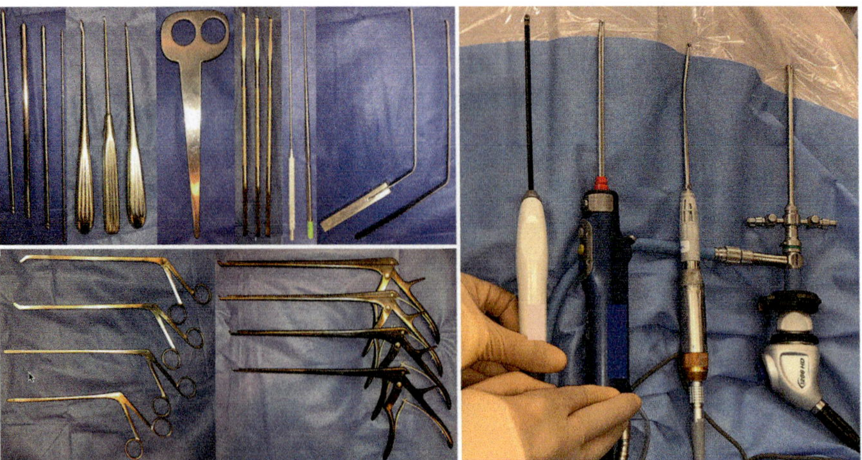

Fig. 30.1 Various surgical tools used in UBE

Surgical Technique

The main objective of biportal endoscopy is to achieve a successful decompression of the neural elements through a technique associated with less physiological stress for the patient with a thoracolumbar burst fracture and familiar with the surgeon.

Thoracolumbar burst fractures usually present with bone fragments invading the spinal canal or other sites in the ventral epidural space. The unilateral biportal endoscopic (UBE) paramedian approach is appropriate for decompressing the central canal and lateral recesses. Part of the success of this technique consists of the correct triangulation of both ports. The triangulation must be directed towards the target.

The biportal endoscopic approach requires a pair of incisions for the endoscope and to introduce the surgical instruments. In a paramedian approach, the skin is incised medial to the superior and inferior pedicles of the index level. The rostrocaudal location of incisions is modified according to the location of the pathology within the spinal canal.

The endoscope is inserted through the caudal incision in a right-sided approach done by a right-handed surgeon. For approaching the left side, this is contrary. Both incisions are planned with the aid of the fluoroscope in AP and lateral views (Fig. 30.2). Subsequently, the surgeon will place the dilators through each incision to triangulate them and feel the bone surfaces and the interlaminar space (Fig. 30.3).

After setting both ports properly, the endoscope is introduced to co-locate the surgical instruments in the interlaminar space and confirm the adequate flow of saline, which enters through the optical system and exits through the working channel. Then, the soft tissue overlying the bone landmarks is removed using pituitary forceps or the radiofrequency probe. The bone references usually are the spinolaminar junction, the lamina (inferior edge from superior lamina or superior edge from inferior lamina), or the medial border of the facet joint (Fig. 30.4).

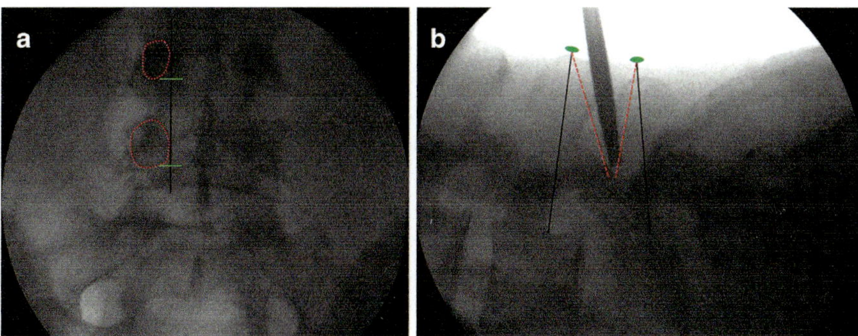

Fig. 30.2 Intraoperative images obtained with the C-arm in a patient with an A3-type L5 burst fracture. (**a**) Paramedian approach planned in an AP view. The red dotted circles represent the L4 and L5 right-side pedicles. The medial pedicle was drawn with a black vertical line. The green parapedicular lines represent the incisions. (**b**) In the lateral fluoroscopic projection, the red dotted lines represent the trajectory of both ports. This case requires addressing the approach to L5 lamina

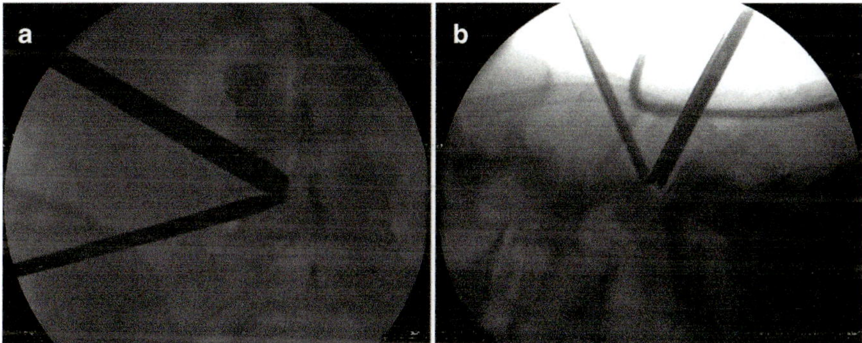

Fig. 30.3 Paramedian right-sided L4–L5 UBE approach. (**a**) AP view. (**b**) Lateral view

Fig. 30.4 Useful bone references in UBE. A, spinolaminar junction; B and B′, lamina; C, medial border of the facet joint

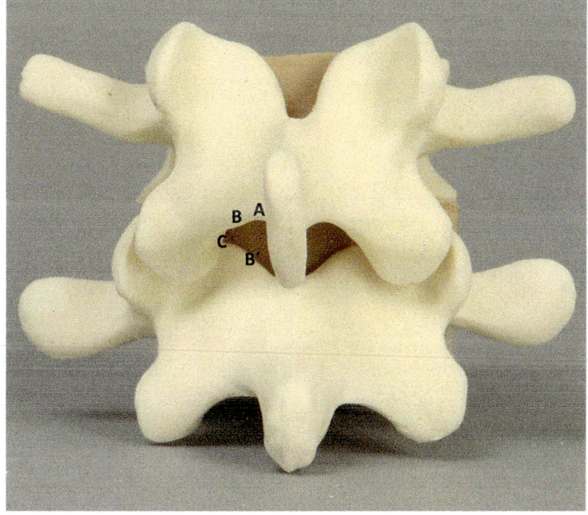

One of the advantages of unilateral biportal endoscopic surgery is a target-addressed technique. Usually, the biportal endoscopic procedure starts by drilling the spinolaminar junction of the cranial lamina. However, the decompression can start by undercutting the inferior lamina or the ipsilateral recess. If the case requires a bilateral decompression, bone removal can be done circumferentially, and for passing to the contralateral side, the base of the spinous process of the cranial lamina should be drilled. During bone decompression, the over-the-top technique helps preserve the neural elements by using the yellow ligament as a protective barrier before removing it.

After sufficient bone removal, the yellow ligament attachments are identified, and it is removed with Kerrison rongeur of different sizes. However, it is advisable to be careful with flavectomy due to possible adhesions between the ventral aspect of the yellow ligament and the dura through meningovertebral ligaments, located mainly in the midline and ventral epidural space, which, when pulled aggressively, could cause a dural tear.

The endpoint of decompression is accomplished when the surgeon can mobilize neural elements freely. Depending on each case, other maneuvers than biportal endoscopic decompression can be used, such as retropulsed bone fragment removal located in the ventral epidural space, transcorporeal vertebroplasty under direct endoscopic vision, or segmental stabilization through various types of fixations (short, long transpedicular, etc.) (Videos 30.1 and 30.2).

Illustrated Cases

Case 1

A 28-year-old male with no history of other diseases suffered a car accident. The patient presented with severe lower back pain (LBP) managed with opioids in the hospital's emergency room with incomplete relief of his misery. The neurological examination revealed right-leg numbness and severe (3/5) right-ankle dorsiflexion weakness.

An incomplete L5 burst fracture with only the superior endplate comminuted and a retropulsed bone fragment within the spinal canal was identified in the computed tomography (CT) scan and magnetic resonance imaging (MRI) of the lumbar spine obtained at the hospital admission. According to AO Spine Thoracolumbar Spine Injury Classification, the injury was classified as L5 incomplete burst fracture type A3, with radicular impairment N2 (Fig. 30.5a–d).

After 8 h under surveillance, the patient did not show any clinical improvement neither in LBP nor in loss of the strength of the right-ankle dorsiflexion. Therefore, a unilateral biportal endoscopic (UBE) decompression of L4–L5, including the right-sided lateral recess and central canal plus spinal stabilization through a transcorporeal vertebroplasty under endoscopic visualization and a short transpedicular fixation L4–S1, was proposed to the patient who accepted signing the informed consent. The intraoperative findings included traumatic damage in the L5 traversing

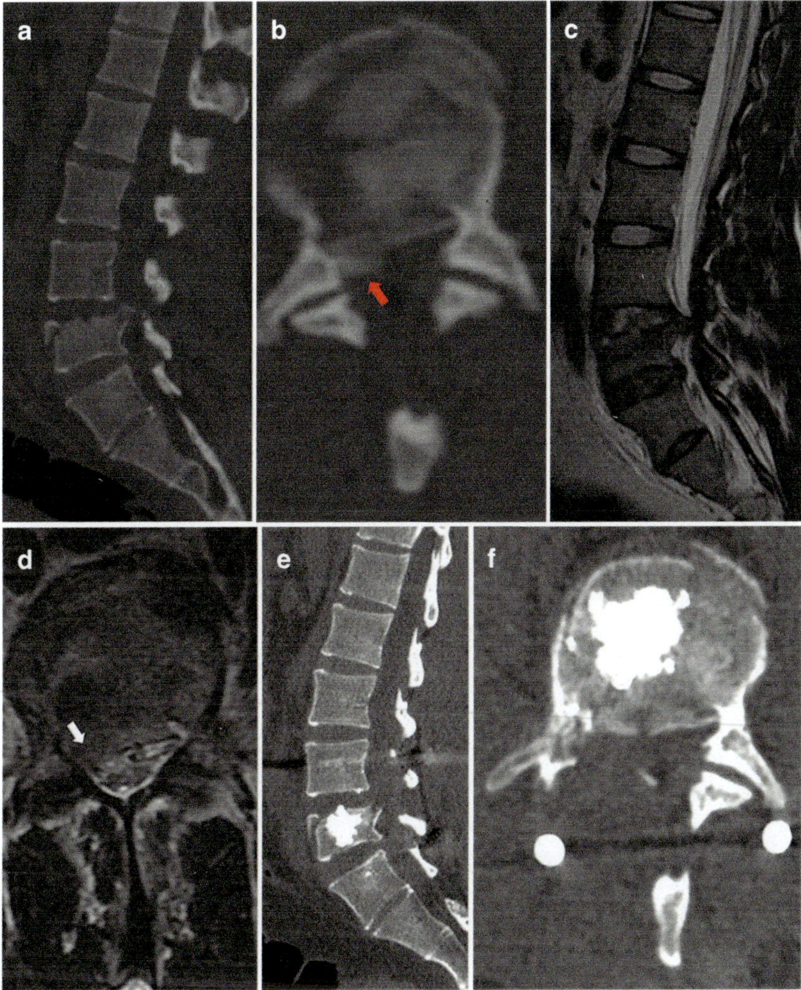

Fig. 30.5 Case 1 illustrations. (**a**) Sagittal view of preoperative lumbar CT scan. (**b**) Axial view of L5 on the preoperative CT scan. The red arrow points to the fractured bone located in the right-sided lateral recess. (**c**) Sagittal view of the preoperative lumbar MRI. The retropulsed bone fragment at L4–L5 occupying the spinal canal is noted. (**d**) Axial view of L5 on the preoperative MRI. The spinal canal stenosis is evident, and the white arrow points to the right side's bone particle within the lateral recess. (**e**) Sagittal view of postoperative lumbar CT scan. Vertebral augmentation can be observed at L5. (**f**) Axial view of L5 on the postoperative CT scan. Sufficient bone decompression was achieved through the UBE technique. (**g**) Postoperative lumbar CT scan reconstructed showing the short-length transpedicular fixation at L4–S1. (**h**) Two-year follow-up lumbar MRI shows spinal canal decompressed and no postoperative kyphosis. (**i**) Axial view of the postoperative lumbar MRI with adequate decompression of neural elements on the fracture site

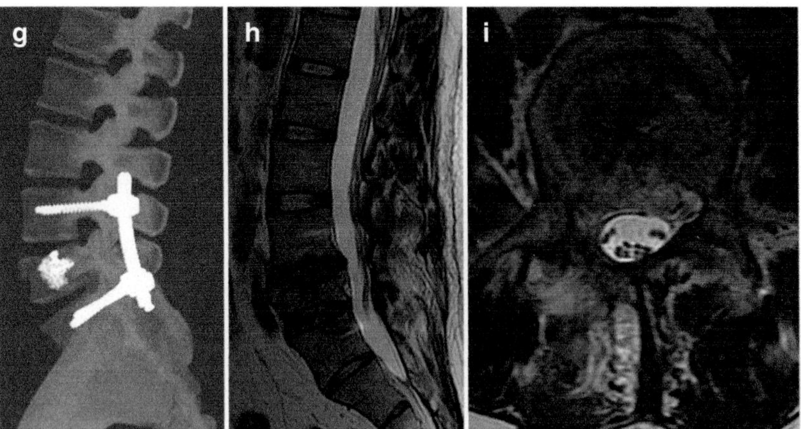

Fig. 30.5 (contnued)

nerve on the right side with a bone spike from the L5 posterior wall. Nonsurgical complications were reported. The estimated blood loss (EBL) was 30 mL with an operative time of 120 min. The drain left in the epidural space was removed the following day before hospital discharge with <7 mL of collected fluid. The patient did not require opioids after the surgery, and postoperative pain control was achieved with NSAIDs. The patient was discharged a day after surgery.

The immediate postoperative VAS score for back pain improved from 9 to 2. Numbness of the right leg also improved significantly after the surgery. The strength of the right-ankle dorsiflexion recovered partially from 3/5 to 4/5 after surgery. However, the patient could walk without assistance the day after the procedure. The postoperative lumbar CT scan showed proper transpedicular fixation of L4 and S1 with bone cement augmentation at the L5 vertebral body. The 2-year follow-up imaging workout demonstrated sufficient decompression of neural elements with no kyphotic deformity of the lumbar spine (Fig. 30.5e–i; Video 30.1).

Case 2

A 51-year-old female with a recent car accident history presented with severe back pain in the upper lumbar region and an inability to stand up. The patient also complained of severe numbness in the perianal area and both legs. Physical examination revealed nonspecific paresthesia of the perianal site and both legs, without impaired strength of the legs and severe pain on direct palpation of the thoracolumbar junction. The patient was treated with opioids to reduce her pain without success.

CT scan and MRI of the lumbar spine showed an incomplete L1 burst fracture, with height collapse of the vertebral body and only comminution of the superior endplate. A retropulsed fragment at T12–L1 was observed. This injury was classified as an incomplete burst fracture of L1, which according to the AO Spine Thoracolumbar Spine Injury Classification was type A3–N3 (Fig. 30.6a–d).

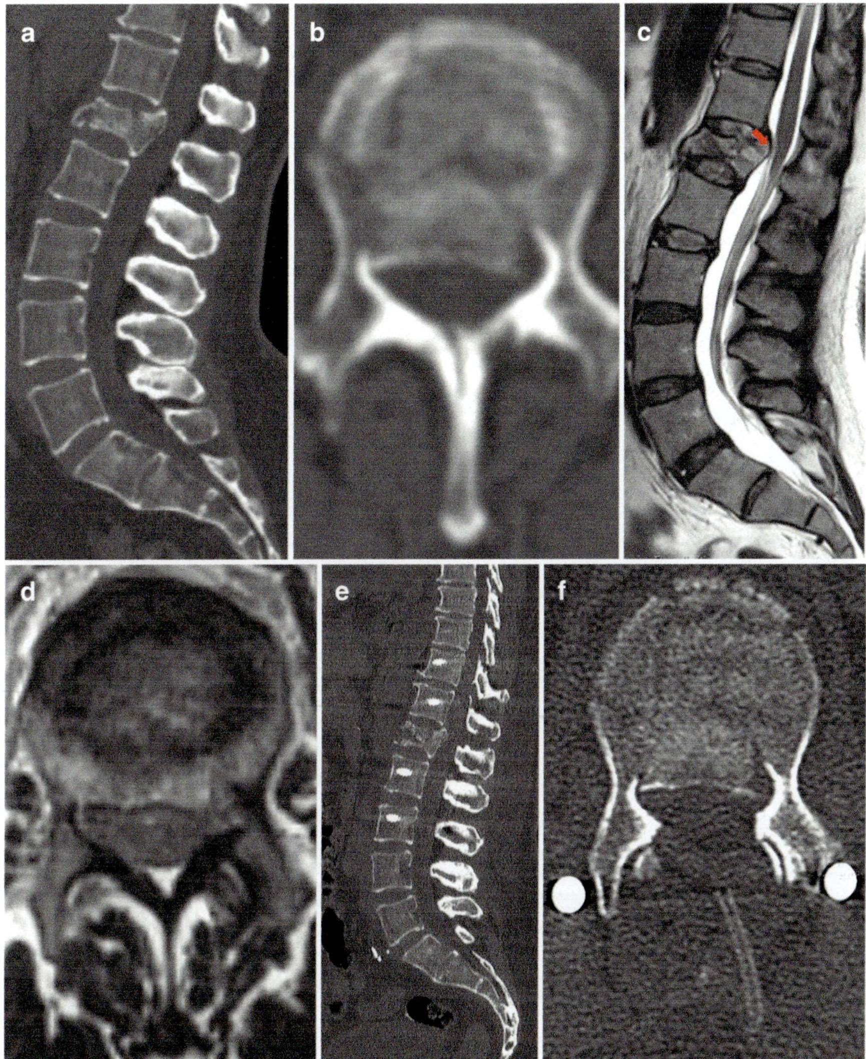

Fig. 30.6 Case 2 illustrations. (**a**) Sagittal view of preoperative lumbar CT scan. (**b**) Axial view of L1 on the preoperative CT scan. Retropulsion of the L1 posterior wall is observed. (**c**) Sagittal view of the preoperative lumbar MRI. The posterior wall of L1 contacts the ventral surface of the medullary cone (red arrow). (**d**) Axial view of L1 on the preoperative MRI. The central stenosis is evident. (**e**) Sagittal view of postoperative lumbar CT scan. After surgery, an increased height of L1 is observed, and sagittal alignment is preserved. (**f**) Axial view of L1 on the postoperative CT scan. Sufficient decompression was achieved through the UBE technique

After 12 h of evolution, the patient did not show any clinical improvement. Therefore, a posterior bilateral decompression of T12–L1 through a biportal endoscopic approach and transpedicular fixation due to the thoracolumbar junction location of the fracture was offered. The patient accepted the procedure and signed the informed consent.

The surgery lasted for 110 min, with an EBL of 40 mL. No intraoperative complications were reported. The paresthesia in the perianal region and legs disappeared, and the back pain improved from a VAS of 10/10 to 1/10 immediately after surgery. The patient did not require postoperative opioids, and NSAIDs were used to control postoperative pain. The patient was discharged on the second day after her procedure.

The postoperative CT scan demonstrated sufficient bilateral decompression of the central spinal canal at the T12–L1 with restitution of vertebral collapse in L1 (Fig. 30.6e, f). In addition, the postoperative images showed an adequate transpedicular construct in T10, T11, L2, and L3 without thoracolumbar kyphosis (Fig. 30.7; Video 30.2).

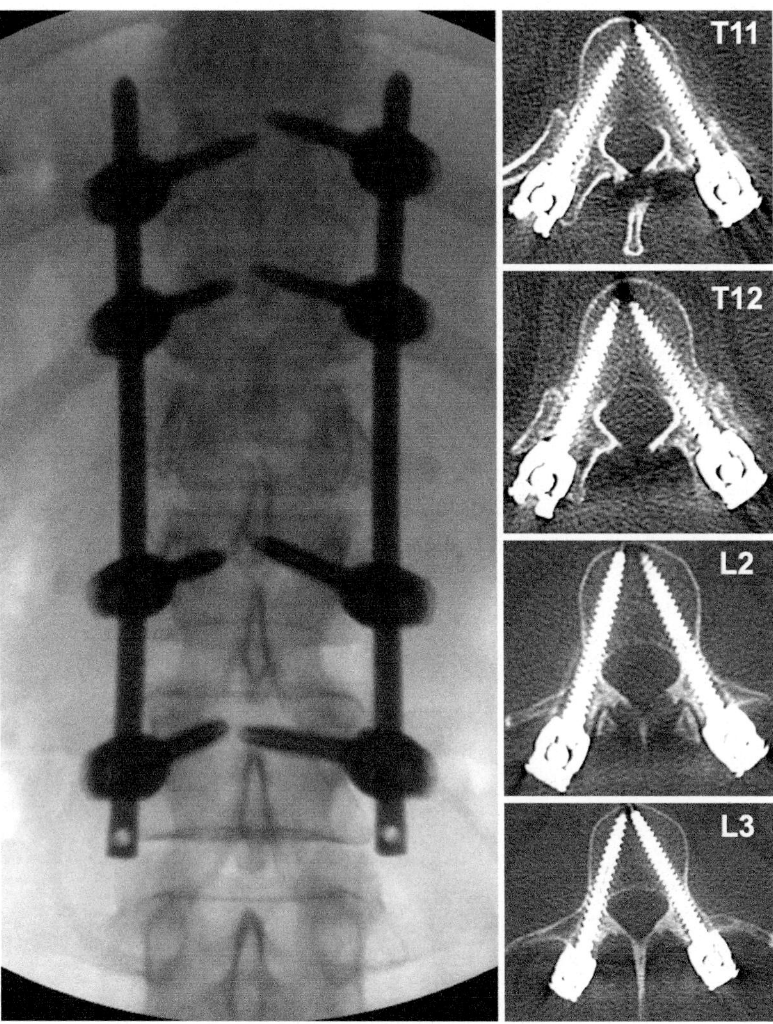

Fig. 30.7 Transpedicular fixation from T11 to L3 from Case 2

Discussion

It is important to remember that 10–20% of thoracolumbar fractures are burst, and 52% occur at the thoracolumbar junction, as Case 2 presented. However, L5 burst fractures such as Case 1 are not frequent and have an approximate incidence of 1.2% [14, 15].

Thoracolumbar burst fractures are commonly seen in daily clinical practice. They usually result from an axial load that produces a compressive force on the vertebral body, especially from trauma in young individuals or falls in senile patients with osteoporosis. The AO Spine Thoracolumbar Spine Injury Classification System has classified these types of fractures as A3 and A4, depending on whether one or both endplates have comminution.

These fractures are associated with bony encroachment to the spinal canal, which may or may not cause compression of the spinal cord, medullary cone, cauda equina, or nerve roots.

In both cases presented in this chapter, the clinical neurological impact caused by the bone fragment located in the spinal canal was identified. In Case 1, a piece of bony spike injured the right-sided L5 nerve root; it was observed through the endoscope. In Case 2, the patient showed sensitive neurological disturbances in the perianal region secondary to stenosis at the level of the medullary cone.

Direct decompression of the neural elements in both scenarios was the reason for performing the biportal endoscopic technique. However, it is essential to note that decompression was not the only goal in the treatment but also the stabilization of the fracture and the resulting kyphosis prevention. For this reason, both cases were treated with other procedures. Therefore, not all thoracolumbar burst fractures will require direct decompression of the neural elements. Hence, the role of biportal endoscopic surgery in this pathology is well defined.

The benefits observed in patients with burst fractures who underwent early decompression (less than 24 h) have also been reported: (1) early mobilization, (2) decreased back pain and less consumption of painkillers, and (3) decrease in respiratory morbidity, length of stay in the ICU, hospital stay, and total mortality rate.

Some arguments do not coincide with early decompression, such as the impact of a second trauma related to the surgery. It is poorly tolerated by the patient, performing the surgery in a suboptimal state or with limited resources and suboptimal planning, among others [3].

The authors consider that both criteria are valid. Still, in the context of neurological deterioration and with an optimal patient state, it is feasible to offer minimally invasive techniques with a minimal impact on the patient's general condition, such as biportal endoscopic decompression and other fixation methods.

Different studies of thoracolumbar burst fractures show that early fixation between 24 and 72 h, with or without spinal cord injury, reduces the total complication rate, time of hospital stay and in ICU, number of days with a ventilator, respiratory morbidity, and infections among other advantages [16–19]. However, the recommendation of how soon the decompression of the neural elements should be in thoracolumbar burst fractures remains controversial because the answer is based on the extrapolation of the results seen in patients with SCI, where decompression is recommended before 24 h after trauma, which is beneficial and could also possibly be helpful for patients with thoracolumbar burst fractures with severe root compression.

The fact is that most surgeons prefer to offer surgical treatment to patients with thoracolumbar burst fractures with neurological deterioration to treat instability, restore sagittal balance, prevent deformity, decrease back pain, allow rapid mobilization out of bed, and release the neural elements [20].

From this perspective, endoscopic surgery provides well-known benefits, like all those related to minimally invasive spinal techniques, which can benefit patients with trauma and low tolerance to other surgery-related trauma [21, 22].

Specifically, applying the unilateral biportal endoscopic (UBE) technique in trauma allowed successful direct decompressions of the dural sac and the traversing nerves. In addition, UBE is a target-addressed technique; therefore, the injury to paraspinal structures is minimal. Also, familiarity with the anatomy seen through the endoscope is similar to that observed through the microscope.

However, it is paramount to clarify that it is necessary to have experience in the UBE technique before performing trauma cases; in addition, planning is relevant because, as mentioned, decompression is only part of the therapeutic process; other methods must be contemplated and applied if required depending on the case.

The authors note that the leading role of the UBE in thoracolumbar burst fractures is the decompression of the neural elements under direct visualization, magnification, and illumination offered by the endoscope with continuous irrigation.

However, it is crucial to point out that the data obtained on applying water-based endoscopic techniques, including UBE, to spinal trauma come from anecdotal case series done by KOLs in endoscopic surgery [23, 24]. Therefore, studies with proper methodology contrasting the benefits of biportal endoscopic surgery with those derived from conventional techniques are necessary to know the value of UBE applied to thoracolumbar burst fractures.

Tips, Pearls, and Pitfalls

- The correct execution of the triangular approach is crucial. A tip is to make the working channel first. Then, the inserted dilator must be directed towards the bone landmark. Subsequently, the dilator for the endoscopic channel is introduced, and it will be easier only to find the working canal already located in the bone reference.
- Always confirm your location with the AP and lateral views to avoid wrong-level surgery.
- Before beginning decompression, it is advisable to confirm the correct inflow and outflow of continuous irrigation through the system created by the two ports.
- It is advisable to perform decompression sequentially, first the bone elements, using the over-the-top technique, and then the yellow ligament.
- If the ventral lumbar epidural space is to be explored, it is imperative to free the neural elements. Excessive retraction of the neural elements should always be avoided.

- The surgeon must be careful when removing bone fragments located in the ventral epidural space since doing so may damage the ventral surface of the dural sac.
- Patients with thoracolumbar burst fractures that present symptoms of progressive neurological deterioration, and coinciding with the compressive imaging findings, are the best candidates to offer direct decompression.
- Complications of direct neural decompression in thoracolumbar burst fractures are similar to those seen in lumbar spinal stenosis decompression. However, there are certain exceptions, for example, dural tears secondary to bone fragments in the epidural space. Sometimes, it is better not to remove them as they can damage the dura. Correct planning with CT scan and MRI is vital to identify them before surgery. Direct dorsal decompression is usually sufficient in some cases, and other techniques can correct traumatic bone defects.
- Bleeding is often of concern, especially in UBE. If this happens, the hydrostatic pressure can intermittently rise to more than 30 mmHg. This will allow locating the specific bleeding site. The radiofrequency probe, bone wax, or different hemostatic products can be used for hemostasis.
- Other complications related to the biportal endoscopic technique are residual epidural hematoma, which can be avoided by performing adequate hemostasis as already mentioned and placing a drain at the end of the surgery in the epidural space.
- Nerve injury, with emphasis on decompression of the spinal cord: Exploring the dorsal and ventral epidural space in lumbar burst fractures is feasible. However, this is not recommended for the thoracic spine, especially in high levels, due to the possibility of injury to the spinal cord by manipulation. The use of other techniques is recommended in thoracic burst fractures.
- Paraspinal soft-tissue edema is often associated with an inadequate approach with poor drainage from continuous saline irrigation. Therefore, before beginning endoscope use, it is advisable to confirm a correct inflow and outflow of solution through both ports.
- Incomplete decompression is especially common when there is insufficient experience with biportal endoscopic procedures. It is highly recommended to get orient with the C-arm to confirm the endpoints of decompression.

Conclusion

The role of biportal endoscopic surgery in thoracolumbar burst fractures is very well defined: decompression of the neural elements in situations that put them at risk, such as bone fragments in the canal. However, despite this being feasible, other techniques must be considered to meet the goals required in each case. Dorsal decompression may be possible in thoracic cord compression, but not spinal cord manipulation to explore the epidural space. More formal studies are necessary to clarify the benefit of the UBE technique in spinal trauma.

References

1. Vaccaro AR, Oner C, Kepler CK, et al. AOSpine thoracolumbar spine injury classification system: fracture description, neurological status, and key modifiers. Spine (Phila Pa 1976). 2013;38(23):2028–37.
2. Kepler CK, Vaccaro AR, Koerner JD, et al. Reliability analysis of the AOSpine thoracolumbar spine injury classification system by a worldwide group of naïve spinal surgeons. Eur Spine J. 2016;25(4):1082–6.
3. Kato S, Murray JC, Kwon BK, Schroeder GD, Vaccaro AR, Fehlings MG. Does surgical intervention or timing of surgery have an effect on neurological recovery in the setting of a thoracolumbar burst fracture? J Orthop Trauma. 2017;31(Suppl 4):S38–43.
4. Krompinger WJ, Fredrickson BE, Mino DE, Yuan HA. Conservative treatment of fractures of the thoracic and lumbar spine. Orthop Clin North Am. 1986;17(1):161–70.
5. Tezer M, Erturer RE, Ozturk C, Ozturk I, Kuzgun U. Conservative treatment of fractures of the thoracolumbar spine. Int Orthop. 2005;29(2):78–82.
6. da Silva OT, Joaquim AF. Burst fractures in the thoracolumbar junction: what do we know about their treatment? Arch Neurosci. 2016;3(4):e39949. https://doi.org/10.5812/archneurosci.39949.
7. Winklhofer S, Thekkumthala-Sommer M, Schmidt D, et al. Magnetic resonance imaging frequently changes classification of acute traumatic thoracolumbar spine injuries. Skelet Radiol. 2013;42(6):779–86.
8. Hitchon PW, Torner JC, Haddad SF, Follett KA. Management options in thoracolumbar burst fractures. Surg Neurol. 1998;49(6):619–27.
9. Tropiano P, Huang RC, Louis CA, Poitout DG, Louis RP. Functional and radiographic outcome of thoracolumbar and lumbar burst fractures managed by closed orthopaedic reduction and casting. Spine (Phila Pa 1976). 2003;28(21):2459–65.
10. Moller A, Hasserius R, Redlund-Johnell I, Ohlin A, Karlsson MK. Nonoperatively treated burst fractures of the thoracic and lumbar spine in adults: a 23- to 41-year follow-up. Spine J. 2007;7(6):701–7.
11. Weninger P, Schultz A, Hertz H. Conservative management of thoracolumbar and lumbar spine compression and burst fractures: functional and radiographic outcomes in 136 cases treated by closed reduction and casting. Arch Orthop Trauma Surg. 2009;129(2):207–19.
12. Joaquim AF, Patel AA, Schroeder GD, Vaccaro AR. A simplified treatment algorithm for treating thoracic and lumbar spine trauma. J Spinal Cord Med. 2019;42(4):416–22.
13. Scheer JK, Bakhsheshian J, Fakurnejad S, Oh T, Dahdaleh NS, Smith ZA. Evidence-based medicine of traumatic thoracolumbar burst fractures: a systematic review of operative management across 20 years. Global Spine J. 2015;5(1):73–82.
14. Kao FC, Hsieh MK, Yu CW, et al. Additional vertebral augmentation with posterior instrumentation for unstable thoracolumbar burst fractures. Injury. 2017;48(8):1806–12.
15. Sahin S, Resnick DK. Minimally incisional stabilization of unstable L5 burst fracture. J Spinal Disord Tech. 2005;18(5):455–7.
16. Bliemel C, Lefering R, Buecking B, et al. Early or delayed stabilization in severely injured patients with spinal fractures? Current surgical objectivity according to the Trauma Registry of DGU: treatment of spine injuries in polytrauma patients. J Trauma Acute Care Surg. 2014;76(2):366–73.
17. Frangen TM, Ruppert S, Muhr G, Schinkel C. The beneficial effects of early stabilization of thoracic spine fractures depend on trauma severity. J Trauma. 2010;68(5):1208–12.
18. Kerwin AJ, Frykberg ER, Schinco MA, Griffen MM, Murphy T, Tepas JJ. The effect of early spine fixation on non-neurologic outcome. J Trauma. 2005;58(1):15–21.
19. Schinkel C, Frangen TM, Kmetic A, Andress HJ, Muhr G, German Trauma Registry. Timing of thoracic spine stabilization in trauma patients: impact on clinical course and outcome. J Trauma. 2006;61(1):156–60.

20. Rabb CH, Hoh DJ, Anderson PA, et al. Congress of Neurological Surgeons systematic review and evidence-based guidelines on the evaluation and treatment of patients with thoracolumbar spine trauma: operative versus nonoperative treatment. Neurosurgery. 2019;84(1):E50–2.
21. Warhurst M, Hartman J, Granville M, Jacobson RE. The role of minimally invasive spinal surgical procedures in the elderly patient: an analysis of 49 patients between 75 and 95 years of age. Cureus. 2020;12(3):e7180.
22. Safaee MM, Shah V, Tenorio A, Uribe JS, Clark AJ. Minimally invasive pedicle screw fixation with indirect decompression by ligamentotaxis in pathological fractures. Oper Neurosurg (Hagerstown). 2020;19(2):210–7.
23. Quillo-Olvera J, Quillo-Olvera D, Quillo-Reséndiz J, Barrera-Arreola M. Unilateral biportal endoscopic-guided transcorporeal vertebroplasty with neural decompression for treating a traumatic lumbar fracture of L5. World Neurosurg. 2020;144:74–81.
24. Kang MS, Heo DH, Chung HJ, et al. Biportal endoscopic posterior lumbar decompression and vertebroplasty for extremely elderly patients affected by lower lumbar delayed vertebral collapse with lumbosacral radiculopathy. J Orthop Surg Res. 2021;16(1):380.

Chapter 31
Complications Associated with Unilateral Biportal Endoscopic Spine Surgery

Rajeesh George, Pang Hung Wu, and Gamaliel Tan Yu Heng

Abbreviations

BESS	Biportal endoscopic spinal surgery
CSF	Cerebrospinal fluid
ICP	Intracranial pressure
IDT	Incidental dural tear
LC-CUSUM	Learning curve cumulative summation test
LDH	Lumbar disc herniation
LF	Ligamentum flavum
PSEH	Postoperative spinal epidural hematoma
UBE	Unilateral biportal endoscopy
ULBD	Unilateral laminotomy for bilateral decompression

Introduction

Percutaneous endoscopic surgery is becoming one of the most common procedures for lumbar disc herniation (LDH), lumbar spinal stenosis, and also fusion. It is a minimally invasive procedure that includes a small incision, low blood loss, and early discharge [1, 2]. Uniportal endoscopic spinal surgery is performed through a

Dr. Rajeesh George and Dr. Pang Hung Wu contributed equally to this work as first authors.

R. George · P. H. Wu (✉) · G. T. Y. Heng
National University Health System, Juronghealth Campus, Department of Orthopaedic Surgery, Ng Teng Fong General Hospital, Singapore, Singapore
e-mail: rajeesh_george@nuhs.edu.sg; wupanghung@gmail.com; gamaliel_tan@nuhs.edu.sg

J. Quillo-Olvera et al. (eds.), *Unilateral Biportal Endoscopy of the Spine*,
https://doi.org/10.1007/978-3-031-14736-4_31

single portal involving light source, irrigation, visualization, and instrumentation. There are technical difficulties that may be encountered by surgeons using a single portal, which are particularly relevant in severe stenosis or in cases in need of bilateral decompression [3–6]. Furthermore, surgeons need to be familiar with the full endoscopic technique, which requires a steep learning curve. Unilateral biportal endoscopic spinal surgery (UBE), referred to with different names in reported studies, is the combination of integrated open and endoscopic spinal surgery, which can lessen the impact of the limitations [7–9].

It is a minimally invasive spinal surgery that has several advantages, such as less postoperative pain and early return to the activities of daily living [10]. It is a variant of arthroscopic surgery that can preserve paravertebral muscles and is less invasive to bone and ligamentous structures since smaller incisions are made. Since Kambin and Brager [11] first introduced spinal surgery with the arthroscopic system for disc herniation, it has been applied to various pathologies in spinal surgery. Thus, this approach has been widely applied in decompressive laminotomy, fusion surgery, and degenerative and even tumorous conditions [12, 13].

UBE has its own unique advantages. It provides excellent magnification and illumination compared with conventional endoscopy owing to the use of arthroscopic instruments that are used in knee and shoulder surgery. Additionally, a wider view can be provided by free handling of endoscopic instruments, avoiding the narrow field of vision provided by a conventional endoscope [14]. UBE is not confined by the working tube or the working channel. With continuous high-pressure normal saline irrigation and a high-definition arthroscope, the surgeon can do very precise decompression in a clear and magnified surgical field [15].

As the number of procedures using this technique has increased, characteristic side effects have arisen, such as water-related problems and incomplete manipulation due to instrument constraints, other than the inherent disadvantage of repetitive radiation exposure due to lack of three-dimensional orientation. Additionally, insufficient disc removal, incidental dural tear, difficulty in controlling bleeding, and a steep learning curve are considered drawbacks to the procedure. However, continuous technical developments have been noted in this surgical approach due to advancements in surgical tools and availability of enhanced high-definition video equipment and have helped to mitigate some of the complications associated with the procedure. Here, we discuss our method of doing UBE and the complications associated with this technique.

Surgical Techniques

We are describing here our method for decompression for a single level for lumbar spinal stenosis using the UBE technique. Variations can be tailored to the procedure at hand and the side of the procedure. Neuromonitoring is routinely used. After induction of general anesthesia, the patient is placed prone with the abdomen free over the radiolucent table. The skin and the surgical field are prepared in the usual manners. UBE surgery is performed under continuous normal saline irrigation. It is critical to ensure that the final layer of draping is waterproof and a smooth drainage system for the saline outflow is properly set up. Without these precautions, the patient may be soaked by the cold normal saline and complicated with hypothermia.

In order to obtain a true anterior-posterior image, the fluoroscope should be tilted parallel to the disc space. We would recommend tilting the table instead to get the endplates parallel rather than tilting the fluoroscope. The spinal levels of interest are determined using biplanar fluoroscopy and marked on the skin. UBE decompression requires two small incisions through the deep fascia: a smaller one about 5–6 mm for insertion of arthroscope and continuous normal saline irrigation and a larger one about 8–10 mm for the outflow of normal saline, which is used as the instrument portal (Fig. 31.1).

An arthroscopic system with either a 0° or 30° scope is essential. The initial target area for decompression is at the spinolaminar junction (the junction of spinous process and lower laminar margin of superior vertebra). The two skin incisions are usually located along the medial pedicle line, separated by 2–3 cm (Fig. 31.1).

The left-sided approach is preferred for right-hand-dominant surgeons. In the right-sided approach, the working portal was made 0.5 cm distal compared with that in the left-sided approach. The viewing portal was made vertically 1 cm proximal (left-sided approach) and distal (right-sided approach) from the working portal.

We use serial dilators up to 10 mm to split the paraspinal muscles, enlarge the instrument portal, and gently detach the soft tissues of the interlaminar space with a periosteal elevator. With the inflow of normal saline, a small space is created and ready to use. With meticulous hemostasis, the whole surgical procedure can be performed in a clear and magnified surgical field. Hemostasis for bleeding from small epidural veins and oozing from bones can be achieved by adjusting the inflow hydrostatic pressure and control of outflow.

Bleeding from soft tissues and larger epidural veins can be cauterized efficiently by a radiofrequency wand. Bone wax is useful for stopping more severe bleeding from cancellous bone. We always start the decompression from the spinolaminar junction using an electric high-speed diamond bur of 3 or 4 mm in diameter.

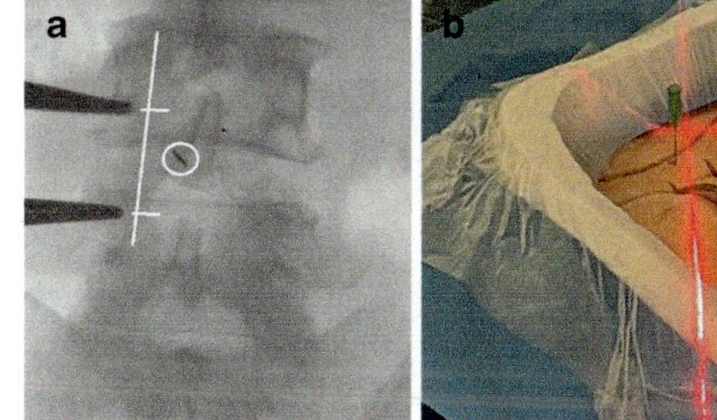

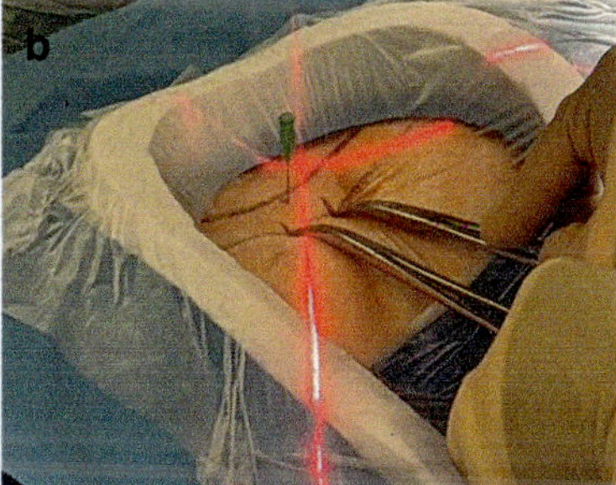

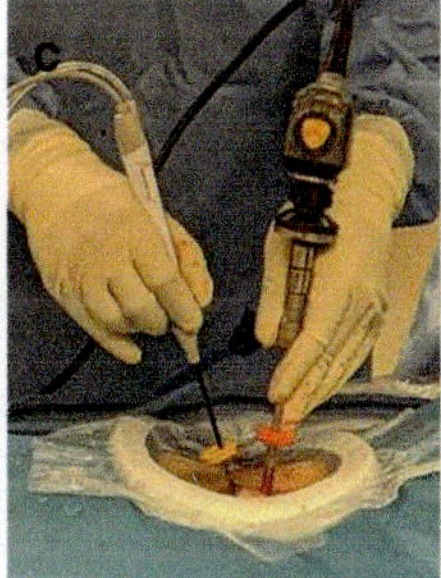

Fig. 31.1 (**a**) The circle indicates the initial targeting area, the spinolaminar junction. The skin incisions are located along the medial pedicle line, separated by 2–3 cm. (**b**) Skin marking of two portals. (**c**) The photograph demonstrates the triangulation of the endoscope and instruments

The decompression procedures are performed according to the following steps:

1. Drill the ipsilateral lamina from its lower margin cranially until the origin of ligamentum flavum is exposed.
2. Drill the upper laminar margin of the lower vertebra and then detach the ligamentum flavum from its caudal attachment.
3. Perform ipsilateral decompression by drilling the medial margin of the ipsilateral lamina and facet joints. The facet drilling should be very conservative to preserve the facet joint as much as possible.
4. Remove the superficial layer of ligamentum flavum and preserve the deep layer as a protector.
5. Drill the undersurface of the contralateral lamina until the lateral recess is almost reached. Note that the ligamentum flavum must be preserved as a protector for underlying neural tissue. In the cases of severe stenosis, the spinous process and facet joints are usually hypertrophic and deformed.
6. Removing more bone from the base of the spinous process would widen the laminotomy window and provide easier access to the contralateral lateral recess.
7. Remove the ipsilateral half of the ligamentum flavum, free the ipsilateral traversing nerve root, and check residual stenosis.
8. Separate the ligamentum flavum from the undersurface of the contralateral lamina using a blunt neural dissector.
9. Separate the contralateral ligamentum flavum from its attachment on the lamina, and decompress the contralateral lateral recess and foramen using a small and curved Kerrison punch.
10. Remove the contralateral half of the ligamentum flavum, and decompress the lower surface of the contralateral facet joint to free the contralateral traversing nerve root; perform hemostasis and closure. No drain is inserted.
11. The patient is usually discharged the same day after physiotherapy clearance.

Complications

The overall mean incidence of the complication rate of UBE is close to 6.7% (0–13.8%) [13], and most complications are root injury, dural tear, and incomplete decompression. Postoperative headache, postoperative hematoma, and transient paresthesia are the other less common complications. Iatrogenic hydroperitoneum has also been reported after the ventral approach to the psoas muscle during transforaminal decompression.

One of the noteworthy features of UBE is that postoperative infection, a relatively common complication of conventional lumbar spinal surgery, has not been commonly reported. Most of the perioperative complications occurred at the beginning of the learning curve.

Incidental Dural Tear (IDT)

IDT is one of the most common complications in microscopic spine surgery, and the reported incidence of IDT is 0.5–18% in lumbar spinal surgery and 2.9% in UBE [16–21]. IDT is considered a minor complication due to the small risk of neurological sequelae when it is well treated. Nevertheless, it may cause chronic lower back pain because proper IDT repair may require greater muscle dissection or wider laminectomy. Sometimes, a surgeon opts to reduce surgery time for an IDT, risking incomplete decompression of the spine. Furthermore, if an IDT is not managed appropriately, further complications such as pseudomeningocele due to cerebrospinal fluid (CSF) leakage, surgical site infection, or meningitis could occur. These complications lead to increased physical and financial burdens to the patient [19].

There are different ways a surgeon can cause a dural tear. The majority of dural tears occur while using a Kerrison rongeur for laminectomy of the ipsilateral or contralateral lower lamina or flavectomy of a deep layer of ligamentum flavum (LF) at the midline. It can also occur while using a curette and while using a burr. Unpracticed handling of muscle serial dilators, slipped tapping of an osteotome, and inattentive clamping of pituitary forceps are other causes of IDT. Most cases of IDT happen while performing surgery under a blurred visual field obscured by small epidural bleeding or laminectomized cancellous bone. Adhesiolysis of scar tissue using a curette on the dura from the lamina for revision surgery is also one of the causes of IDT.

Thus, the first preventive strategy of IDT is to make a clear surgical field to see the structural margin clearly by keeping the saline output fluent and controlling small bleeds from epidural small vessels by small-headed radiofrequency and laminectomized bone bleeds by sealing with bone wax [22].

Two surgical procedures are the common causes of large durotomies and surgical practice related to small dural defects. With curettage, dural tears (mean size, 9.33 mm) occur. An incorrect direction of the osteotome can also cause a large dural tear. The edge of the osteotome includes both sharp and smooth parts. The sharp part is essential for osteotomy but can cause dural tears. The sharp part of the osteotome must always be directed laterally. Second, unnecessary removal of small particles with pituitary forceps (7.33 mm) can cause large defects. Because of the high magnification, small bone ligament and ligament particles must be removed. However, they will usually not be symptomatic but, rather, will adhere to the dura, such that their removal can result in large longitudinal dural tears. Small dural tears were related to miscellaneous procedures with the Kerrison punch (5.7 mm) and drills (5.4 mm) [23].

According to the location, IDTs most commonly occur during flavectomy in the central area of the spinal canal. The central area of the dura is connected to a few lines of fibrous tissue under the LF, and it is covered and hidden by epidural fat. Infused saline compresses both sides of the dura so that the center of the dura is folded and appears as a central folding. If a central dural folding goes unnoticed while inputting a Kerrison punch or curette under the epidural fat at the midline for a flavectomy, direct injury of the dura at the midline may occur. To prevent IDT around the central dural folding during flavectomy, instruments should be inserted above the epidural fat layer no further without clear visibility of the structural margins [22].

The LF can be divided into two layers: the superficial layer above the lower lamina level and the deep layer at the same and below the level of the lower lamina. To make a sufficient working space and inspect the bony margin, the superficial layer of the LF should be removed before laminectomy. However, removal of the deep layer should be postponed till the completion of the laminectomy to protect the dura. This is especially important when using a high-speed burr so that its head does not directly injure the dural membrane. The peripheral fibrous band and vessel bundles of the dura may be dragged and wound around the neck of a rolling burr, causing a larger flap tear. Therefore, it is suggested to preserve the deep layer of the LF during laminotomy using a burr. If the deep layer of the LF were fully removed before finishing the laminotomy, a piece of Cottonoid could be inserted under the proximal lamina and made long enough to cover the dura briefly while using the burr, especially at the contralateral proximal corner. Any protective Cottonoid covering should be located at least 1 cm proximally beneath the proximal lamina to prevent it from being swept away by the saline flow [22].

Currently, primary repair of a dural tear is the gold standard for treating IDT during conventional spinal surgery [13, 18]. Endoscopic spine surgery, however, has no standard treatment protocol to cope with IDT. Common strategies include conversion to open repair with discontinuation of minimally invasive spine surgery or conservative management with a delayed decision depending on the state of sequelae. Because UBE is a new technique, surgeons must struggle to overcome the learning-curve period of an unfamiliar endoscopic view that is underwater.

One of the strategies of dealing with an IDT is to determine the size, location, and morphology of the dural tear. The tears can be classified by size (small-sized tear of <1 cm or large-sized tear of ≥1 cm), location (center-midline, or lateral side), and morphology (slit tear or flap tear). Treatment methods include patch compression method, dural repair using vascular clips, immediate open repair, or delayed conversion to open repair [22, 23].

According to the location of the tear, Zone 1 refers to the dura over the exiting nerve root and includes shoulder lesions under the lower margin of the upper pedicle. Zone 2 refers to the path of the thecal sac but excludes the axilla of the exiting nerve junction and the shoulder of the traversing nerve between the upper and lower pedicle. Zone 3 refers to the traversing nerve root and includes the axillar junction with the thecal sac above the upper margin of the lower pedicle (Fig. 31.2). The size of a dural tear could be estimated before repair using a surgical instrument of specified length, normally a 3 mm Kerrison punch or a 5 mm hook dissector.

The patch compression method was applied for small IDTs of <1 cm. Gelfoam was cut into two pieces of 1 cm. A piece of TachoSil is patched on the tear site, and Gelfoam is placed over it. Meticulous control for small bleeding from peripheral muscle ends was performed using small-headed radiofrequency. Leaving only a small amount of hematoma is enough to decrease dural pulsation by compressing the patched site.

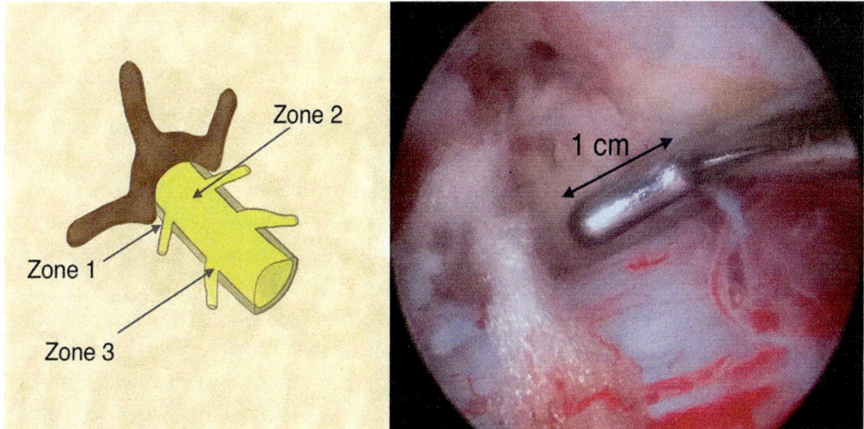

Fig. 31.2 Depicting the zones of dural tear and estimating the size of tear using standard blunt nerve probe

Most of our surgical wounds could not be sutured tightly at the muscle layer through small endoscopic wounds, so the subcutaneous fascia was closed by the continuous suture method using absorbable thread (sized 3.0 with a small needle) and skin was sealed again with SSC dressing with no drain indwelling. The same was followed for cases complicated by IDT. Ambulation was permitted when the patient had no complaint of moderate-to-severe headache after 48 h of bedrest. Intravenous antibiotics were used for two more doses and stopped.

A larger 1 cm dural tear or flap tear of <10 mm could be closed with a few stitches using a vascular clip. First, the durotomy area should be fully exposed from the proximal to the distal dural tear margin. Epidural fat tissue is removed for clear exposure of the dural tear margin. In the presence of extradural herniation of nerve rootlets in the dural tear area, herniated nerve rootlets were eased back intradurally using dissectors. One or two pieces of Gelfoam were inserted to protect the nerve rootlets via the dural tear area. A temporary approximation of dural tear leaflets was performed using pituitary forceps. Nonpenetrating clips were used with a gap of 1–2 mm. Medium-sized clips were used. After dural clipping, TachoSil was applied over the clipping area.

In the event of failed temporary approximation of durotomy leaflets, one can consider an additional third portal as a second working portal with the help of an assistant who held the endoscope, an operator performed dural repair using two hands. The first hand was used to manipulate pituitary forceps for approximation of the dural tear area, and the other hand was used to apply clips.

No drain was put, but putting a drain to prevent postoperative hematoma is an option. A drainage catheter is usually removed on day 1 after surgery. Finally, we recommend bedrest ranging from 3 to 5 days after surgery. If the repair is not satisfactory, open repair is recommended [24].

Postoperative Headache, Postoperative Hematoma, Transient Paresthesia

The surgeon must remain aware of the potential for an increase in intracranial pressure (ICP) during UBE surgery, which may lead to headaches, seizures, or even death. The mechanism of ICP elevation is thought to be a cranial shifting of CSF rather than the direct movement of the irrigation fluid itself. The most common symptoms of increased ICP are headache, papilledema, vomiting, neck stiffness, tinnitus, extremity paresthesia, low back pain, and gait ataxia.

There are some precautions one needs to consider when performing UBE. Maintain the lowest irrigation pressure needed to obtain endoscopic visualization. When making the working space, it is considered safe to elevate the irrigation pressure. However, after the epidural space is exposed, one must try to keep the irrigation pressure low [25].

Ensuring that the irrigation fluid is not stagnant and maintaining continuous outflow enable continued clean endoscopic visualization and minimize the possibility of neurological complications caused by elevations in ICP [25].

Special consideration should be taken for the patients with intracranial pathology before surgery. In patients who have intracranial pathologies such as pseudotumor, hydrocephalus, or other space-occupying lesions, there will be a loss or alteration in intracranial compliance that will have an effect on the autoregulatory mechanism of ICP. Therefore, these patients may show unexpected increases in ICP. Although such conditions are not considered to be absolute contraindications, it is necessary to take great care with these patients before performing UBE [25].

Turbid water and an obscure field due to failure of bleeding control and continuous irrigation may lead to the abovementioned complications for surgeons not familiar with the technique and visual field. Rather than attempting to obtain a clear view by increasing the infusion pressure, it is more sensible to attempt facilitating outflow by applying for an extension or crosscut of the fascia incision through the working portal. A clear visual field obtained through smooth continuous irrigation with good outflow can prevent the complications mentioned here.

Epidural Hematoma

Epidural bleeding due to vessel injury has a rate of only 0.6% for the uniportal technique [1, 26]. The overall radiologic postoperative spinal epidural hematoma (PSEH) after UBE was 23.6%, which was lower than open conventional surgery [27]. Symptoms of PSEH include flaccid or spastic paralysis if occurred at cord level, and paralysis, radicular pain, or bladder dysfunction if occurred at the lumbar level, usually observed within 24 h after surgery [28]. Mild PSEH symptoms without neurologic deterioration usually resolve within 3 weeks after surgery, and radiologic regression occurs spontaneously within 3 months after surgery [29]. Another study reported a rate of 1.9% for symptomatic epidural hematomas in UBE, with related factors being female sex, age, anticoagulation factors, and use of a water infusion pump [27]. High water pressure can improve visibility for the surgeon but can hide small bleeding (Fig. 31.3).

Hematomas were prevalent during the early stage of the learning curve. This implies that with more experience and meticulous control of bleeding, this complication can be reduced. Bone bleeding and superficial bleeding can be controlled by a radiofrequency wand, and epidural bleeding can be controlled by small-headed radiofrequency.

Using a dry scope to look for bleeders at the end of the procedure is also a good practice to prevent this complication. When the surgeon is able to maintain low water pressure, this preserves muscle integrity, and placement of the blood drainage bag could be avoided. Because the prognosis of epidural hematomas is related to motor function [30], repetitive neurologic examinations with conservative treatment are crucial. The surgical timing of spinal epidural hematoma evacuation is controversial. A number of authors have reported that neurologic outcome is better in earlier surgical intervention within 12 h after the onset of symptoms or within 6 h of maximum neurologic deficit, recommending immediate surgical evacuation [29].

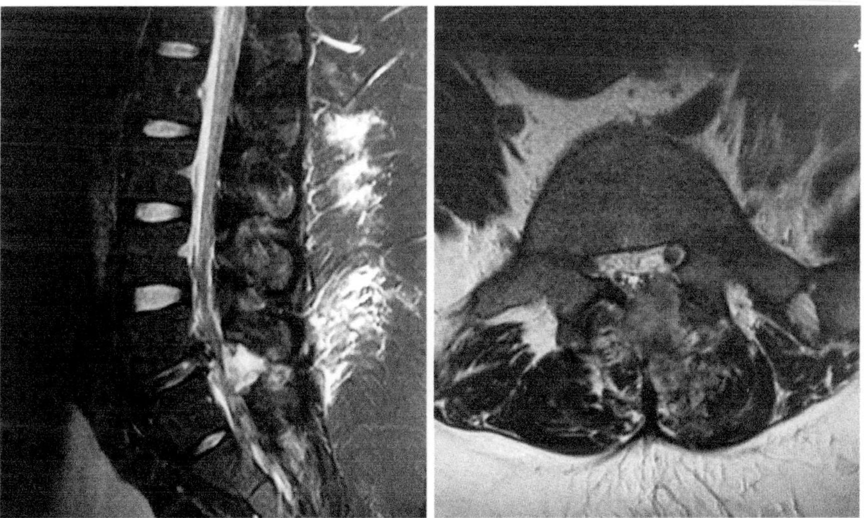

Fig. 31.3 T2-TIRM and T2-weighted axial MRI images showing epidural hematoma at L4–L5 post-UBE surgery

Recurrence of Intervertebral Disc Herniation

The reported rate of recurrences was 2.5% within 1 year of follow-up. Furthermore, the rate of recurrence was not higher than that in conventional treatment, and the early (first 50) and later cases did not show significant differences in the rate of recurrence, implying that skill level does not affect recurrence. Sufficient laminectomy and disc removal can decrease the incidence of recurrence and associated pain [28]. We measure adequate decompression when we can see the bilateral traversing nerve roots probing the foramen to ensure sufficient space for the nerve root and adequate pedicle-to-pedicle space. The advantage of endoscopy is the ability to look over to the contralateral side and see the contralateral nerve root.

Incomplete Decompression

Incomplete decompression is a condition with persistent remnant postoperative pain and is a common factor for a poor prognosis in endoscopic spine surgery [31]. This condition is correlated with degenerative changes, including hypertrophied facet, calcified disc, and high upward migration of disc material, in the uniportal technique [32]. In UBE, for discectomy, we rely on the assistant to use the nerve root retractor to safely access the disc and do discectomy. Compared to that for the uniportal transforaminal technique, UBE can access upward and downward migrated discs freely. However, physicians must hold the endoscope during the procedure, as root retraction is not easy for disc removal. This is likely the reason why the early stage of the learning curve in the few reported studies shows unsuccessful outcomes [33]. The development of instruments, such as a rotating retractor above the arthroscope, may help in avoiding these problems. Blurred vision due to intraoperative bleeding is one of the shortcomings of UBE and can cause incomplete decompression. Meticulous control of the bone and ligament level, control of the systolic blood pressure (under 100 mmHg), and intermittent use of bone wax and Gelfoam can remedy this complication. As mentioned before, we measure adequate decompression when we can see the bilateral traversing nerve roots probing the neural foramen to ensure sufficient space for the nerve root and adequate pedicle-to-pedicle space. The advantage of endoscopy is that we can look over to the opposite side and see the contralateral nerve root.

Iatrogenic Instability (Pars Interarticularis Fracture)

The rate of iatrogenic spondylolisthesis after open laminectomy is reported as 3.95–9.5% [34, 35]. The facet joint complex (including the synovial facet joint and the joint capsule) is the most important among the posterior stabilizing structures.

Biomechanical tests have demonstrated that more than 50% of facet joint destruction can lead to segmental instability [36]. All the minimally invasive approaches aim to obtain adequate decompression while preserving the integrity of the facet joint complex. Extensive drilling of the facet joint and a smaller disc space height are risk factors for this condition. Because UBE minimizes the muscle dissection and preserves the zygapophyseal joint (in contrast to an open technique), the rate of this condition is as low as 0.6%. However, anatomic characteristics of the patient can produce this condition, and the use of a Kerrison punch for undercutting of the facet joint is recommended for its prevention. Unilateral facet joint violation does not usually require surgery [4]. However, for progressive spondylolisthesis and uncontrollable back and leg pain, open or endoscopic interbody fusion can be considered. Careful bone removal during surgery and prevention are the only ways to reduce this complication.

When performing bilateral decompression through unilateral laminotomy, the approach-side facet joint destruction is always a concern. Facet undercutting has been suggested to avoid excessive facet joint destruction. Using curved instruments including osteotomes, Kerrison punches, and high-speed drills might help reduce facet destruction [37]. However, such techniques were difficult for open, tubular retractor-assisted or microendoscopic approaches because the surgeon's visual point remained outside of the patient's body or outside of the lamina. With an endoscopic approach, especially UBE, the surgeon's visual point can be advanced inside of the lamina or into the contralateral lateral recess and the contralateral foramen. This feature enables a precise check of the offending pathological structures without visual limitation. If a 30° endoscope is used, the visual field would be even wider.

The reported facet joint preservation was 92.9% on the contralateral side and 84.2% on the approach side. It is unavoidable that facet joint destruction is more severe on the approach side [38, 39]. For patients with severe stenosis, the spinous process and facet joints usually become hypertrophic and deformed. These deformities make the space between the spinous process and the facet joint very narrow. Bilateral decompression via unilateral laminotomy then becomes very difficult and may result in excessive destruction of the ipsilateral facet joint. Two modified approach techniques may solve these problems. First, do the contralateral side decompression to create space for the neural tissue to mobilize contralaterally. Second, remove more bone at the base of the spinous process for easier sublaminar decompression and getting access to the contralateral recess. These modified techniques shift the laminotomy window contralaterally and minimize drilling on the ipsilateral lamina and facet joint.

CSF Leakage, Ascites, and Edema

The reported rate of postoperative CSF leakage is 3–27% for the open technique [40] and 1.1% for the uniportal technique [41]. The reported rate of postoperative CSF leakage in UBE was 0.6%. This is because UBE can preserve the back muscles, which play a role in preventing continuous leakage. On the other hand, while ascites after endoscopic operation have not been previously reported, the biportal technique demonstrated this complication. Multifidus muscle edema due to water circulation has already been reported [42] and is suspected to have the same mechanism. This can be attributed to the use of a broader radiofrequency coagulator than that used in the uniportal technique for muscle dissection. Careful dissection and proper size selection of the coagulator can prevent this complication.

Infection

The rate of postoperative infections is estimated to be 0.65% for the open technique [40], and the postoperative infection rate for endoscopic surgery has not yet been widely reported. Endoscopic surgery is associated with minimal risk of infection because a continuous irrigation system is used during the procedure, but the possibility of infection should always be considered, and aseptic procedures should be stressed.

Learning Curve

The "learning curve" is defined as the improvement in surgical procedure performance with increasing experience and training. Conventionally, the learning curve for surgical techniques was evaluated by investigation of the mean operative time, hospital stay, bleeding rate, and complication rate [18, 43]. However, these measures cannot define surgical competency. The LC-CUSUM analysis is a good statistical method for surgeons to determine when adequate performance can be reached in surgical procedures [44]. To monitor the learning curve, Biau and Porcher and Biau et al. [44] introduced the learning curve cumulative summation test (LC-CUSUM), which was specifically designed to monitor a process from an out-of-control to an in-control state. The LC-CUSUM is a modified statistical tool of the CUSUM analysis, designed to monitor a process over time and detect inadequate performance. The level of performance allows for the determination of when proficiency has been achieved [45].

In the reported studies, the technique of UBE for lumbar decompressive laminectomy reached an adequate operative time at the 58th operation compared with ULBD performed by a senior surgeon. In the late operative period (after 31 cases), the mean operative time was significantly lower than that in the early period (30 cases). It was also lower than the mean operation time of ULBD (reference operative time, 75 min) [14]. A substantial learning period might be required before adequate performance is achieved for lumbar decompressive laminectomy via BESS. The LC-CUSUM analysis can be used for self-monitoring of a process when aiming to achieve surgical technical competency.

Discussion

The use of biportal arthroscopy for spinal surgery was first reported in 1996 [43]. UBE is considered to be a new method that combines the advantages of the microscope and interlaminar endoscopic spinal surgery. One portal provides an endoscopic field of view and continuous irrigation, and the other portal is used for instrument manipulation. On the one hand, the advantages of UBE include increased surgical movement of instruments with the independent visualization and working portals, good and wide field of visualization to unrestricted-access contralateral and foraminal areas, less bleeding because of continuous irrigation, and a reduced armamentarium because ordinary arthroscopy and spinal instruments can be used [17, 18, 20, 35, 36]. On the other hand, it requires the basic techniques of arthroscopy, initial manipulation of detaching some muscles for a potential space, keeping irrigation outflow, taking care of the use of radiofrequency, and a longer operative time [13, 21].

As the number of procedures using this technique has increased, characteristic side effects have arisen, such as water-related problems and incomplete manipulation due to instrument constraints, other than the inherent disadvantage of repetitive radiation exposure due to lack of three-dimensional orientation. Additionally, insufficient disc removal, difficulty in controlling bleeding, and a steep learning curve are considered drawbacks to the procedure. However, continuous technical developments have been noted in this surgical approach due to advancements in surgical tools and availability of enhanced high-definition video equipment.

The overall rate of unsuccessful outcomes was 10.29%, and after the initial period of learning, the rate was 5.60%. Primary causes (incidence higher than 1%) were hematomas, lesion recurrence, incomplete decompression, and dural tears. Secondary causes (incidence lower than 1%) were instability, ascites, and infection. These factors have different characteristics and an impact on patient satisfaction [33].

IDT is one of the most common complications in microscopic spine surgery, and the reported incidence of IDT is 0.5–18% in lumbar spinal surgery and 2.9% in BESS [7–12]. The first preventive strategy of IDT is to make a clear surgical field. One of the strategies of dealing with an IDT is to determine the size, location, and morphology of the dural tear and deal with the tear accordingly. The management varies from TachoSil patch repair and nonpenetrating vascular clips to open repair.

Turbid water and an obscure field due to failure of bleeding control and continuous irrigation may lead to postoperative headache, postoperative hematoma, and transient paresthesia for surgeons not familiar with the technique and visual field. One should try to obtain a clear view by applying for an extension or crosscut of the fascia incision through the working portal. A clear visual field obtained through smooth continuous irrigation can prevent the above complications.

The reported rate of symptomatic epidural hematomas in UBE is around 1.9%. Meticulous control of bleeding through radiofrequency probe and wand and bone wax helps to prevent this complication. Dry scope at the end of the procedure to look for bleeders is also a good technique to avoid this complication.

Inadequate decompression and inadequate disc removal are also known complications and contribute to patient dissatisfaction and financial burden. Meticulous hemostasis, stepwise decompression, identifying the landmarks after complete decompression, and overcoming the learning curve are a few of the methods to avoid this complication.

Iatrogenic instability (pars interarticularis fracture) is a rare complication with an incidence of 0.6% in reported studies. Extensive drilling of the facet joint and a smaller disc space height are risk factors for this condition. Paying a close look at the anatomic characteristics of the patient and the use of a Kerrison punch for undercutting of the facet joint are recommended for its prevention.

Conclusion

UBE is a minimally invasive spinal surgery for the direct decompression of neural elements with dynamic handling of instruments under a clear view while reducing muscle dissection and damage to the posterior lumbar structures. It can be considered as the next generation of surgical development after open lumbar surgery and microscopic spinal surgery, with results comparable to the results of those surgical techniques other than conventional endoscopic spinal surgery with the use of one portal. However, it comes with its own range of complications and challenges. Some of the complications are unique and so are the treatment for these complications. These risks should be considered and explained to the patient before performing UBE. We would recommend continuing to watch out for future prospective studies with controlled treatment protocols and long-term follow-up periods (longer than 3 years) to elucidate the long-term prevalence and outcomes.

References

1. Mayer HM, Brock M, Berlien HP, Weber B. Percutaneous endoscopic laser discectomy (PELD). A new surgical technique for non-sequestrated lumbar discs. Acta Neurochir Suppl (Wien). 1992;54:53–8.
2. Ruetten S, Komp M, Merk H, Godolias G. Full-endoscopic interlaminar and transforaminal lumbar discectomy versus conventional microsurgical technique: a prospective, randomized, controlled study. Spine (Phila Pa 1976). 2008;33(9):931–9.
3. Choi I, Ahn JO, So WS, Lee SJ, Choi IJ, Kim H. Exiting root injury in transforaminal endoscopic discectomy: preoperative image considerations for safety. Eur Spine J. 2013;22(11):2481–7.
4. Kim SK, Kang SS, Hong YH, Park SW, Lee SC. Clinical comparison of unilateral biportal endoscopic technique versus open microdiscectomy for single-level lumbar discectomy: a multicenter, retrospective analysis. J Orthop Surg Res. 2018;13(1):22.
5. Nakagawa H, Kamimura M, Uchiyama S, Takahara K, Itsubo T, Miyasaka T. Microendoscopic discectomy (MED) for lumbar disc prolapse. J Clin Neurosci. 2003;10(2):231–5.
6. Nowitzke AM. Assessment of the learning curve for lumbar microendoscopic discectomy. Neurosurgery. 2005;56(4):755–62. discussion 762

7. Eun SS, Eum JH, Lee SH, Sabal LA. Biportal endoscopic lumbar decompression for lumbar disk herniation and spinal canal stenosis: a technical note. J Neurol Surg A Cent Eur Neurosurg. 2017;78(4):390–6.
8. Hwa Eum J, Hwa Heo D, Son SK, Park CK. Percutaneous biportal endoscopic decompression for lumbar spinal stenosis: a technical note and preliminary clinical results. J Neurosurg Spine. 2016;24(4):602–7.
9. Kim JE, Choi DJ. Unilateral biportal endoscopic decompression by 30° endoscopy in lumbar spinal stenosis: technical note and preliminary report. J Orthop. 2018;15(2):366–71.
10. Park SM, Kim GU, Kim HJ, Choi JH, Chang BS, Lee CK, et al. Is the use of a unilateral biportal endoscopic approach associated with rapid recovery after lumbar decompressive laminectomy? A preliminary analysis of a prospective randomized controlled trial. World Neurosurg. 2019;128:e709–e18.
11. Kambin P, Brager MD. Percutaneous posterolateral discectomy. Anatomy and mechanism. Clin Orthop Relat Res. 1987;223:145–54.
12. Kang SS, Lee SC, Kim SK. A novel percutaneous biportal endoscopic technique for symptomatic spinal epidural lipomatosis: technical note and case presentations. World Neurosurg. 2019;129:49–54.
13. Lin GX, Huang P, Kotheeranurak V, Park CW, Heo DH, Park CK, et al. A systematic review of unilateral biportal endoscopic spinal surgery: preliminary clinical results and complications. World Neurosurg. 2019;125:425–32.
14. Park SM, Kim HJ, Kim GU, Choi MH, Chang BS, Lee CK, et al. Learning curve for lumbar decompressive laminectomy in biportal endoscopic spinal surgery using the cumulative summation test for learning curve. World Neurosurg. 2019;122:e1007–e13.
15. Pao JL, Lin SM, Chen WC, Chang CH. Unilateral biportal endoscopic decompression for degenerative lumbar canal stenosis. J Spine Surg. 2020;6(2):438–46.
16. Bosacco SJ, Gardner MJ, Guille JT. Evaluation and treatment of dural tears in lumbar spine surgery: a review. Clin Orthop Relat Res. 2001;389:238–47.
17. Cammisa FP Jr, Girardi FP, Sangani PK, Parvataneni HK, Cadag S, Sandhu HS. Incidental durotomy in spine surgery. Spine (Phila Pa 1976). 2000;25(20):2663–7.
18. Choi DJ, Choi CM, Jung JT, Lee SJ, Kim YS. Learning curve associated with complications in biportal endoscopic spinal surgery: challenges and strategies. Asian Spine J. 2016;10(4):624–9.
19. Epstein NE. The frequency and etiology of intraoperative dural tears in 110 predominantly geriatric patients undergoing multilevel laminectomy with noninstrumented fusions. J Spinal Disord Tech. 2007;20(5):380–6.
20. Guerin P, El Fegoun AB, Obeid I, Gille O, Lelong L, Luc S, et al. Incidental durotomy during spine surgery: incidence, management and complications. A retrospective review. Injury. 2012;43(4):397–401.
21. Tafazal SI, Sell PJ. Incidental durotomy in lumbar spine surgery: incidence and management. Eur Spine J. 2005;14(3):287–90.
22. Kim JE, Choi DJ, Park EJ. Risk factors and options of management for an incidental dural tear in biportal endoscopic spine surgery. Asian Spine J. 2020;14(6):790–800.
23. Park HJ, Kim SK, Lee SC, Kim W, Han S, Kang SS. Dural tears in percutaneous biportal endoscopic spine surgery: anatomical location and management. World Neurosurg. 2020;136:e578–e85.
24. Kim HS, Raorane HD, Wu PH, Heo DH, Sharma SB, Jang IT. Incidental durotomy during endoscopic stenosis lumbar decompression: incidence, classification, and proposed management strategies. World Neurosurg. 2020;139:e13–22.
25. Kang T, Park SY, Lee SH, Park JH, Suh SW. Assessing changes in cervical epidural pressure during biportal endoscopic lumbar discectomy. J Neurosurg Spine. 2020:1–7. https://doi.org/10.3171/2020.6.SPINE20586.
26. Mayer HM, Brock M. Percutaneous endoscopic lumbar discectomy (PELD). Neurosurg Rev. 1993;16(2):115–20.

27. Kim JE, Choi DJ, Kim MC, Park EJ. Risk factors of postoperative spinal epidural hematoma after biportal endoscopic spinal surgery. World Neurosurg. 2019;129:e324–e9.
28. Anno M, Yamazaki T, Hara N, Ito Y. The incidence, clinical features, and a comparison between early and delayed onset of postoperative spinal epidural hematoma. Spine (Phila Pa 1976). 2019;44(6):420–3.
29. Ikuta K, Tono O, Tanaka T, Arima J, Nakano S, Sasaki K, et al. Evaluation of postoperative spinal epidural hematoma after microendoscopic posterior decompression for lumbar spinal stenosis: a clinical and magnetic resonance imaging study. J Neurosurg Spine. 2006;5(5):404–9.
30. Lawton MT, Porter RW, Heiserman JE, Jacobowitz R, Sonntag VK, Dickman CA. Surgical management of spinal epidural hematoma: relationship between surgical timing and neurological outcome. J Neurosurg. 1995;83(1):1–7.
31. Singh V, Manchikanti L, Benyamin RM, Helm S, Hirsch JA. Percutaneous lumbar laser disc decompression: a systematic review of current evidence. Pain Physician. 2009;12(3):573–88.
32. Zhao XL, Fu ZJ, Xu YG, Zhao XJ, Song WG, Zheng H. Treatment of lumbar intervertebral disc herniation using C-arm fluoroscopy guided target percutaneous laser disc decompression. Photomed Laser Surg. 2012;30(2):92–5.
33. Kim W, Kim SK, Kang SS, Park HJ, Han S, Lee SC. Pooled analysis of unsuccessful percutaneous biportal endoscopic surgery outcomes from a multi-institutional retrospective cohort of 797 cases. Acta Neurochir. 2020;162(2):279–87.
34. Heindel P, Tuchman A, Hsieh PC, Pham MH, D'Oro A, Patel NN, et al. Reoperation rates after single-level lumbar discectomy. Spine (Phila Pa 1976). 2017;42(8):E496–501.
35. Ramhmdani S, Xia Y, Xu R, Kosztowski T, Sciubba D, Witham T, et al. Iatrogenic spondylolisthesis following open lumbar laminectomy: case series and review of the literature. World Neurosurg. 2018;113:e383–e90.
36. Moliterno JA, Knopman J, Parikh K, Cohan JN, Huang QD, Aaker GD, et al. Results and risk factors for recurrence following single-level tubular lumbar microdiscectomy. J Neurosurg Spine. 2010;12(6):680–6.
37. Guiot BH, Khoo LT, Fessler RG. A minimally invasive technique for decompression of the lumbar spine. Spine (Phila Pa 1976). 2002;27(4):432–8.
38. Dohzono S, Matsumura A, Terai H, Toyoda H, Suzuki A, Nakamura H. Radiographic evaluation of postoperative bone regrowth after microscopic bilateral decompression via a unilateral approach for degenerative lumbar spondylolisthesis. J Neurosurg Spine. 2013;18(5):472–8.
39. Matsumura A, Namikawa T, Terai H, Tsujio T, Suzuki A, Dozono S, et al. The influence of approach side on facet preservation in microscopic bilateral decompression via a unilateral approach for degenerative lumbar scoliosis. Clinical article. J Neurosurg Spine. 2010;13(6):758–65.
40. Ishikura H, Ogihara S, Oka H, Maruyama T, Inanami H, Miyoshi K, et al. Risk factors for incidental durotomy during posterior open spine surgery for degenerative diseases in adults: a multicenter observational study. PLoS One. 2017;12(11):e0188038.
41. Ahn Y, Lee HY, Lee SH, Lee JH. Dural tears in percutaneous endoscopic lumbar discectomy. Eur Spine J. 2011;20(1):58–64.
42. Ahn JS, Lee HJ, Park EJ, Kim SB, Choi DJ, Kwon YS, et al. Multifidus muscle changes after biportal endoscopic spinal surgery: magnetic resonance imaging evaluation. World Neurosurg. 2019;130:e525–e34.
43. Wang H, Huang B, Li C, Zhang Z, Wang J, Zheng W, et al. Learning curve for percutaneous endoscopic lumbar discectomy depending on the surgeon's training level of minimally invasive spine surgery. Clin Neurol Neurosurg. 2013;115(10):1987–91.
44. Biau DJ, Williams SM, Schlup MM, Nizard RS, Porcher R. Quantitative and individualized assessment of the learning curve using LC-CUSUM. Br J Surg. 2008;95(7):925–9.
45. Biau DJ, Porcher R. A method for monitoring a process from an out of control to an in control state: application to the learning curve. Stat Med. 2010;29(18):1900–9.

Chapter 32
Perioperative Care in Unilateral Biportal Endoscopic Spine Surgery

Matthew Sebastian, Pang Hung Wu, Shuxun Lin, Rajeesh George, and Gamaliel Tan Yu Heng

Abbreviations

AP	Anteroposterior
CT	Computed tomography
DVT	Deep vein thrombosis
LOS	Length of hospital stay
MAC	Monitored anesthesia care
MRI	Magnetic resonance imaging
MRSA	Methicillin-resistant *Staphylococcus aureus*
NSAIDs	Nonsteroidal anti-inflammatory drugs
ODI	Oswestry Disability Index
PCA	Patient-controlled analgesia
PE	Pulmonary embolism
PONV	Postoperative nausea and vomiting
POUR	Postoperative urinary retention
SSI	Surgical site infections
TLIP	Thoracolumbar interfacial plane
UBE	Unilateral biportal endoscopy
VAS	Visual analog scale

M. Sebastian · P. H. Wu (✉) · S. Lin · R. George · G. T. Y. Heng
National University Health System, Juronghealth Campus, Department of Orthopaedic Surgery, Ng Teng Fong General Hospital, Singapore, Singapore
e-mail: mattistian@gmail.com; wupanghung@gmail.com; shuxun_lin@nuhs.edu.sg; rajeesh_george@nuhs.edu.sg; gamaliel_tan@nuhs.edu.sg

J. Quillo-Olvera et al. (eds.), *Unilateral Biportal Endoscopy of the Spine*, https://doi.org/10.1007/978-3-031-14736-4_32

Introduction

Degenerative lumbar spinal conditions are a common indication for spinal surgery in the elderly population [1]. With the evolution of minimally invasive spine surgery, endoscopic decompression with or without concomitant fusion is gaining popularity as the preferred surgical modality in our practice.

Perioperative care in unilateral biportal endoscopic spine surgery (UBE) is as vital as with any open spine procedure. The preoperative, intraoperative, and postoperative chain of events has profound effects on the eventual outcome of the surgery. The continuum of care begins at the patient's first visit to the clinic and extends long after surgery. Other than the specific surgical indications and assessment of the patients described in our previous chapter, we ought to be aware of coexisting medical problems and their implications, commonly used anesthetic techniques, potential postoperative complications, prophylactic measures, and rehabilitation protocols that aim at minimizing postoperative morbidity.

This chapter provides an overview of these issues.

Preoperative Care

Preoperative care involves the identification of the premorbid functional status of the patient and medical comorbidities, which may adversely affect surgical risk and prolong the length of hospital stay. We do preoperative counseling to adjust patients' postoperative expectations; optimizing these risk factors ensures enhanced recovery after surgery improves patients' satisfaction after the operation and early rehabilitation (Fig. 32.1).

Clinical Presentation and Assessment

Patient selection is of utmost importance in any surgery and particularly UBE as well to ensure the best clinical outcomes. Indications for surgical management of lumbar degenerative disease in UBE are similar for open lumbar decompression and fusion. We evaluated the clinical symptoms by measurement of visual analog scale (VAS) and Oswestry Disability Index (ODI). We carefully documented claudication distance and timing. The overall clinical outcome is evaluated using the MacNab score.

Radiographs (erect lumbosacral spine AP/lateral views and flexion-extension views) and corresponding MRI scans are obtained preoperatively for all surgical patients (Fig. 32.2). We tend to include cases for less than 30° coronal deformity and sagittal balanced patients for decompression surgery.

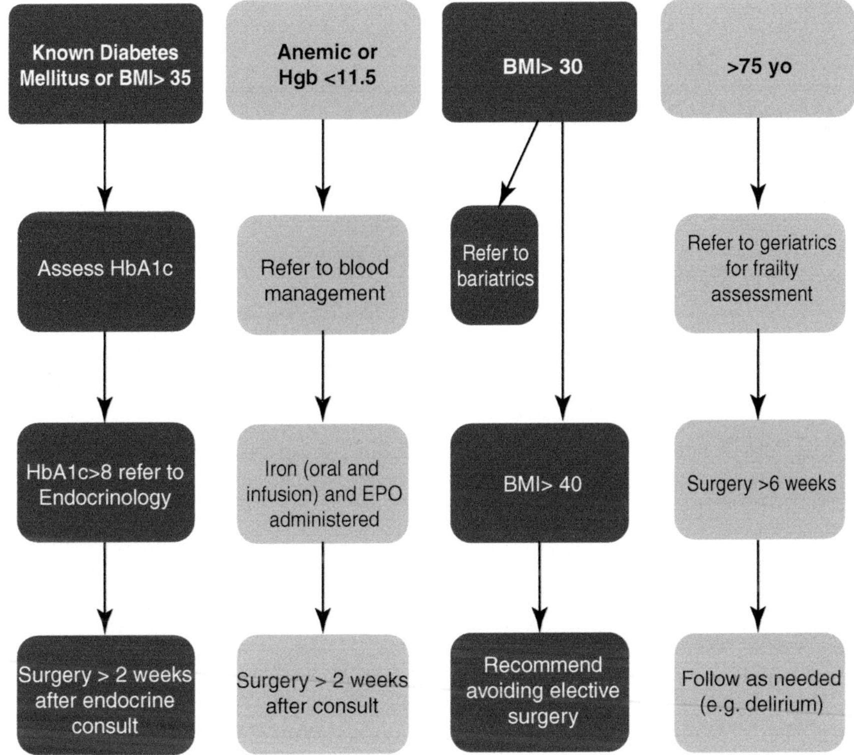

Fig. 32.1 Patient selection for UBE

MRI: We evaluate the areas requiring decompression marked by five levels of axial-cut line evaluation—namely just below the pedicle of cephalad vertebra, superior endplate, mid-disc, lower endplate cut, and above the pedicle of caudal vertebra cuts; this helps us to evaluate how extensive is the decompression surgery required (Fig. 32.3).

Additional CT scans help in the assessment and complement MRI for grading of foramen stenosis and preoperative planning. Comparing corresponding segmental images on CT and MRI scans helps to differentiate between bony and ligamentous contributions to spinal stenosis. Some surgeons recommend surgical treatment for only patients with stenotic lesions (whether due to bony stenosis, extruded disc herniation, or contained disc bulge) producing a neuro-foraminal width of 3 mm or less on the sagittal MRI and CT cuts or lateral recess height of 3 mm or less on the axial MRI and CT cuts [2].

One must ensure that imaging findings are consistent with clinical symptoms in terms of pain location or affected root nerve. Selective nerve root block is helpful as a therapeutic and diagnostic tool to identify the specific nerve root compressed.

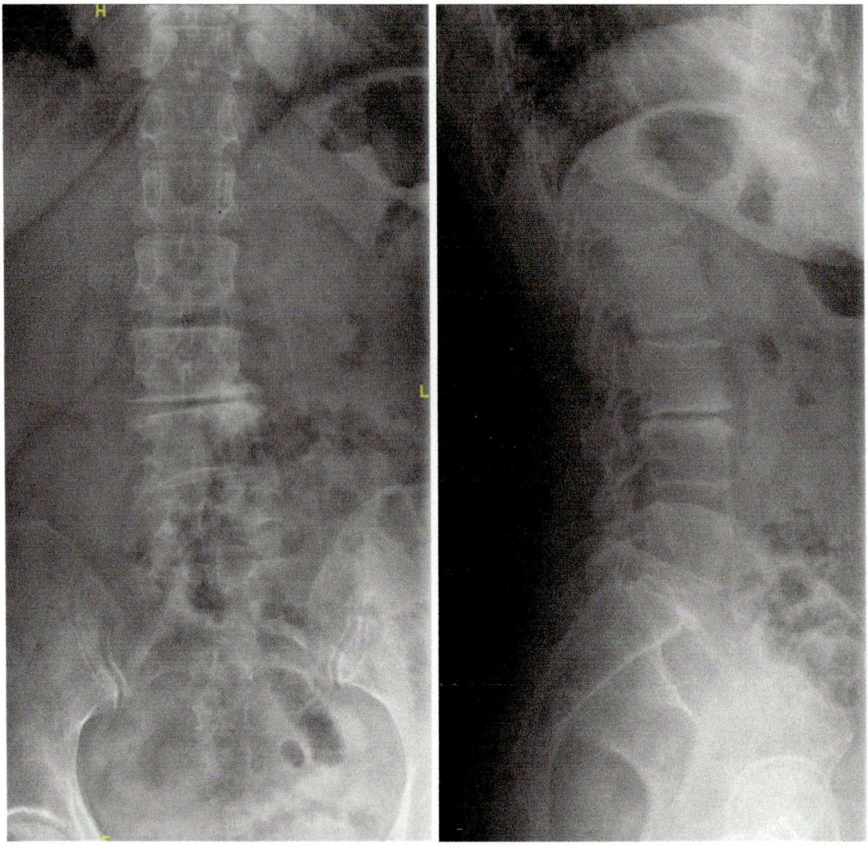

Fig. 32.2 Multilevel degenerative changes seen, most severe between L3 and L4 with endplate sclerosis and scoliosis <30°

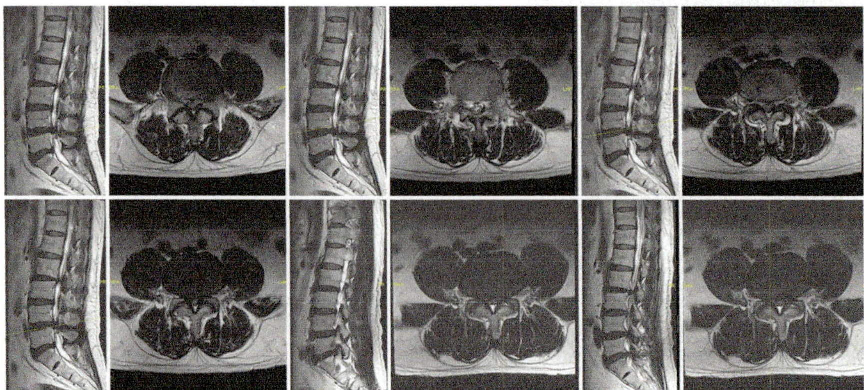

Fig. 32.3 At the L4–L5 level, a combination of diffuse disc bulge, ligamentum flavum, and facet joint hypertrophy resulting in severe spinal canal stenosis and severe bilateral lateral recess stenosis with mild-to-moderate neural foraminal narrowing. Sagittal cut evaluation is important to decide the route of approach—for extraforaminal, extraforaminal, foraminal (for far-lateral approach), lateral recess, and central (for inter-laminar approach)

A provocative discogram is a useful tool that aids in identifying pain generators in patients with uncertain or non-correlating clinical condition after an MRI scan [3]. Discogram can be a useful tool for the diagnostic evaluation of discogenic pain (Fig. 32.4).

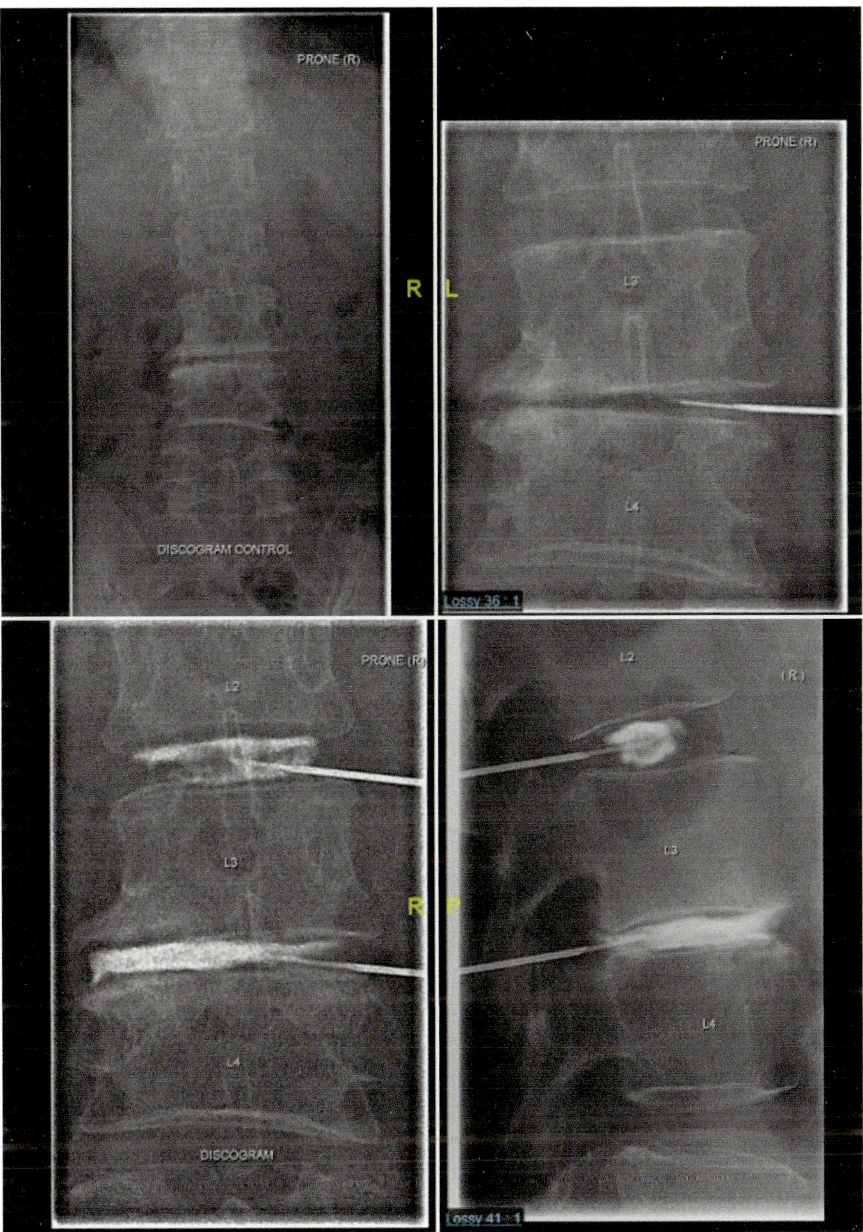

Fig. 32.4 Prior to the discogram, the pain grade was 4/10 which increased to 6/10 (back and right buttock pain) after injecting 2 mL radio-opaque dye between L3 and L4. This pain was not reproduced on provoking the immediately higher level

Symptomatic degenerative lumbar canal stenosis with failed conservative management is suitable for endoscopic decompression with concomitant fusion procedure in patients with spinal instability. In our practice, indications for biportal decompression are 1–3 levels of stenosis and grade 1 spondylolisthesis.

Biportal fusion: Indications are the same as open fusion; we perform UBE fusion for up to three levels. More levels of decompression are possible but may lead to prolonged operative time. We aim to complete UBE-related surgeries within 3 h to optimize the benefit of UBE as a minimally invasive procedure. If more time requirement and more levels of UBE are to be performed, we suggest a discussion with the patient and anesthetic team to adjust their expectation in these cases.

Clinical and Radiological Factors Predictive of Conservative Failure

The most common indication for surgery is failure to improve with conservative treatment [4]. Most of the predictive indicators are based on the MRI scan. Out of these factors, the commonly used one is the ratio between anterior-posterior fragment size and dura thecal sac size. It has been found that in patients with equal AP diameters of the disc fragment and thecal sac, conservative therapy will most likely be futile. Other criteria predictive of conservative treatment failure include cerebral spinal fluid flow blockage and a herniation disc location that is closer to the foramen further from the midline. The foramen ratio of normal in comparison to the side of the foramen with disc herniation is also predictive of necessity in surgery. Pfirrmann grade higher than 2 is generally a positive prognostic factor for surgery [5].

The main indication for spinal fusion is similar to that of spinal decompression, but with additional concomitant instability either as a complication of the disease process or as iatrogenic caused by the surgery itself. It can also be performed for degenerative disc disease without spinal stenosis. However, it should be done with a stringent indication of selected cases that have failed most if not all forms of conservative management [6].

Imaging guidelines for selecting patients for endoscopic decompression:

We have modified the exclusion criteria applied by Li et al. to include up to three levels of lumbar decompression without fusion [7]:

1. If imaging is suggestive of two-segment stenosis and clinical manifestations are of two-segment stenosis, the patients are considered as having two-segment stenosis.
2. Patients are considered as having two-segment stenosis if the symptoms are restricted to the innervated areas of two segments even though imaging shows three or more segment stenosis.

3. If CT and MRI show three or more segment stenosis, but the clinical symptoms and signs are not correlating with the involved segments, and none of the segments could be ruled out for inducing the disease, the patients may not have a satisfactory outcome postoperatively.

However, if in doubt, we tend to decompress all the levels of stenosis at the same setting.

Schizas scale is the recommended tool to measure spinal stenosis on MRI. In the Schizas system, grade A stenosis is the mildest, with abundant CSF inside the dural sac. There are four subgroups within grade A. In grade B stenosis, the rootlets occupy the entire dural sac but can still be individualized. In grade C, no rootlets can be recognized, but epidural fat can be visualized dorsally. Lastly, in grade D, the thecal sac is obliterated, and no epidural fat, CSF, or individual rootlets are visible. The degree of stenosis is evaluated at the level of the mid-disc, the cranial portion of the disc, and the caudal portion of the disc [8].

Obesity

The use of soft-tissue retractors may not be efficient enough for optimal visualization during open lumbar procedures owing to excessive soft-tissue girth. However, obese patients with degenerative lumbar spine may benefit the most from an endoscopic procedure as this is known to minimize the number of complications among obese patients [9].

Revision Surgery

Altered anatomy and scar tissue as a result of previous lumbar surgery pose a significant challenge for a minimally invasive approach, even more for open surgical procedures. Transforaminal endoscopic discectomy and foraminotomy have been described for lumbar radiculopathy in the setting of a previous instrumented spinal fusion [10].

Considerations are made for using a different route of approach, i.e., transforaminal (paraspinal) approach for a previous interlaminar decompression and vice versa. If the same approach is used, a preoperative CT scan is performed to evaluate the area of docking and the competency of the facet joint. There is a higher risk of dural tear and neural complications in revision than primary surgery; advice is given to the patient to adjust expectations and about the possible risk of conversion to open surgery.

Education and Counseling

Preoperative education and counseling can influence patient expectations and postoperative satisfaction levels [11]. The uncertainty of outcomes can contribute to preoperative anxiety, which may have unfavorable effects on the surgical outcome. Combining preoperative education with consistent written patient information materials complemented with videos of the proposed surgery will be beneficial in allaying surgery and rehabilitation-related apprehension [12].

Cessation of Smoking and Alcohol

Smoking tobacco and consumption of alcohol are risk factors for perioperative and postoperative complications including delayed spinal fusion, pseudoarthrosis, delayed wound healing, pulmonary and cardiovascular complications, and deep vein thrombosis, thus contributing to potentially avoidable morbidity and mortality [13].

Cessation of smoking for 4 weeks is advised to reduce postoperative respiratory and wound complications. Nicotine replacement therapy is usually combined with intensive counseling to motivate patients as they need to continue the cessation postoperatively as well as to avoid complications including but not limited to recurrence of lumbar disc herniation and pseudoarthrosis. Behavioral interventions, disulfiram, and benzodiazepines are used in programs targeted at alcohol consumption cessation or control [14].

Pre-rehabilitation

Pre-rehabilitation has been described as enhancing functional capacity before surgery to accelerate return to function following surgery. It combines exercise, nutrition therapy, and psychological preparation. Currently, there is insufficient evidence to ascertain if it improves postoperative recovery and outcomes in lumbar spine surgery [15]. However, this may prove beneficial particularly in the elderly population scheduled to undergo UBE [16]. It could help by decreasing the postoperative pain and length of hospital stay (LOS).

Pre-anesthetic Medication

Nonanalgesic medication: IV fluid administrated preoperatively reduces perioperative nausea, dizziness, and drowsiness.

Preoperative analgesics on the day of surgery:

1. High-dose oral NSAIDs: In the case of fusion surgeries, this is not ubiquitously recommended. However, an association of NSAIDs with an increased incidence of impaired osteogenesis and pseudoarthrosis after spinal fusion is not proven yet.
2. Acetaminophen (1000 mg).
3. Sustained-release oxycodone to be avoided in multimodal opioid-sparing analgesia strategy.
4. Other pain medications that may benefit patients include:
   (a) Preemptive analgesia: Gabapentin (600 mg) combined with NSAIDs
       Gabapentin has been associated with reductions in pruritus, nausea, and vomiting.
   (b) Pregabalin (100–150 mg) [17, 18]
       Sedative or anxiolytic drugs are to be avoided to prevent the risk of neurocognitive impairment [19].

Nutritional Supplementation

Malnutrition has been well established as a risk factor for poor surgical outcomes in general. It is prudent to offer preoperative nutritional interventions to such patients. Body mass index, blood tests, and standardized nutritional scoring systems are useful in diagnosing malnutrition in prospective patients for surgery. Decreased albumin, transferrin levels, and low lymphocyte count are predictors of increased risk of surgical site infections, postoperative complications, increased length of hospital stay (LOS), subsequent readmission rates, and mortality following spinal surgery. Treatment of malnutrition consists of referral to a dietician who may help with dietary advice and meal fortification with protein and prescribe nutritional supplements. The clinical benefit of carbohydrate loading in spinal surgery remains controversial, and there appears to be a lack of consensus for a specific recommendation [20].

Intraoperative Care

Detailed procedural steps are beyond the scope of this chapter; some pointers of intraoperative care are made here to highlight our practice to optimize good perioperative outcomes.

Antimicrobial Prophylaxis and Skin Preparation

Currently, there is a lack of a universally followed guideline for antibiotic prophylaxis/antiseptic of choice for minimally invasive spinal surgery. Preoperative screening and eradication of methicillin-sensitive or methicillin-resistant *Staphylococcus aureus* (MRSA) are advised to reduce surgical site infections (SSIs) in noncarriers compared to carriers. A combination of topical chlorhexidine and intranasal mupirocin is effective in reducing *S. aureus*-associated SSIs. Alcohol-based agents are superior to aqueous solutions for skin antisepsis. By allowing povidone-iodine to dry for several minutes before spine surgery, bacterial load on the skin can be significantly reduced [20].

Broad-spectrum antibiotic (first-generation cephalosporin) like cephazolin which covers *S. aureus*, 30 min to 1 h before skin incision with redosing every 4 h during longer surgeries, is widely accepted and followed. Antiseptic dressing the night before surgery was associated with a reduction in SSI after orthopedic surgery, but this is yet to be studied in spine surgery [21].

One of the main advantages of MIS including UBE is that the risk of SSI is very low in itself. A significant sevenfold reduction in SSIs was noted when comparing MIS with open surgery. This significance was also demonstrated with a tenfold reduction for procedures involving decompression alone [22].

Positioning and Intraoperative Setup

The patient is placed into a prone position on a surgical table (Fig. 32.5) or Wilson frame with the abdomen hanging freely. This reduces intra-abdominal pressure and prevents secondary venous congestion. The arms are abducted, the elbows are flexed at 90°, and the bony prominences are padded appropriately. A chest roll may be placed to maximize the lumbar lordosis if using Jackson table. The surgeon should be positioned on the side of the pathology while the fluoroscope, monitor, and microscope are placed on the contralateral side. Neuro-monitoring is optional; it is commonly performed in our institution.

Urinary Catheterization

Prolonged urinary drainage is associated with complications such as urinary tract infections, surgical site infections, and postoperative urinary retention (POUR) following spine surgery, which in turn increases the risk of sepsis and LOS. Limited urinary catheterization in patients undergoing spine surgery and discontinuing catheters within a few hours after surgery can potentially avoid such complications and encourage early patient ambulation [20–23]. We do not routinely use urinary catheterization in UBE unless clinically indicated for prolonged surgery.

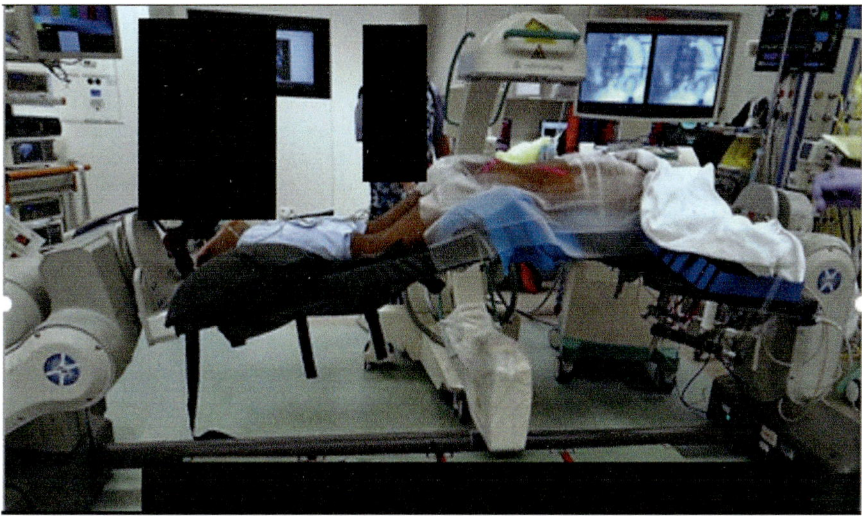

Fig. 32.5 Patient positioning

Thromboprophylaxis

The incidence of pulmonary embolism (PE) and symptomatic deep vein thrombosis (DVT) in elective spine surgery is low at 0.9% and 0.7%, respectively. There is no statistically significant difference between chemoprophylaxis and mechanoprophylaxis to prevent DVT and PE [24]. Mechanical thromboprophylaxis using calf pumps/foot pumps for intermittent pneumatic compression is recommended [25]. Early ambulation postoperatively is to be encouraged.

Intraoperative Anesthesia

Monitored anesthesia care (MAC) may be adequate for single-level procedures with an estimated surgical time of 30–90 min. Short-acting anesthetic agents may be used, and avoid the use of opioids intraoperatively as well. Local anesthesia with/without sedation and low-dose epidural anesthesia would be a better choice for the standard MIS lumbar fusion technique. The possibility of local anesthesia offers an additional benefit for elder patients, especially with systemic diseases [26]. Perform generous infiltration of lidocaine 1% with bupivacaine 0.25%. The surgical incision site is recommended to reduce the patient's analgesic requirements.

Our preference is the following: pre-op infiltration: 10 mL of bupivacaine with adrenaline and postoperative 0.5% infiltration of portal wounds.

Muscle relaxants should be avoided if possible as this may hinder early and efficient postoperative mobilization [23].

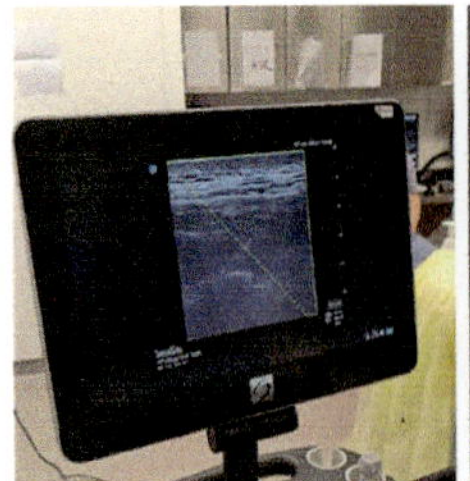
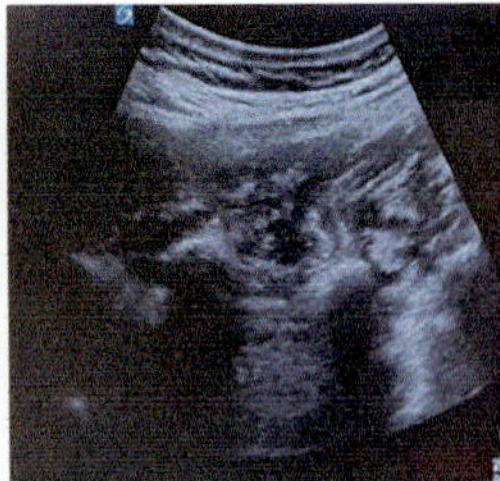
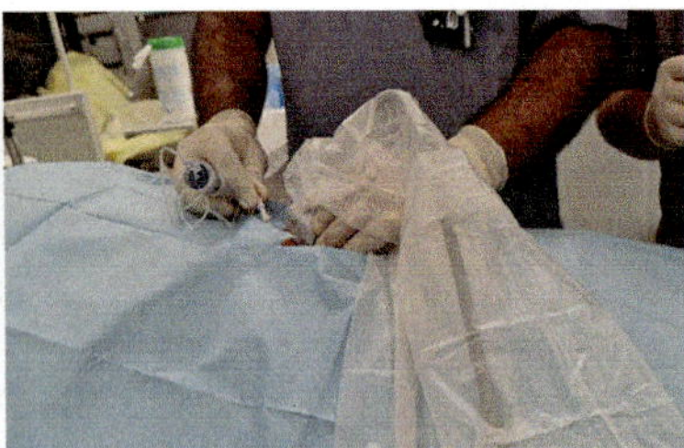

Fig. 32.6 Anesthetist performing ultrasound-guided TLIP block: Local anesthetic is injected into the fascial plane between the multifidus muscle and longissimus muscle at the upper level of the lumbar vertebrae intended for decompression

Regional blocks: Erector spinae plane block, quadratus lumborum, and thoracolumbar interfacial plane (TLIP) blocks have been described. Only the TLIP block has been evaluated for lumbar fusion, which can be extended to UBE, particularly lumbar fusion surgery [27]. This aids in early pain-free postoperative mobilization (Fig. 32.6).

Intraoperative Hypothermia

Intraoperative hypothermia is to be avoided as it increases the risk of cardiac complications, shivering, and prolonged LOS. Normothermia can be ensured by the use of warmed infusion liquids, warm irrigation fluids, rewarming, and forced air-warming blankets and devices [28, 29].

Intravenous Tranexamic Acid

Prevention and control of intraoperative bleeding from bone or epidural vessels are important to ensure a bloodless surgical field during UBE procedures. Intravenous administration of tranexamic acid ensures this (stat dose preoperatively and maintenance dose intraoperatively). IV tranexamic acid is contraindicated in the previous history of cardiovascular surgery, previous history, or high risk of thromboembolic disease, subarachnoid hemorrhage, and renal impairment [30].

Postoperative Care

Postoperative Nausea and Vomiting (PONV)

PONV results in varying degrees of dehydration, thus impacting the early return of adequate nutrition intake, increasing intravenous fluid administration postoperatively, and lengthening hospital stay. Major risk factors are the previous history of PONV, motion sickness, and female gender. These can be treated by serving appropriate antiemetic medications [20].

Wound Care

Endoscopic portal closure with absorbable suture (Vicryl 1/0, 2/0/, 3/0) with tissue glue or surgical skin closure with a waterproof dressing (Fig. 32.7): Injection of slowly releasing, long-acting liposomal bupivacaine into the wound before closure may be effective for controlling postoperative pain.

Rehabilitation

Early mobilization following spinal surgery and other major procedures has been linked to reduced morbidity and LOS [31]. Early mobilization has been shown to reduce respiratory complications, improve functional capacity, and reduce thromboembolic events. Mobilization may be started as early as 2 h after surgery under the supervision of a trained physiotherapist without restriction to resume daily activities. Furthermore, early commencement of physical therapy in spine surgery patients has been shown to facilitate early return to functional activity. Early involvement of physical therapists, especially in high-risk patients (chronic low back pain), may expedite postoperative mobilization. The patient is safe for discharge after

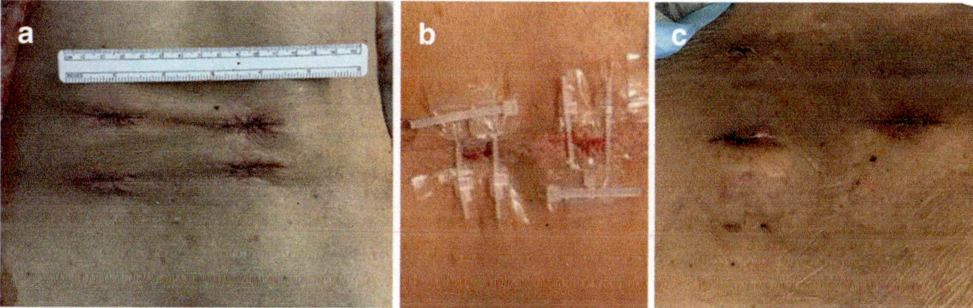

Fig. 32.7 Progression of wound healing. (**a**, **b**) Endoscopic portal closure with surgical skin closure. (**c**) Wound healing after 2 weeks postoperatively

supervised physiotherapy and ensuring independent transfer and walking. Patients are advised to stay away from work and avoid driving for the first 3 weeks after surgery [20, 23]. Postoperative brace: Not routinely recommended. Postoperative spinal orthosis did not affect clinical outcome scores and lumbar fusion rates in MIS lumbar fusion surgery (Table 32.1) [32].

Table 32.1 Biportal Early Staged Therapy Program by Ng Teng Fong General Hospital Designed by Dr. Pang Hung Wu

Timing	Purpose	Treatment points	Notes	Basic exercises	Selective actions
1–3 days	Postoperative pain relief, gradual initiation of therapy, and mobilization	Bed rest with periodic turning under adequate analgesia cover. Active and active-assisted range of lower limb joints. Mobilization at home is encouraged	Assess neurological status. Tailor therapy as per early postoperative assessment	Passive straight leg-raising exercises	Bridge support (Single bridge)
4 days to 2 weeks	Rehabilitate pelvic bridge function and strengthen lumbosacral antigravity muscles	Active and passive exercises for the lower limbs in bed, straight leg-raising training, and isometric contraction training for lumbar extensors. A lumbosacral brace may be used to sit-to-stand exercise for about 10 min 2–3 times a day. Mobilization near neighborhood	Therapy to be limited as allowed by pain after administering analgesics. Patient graduates to next level of exercise and rehabilitations after successfully completing this level	Bridge support (single bridge/ double bridge)	Horizontal arch movement and supine curly hug exercise
2–3 weeks	Enhance mobilization of lumbar spine	A lumbosacral brace is used for indoor walking coupled with moderate-intensity exercise for the lower limbs beyond neighborhood as tolerated	The patients who successfully complete this level are safe for home. Analgesics are not used	Bridge support Supine arch motion Supine curly hug exercise	Prone upper-limb-support stretching exercise

Table 32.1 (continued)

Timing	Purpose	Treatment points	Notes	Basic exercises	Selective actions
4–6 weeks	Light core muscle strengthening and transition to daily activities	With a protective lumbosacral support, patient is encouraged to return to the community and get back to starting daily life activities without completing it and nonphysical work. Increase the walking distance to further improve endurance of lower limbs. Hard physical labor is to be avoided	Gradually wean off brace during exercise. Avoid weight bearing on the waist and straight leg-bending activities, learn correct sitting posture	Bridge support Supine arch motion Supine curly hug exercise Prone upper limb support and stretching exercise	Forward bending Supine leg lift
6–12 weeks	To graduate and complete daily activities independently. General work permitted	Gradually participate in general work with waist protection Gradually perform strength training for the core muscle groups of the spine	Avoid physical labor and weight bearing on the waist	Supine arch motion Supine curly hug exercise Prone upper limb support and stretching exercises	Sit forward and bend your legs Pelvic alternate pronation exercise
12–24 weeks	No restriction of daily activities	Allowed to discontinue brace and participate in general work. Graduate to moderate-intensity core muscle strengthening	Avoid strenuous exercise and heavy load/ weight bearing	Prone upper limb support and stretching exercises Supine leg lift Lateral pelvic-strengthening exercise Crawling training Cycling and strengthening exercises	

Opioid-Sparing Multimodal Analgesia

Acetaminophen (paracetamol) is a basic part of perioperative multimodal pain management and is used widely, either orally or intravenously. Multimodal opioid-sparing techniques are recommended. Alternatives for opioid-sparing analgesia include acetaminophen, gabapentin, and NSAIDs; morphine PCA is preferred in cases where postoperative pain is not controlled by a combination of acetaminophen and NSAIDs [33]. In the case of multilevel endoscopic surgeries, epidural injection or epidural PCA therapy may be useful for controlling postoperative pain; this may however not be warranted for single-level UBE lumbar fusion [34, 35].

Use of Drains

We do not use drains routinely in UBE as we perform UBE as ambulatory procedures. The risk of developing postoperative epidural hematoma in patients who underwent single-level UBE was found to be 24.7%, out of which up to 5% of patients may be symptomatic (Fig. 32.8). Revision surgery is recommended in case of symptomatic patients (motor neurological deficit) with canal encroachment >50% on MRI scan [36].

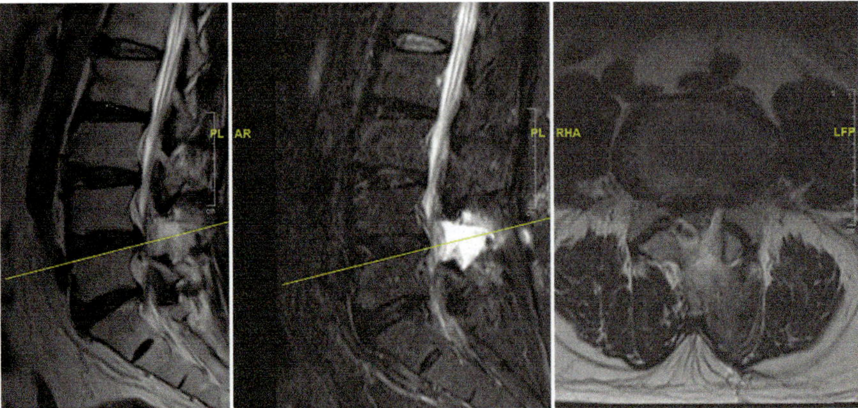

Fig. 32.8 MRI of the lumbar spine following left L4/L5 endoscopic decompression. The fluid collection was seen at the surgical bed without rim enhancement. A relatively common imaging feature displaying early post-decompression findings. In this patient, there was an inadvertent dural tear repaired endoscopically with patch blocking repair technique

Follow-Up

Telemedicine phone/internet face-to-face interviews are performed on follow-up of 2 days and 7 days postoperatively and wound inspection in the clinic after 2 weeks. Further, follow up after 3 months, 6 months, and 1 year postoperatively with documentation of functional outcome scores. Digital questionnaires may be used prior to clinic visits for monitoring and audit. It is advisable to keep a low threshold for close clinical follow-up and readmission, especially in the early postoperative period, and patients should be encouraged to call in case of any uncertainties [23].

Conclusion

Despite being a minimally invasive option, biportal endoscopic surgery (UBE) must be applied with all perioperative measures and care to obtain adequate clinical results. Therefore, this chapter's recommendations are routinely carried out considering the biportal endoscopic technique as an excellent surgical procedure and potentially associated with collateral effects and complications like any other spinal surgery.

References

1. Weinstein JN, et al. Surgical versus nonsurgical therapy for lumbar spinal stenosis. N Engl J Med. 2008;358(8):794–810. https://doi.org/10.1056/NEJMoa0707136.
2. Lewandrowski K-U. Incidence, management, and cost of complications after transforaminal endoscopic decompression surgery for lumbar foraminal and lateral recess stenosis: a value proposition for outpatient ambulatory surgery. Int J Spine Surg. 2019;13(1):53–67. https://doi.org/10.14444/6008.
3. Bini W, Yeung AT, Calatayud V, Chaaban A, Seferlis T. The role of provocative discography in minimally invasive selective endoscopic discectomy. Neurocirugia (Astur Spain). 2002;13(1):27–31.; discussion 32. https://doi.org/10.1016/s1130-1473(02)70646-5.
4. Storm PB, Chou D, Tamargo RJ. Surgical management of cervical and lumbosacral radiculopathies: indications and outcomes. Phys Med Rehabil Clin N Am. 2002;13(3):735–59. https://doi.org/10.1016/s1047-9651(02)00014-1.
5. Motiei-Langroudi R, Sadeghian H, Seddighi AS. Clinical and magnetic resonance imaging factors which may predict the need for surgery in lumbar disc herniation. Asian Spine J. 2014;8(4):446–52. https://doi.org/10.4184/asj.2014.8.4.446.
6. Wu PH, Kim HS, Jang I-T. Intervertebral disc diseases PART 2: A review of the current diagnostic and treatment strategies for intervertebral disc disease. Int J Mol Sci. 2020;21(6):E2135. https://doi.org/10.3390/ijms21062135.
7. Li L, et al. Clinical effect evaluation and correlation between preoperative imaging parameters and clinical effect of endoscopic transforaminal decompression for lumbar spinal stenosis. BMC Musculoskelet Disord. 2020;21(1):68. https://doi.org/10.1186/s12891-020-3076-0.

8. Schizas C, et al. Qualitative grading of severity of lumbar spinal stenosis based on the morphology of the dural sac on magnetic resonance images. Spine. 2010;35(21):1919–24. https://doi.org/10.1097/BRS.0b013e3181d359bd.
9. Hudak EM, Perry MW. Outpatient minimally invasive spine surgery using endoscopy for the treatment of lumbar spinal stenosis among obese patients. J Orthop. 2015;12(3):156–9. https://doi.org/10.1016/j.jor.2015.01.007.
10. Telfeian AE. Endoscopic foraminotomy for recurrent lumbar radiculopathy after TLIF: technical report. Surg Neurol Int. 2015;6:62. https://doi.org/10.4103/2152-7806.155261.
11. Kong C-B, Jeon D-W, Chang B-S, Lee JH, Suk K-S, Park J-B. Outcome of spinal fusion for lumbar degenerative disease: a cross-sectional study in Korea. Spine. 2010;35(15):1489–94. https://doi.org/10.1097/BRS.0b013e3181c49fd0.
12. Burgess LC, Arundel J, Wainwright TW. The effect of preoperative education on psychological, clinical and economic outcomes in elective spinal surgery: a systematic review. Healthcare. 2019;7(1):E48. https://doi.org/10.3390/healthcare7010048.
13. Hermann PC, et al. Influence of smoking on spinal fusion after spondylodesis surgery: a comparative clinical study. Technol Health Care. 2016;24(5):737–44. https://doi.org/10.3233/THC-161164.
14. Oppedal K, Møller AM, Pedersen B, Tønnesen H. Preoperative alcohol cessation prior to elective surgery. Cochrane Database Syst Rev. 2012;7:CD008343. https://doi.org/10.1002/14651858.CD008343.pub2.
15. Janssen ERC, Punt IM, Clemens MJ, Staal JB, Hoogeboom TJ, Willems PC. Current prehabilitation programs do not improve the postoperative outcomes of patients scheduled for lumbar spine surgery: a systematic review with meta-analysis. J Orthop Sports Phys Ther. 2021;51(3):103–14. https://doi.org/10.2519/jospt.2021.9748.
16. Delgado-López PD, Rodríguez-Salazar A, Castilla-Díez JM. 'Prehabilitation' in degenerative spine surgery: a literature review. Neurocirugia (Astur: Engl Ed). 2019;30(3):124–32. https://doi.org/10.1016/j.neucir.2018.11.008.
17. Buvanendran A, Thillainathan V. Preoperative and postoperative anesthetic and analgesic techniques for minimally invasive surgery of the spine. Spine. 2010;35(26 Suppl):S274–80. https://doi.org/10.1097/BRS.0b013e31820240f8.
18. Soffin EM, et al. Opioid-free anesthesia within an enhanced recovery after surgery pathway for minimally invasive lumbar spine surgery: a retrospective matched cohort study. Neurosurg Focus. 2019;46(4):E8. https://doi.org/10.3171/2019.1.FOCUS18645.
19. By the American Geriatrics Society 2015 Beers Criteria Update Expert Panel. American Geriatrics Society 2015 updated Beers Criteria for potentially inappropriate medication use in older adults. J Am Geriatr Soc. 2015;63(11):2227–46. https://doi.org/10.1111/jgs.13702.
20. Debono B, et al. Consensus statement for perioperative care in lumbar spinal fusion: Enhanced Recovery After Surgery (ERAS®) Society recommendations. Spine J. 2021;21(5):729–52. https://doi.org/10.1016/j.spinee.2021.01.001.
21. Eiselt D. Presurgical skin preparation with a novel 2% chlorhexidine gluconate cloth reduces rates of surgical site infection in orthopaedic surgical patients. Orthop Nurs. 2009;28(3):141–5. https://doi.org/10.1097/NOR.0b013e3181a469db.
22. Mueller K, Zhao D, Johnson O, Sandhu FA, Voyadzis J-M. The difference in surgical site infection rates between open and minimally invasive spine surgery for degenerative lumbar pathology: a retrospective single center experience of 1442 cases. Oper Neurosurg (Hagerstown Md). 2019;16(6):750–5. https://doi.org/10.1093/ons/opy221.
23. Staartjes VE, de Wispelaere MP, Schröder ML. Improving recovery after elective degenerative spine surgery: 5-year experience with an enhanced recovery after surgery (ERAS) protocol. Neurosurg Focus. 2019;46(4):E7. https://doi.org/10.3171/2019.1.FOCUS18646.
24. Mosenthal WP, et al. Thromboprophylaxis in spinal surgery. Spine. 2018;43(8):E474–81. https://doi.org/10.1097/BRS.0000000000002379.
25. Epstein NE. Efficacy of pneumatic compression stocking prophylaxis in the prevention of deep venous thrombosis and pulmonary embolism following 139 lumbar laminectomies with

instrumented fusions. J Spinal Disord Tech. 2006;19(1):28–31. https://doi.org/10.1097/01.bsd.0000173454.71657.02.

26. Wu J, et al. Percutaneous endoscopic lumbar interbody fusion: technical note and preliminary clinical experience with 2-year follow-up. Biomed Res Int. 2018;2018:5806037. https://doi.org/10.1155/2018/5806037.
27. Christopher S, Gopal TVS, Vardhan V. Thoracolumbar interfascial plane block, way forward for awake endoscopic laminectomies. Indian J Anaesth. 2020;64(5):436–7. https://doi.org/10.4103/ija.IJA_915_19.
28. Jin Y, Tian J, Sun M, Yang K. A systematic review of randomised controlled trials of the effects of warmed irrigation fluid on core body temperature during endoscopic surgeries. J Clin Nurs. 2011;20(3–4):305–16. https://doi.org/10.1111/j.1365-2702.2010.03484.x.
29. Moola S, Lockwood C. Effectiveness of strategies for the management and/or prevention of hypothermia within the adult perioperative environment. Int J Evid Based Healthc. 2011;9(4):337–45. https://doi.org/10.1111/j.1744-1609.2011.00227.x.
30. Lu VM, Ho Y-T, Nambiar M, Mobbs RJ, Phan K. The perioperative efficacy and safety of antifibrinolytics in adult spinal fusion surgery: a systematic review and meta-analysis. Spine. 2018;43(16):E949–58. https://doi.org/10.1097/BRS.0000000000002580.
31. Ne E. A review article on the benefits of early mobilization following spinal surgery and other medical/surgical procedures. Surg Neurol Int. 2014;5(Suppl):3. https://doi.org/10.4103/2152-7806.130674.
32. Ma H-H, et al. Postoperative spinal orthosis may not be necessary for minimally invasive lumbar spine fusion surgery: a prospective randomized controlled trial. BMC Musculoskelet Disord. 2021;22(1):619. https://doi.org/10.1186/s12891-021-04490-4.
33. Walker CT, et al. Implementation of a standardized multimodal postoperative analgesia protocol improves pain control, reduces opioid consumption, and shortens length of hospital stay after posterior lumbar spinal fusion. Neurosurgery. 2020;87(1):130–6. https://doi.org/10.1093/neuros/nyz312.
34. Ong CK-S, Lirk P, Seymour RA, Jenkins BJ. The efficacy of preemptive analgesia for acute postoperative pain management: a meta-analysis. Anesth Analg. 2005;100(3):757–73. https://doi.org/10.1213/01.ANE.0000144428.98767.0E.
35. Heo DH, Park CK. Clinical results of percutaneous biportal endoscopic lumbar interbody fusion with application of enhanced recovery after surgery. Neurosurg Focus. 2019;46(4):E18. https://doi.org/10.3171/2019.1.FOCUS18695.
36. Kim J-E, Choi D-J, Park EJ. Evaluation of postoperative spinal epidural hematoma after biportal endoscopic spine surgery for single-level lumbar spinal stenosis: clinical and magnetic resonance imaging study. World Neurosurg. 2019;126:e786–92. https://doi.org/10.1016/j.wneu.2019.02.150.

Chapter 33
How to Establish the Unilateral Biportal Endoscopic Surgery in the Surgeons' Daily Practice

Sheung-Tung Ho, Tsz-King Suen, and Yip-Kan Yeung

Abbreviations

ACDF	Anterior cervical decompression and fusion
APECD	Anterior percutaneous endoscopic cervical discectomy
BMI	Body mass index
CK	Creatine kinase
CRP	C-reactive protein
CSF	Cerebral spinal fluid
ERAS	Enhanced recovery after surgery
HbA1c	Glycated haemoglobin
IELD	Interlaminar endoscopic lumbar discectomy
MED	Microendoscopic discectomy
MIS	Minimally invasive
MISS	Minimally invasive spine surgery
MRI	Magnetic resonance imaging
ODI	Oswestry Disability Index
PCF	Posterior cervical foraminotomy
PRCT	Prospective randomized controlled trial
PSEH	Post-operative spinal epidural haematoma
TELD	Transforaminal endoscopic lumbar discectomy

S.-T. Ho (✉) · Y.-K. Yeung
Department of Orthopaedics & Traumatology, Caritas Medical Centre, Hong Kong SAR, China
e-mail: drhosheungtung@gmail.com; yyk028@ha.org.hk

T.-K. Suen
Hong Kong Baptist Hospital, Hong Kong SAR, China
e-mail: aarsuen@gmail.com

J. Quillo-Olvera et al. (eds.), *Unilateral Biportal Endoscopy of the Spine*,
https://doi.org/10.1007/978-3-031-14736-4_33

TLIF	Transforaminal lumbar interbody fusion
UBE	Unilateral biportal endoscopy
ULBD	Unilateral laminotomy for bilateral decompression
VAS	Visual analogue scale

Introduction

With the advent of endoscopy technology, computer image guidance, spine implants and fusion devices, and surgical techniques (e.g. percutaneous pedicle screw fixation, lumbar interbody fusion), spine operations can now be performed through minimally invasive techniques with smaller incisions, increased visualization, less blood loss and quicker return to daily activities. Minimally invasive spine surgery (MISS) is widely used and demonstrates its advantages over open spine surgery in many lumbar disorders. Recently, the scope of MISS has expanded to include cervical spine surgery [1] and adult spine deformity [2]. MISS will continue to innovate and evolve over the coming years.

The demand of MISS is forecast to grow at a compound annual growth rate of 4.8% during the period 2020–2025 [3]. North America and Europe dominate the demand, but Asia Pacific region is estimated to grow at the fastest rate. On the one hand, the market demand or service gap is well validated. On the other hand, spine surgeons are motivated to practise MISS aiming to master new technical skills, to achieve better clinical outcomes and to meet their patient demand.

The Paradigm Shift from Open Spine Surgery to Minimally Invasive Spine Surgery

An increasing percentage of MISS has been observed to replace open spine surgery in the recent decade. Nearly 75% of all spinal surgeries can be performed with complete or partial use of MISS over conventional open techniques [4]. Indeed, with more experience in specialized centre, up to 97% of lumbar degenerative spinal conditions can be done by endoscopic surgery replacing open and microscopic minimally invasive surgery [5].

Lumbar Disc Herniation

Lumbar disc herniation affects 1–3% of population in their lifetime. About 10% of people have sufficient pain after 6 weeks, and then need to consider surgery [6]. Open microscopic discectomy was once regarded as the gold standard of lumbar discectomy. Several meta-analyses revealed that there is no difference in pain, functional outcome, complication rate and reoperation reported after tubular microendoscopic discectomy or transforaminal endoscopic lumbar discectomy (TELD) versus open microscopic discectomy [7–9]. However, endoscopic lumbar discectomy has a shorter operation time, less estimated blood loss, shorter hospital stay and higher patient satisfaction [7, 8]. Compared with open microscopic discectomy and micro-endoscopic discectomy (MED), TELD gave the best visual analogue scale (VAS) scores for wound pain and back pain in a retrospective comparative study of 192 patients with minimal 2-year follow-up [10]. Another retrospective matched cohort study comparing TELD with open microscopic discectomy demonstrated significant advantages in back pain, operation time, blood loss, hospital stay and return to work (14 vs. 29 days) in young adults (age 20–25) [11, 12].

Lumbar Spinal Stenosis

The prevalence of lumbar spinal stenosis in adults is high. The estimated mean prevalence is 11% based on clinical diagnosis in general population and 25–39% in patients from primary or secondary care [13]. Although a substantial proportion of patients remained unchanged for up to 8 years of follow-up, about 15% had worsened symptoms [14]. Those with severe baseline symptoms, severe stenosis and degenerative spondylolisthesis tend to require surgery. Lumbar spinal stenosis is the most common cause of lumbar spine surgery in elderly aged over 65 years [15]. A prospective cohort 10-year study of symptomatic lumbar spinal stenosis showed that outcomes for patients randomized for surgery were considerably better than for those randomized for conservative treatment [16].

Again, MISS is favoured over conventional open surgery for lumbar spinal stenosis. Minimally invasive unilateral laminotomy for bilateral decompression (ULBD) is the preferred surgical treatment for lumbar spinal stenosis. A systemic review and network meta-analysis of clinical studies showed that minimally invasive ULBD performs better in decreasing the visual analogue scale (VAS) scores for back and leg pain compared with conventional decompressive laminectomy [17]. A prospective randomized controlled trial (PRCT) demonstrated that full endoscopic interlaminar decompression adopting a unilateral approach provided the same clinical results compared to the conventional microsurgical bilateral laminotomy, but the rate of complications and revision was significantly reduced [18]. A meta-analysis of lumbar endoscopic ULBD showed significant improvement in Oswestry Disability Index (ODI) and VAS scores for leg and back pain, exceeding the criteria of minimal clinically important difference [19].

Lumbar Degenerative Spondylolisthesis

For lumbar spinal stenosis associated with stable low-grade degenerative spondylolisthesis, minimally invasive (MIS) ULBD is less destabilizing than open laminotomy. A meta-analysis revealed no slip progression (0% vs. 72%), lower secondary fusion rate (3.3% vs. 12.8%) and lower total reoperation rate (5.8% vs. 16.3%) in MIS ULBD, compared to open laminotomy [20]. Another meta-analysis showed that concomitant low-grade degenerative spondylolisthesis does not influence the outcome of decompression alone in degenerative lumbar spinal stenosis, especially when a minimally invasive procedure was performed and patients do not have predominant symptoms of mechanical back pain [21]. Thus, minimally invasive ULBD, including UBE ULBD, may spare lumbar fusion in degenerative spinal stenosis with concomitant stable low-grade spondylolisthesis.

For lumbar spinal stenosis with spondylolisthesis requiring transforaminal lumbar interbody fusion (TLIF), meta-analysis showed that MIS TLIF has reduced blood loss and length of hospital stay, but increased radiation exposure time than open TLIF. No significant difference is found in back and leg pain and ODI scores between MIS and open TLIF at final follow-up [22]. There are trends towards few complications (11.3% vs. 14.2%, $P = 0.05$) [22] and similar fusion rate (94.8% vs. 90%) [23]. Another meta-analysis revealed that open TLIF has significantly more blood loss by 383 mL, 1.2 day longer hospital stay and 3.8 times higher risk of dural tear and a trend towards higher post-operative wound infection rates (4.5% vs. 2.4%) and an inferior improvement of ODI score (39.3 vs. 44.1) compared to MIS TLIF [24]. A meta-analysis of six studies of 480 patients revealed no significant difference in clinical efficacy (ODI and VAS scores for leg and back, fusion rate) and safety (complications, reoperation) between endoscopic TLIF and MIS TLIF, but endoscopic TLIF has a longer operative time, less intraoperative blood loss and shorter hospital stay [25].

Thoracic Disc Herniation

Symptomatic thoracic disc herniation is very rare, constituting only 0.15–1.8% of all surgically treated disc herniation [26]. The least invasive thoracic discectomy is posterolateral endoscopy for soft and lateralized thoracic disc herniation. Central thoracic disc herniation, giant thoracic disc herniation with more than 40% spinal canal occupation, severe disc narrowing, thoracic ossification of posterior longitudinal ligament, and hard or calcified disc not amendable to other approaches require transthoracic approach via thoracoscope or retropleural mini-thoracotomy [26–28]. It is interesting to note that endoscopic treatment of thoracic disc herniation was first reported in 2012 using an ipsilateral two-portal arthroscopy for decompression and interbody fusion [29] after cadaver study in 1994 [30]. This is well before the report of current posterolateral endoscopic approaches, namely transpedicular [31] and transforaminal endoscopic thoracic discectomy [32].

Cervical Disc Herniation

Anterior cervical decompression and fusion (ACDF) or anterior decompression disc replacement is the standard treatment for cervical radiculopathy secondary to lateral cervical disc herniation or foraminal stenosis. MISS for cervical disc herniation includes minimally invasive anterior foraminotomy [33], anterior percutaneous endoscopic cervical discectomy (APECD) [34], MIS posterior cervical foraminotomy (PCF) and endoscopic PCF. Again, both APECD and minimally invasive PCF provide the typical benefits over conventional open surgery. The 5-year outcomes of APECD were comparable to open ACDF, but APECD had a reduced operative time, hospital stay and earlier return to work for treating soft cervical disc herniation in a comparative cohort study [35]. Compared to ACDF, PCF results in significantly greater improvement in VAS-arm scores and similar improvements in VAS-neck and Neck Disability Index scores in a meta-analysis of minimally invasive PCF [36] or endoscopic PCF [37]. The clinical success rate of minimally invasive PCF and open PCF is of no difference statistically [38]. PCF avoids the anterior neck vital structures and preserves motion segment compared to ACDF. Furthermore, in 3D finite element model, PCF has better biomechanical performance than ACDF [39] and also APECD [40]. Thus, minimally invasive PCF or endoscopic PCF may be an effective alternative for treating cervical disc herniation.

Minimally Invasive Spine Surgery in High-Risk Patients

The incidence of medical comorbidities, complications secondary to post-operative immobility, post-operative blood loss and infection increase after open spine surgery as patients are older. A comparative study showed that MISS in degenerative lumbar spine is associated with significantly lower operative time, estimated blood loss and length of stay, and a trend of lower complication rates, readmissions or reoperations and better pain improvement than open surgery in elderly [41]. No difference is observed in adverse events after MI lumbar interbody fusion for all age groups [42]. MISS for lumbar spine in elderly is both safe and highly effective [43]. With aging population and a strong desire for elderly to remain physically active, MISS is gaining popularity over open surgery in elderly. In well-selected cases, many different MISS may be performed in elderly aged ≥75 under local anaesthesia with minimal risk [44].

The prevalence of obesity and diabetes has been steadily increasing worldwide. Obesity poses many challenges along the whole patient journal to spine surgeons. Open lumbar spine surgery in obese patients has been associated with higher complication and reoperation rate [45]. Body mass index (BMI) >35 is a known risk factor of surgical site infection after spinal surgery [46]. MISS for lumbar spine in overweight patients with BMI >25 does not have increased perioperative complications [47]. Endoscopic lumbar stenosis decompression is safe and effective in patients with BMI ≥30 [48]. Minimally invasive TLIF has equivalent efficacy to open TLIF in obese patients, but a lower blood loss, lower complication rate and shorter length of hospital stay, as revealed in a meta-analysis [49]. No significant difference in post-operative complication and reoperation between obese and non-obese patients undergoing MISS is shown in two meta-analyses [45, 50]. MISS may offer comparable outcomes and may be preferred in obese patients.

Diabetes is a known risk factor for surgical site infection after spinal surgery [46]. The prevalence of diabetics undergoing degenerative spine surgery had been increasing significantly from 2002 to 2011 [51, 52]. Diabetic patients have increased risk of acute complications of different magnitudes, depending on the extent of control of blood sugar level after degenerative lumbar and cervical spine surgery [51, 52]. Two observational studies showed that MISS does not pose higher risk of complication in diabetic patients compared with non-diabetic patients in lumbar spine decompression [53] and lumbar interbody fusion [54].

Smoking is associated with surgical site infection, post-operative wound complications, non-union and worse outcomes after spinal surgery [55]. A prospective cohort of smokers did not show an increased risk of perioperative complications in minimally invasive lumbar spine fusion surgery [56].

Elderly, obese patients, diabetics and smokers have higher complication rate after open spinal surgery. Apart from age, other factors are potentially modifiable. Supervised weight loss programme should be tried. Surgical management is indicated for patients with BMI ≥40 or ≥35 with obesity-associated comorbidity [57]. Bariatric surgery may mitigate the worse outcomes associated with severe obesity (BMI >40). Prior bariatric surgery in this patient group is associated with lower overall complication rates, including device-related complications, deep vein thrombosis and haematomas after thoracolumbar spine surgery [58] and lower complications and in-hospital mortality after spine fusion surgery [59]. Diabetes screening and HbA1c level should be done. Optimizing preoperative glucose management with glycated haemoglobin (HbA1c) <7% may improve outcomes as preoperative HbA1c >7% is associated with significantly higher wound complications [60]. Smokers are strongly recommended to quit smoking 4–8 weeks before spine surgery and 6 months after spinal fusion surgery [61]. If spinal surgery is indicated, MISS could be advantageous in these high-risk patient groups.

Zone of Benefit of Minimally Invasive Spine Surgery (MISS)

The current benefits of MISS can be illustrated by plotting the complexity of the thoracolumbar procedures against their invasiveness (Fig. 33.1) [62]. The zone of benefit with MISS currently lies within the treatment of pathologies ranging from lumbar disc herniation to moderate deformities up to approximately five levels. Another zone of benefit of MISS would be in high-risk patients, such as elderly, obese patients, diabetics and smokers. These high-risk patients have increased complications with open spine surgery, which may be mitigated by MISS.

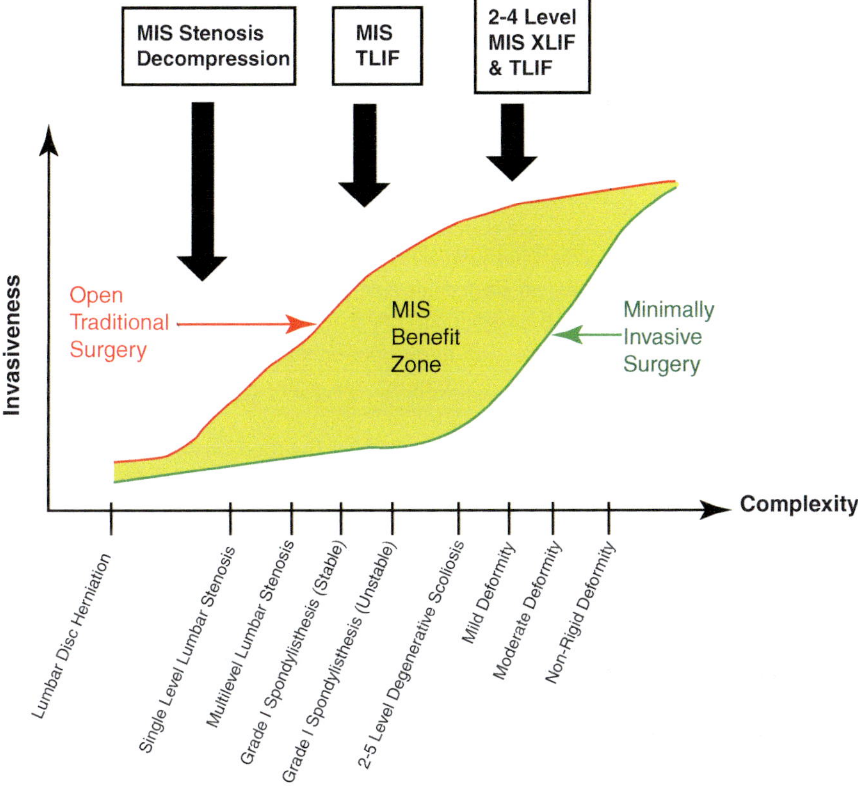

Fig. 33.1 Comparison between level of complexity and invasiveness in minimally invasive spine surgery versus open surgery [63]

Merits of Unilateral Biportal Endoscope (UBE)

Mayer divided the scope of MISS broadly into either an access technique or an access and target surgery [63]. Among the access and target spine surgery, tubular microscopic or endoscopic surgery, uniportal endoscopic surgery and biportal endoscopic surgery are the three common forms of MISS, of which the inherent differences are reviewed by Wu [64].

The lens and light sources in tubular microendoscopic surgery are outside the body far away from the target, whereas the lens and light source in endoscopic surgery is inside the body at the tip of the endoscope right at the target. Unlike microscope-assisted surgery, which requires hands-off time from handling instruments to achieve each view, endoscopic spine surgery allows mobility for real-time views without being time consuming. The magnification offered by endoscope may be adjusted by varying the distance of endoscope from the target. Zooming in close to the target can see the lesion in detail. Because of high resolution and zoom-in effect, control of micro-bleedings from bone or capillaries is possible. Both uniportal and biportal endoscopes give excellent magnification, clear visualization with constant fluid irrigation and significant more reliable identification of anatomic structures with high-definition digital camera compared to microscopic view in tubular assisted spine surgery [65].

The basic medium for tubular microendoscopic surgery is air; frequent suction and use of bipolar and monopolar diathermy are required for haemostasis and water irrigation for the clearance of operating field. The basic medium for endoscope is water, which can make a clean operative field via washout of blood and bone dust. Constant fluid irrigation plays an important role in reducing the risk of infection. Indeed, the infection rate of UBE spinal surgery is very low. A review of 14 studies reported no instance of spinal infection in 648 patients after UBE for lumbar spinal stenosis [66]. Of UBE TLIF, only one infection was reported among 290 patients of 8 series [67–74].

UBE gives a wide area of vision. Visualization of the tip of instrument in uniportal full endoscopic surgery is by rotating the endoscope, whereas UBE gives a boarder helicopter point of view when instruments are introduced from the working portal. UBE working portal allows the use of instruments of bigger size with less limitation of angle of instruments versus the limited angle of small instruments in the small-sized working channel in uniportal full endoscope. The floating relation between visual and working portal allows flexible instrument manipulation to target the pathology. Two smaller instruments can be at the same time through the working portal in UBE versus the "one-instrument-at-a-time technique" in uniportal full endoscopic spine surgery. Exchange of visual and working portal may be done if deemed necessary. Song et al. reported successful two cases of bilateral foraminal decompression via contralateral approach bilaterally without additional skin incision or surgical trajectory by switching the surgeon's position and primary two portals of UBE [75].

UBE may be viewed as an endoscope-assisted microsurgery, implying conversion of microsurgery into endoscopic surgery. The working portal of UBE may be one or even more than one (e.g. third portal for approximation of dural tear leaflets in endoscopic dural repair). The working portal can be maintained by a complete sheath, semi-tubular sheath of different size to accommodate small and large instruments or none. With a semi-tubular sheath, the soft and free part works as open surgery, and the rigid and retractor part acts as tubular surgery. The semi-tubular system has a big benefit, that is, there is no visual or motion limitation, so UBE can have the same indications as open surgery, but in a less or minimally invasive way.

In short, UBE has the advantages of excellent magnification and visualization for complete decompression of neural elements, very low infection rate related to water irrigation, less constraints of size and manoeuvrability of instruments and even exchange of visual and working portal. These all allow UBE to have different approaches and versatile indications in spinal surgery.

Versatile Indications

UBE has been successfully applied on various disorders. UBE posterior cervical foraminotomy (PCF) is indicated in patients with cervical radiculopathy due to foraminal stenosis with or without paracentral or foraminal cervical soft-tissue disc protrusion. Park JH et al. reported a case series of 13 patients with cervical foraminal soft-tissue disc protrusion who were successfully treated with UBE PCF discectomy with UBE technique [76]. Song KS and Lee reported the inclinatory cervical laminotomy using UBE techniques in seven patients with cervical foraminal stenosis with or without paracentral or foraminal disc protrusion to provide successful decompression as far as the distal part of foramen with better operative view and more easy manipulation [77]. The advantages of UBE over traditional PCF include wider operative view, easy identification of perineural fat on an axillar area of exiting root, more effective preservation of facet joint and dorsal portion of facet capsule by tunnel-shaped foraminotomy and unconstrained use of instruments [77]. UBE has also been attempted in treating cervical spondylotic myelopathy. Kim J et al. successfully performed neural decompression at C5–C6–C7 levels using biportal endoscopic unilateral laminotomy with bilateral decompression for the treatment of cervical spondylotic myelopathy [78]. However, the main applications of UBE are lumbar canal decompression for lumbar disc herniation or lumbar spinal stenosis and lumbar interbody fusion.

Indications of UBE lumbar discectomy include lumbar disc herniation [79, 80], recurrent disc herniation [81], high-grade migrated disc [82], bilateral or huge disc herniation [83] and far-lateral lumbar disc herniation [84]. Indications of UBE lumbar spine decompression include central lumbar spinal stenosis [66, 85, 86] and foraminal stenosis [87]. Extended indications include lumbar interbody fusion [67–74, 88, 89]. UBE techniques can also be applied to remove epidural space-occupying lesions, such as epidural abscess [90] and epidural lipomatosis [91]. The excellent visualization of operative field with UBE greatly facilitates decompression of neural elements. Kang MS et al. reported a series of 18 extremely elderly (aged ≥75) patients affected by lower lumbar delayed vertebral collapse with lumbosacral radiculopathy treated by posterior decompression assisted with UBE, combined with anterior column stabilization by vertebroplasty under epidural anaesthesia [92]. UBE-assisted neural decompression is also illustrated in two case reports, namely treatment in an unexpected complication after minimally invasive TLIF [93] and endoscopic guided transcorporeal vertebroplasty for traumatic L5 incomplete burst fracture [94].

UBE allows interlaminar or extraforaminal surgical approaches to spine. Interlaminar approach is used for lumbar discectomy or lumbar canal decompression. Extraforaminal approach is used for foraminal lesions or stenosis [87, 95, 96], particularly at L5/S1 and far-lateral disc herniation [84, 97] and far-lateral facet cyst [98].

For endoscopic lumbar discectomy, transforaminal or interlaminar approach does not give any difference in lumbar disc herniation recurrence, hospital stay, ODI scores, VAS scores, Japanese Orthopaedic Association (JOA) scores and MacNab criteria at the final follow-up in a meta-analysis [12]. IELD is generally favoured in high-grade migrated disc [82], calcified disc herniation and associated central stenosis. Even for less experienced surgeons, IELD obtains satisfactory results for high migrated disc [99]. Biportal IELD gains popularity over uniportal TELD in managing disc herniation at L5/S1. Transforaminal approach to L5/S1 is limited by high iliac crest, hypertrophy of L5/S1 facet and naturally narrower L5/S1 foramen. A meta-analysis revealed that both IELD and TELD have comparable clinical efficacy and safety, but IELD is significantly associated with shorter fluoroscopy time and operative time, but a higher dural tear rate than TELD [19]. Foraminoplasty is required in all cases in high iliac crest cases when the iliac crest is above the mid-L5 pedicle on lateral radiography [100]. IELD is preferred for axillary disc herniation and downward migrated disc, especially high-grade migration [101].

A multicentre, retrospective study of 141 patients who underwent single-level discectomy showed that both UBE and open microsurgery for lumbar discectomy yielded similar clinical results, including pain control, functional disability, patient satisfaction, complications and rate of surgical conversion [80]. In that study, UBE had less estimated blood loss and shorter length of hospital stay but had a significant longer operative time than open microsurgery [80]. Among endoscopic discectomy, based on perioperative change of creatine phosphokinase (CK) and C-reaction protein (CRP) levels, TELD is the least invasive technique, followed by uniportal IELD and biportal IELD [102]. Although UBE IELD is more invasive than uniportal TELD in terms of perioperative change of CK and CRP levels, the changes of multifidus muscle injury and atrophy on MRI after UBE show a tendency to reverse within several months [103]. On the other hand, the duration and level of radiation exposure are the highest in TELD, less in biportal IELD and least in microendoscopic discectomy; the difference between the groups is highly significant [104]. It seems that the less of invasiveness in discectomy, the greater the exposure to radiation.

For lumbar spinal stenosis, UBE is a viable alternative to microscopic technique with similar operative time, clinical outcomes and complications, as concluded in two meta-analyses [105, 106]. Heo DH et al. reported that functional outcomes (VAS score for back pain and leg pain ODI score) at the final follow-up were similar among tubular microsurgery and unipolar or bipolar endoscopy, but UBE achieved significantly more dural expansion and lower angle of facetectomy than uniportal endoscopy in lumbar decompression in a retrospective comparative study [107]. Another retrospective comparative study showed that UBE ULBD was associated with significantly less VAS at back at 2 months than microscopic ULBD [108]. UBE ULBD had advantages over microendoscopic ULBD in terms of postoperative segmental instability, pain control and serum CK and CRP in another retrospective study [109]. Two PRCT showed similar outcomes as microscopic surgery, but UBE decompression resulted in rapid pain recovery, less pain, lower fentanyl usage and early discharge in symptomatic lumbar spine stenosis [110, 111]. Another PRCT showed statistically superior clinical outcomes post-operatively up to 2-year follow-up in ODI score, Zurich Claudication Questionnaire and percentage of excellent results according to modified MacNab criteria in UBE compared to tubular micro-endoscopy for single-level degenerative lumbar spinals stenosis [112]. UBE has advantages over uniportal endoscopy in decompression for lumbar foraminal stenosis, with less risk of injury to the existing nerve root, a wider working space and exposure not limited by the hypertrophied sacral ala in far-lateral stenosis at L5/S1 [113].

UBE may be more favourable than other MISS ULBD in facet preservation in the treatment of spinal stenosis and less risk of post-operative segmental instability. Stenotic dural areas were significantly expanded in all three minimally invasive ULBD (microscopy, uniportal endoscopy or UBE), but UBE had significant higher mean dural expansion and significant lower mean angle of facetectomy than uniportal endoscopy and microendoscopy for lumbar central stenosis in a retrospective study [107]. The facet joint preservation by UBE ULBD was 84.2% on the approach side and 92.9% on the contralateral side in a series of 81 patients with lumbar spinal stenosis (12 had associated spondylolisthesis) [114]. Another retrospective analysis revealed a significantly lower bone resection area in 3D CT scan (1 cm^2 vs. 1.5 cm^2) and higher facet preservation rate (86% vs. 78% on the approach side and 85% vs. 94% on the contralateral side) for UBE compared to microendoscopic technique [115]. Compared with conventional microscopic ULBD, the percentage of change in preoperative and post-operative horizontal displacement of the operated level on standing flexion/extension was significantly less in UBE group (0.28% vs. 2.92%) [109].

In lumbar spinal stenosis with significant and symptomatic unilateral radiculopathy, decompression of lateral recess or foraminal stenosis preferably via the contralateral side is well documented in tubular microscopic decompression [116] or uniportal endoscopic decompression [117]. Similarly, through the interlaminar window, contralateral approach may be used in UBE for decompression of contralateral lesions. The contralateral approach enables better preservation of facet joint in dealing with lesions in lateral recess or foraminal zone. Park JH et al. reported contralateral keyhole UBE surgery for ruptured lumbar disc in 27 patients with only a 4.9% reduction rate of facet joint plane [118]. The authors listed suitable indications of contralateral keyhole biportal endoscopic surgery as down-migrated ruptured disc on paracentral and foraminal area, and upper lumbar levels with more vulnerable facet joint from ipsilateral laminectomy [118]. Two reports on 23 patients with lumbar facet cyst demonstrated the feasibility of treatment with a contralateral sublaminar approach using UBE to minimize iatrogenic facet violation and trauma to posterior muscular and ligamentous structures [119, 120]. UBE decompression via a contralateral approach is particularly useful in asymmetric spinal stenosis [121]. For lateral stenosis arising from narrowed foramen or ruptured disc on the concave side of degenerative scoliosis, vertebral rotation and lateral deviation of ipsilateral spinous process, ossification of interspinous ligament, facet hypertrophy and overhanging all contribute to the severe restriction on viewing and accessing the pathological site. Contralateral approach provides a wider access and wider arc of motion.

Decompression is achieved via leverage on the normal side of facet joint, instead of working over an inverted facet edge with difficult docking. The trajectory allows undercutting of superior articular process with more facet joint preserved on the pathological site. In contralateral approach, paraspinal muscles and medial branch of dorsal rami supplying the multifidus muscles are relatively spared. Preservation of paraspinal muscles and facet joints on the pathological side is crucial in non-fusion minimally invasive lumbar spine decompression. Decompression of spinal stenosis at two levels (lateral recess and cranial level foraminal compression) is feasible via a single interlaminar window using a contralateral approach [122].

Common indications for UBE extraforaminal lumbar interbody fusion are (1) grade 1 or 2 degenerative or isthmic spondylolisthesis, (2) recurrent disc herniation or (3) central or foraminal stenosis with instability. Over 200 cases of biportal endoscopic lumbar interbody fusion have been published since 2017 [123]. The overall complications ranged from 4.3% to 14.3%. Incidental durotomy rate was 3.3%. The radiographic fusion rate at 1 year ranged from 78% to 91%. UBE TLIF has favourable clinical outcomes and fusion rate but significantly less intraoperative blood loss, reduced immediate post-operative back pain, reduced hospital stay and time to ambulation compared to minimally invasive TLIF [123]. UBE TLIF allows better endplate preparation under endoscopic guidance, large volume of fusion material (autograft, demineralized bone matrix), release of medial part of contralateral facet and large-sized cage for disc space distraction and reduction of spondylolisthesis in restoring segmental lordosis [124]. At L4/5 and L5/S1 levels where the disc length between the lateral border of dura and the existing nerve is 16 mm or larger, a large oblique lumbar interbody fusion (OLIF) cage may be inserted during UBE TLIF [89]. However, the UBI TLIF is more difficult to perform with a longer operation time [123, 124].

In summary, UBE is a good alternative to other MISS in the management of lumbar spine disorders. Among the tubular microsurgery, uniportal endoscopy and biportal endoscopy, clinical outcomes after UBE are not inferior to other types of MISS.

Favourable Learning Curve

UBE has a relatively short learning period, wherein the learner can master the skills or tasks in a relatively short time. UBE has merits over uniportal technique; it allows a wider range of view with free handling of basic instruments available in open spine surgery. For those with experience in open spine surgery, the overall technical performance may not be too difficult. UBE technique should be familiar to many orthopaedic surgeons who already master the joint arthroscopic techniques. UBE has the least number of cases to achieve a maximal level of performance (asymptote) in lumbar discectomy. The asymptote was 14 by UBE discectomy [81], 25–30 by tubular microendoscopic discectomy [125, 126] and 33 by TELD [127]. For L5/S1 interlaminar discectomy, proficiency can be reached reasonably fast [128], and the case number cut-off for proficiency was 18 in uniportal percutaneous endoscopic discectomy, compared with 10 in open microscopic discectomy [129]. The learning curve for uniportal transforaminal endoscopic discectomy is quite conflicting between different studies. One study reported that it took 60–80 cases to achieve a constant and close-to-average operative time, 60 cases for a confident identification of the exiting and traversing nerve roots and 80 cases for a proper foraminoplasty [130]. Another study reported that a steady operation time was reached by 35 cases [131].

The learning curve of UBE for lumbar decompression is comparable to that of other MISS. The operative time plateaued following 50 cases [132], and the intraoperative blood loss stabilized after the first 30 cases [133] in microendoscopic decompression surgery for lumbar spinal stenosis. The learning curve cumulative summation test signalled competency for UBE decompressive laminectomy at the 58th case [134]. It took 100 cases for the operative time to reach a plateau by percutaneous uniportal endoscopic decompression [135].

For minimally invasive TLIF, the number of cases required to achieve the proficiency of operative time was reported as 14, 15, 30 and 44 in different studies [136–139]. Higher complication rate occurred in the early cases. The overall complication rate was 12.67% but can reach 33% in the initial 12 cases before 50% learning milestone [140]. In another retrospective study, complication rate plateaued after 43 cases with 18.6% in the first 43 cases dropped to 3.9% in the latter 76 cases [141]. For UBE TLIF, it required approximately 34 cases to reach stable operative time and an adequate performance level [142].

Start-Up of UBE Practice

Wu PH proposed an octagonal model of considerations in the set-up of an equipment-based surgical practice [143]. He listed eight factors to consider in setting up a sustainable endoscopic spine surgery practice: (1) surgical expertise; (2) continuing medical education; (3) anaesthetic expertise; (4) administrative and nursing support; (5) cost of equipment; (6) support for provision and maintenance of endoscopic equipment; (7) patients' need, concerns and expectation; and (8) post-operative care service.

Before the set-up of practice, attaining surgical expertise and overcoming the learning curve of UBE are the first and most important. From the surgical perspective, at least two surgeons with interest in UBE spine surgery working together are better than solo practice. It is always better to have backup. To prepare the introduction of MISS to my department in a public hospital, several surgeons interested in MISS were sponsored to attend spine workshops including the Asian Academy of Minimally Invasive Spine Surgery Course in Pune, AO Davos Spine Course, AOSpine Advanced Specimen Course in Muttenz, RIWOspine Endoscopic Course, International MISS Course by Wooridul Hospital and hands-on workshop organized by the Korean Neurosurgical Society. Overseas observation/attachment to MISS experts included Sebastian Ruetten of St. Anna Hospital, Germany; William Smith of Western Regional Brain and Spine Centre, USA; Muneto Yoshida of Wakayama University Hospital and Fujio Ito of Aichi Hospital, Japan; Jin-Sung Kim of Seoul St. Mary's Hospital; and Cheul-Woong Park of Daejeon Woori Hospital, Korea. One staff surgeon completed a 1-year spine fellowship in Australia and received a corporate scholarship in MISS from the Hospital Authority, Hong Kong. Three staffs were awarded short-term AOSpine Asia Pacific fellowship to attach spine centres in Asia Pacific region. Of course, the best is to have a proctor with considerable experience and reputation in the field to provide training and supervision in the initial cases. This was not feasible as our department is one of the early adopters of UBE in our local orthopaedic fraternity. Although UBE spine surgery can be done without assistant, our practice is to have surgeons work in pairs or together, rather than solo practice with trainees. Each serves alternatively as chief surgeon and assistant to assess the skills and to provide feedback to each other (reciprocal proctoring). To learn and teach may be the best way to attain surgical proficiency in a relatively short time. It should be noted that learning curve and training needs apply not only for the surgeon, but also for the whole clinical team including anaesthetists, operative theatre nurses and ward nurses.

Anaesthetist support is particularly important for MISS. Local anaesthesia and epidural anaesthesia allow rapid recovery after surgery and same-day discharge in selected cases. Moderate sedation is the best depth of sedation for MISS as the patient responds purposefully to verbal commands and to irritation of endoscopy instrument to neural tissue before the actual neural injury, while spontaneous ventilation and no intervention are required to maintain a patent airway. Awake lumbar endoscopic discectomy was achieved in the setting of COVID-19 with same-day discharge and no intraoperative complications or readmission [143]. Awake TLIF without general endotracheal anaesthesia under conscious sedation, long-acting local analgesia, endoscopic visualization, an expandable interbody device, recombinant human bone morphogenetic protein and percutaneous instrumentation were technically and clinically feasible [144]. Combination of conscious sedation epidural anaesthesia with half-diluted local anaesthetics under fluoroscopic guidance and monitoring of capnogram is a safe and feasible anaesthesia for patients with all ages and an ASA class III or less undergoing lumbar spine surgery less than 4 h in procedural length [145]. The procedures done include endoscopic decompression, open decompression and open posterior spinal fusion. Awake spine surgeries reported in the literature include lumbar spinal decompression, anterior cervical discectomy and fusion, lumbar fusion and dorsal column stimulator placement [146]. It provides live neural feedback during surgery and reduces the side effects associated with general anaesthesia. The use of awake MISS is an option for patients who are otherwise not eligible for general anaesthesia.

Evidence-based information on MISS and UBE spine surgery, particularly the clinical effectiveness and patient safety, should be promulgated. Besides preparing the surgical team, support from colleagues (even surgeons not performing the operation) and prior approval from hospital administration are needed. Introduction of innovative or new procedures may require approval from the relevant clinical governance body for planning and adoption. The Safe Introduction of New Procedures/Technology (HAMSINP) in Hong Kong, New Interventions and Procedures Advisory Group (NIPAG) in the UK and Australian Safety and Efficacy Register of New Interventional Procedures are some examples. The reasons of introduction, intended benefits, potential impact over existing practice, risk assessment and possible complications, summary of supporting evidence and implementation issues and quality control (particularly patient safety) should be delineated. Credentialing is a good way to gain confidence from the hospital administration and other stakeholders including orthopaedic surgeons and patients.

The cost of equipment and instrument delivery are important implementation issues. The cost recovery depends on surgical volume minus the costs of maintenance and updates. Fortunately, the cost needed to start biportal endoscopic surgery is lower than that of uniportal endoscopic spine surgery [143]. Uniportal endoscopic spine surgery requires specific endoscopes and dedicated instruments in each type of endoscopic approach, whereas many of the UBE spine surgery instruments may be adopted from instruments already used and available in other orthopaedic subspecialty; for example, joint arthroscopic surgery and open spine surgery, 4 mm 30° large joint arthroscope and camera system, radiofrequency energy system and water pressure system from arthroscopic surgery may be used. Many conventional open spine instruments, such as Kerrison rongeur, curette and pituitary forceps, can be used. Other than that, there are little specialized instruments; 0° arthroscope is specific for UBE visualization. On the other hand, 30° arthroscope may be favoured in L5/S1 foraminal decompression and severe lumbar stenosis decompression. Extraforaminal approach using UBE with a 30° arthroscope allows a better view of working space on the transverse process and inner and distal area of pedicle for optimal subpedicular decompression at the junction of transverse process and pedicle [87]. The 30° arthroscope offers a wider view by rotation of scope, and the ablated extent of lamina may be less in the decompression of severe spinal stenosis [147]. The conventional arthroscopic radiofrequency energy system may be used in the initial working portal at multifidus triangle on the surface of lamina between multifidus and interspinales lumborum. A low-energy radiofrequency ablator is strongly recommended for haemostasis in the true working epidural space to minimize thermal injury to neural tissues. Serial dilator, muscle detacher, specially designed angled curettes, rotatory Kerrison rongeur, angled osteotome and curved chisels are helpful gadgets for smooth surgery. Other specialized instruments specific to UBE include scope retractor for dural protection and endoscopic knot pusher for dural repair [148].

Spine surgery is a high-cost surgery. The initial set-up cost of MISS is high, and there are consumables and replacement or repair of broken endoscope or instruments. For example, the average operative cost of uniportal endoscopic TELD was about US $1430 per case, including $1067 for disposable bipolar forceps and single-use drill bar and $362 for the cost of equipment breakage per case, sharing for 295 cases in Japan [149]. From the hospital administration prospective, besides clinical effectiveness, cost-effectiveness is another implementation issue to consider. Cost-effectiveness depends on whether the upfront cost of instrument, longer initial operative time and steep learning curve may be offset by lower complication rate or reoperation rate, shorter hospital stay and more rapid return to work. Studies showed that endoscopic discectomy was associated with cost saving compared with conventional microdiscectomy [150], and tubular microdiscectomy [151] but tubular endoscopic multilevel laminectomy [152] were not associated with cost saving compared with equivalent open spine surgery. However, minimally invasive lumbar decompression may theoretically mitigate the risk of iatrogenic instability and adjacent segment disease in the long term. Meta-analysis showed that minimally invasive TLIF is associated with significant reduced hospital cost compared to open TLIF [153]. This may be explained by the fact that minimally invasive TLIF is associated with lower medical complication rate, though with a similar rate of surgical complications compared with open posterior lumbar fusion [154]. The cost saving is related to the shorter hospital stay, reduced blood loss, fewer complications and increased health-related quality of life (HRQOL) compensated for potential higher upfront cost of MISS implants and surgery equipment for one- or two-level lumbar spinal fusion [155].

Patient preoperative expectation has a high impact on patient satisfaction and patient-reported outcomes after spine surgery. High preoperative expectations appear to be associated with higher satisfaction and patient-reported outcomes for lumbar disc herniation, but not for lumbar spinal stenosis [156]. Patient expectations frequently exceed the actual outcome, creating an expectation-actuality discrepancy, and a larger expectation-actuality discrepancy portends lower satisfaction [156]. Such expectation-actuality discrepancies are often magnified by some biased or invalid information on the internet or social media and the eye-catching media coverage of successful cases in the application of advanced technology leading to higher patient expectation and sometimes unrealistic patient expectation. This is particularly valid in minimally invasive spine surgery. The patient may misinterpret that minimally invasive surgery is an equivalent to smaller skin incision, less pain and fewer complications. Furthermore, wide discrepancies between the patient and surgeon regarding the expected result of spine surgery were documented, and patients consistently had higher expectations than the surgeons, especially for back or neck pain and function [157]. The more the amount of improvement expected preoperatively and the more preoperative expectations, the lower the proportion of expectation fulfilled [158]. Fulfilment of expectations is an important outcome of spine surgery. Patient expectations have to be considered. Unrealistic expectations have to be addressed before making a final decision for surgery. Shared decision and alignment of realistic expectations prior to surgery are as important as the explanation of association between spinal problem and neurological deficit and the expected improvement in pain and function after surgery.

It would be best if MISS can be incorporated as part of the ERAS programme, which is a multimodal, multidisciplinary approach to optimize the post-operative recovery process through preoperative, perioperative and post-operative interventions [159]. Optimization of preoperative medical conditions, e.g. body weight control, smoking cessation, anaemia correction (oral or intravenous iron supplementation), stabilization of blood sugar, screening and correction of vitamin

D insufficiency and enhancement of bone mineral density, nutritional enhancement calls support from medical colleagues, nurses and dietitians. Multidisciplinary protocol for preoperative, intraoperative and post-operative workup and care can improve patient outcomes while reducing complications, cost and hospital stay [160]. Preoperative patient education programme and alignment of patient expectation by the surgeon and nursing team enhance the surgical experience and patient satisfaction. The use of tranexamic acid helps to reduce blood loss [161]. Perioperative multimodal analgesia and MIS reduce the pain experience and facilitate early mobilization and rapid rehabilitation and likely early discharge and better cost-effectiveness. Post-operative early mobilization, deep-breathing diaphragm mobilization exercise, incentive spirometry use (ten times per hour while awake) [162] and optimal glycaemic control (7.7–11.1 mmol/L) contribute to the prevention of post-operative complications. Studies demonstrated that ERAS protocols do accelerate return of function, minimize post-operative pain, reduce length of stay and ensure cost saving in spine surgery [163]. The benefits of ERAS are also evident in two longitudinal cohort comparative studies after implementation of ERAS in minimally invasive TLIF [164, 165]. Another study compared UBE TLIF with ERAS with microscopic TLIF without ERAS [69]. UBE TLIF group had significantly lower estimated blood loss and lower post-operative back pain on days 1 and 2 with similar fusion rate [69].

Monitoring of Own Learning Curve

The knowledge and judgement of MIS spine surgery are more easily acquired through clinical meetings or spine courses or workshops. In a global survey of endoscopic spine surgeons, the main sources of knowledge were learning in small meetings (57.3%), attending workshops (63.1%), and national and international conferences (59.8%) [166]. Didactic lectures provide evidence-based information and theoretical basis in disease-based approach more often than technology-driven approach. The dexterity involved is more difficult to master. The limited access and unfamiliar orientation of operative field, the use of microsurgical instruments and a limited ability of the tutor to assist in the small surgical field all are significant obstacles in the learning of dexterity skills related to MIS. Surgical skill workshops, particularly cadaver workshops, and short-term fellowship or observership are useful. Attending workshops, both simulation based and cadaver based, helps early orientation of MISS. Friends and colleagues who have incorporated MISS into practice seem to be the best teachers in guidance through the learning curve.

Learning curve is the correlation between a surgeon's performance on a new procedure and the number of attempts of time required to complete the task. This can be represented by a graph of the performance against the learning efforts (or number of attempts). In MISS, learning curve is usually measured by the surgical time and occurrence of complications against the chronological case numbers [167]. Falavigna et al. listed many variables that may be used to assess the dexterity during the MIS spine surgery training [168]. These include operative time, established blood loss, operative complications, need for conversion to open approach, duration of intraoperative X-ray use, length of hospital stay, radiological outcomes such as adequate decompression and fusion rate, and clinical and neurological outcomes. In this list, I would suggest that we may use the volume of irrigation fluid used in the UBE as another assessment parameter. Without prospective auditing or objective evaluation, one may overlook one's incompetence and deficit.

The duration of learning curve is much affected by the prior surgical experience and skills. Experienced spine surgeon in open surgery has good knowledge on the anatomy and spine pathology and good judgement on the rationale for spine surgery, which are the basic principles of open spine surgery and MISS as well. Furthermore, there are occasions when MISS may have to convert to open surgical should difficulties or complications arise. So it would seem that an experienced spine surgeon in open surgery may be more ready to pick up MISS. On the other hand, high productivity and proficiency in open surgery may be negative impact factors on the establishment of MISS. There is not only the time and effort in learning new surgical skills, but also longer operative time and higher complication in the initial learning curve. Replacing traditional time-proven open spinal surgeries with endoscopic spinal surgeries may put the surgeons' reputation at risk and have an additional negative impact on his/her practice due to reduced revenue [169]. The mentorship and proctorship approach is useful in helping traditionally trained spine surgeons to integrate endoscopic spine surgery into their well-established practice, a significant improved outcome after 15 cases of endoscopic lumbar decompression [169]. Under the close guidance of an endoscopic master spine surgeon, the endoscopic learning curve may be comprehended by the experienced traditionally trained spine surgeon in approximately 15 lumbar decompression cases. During this initial 15-case learning curve, clinical outcomes with endoscopy may be slightly inferior to open laminectomy but may ultimately improve to equivalent levels. Ransom NA et al. suggested employing diagnostic prognosticators and practising selective blocks, discogram and epidurograms when barriers of surgical skills are overcome and then proceed to lumbar spine endoscopy from simple to more complex cases [169].

UBE spine surgery may be regarded as a form of arthroscopic assisted MISS. Arthroscopic surgery requires hand-eye coordination, triangulation and ability to work in three dimensions, guided by two-dimensional visual information. Structured training programme, e.g. Fundamentals of Arthroscopic Surgery Training (FAST), and arthroscopic skill assessment tool, e.g. Arthroscopic Surgical Skill Evaluation Tool (ASSET) [170–172], have been practised in joint arthroscopy surgery. Stimulation training programme improves arthroscopic skills significantly [173, 174], particularly in arthroscopic probing and triangulation skills with significantly decreased task completion times and increased efficiency of movement [175]. Previous training and experience in arthroscopic surgery would be an advantage. It would be beneficial for a spine surgeon to learn also arthroscopic surgery in knee and shoulder during their trainee or junior specialist stage to prepare for MISS.

Training on cadaver or stimulators may be the best learning strategy of dexterity in MIS spine surgery. The use of high-fidelity spine simulators for MIS spine surgery has been incorporated in AOSpine Davos course since 2016. Although the utilization of virtual reality (VR) technology in surgical training is less than 10 years, VR-based simulators prove their success in assessing and training surgical skills in spine surgery. VR simulators have been used in pedicle screw placement, vertebroplasty, posterior cervical laminectomy and foraminotomy, lumbar puncture, facet joint infection and spinal needle insertion and placement [176]. VR simulators routinely outperformed traditional methods of training for MIS spine surgery including pedicle screw insertion. Surgical simulator has been used to improve clinical results in early follow-up for both vertebroplasty and percutaneous endoscopic lumbar discectomy with reported patient outcome measures [177].

Self-direction and reflection are the keys of lifetime continuous learning. It is of paramount importance for the surgeon to monitor his/her own learning curve and so to adjust the progression of the complexity of MISS without scarifying the safety within the constraint of resources (e.g. operation theatre time). The monitoring of learning curve enables selection of cases matching the ladder of progression of endoscopic surgery. An endoscopic ladder of competence progression model based on interaction with neural elements and handling of endoscopic equipment, soft-tissue dissection and bony decompression, presence of vascular structures, low tolerance of neutral retraction and devices to be inserted in addition to decompression was proposed [64]. Primary ladder cases include transforaminal endoscopic lumbar discectomy, interlaminar endoscopic lumbar discectomy and left-sided UBE for right-handed surgeon. For right-handed surgeon, left-side L4/5 UBE surgery is a good start for the first few cases. The secondary ladder cases include bilateral decompression for lumbar spinal stenosis, discectomy of highly migrated prolapsed intervertebral disc, extraforaminal/posterolateral approach and right-sided UBE surgery for right-handed surgeon. Tertiary ladder cases include operation in cervical or thoracic level and revision cases. Quaternary ladder cases include interbody fusion, revision interbody fusion, anterior endoscopic cervical decompression with total disc replacement and/or cage, and interlaminar contralateral endoscopic lumbar foraminotomy. UBE TLIF requires endplate preparation, and cage insertion via a narrow endoscopic channel constitutes the quaternary ladder. An informal outcome tracking helps in the counselling of patients and shared decision for surgery. A formal monitoring or audits of the outcomes and complications in the initial 20–50 cases are needed to fulfil the demand of clinical governance from various levels (clinical department, hospital administration, local healthcare authorities).

Stay Away from Troubles

Limited operative view, limited working space, lack of depth perception and hand-eye dissociation all make MISS difficult. Learning curve is associated with an increased complication rate. A complication rate of 10.3% (7/68) was reported in the early learning of UBE spine surgery [81]. Dural and root injuries and post-operative epidural haematoma occurred as complications with this new technique. Later series showed a lower complication rate of 6–7%. A systematic review of 556 patients in 11 studies of UBE lumbar decompression revealed a mean overall complication rate of 6.7% (0–13.8%) and an average of 84.3% satisfaction outcomes based on MacNab criteria [178]. In another review of 648 patients in 14 studies of interlaminar decompression, transforaminal decompression and interbody fusion through UBE technique in the PubMed database, complications occurred in 39 cases (6.0%), with 20 cases of dural tear [66]. Post-operative headache occurred in three cases, post-operative haematoma in five, root injury in four, transient paraesthesia in two and post-operative incomplete decompression in four. One case of iatrogenic hydroperitoneum occurred in the retroperitoneal space filled with water after the ventral approach to the psoas muscle during transforaminal decompression [66]. A pooled analysis of unsuccessful outcomes after UBE revealed a patient dissatisfaction rate of 10.3%, contributed by incomplete decompression, post-operative instability, haematoma, ascites, incidental durotomy and local recurrence among 797 patients who underwent UBE surgery [179]. The incidence of haematoma, incomplete operation and incidental durotomy was significantly higher in the first 50 cases than that in later cases [179]. Post-operative instability may result from excessive facetectomy or excision of superior articular process. Ascites may result from inadvertent penetration of psoas muscle with infusion of saline leading to hydro-peritoneum.

Avoiding Complications

Avoiding complications through awareness and anticipation of complications should be the best means of managing complications whenever possible. Patient selection is the key. Select cases' complexity is commensurate with own competence. The complexity of discectomy varies with the location of disc herniation (paracentral, central, foraminal, extent of disc migration), hardness of the disc (soft or calcified) and degree of canal occupation by disc, presence/absence of discal cysts and recurrence status. Leg numbness symptoms last longer in central disc herniation than in paracentral and foraminal disc herniation after surgery [180]. Avoid centrally located disc herniation with high-canal compromised (>50%) or high-grade migrated disc (beyond the posterior marginal disc space) as the failure after endoscopic discectomy from remnant fragments is significantly higher [181]. Recurrent disc herniation after previous open discectomy is not a good case for UBE ILED. TELD is preferred for revision as there is usually no scarring in the translaminar route as in primary discectomy. Avoid conditions with less favourable outcomes after decompression for lumbar stenosis, e.g. loss of lumbar lordosis [182] and presence of degenerative scoliosis (particularly unstable ones with $\geq 3°$ in Cobb angle difference between the supine and standing positions) [183].

Tips and Pearls of UBE

- Prone position with a flexed lumbar spine opens up the interlaminar space. Watertight draping is used to prevent fluid soaking of the patient's body and the possible risk of hypothermia leading to coagulopathy.
- Correct placement of visual and working portal is important [64]. Fluoroscopic verification should be done at the beginning and at intraoperative intervals when orientation is uncertain. Too cephalad position would lead to excessive and unnecessary amount of bony decompression. Too caudal position would lead to inefficiency for working instruments to reach the cephalad ligamentum flavum attachment. Too lateral position would lead to excessive and unnecessary amount of ipsilateral facet dissection and difficulty in reaching the contralateral side. A more lateral entry point is required in patients with high BMI to visualize the contralateral side. The right side has a more caudal docking point than the left side for a right-handed surgeon to limit the amount of cephalad laminotomy for working instrument to gain access to the contralateral side.
- The scope portal is for inflow and working portal for outflow; the two portals may be interchangeable. Working space is a hydrostatic pressure cavity, and water flow is essential for clear visualization. The initial working space is created by triangulation at multifidus triangle on the surface of lamina between multifidus and interspinales lumborum. The true working space is the epidural space. UBE is the art of water flow. Always ensure a good outflow and maintain water pressure below 30 mmHg during surgery. Hong et al. suggested a lower water pressure between 2 and 23 mmHg [184]. Water pressure was significantly lower with rigid cannulation than that without cannulation [184]. Most of the oozing from bone and epidural space can be controlled with less than 25 mmHg hydrostatic pressure [85]. If pressure pump is not used, the hydrostatic pressure can be maintained at 22–29 mmHg when the saline bag is 30–40 cm higher than the portals. There is a linear correlation between the inflow pressure and the cervical epidural pressure [185]. Constant inflow of irrigation without proper outflow will cause fluid to accumulate in the confined spinal canal, which can lead to an increase in epidural hydrostatic pressure and subsequently over-increase in intracranial pressure. Increased irrigation pressure to control bleeding or prolong operative time may cause massive saline infusion, which may lead to rise in epidural pressure. This may result in headache, posterior neck pain and potential complications like seizure, cerebral oedema and neurological dysfunction. Although rare (0.02%), seizure was reported after percutaneous endoscopic lumbar discectomy [186, 187]. All four patients had complained of neck pain before the seizure event [186]. Occurrence of neck pain should be considered as a prodromal sign as neck pain correlates with a highly increased cervical epidural pressure [188]. Both the irrigation infusion pressure and the total volume of fluid may account for the seizure [187].

- Muscle bleeding can be controlled with radiofrequency ablation. Bone bleeding may be controlled with bone wax. Bone wax may not stick to bone surface easily under constant fluid irrigation. Bleeding control from edged bone or epidural small vessels can be done with push-rock method [81]. A piece of geofoam is inserted and packed under the lamina with a freer. A lump of bone wax is then rocked on it and smashed to compress the bleeding site. If the bleeding cannot be controlled with every effort, lowering of diastolic blood pressure to 90–100 mmHg might be helpful in some cases, but increasing the saline pressure is not recommended [81]. That can lead to increased intracranial pressure in the patient and might sometimes cause headache after recovery from anaesthesia or cause a delayed recovery from general anaesthesia with stiff posture or hyperventilation. Excessive pressure from the water pump may elevate epidural pressure and mask bleeding during infusion, which may lead to post-operative epidural haematoma after switching off the pump.
- Last bone work with burr or drill should be completed before complete removal of ligamentum flavum to reduce the risk of durotomy or neural tissue injury. Insufficient dissection of dorsal meningovertebral ligament linking the dorsal thecal sac to ligamentum flavum and lamina may be the main mechanism of dorsal dural injury [189]. Outer layer of ligamentum flavum may be removed by angled curettes. Inner layer of ligamentum flavum should be preserved until bone work is completed. Free mobilization of dural sac and nerve root and correlation of the removal fragments of herniated disc with the size measured on preoperative MRI at the end of discectomy minimize the chance of incomplete removal of herniated disc. For lumbar spinal stenosis, ligamentum flavum is removed until the traversing root is completely exposed. Adequate decompression is achieved when over-decompression is done 2–3 mm lateral from dura margin on disc level, freeing of traversing nerve root at the medial margin of pedicle on lateral recess level and freeing of epidural adhesion between ventral dural surface and dura including nerve root [190].
- The use of drain after MISS is controversial. Closed suction drainage was found to be unnecessary in a retrospective study [191] and another prospective randomized trial [192] in minimally invasive lumbar fusion surgery. In view of the higher incidence of post-operative spinal epidural haematoma after UBE surgery, it is our practice to routinely insert a low suction drain (Jackson-Pratt drain) after the operation.

Incidental Durotomy

Incidental durotomy is the most common intraoperative complication in decompressive surgery for lumbar spinal stenosis [193]. An incidence of 5% was reported from Sweden's National Quality Registry for Spine Surgery in open spine surgery [194]. The incidence ranges from 0.38% to 6% in minimally invasive TLIF [195]. An intraoperative incidence of 8.2% (27/330 patients) was reported in a retrospective series of endoscopic stenosis lumbar decompression [196]. An international survey revealed an incidence of 1.07% (689/64,470) with lumbar endoscopy by 93 surgeons in 21 countries [197]. The incidence of incidental durotomy was 4.1% (range: 2.9–5.8%) in a systematic review of six studies [178]. Two studies published after the systematic review reported an incidence of 3.1% (20/684) [66] and 13.2% (7/53) [189].

Long-term outcome after incidental durotomy was reported as unaffected in 64%, post-operative cerebral spinal fluid (CSF) fistula in 18%, severe radiculopathy with dysaesthesia in 12.4%, sensory loss in 3.4% and motor loss in 2.2% [197]. It should be noted that 45% of surveyed surgeons had no contingency plan and were looking for further training on how to manage the complication [197].

Watertight dural primary repair is crucial and very effective to prevent the development of pseudomeningocele or CSF leakage and should be done whenever possible. The current evidence does not support the use of sealant, which may reduce the rate of CSF leakage [198]. Fortunately, endoscopic surgery or MIS has lower CSF leakage rate compared with open surgery regardless of sealant use [198]. This may be due to the preservation of overlying back muscles and relatively small dead space left after MIS spine surgery. With watertight dural suturing, early mobilization and ambulation do not increase the risk of CSF leakage and associated complications, compared to flat bed rest for 24–48 h in a retrospective analysis [199] and randomized trial [200]. On the other hand, prolong bed rest may be associated with increased medical complications [201].

Unlike open surgery, suturing of dura via a narrow working channel is technically difficult and can be very challenging [202] even with knot pusher for watertight suturing of dura [148]. Suture-less non-penetrating titanium clips are already used in dural repair in open surgery, including MIS spine surgery [203]. Such clip instruments may be inserted through working portal for dural repair and sometimes may require an additional third portal for approximation of dura tear leaflets [204]. Fibrin glue, collagen matrix patch, autologous muscle or fat overlay may be used as alternatives. TachoSil [205] and Hemopatch [206] have been used successfully as dural sealants for incidental durotomy. Whenever direct repair or dural sealing is not possible during MISS, it should be converted to open surgery. Conversion to open repair was deemed necessary in 7.6% [197].

Park HJ et al. retrospectively analysed the 4.5% (29/643) incidental durotomy in UBE spine surgery [207]. Tears located in exiting nerve root (zone 1, 2 cases, 6.9%) were associated with curettage. Tears located in thecal sac (zone 2, 18 cases, 65.1%) were associated with the use of electric drill or pituitary forceps, predominantly occurred during a unilateral approach for bilateral decompression. Tears in traversing nerve root (zone 3, 9 cases, 31%) were associated with the use of Kerrison punch. A treatment algorithm according to anatomic location and size of dural tear was proposed. Dural tear <4 mm was observed with in-hospital monitoring with 24-h bed rest. Dural tear of 4–12 mm was treated with fibrin sealant patch application and in-hospital monitoring with 24-h bed rest. Dural tear >12 mm with regular margin in zone 2 or 3 was treated with non-penetrating titanium clip. Dural tear >12 mm with irregular margin was treated by primary suture after conversion to microsurgery. After repair of dural tear >12 mm, they proposed in-hospital observation >48 h with bed rest, and lumbar drainage was considered.

Post-operative Spinal Epidural Haematoma

Symptomatic post-operative spinal epidural haematoma (PSEH) can occur after lumbar spine surgery. The reported incidence of PSEH ranges from 0.37% (8/2183) [208] to 0.51% (47/9258) [209] after lumbar spine surgery in recent two observational studies. Lumbar PSEH usually presents with unbearable pain, paralysis and bladder dysfunction [208]. Delayed PSEH after 3 days may occur in 0.16% in posterior lumbar spinal surgery [209]. Intraoperative blood loss, prolonged surgical time, high blood pressure, use of non-steroidal anti-inflammatory drugs and concurrent bleeding factors are risk factors for PSEH [210].

There is evidence that clinical and morphometric PSEH occurs more frequently after UBE spine surgery. Compared with conventional spine surgery, the incidence of clinical PSEH requiring revision surgery was 8.4% (8/95) in UBE compared with 1.4% (2/142) in conventional surgery [211]. UBE had high incidence of morphometric PSEH than conventional spine surgery: 87.4% (83/95) vs. 74.6% (106/142) for MRI-positive PSEH and 52.6% (50/95) vs. 28.9% (41/142) for thecal cord compression more than a quarter [211].

PSEH after UBE lumbar decompression surgery was studied by Kim et al. [212–214]. The overall incidence of radiologic PSEH as detected on MRI was 23.1% (176/762) per level of lumbar decompression. The overall rate of symptomatic PSEH requiring evacuation was 1.5% (10/674). Perioperative risk factors included female sex, older age >70 years, preoperative anticoagulant medication, usage of intraoperative water infusion pump and surgery requiring more bone work (laminectomy or interbody fusion) [213]. A comparative study of 206 UBE lumbar decompression through interlaminar approach found that intraoperative use of gelatin-thrombin matrix sealant (Floseal) was associated with a significantly lower occurrence of radiologic PSEH (13.6% vs. 26.4%) and significantly higher satisfactory outcomes according to modified MacNab criteria (87.6% vs. 79.4%) compared with no intraoperative Floseal [214].

Conclusion

Adoption of UBE techniques and implementation into daily practice must be well planned and meticulously prepared. Knowledge and surgical expertise are essential, but service organization and administration are also important. Unilateral biportal endoscopic spine surgery is not without complications. Stringent patient selection, rigid surgical indications, well-executed surgical plan and contingency plan for complications are crucial to ensure optimal patient care.

Acknowledgement We would like to acknowledge the Indian Spine Journal and Dr. Louis Chang in granting the permission to use Fig. 2: Comparison Between Level of Complexity and Invasiveness in Minimally Invasive Surgery Versus Open Surgery by Louis Chang et al. Fundamentals of Minimally Invasive Surgery, published in Indian Spine Journal 2020;3:4–10.

References

1. Skovrlj B, Qureshi SA. Minimally invasive cervical spine surgery. J Neurosurg Sci. 2017;61(3):325–34. https://doi.org/10.23736/S0390-5616.16.03906-0.
2. Wewel JT, Godzik J, Uribe JS. The utilization of minimally invasive surgery techniques for the treatment of spinal deformity. J Spine Surg. 2019;5(Suppl 1):S84–90. https://doi.org/10.21037/jss.2019.04.22.
3. IndustryARC: Minimally Invasive Spine Surgery Market – Forecast (2021–2026). 2019. https://www.industryarc.com/Research/Minimally-Invasive-Spine-Surgery-Market-Research-501896.
4. Del Castillo-Calcaneo J, Navarro-Ramirez R, Gimenez-Gigon M, et al. Principles and fundamentals of minimally invasive spine surgery. World Neurosurg. 2018;119:465–71.
5. Kim HS, Wu PH, Raorane HD, et al. Generation change of practice in spinal surgery: can endoscopic spine surgery expand its indications to fill in the role of conventional open spine surgery in most of degenerative spinal diseases and disc herniation's: a study of 616 spinal cases 3 years. Neurol India. 2020;68(5):1157–65.
6. Jordon J, Konstantinou K, O'Dowd J. Herniated lumbar disc. BMJ Clin Evid. 2009;2009:1118.
7. Ruan W, Feng F, Liu Z, et al. Comparison of percutaneous endoscopic lumbar discectomy versus open lumbar microdiscectomy for lumbar disc herniation: a meta-analysis. Int J Surg. 2016;31:86–92. https://doi.org/10.1016/j.ijsu.2016.05.061.
8. Phan K, Xu J, Schultz K, et al. Full-endoscopic versus micro-endoscopic and open discectomy: a systematic review and meta-analysis of outcomes and complications. Clin Neurol Neurosurg. 2017;154:1–12. https://doi.org/10.1016/j.clineuro.2017.01.003.
9. Zhang B, Liu S, Liu J, et al. Transforaminal endoscopic discectomy versus conventional microdiscectomy for lumbar disc herniation: a systematic review and meta-analysis. J Orthop Surg Res. 2018;13(1):169. https://doi.org/10.1186/s13018-018-0868-0.
10. Liu X, Yuan S, Tian Y, et al. Comparison of percutaneous endoscopic transforaminal discectomy, microendoscopic discectomy and microdiscectomy for symptomatic lumbar disc herniation: minimum 2-year follow-up results. J Neurosurg Spine. 2018;28(3):317–25. https://doi.org/10.3171/2017.6.SPINE172.
11. Ahn SS, Kim SH, Kim DW. Comparison of outcomes of percutaneous endoscopic lumbar discectomy and open lumbar microdiscectomy for young adults: a retrospective matched cohort study. World Neurosurg. 2016;86:250–8. https://doi.org/10.1016/j.wneu.2015.09.047.
12. Huang Y, Yin J, Sun Z, et al. Percutaneous endoscopic lumbar discectomy for LDH via a transforaminal approach versus an interlaminar approach: a meta-analysis. Orthopade. 2020;49(4):338–49. https://doi.org/10.1007/s00132-019-03710-z.
13. Jensen RK, Jensen TS, Koes B, et al. Prevalence of lumbar spinal stenosis in general and clinical populations: a systematic review and meta-analysis. Eur Spine J. 2020;29:2143–63.
14. Johnsson KE, Rosen I, Uden A. The natural course of lumbar spinal stenosis. Clin Orthop Relat Res. 1992;1279:82–6.
15. Deyo RA, Mirza SK, Martin BI, et al. Trends, major medical complications, and charges associated with surgery for lumbar spinal stenosis in older adults. JAMA. 2010;303(13):1259–65. https://doi.org/10.1001/jama.2010.338.

16. Amundsen T, Weber H, Nordal HJ, et al. Lumbar spinal stenosis: conservative or surgical management?: a prospective 10-year study. Spine. 2000;25(11):1424–35. https://doi.org/10.1097/00007632-200006010-00016.
17. Ma H, Hai B, Yan M, et al. Evaluation of effectiveness of treatment strategies for degenerative lumbar spinal stenosis: a systematic review and network meta-analysis of clinical studies. World Neurosurg. 2021;152:95–106. https://doi.org/10.1016/j.wneu.2021.06.016.
18. Komp M, Hahn P, Oezdemir S, et al. Bilateral spinal decompression of lumbar central stenosis with the full-endoscopic interlaminar versus microsurgical laminotomy technique: a prospective, randomized, controlled study. Pain Physician. 2015;18(1):61–70.
19. Lee CH, Choi M, Ryu DS, et al. Efficacy and safety of full-endoscopic decompression via interlaminar approach for central or lateral recess spinal stenosis of the lumbar spine: a meta-analysis. Spine. 2018;43(24):1756–64. https://doi.org/10.1097/BRS.0000000000002708.
20. Scholler K, Alimi M, Cong GT, et al. Lumbar spinal stenosis associated with degenerative lumbar spondylolisthesis: a systematic review and meta-analysis of secondary fusion rates following open vs minimally invasive decompression. Neurosurgery. 2017;80(3):355–67. https://doi.org/10.1093/neuros/nyw091.
21. Wang M, Luo XJ, Ye YJ, et al. Does concomitant degenerative spondylolisthesis influence the outcome of decompression alone in degenerative lumbar spinal stenosis? A meta-analysis of comparative studies. World Neurosurg. 2019;123:226–38. https://doi.org/10.1016/j.wneu.2018.11.246.
22. Hammad A, Wirries A, Ardeshiri A, et al. Open versus minimally invasive TLIF: literature review and meta-analysis. J Orthop Surg Res. 2019;14(1):229. https://doi.org/10.1186/s13018-019-1266-y.
23. Wu RH, Fraser JF, Hartl R. Minimal access versus open transforaminal lumbar interbody fusion: meta-analysis of fusion rates. Spine. 2010;35(26):2273–81.
24. Tan JH, Liu G, Ng R, et al. Is MIS-TLIF superior to open TLIF in obese patients?: a systematic review and meta-analysis. Eur Spine J. 2018;27(8):1877–86. https://doi.org/10.1007/s00586-018-5630-0.
25. Kou Y, Chang J, Guan X, et al. Endoscopic lumbar interbody fusion and minimally invasive transforaminal lumbar interbody fusion for the treatment of lumbar degenerative diseases: a systematic review and meta-analysis. World Neurosurg. 2021;152:e652–368. https://doi.org/10.1016/j.wneu.2021.05.109.
26. Choi G, Pophale CS, Patel B, et al. Endoscopic spine surgery. J Korean Neurosurg Soc. 2017;60(5):485–97. https://doi.org/10.3340/jkns.2017.0203.0014.
27. Bouthors C, Benzakour A, Court C. Surgical treatment of thoracic disc herniation: an overview. Int Orthop. 2019;43(4):807–16. https://doi.org/10.1007/s00264-018-4224-0.
28. Sharma SB, Kim JS. A review of minimally invasive surgical techniques for the management of thoracic disc herniations. Neurospine. 2019;16(1):24–33. https://doi.org/10.14245/ns.1938014.007.
29. Osman SG, Schwartz JA, Marsolais EB. Arthroscopic discectomy and interbody fusion of the thoracic spine: a report of ipsilateral 2-portal approach. Int J Spine Surg. 2012;6:103–9. https://doi.org/10.1016/j.ijsp.2012.02.004.
30. Osman SG, Marsolais EB. Posterolateral arthroscopic discectomies of the thoracic and lumbar spine. Clin Orthop Relat Res. 1994;304:122–9.
31. Jho HD. Endoscopic transpedicular thoracic discectomy. J Neurosurg. 1999;91(2 Suppl):151–6.
32. Choi G, Munoz-Suarez D. Transforaminal endoscopic thoracic discectomy: technical review to prevent complications. Neurospine. 2020;17(Suppl 1):S58–65. https://doi.org/10.14245/ns.2040250.125.
33. Maduri R, Bobinski L, Duff JM. Minimally invasive anterior foraminotomy for cervical radiculopathy: how I do it. Acta Neurochir. 2020;162(3):679–83. https://doi.org/10.1007/s00701-019-04201-y.

34. Tzaan WC. Anterior percutaneous endoscopic cervical discectomy for cervical intervertebral disc herniation: outcome, complications, and technique. J Spinal Disord Tech. 2011;24(7):421–31. https://doi.org/10.1097/BSD.0b013e31820ef328.
35. Ahn Y, Keum HJ, Shin SH. Percutaneous endoscopic cervical discectomy versus anterior cervical discectomy and fusion: a comparative cohort study with a five-year follow-up. J Clin Med. 2020;9(2):371. https://doi.org/10.3390/jcm9020371.
36. Sahai N, Changoor S, Dun CJ, et al. Minimally invasive posterior cervical foraminotomy as an alternative to anterior cervical discectomy and fusion for unilateral cervical radiculopathy: a systematic review and meta-analysis. Spine. 2019;44(24):1731–9. https://doi.org/10.1097/BRS.0000000000003156.
37. Zhang Y, Ouyang Z, Wang W. Percutaneous endoscopic cervical foraminotomy as a new treatment for cervical radiculopathy: a systematic review and meta-analysis. Medicine. 2020;99(45):e22744. https://doi.org/10.1097/MD.0000000000022744.
38. McAnay SJ, Qureshi SA. Minimally invasive cervical foraminotomy. JBJS Essent Surg Tech. 2016;6(2):e23. https://doi.org/10.2106/JBJS.ST.16.00012.
39. Ren J, Li R, Zhu K, et al. Biomechanical comparison of percutaneous posterior endoscopic cervical discectomy and anterior cervical decompression and fusion on the treatment of cervical spondylotic radiculopathy. J Orthop Surg Res. 2019;14(1):71. https://doi.org/10.1186/s13018-019-1113-1.
40. Chen C, Yuchi CX, Gao Z, et al. Comparative analysis of the biomechanics of the adjacent segments after minimally invasive cervical surgeries versus anterior cervical discectomy and fusion: a finite element study. J Orthop Translat. 2020;23:107–12. https://doi.org/10.1016/j.jot.2020.03.006.
41. Yolcu YU, Helal A, Alexander AY, et al. Minimally invasive versus open surgery for degenerative spine disorders for elderly patients: experiences from a single institution. World Neurosurg. 2021;146:e1262–9. https://doi.org/10.1016/j.wneu.2020.11.145.
42. Manson N, Hubbe U, Pereira P. Are the outcomes of minimally invasive transforaminal/posterior lumbar fusion influenced by the patient's age or BMI? Clin Spine Surg. 2020;33(7):284–91. https://doi.org/10.1097/BSD.0000000000001019.
43. Avila MJ, Walter CM, Baaj AA. Outcomes and complications of minimally invasive surgery of the lumbar spine in the elderly. Cureus. 2016;8(3):e519. https://doi.org/10.7759/cureus.519.
44. Warhurst M, Hartman J, Granville M, et al. The role of minimally invasive spinal surgical procedures in the elderly patient: an analysis of 49 patients between 75 and 95 years of age. Cureus. 2020;12(3):e7180. https://doi.org/10.7759/cureus.7180.
45. Goyal A, Elminawy M, Kerezoudis P. Impact of obesity on outcomes following lumbar spine surgery: a systematic review and meta-analysis. Clin Neurol Neurosurg. 2019;177:27–36. https://doi.org/10.1016/j.clineuro.2018.12.012.
46. Fei Q, Li J, Lin J, et al. Risk factors for surgical site infection after spinal surgery: a meta-analysis. World Neurosurg. 2016;95:507–15. https://doi.org/10.1016/j.wneu.2015.05.059.
47. Park P, Upadhyaday C, Garton HJL. The impact of minimally invasive spine surgery on perioperative complications in overweight or obese patients. Neurosurgery. 2008;62(3):693–9.; discussion 693–9. https://doi.org/10.1227/01.neu.0000317318.33365.f1.
48. Hudak E, Perry MW. Outpatient minimally invasive spine surgery using endoscopy for the treatment of lumbar spinal stenosis among obese patients. J Orthop. 2015;12(3):156–9. https://doi.org/10.1016/j.jor.2015.01.007.
49. Othman YA, Alhammound A, Aldahamsheh O, et al. Minimally invasive spine lumbar surgery in obese patients: a systematic review and meta-analysis. HSS J. 2020;16(2):168–76. https://doi.org/10.1007/s11420-019-09735-6.
50. Wang T, Han C, Jiang H, et al. The effect of obesity on clinical outcomes after minimally invasive surgery of the spine: a systematic review and meta-analysis. World Neurosurg. 2018;110:e438–49. https://doi.org/10.1016/j.wneu.2017.11.010.

51. Guzman JZ, Iatridis JC, Skovrlj B, et al. Outcomes and complications of diabetes mellitus on patients undergoing degenerative lumbar spine surgery. Spine. 2014;39(19):1596–604. https://doi.org/10.1097/BRS.0000000000000482.
52. Guzman JZ, Skovrlj B, Shin J, et al. The impact of diabetes mellitus on patients undergoing degenerative cervical spine surgery. Spine. 2014;39(20):1656–65. https://doi.org/10.1097/BRS.0000000000000498.
53. Regev GJ, Lador R, Salame K, et al. Minimally invasive spinal decompression surgery in diabetic patients: perioperative risks, complications and clinical outcomes compared with non-diabetic patients' cohort. Eur Spine J. 2019;28(1):55–60. https://doi.org/10.1007/s00586-018-5716-8.
54. Senker W, Stefanits H, Gmeiner M, et al. The impact of type 2 diabetes on the peri- and postoperative outcomes of minimally invasive fusion techniques in the lumbar spine. J Neurosurg Sci. 2020;64(6):509–14. https://doi.org/10.23736/S0390-5616.18.04467-3.
55. Ho ST. Adverse effects of smoking on outcomes of orthopaedics. J Orthop Trauma Rehabil. 2017;23:54–8.
56. Senker W, Stefanits H, Gmeiner M, et al. The influence of smoking in minimally invasive spinal fusion surgery. Open Med. 2021;16(1):198–206. https://doi.org/10.1515/med-2021-0223.
57. Bray GA, Fruhbeck G, Ryan DH, et al. Management of obesity. Lancet. 2016;387(10031):1947–56. https://doi.org/10.1016/S0140-6736(16)00271-3.
58. Passias PG, Horn SR, Vasquez-Montes D, et al. Prior bariatric surgery lowers complication rates following spine surgery in obese patients. Acta Neurochir. 2018;160(12):2459–65. https://doi.org/10.1007/s00701-018-3722-6.
59. Han L, Han H, Wang L, et al. Prior bariatric surgery is associated with lower complications, in-hospital mortality, and healthcare utilization after elective spine fusion surgery. Surg Obes Relat Dis. 2020;16(6):760–7. https://doi.org/10.1016/j.soard.2019.12.027.
60. Duggan EW, Carlson K, Umpierrez GE. Perioperative hyperglycemia management: an update. Anesthesiology. 2017;126(3):547–60. https://doi.org/10.1097/ALN.0000000000001515.
61. Ho ST. Quit smoking before orthopaedic surgery. J Orthop Trauma Rehab. 2017;23:A1–3.
62. Chang L, Kirnaz S, Castillo-Calcaneo D, et al. Fundamentals of minimally invasive spine surgery. Indian Spine J. 2020;3:4–10. https://doi.org/10.4103/isj_31_19.
63. Mayer M, Mayer F. Fundamental concepts of minimally invasive spine surgery (MISS) and purpose to purse. J Minim Invasive Spine Surg Tech. 2017;2(1):1–6.
64. Wu PH, Kim HS, Choi DJ, et al. Overview of tips in overcoming learning curve in uniportal and biportal endoscopic spine surgery. J Minim Invasive Spine Surg Tech. 2021;6:S84–96. https://doi.org/10.21182/jimisst.2020.00024.
65. Burkhardt BW, Wilmes M, Sharif S, et al. The visualization of the surgical field in tubular assisted spine surgery: is there a difference between HD-endoscopy and microscopy? Clin Neurol Neurosurg. 2017;158:5–11. https://doi.org/10.1016/j.clineuro.2017.04.010.
66. Kim JE, Choi DJ, Park EJJ, et al. Biportal endoscopic spine surgery for lumbar spinal stenosis. Asian Spine J. 2019;13(2):334–42. https://doi.org/10.31616/asj.2018.0210.
67. Heo DH, Son SK, Eum JH, Park CK. Fully endoscopic lumbar interbody fusion using a percutaneous unilateral biportal endoscopic technique: technical note and preliminary clinical results. Neurosurg Focus. 2017;43(2):E8. https://doi.org/10.3171/2017.5.FOCUS17146.
68. Kim JE, Choi DJ. Biportal endoscopic transforaminal lumbar interbody fusion with arthroscopy. Clin Orthop Surg. 2018;10(2):248–52. https://doi.org/10.4055/cios.2018.10.2.248.
69. Hoe DH, Park CK. Clinical results of percutaneous biportal endoscopic lumbar interbody fusion with application of enhanced recovery after surgery. Neurosurg Focus. 2019;46(4):E18. https://doi.org/10.3171/2019.1.FOCUS18695.
70. Park MK, Park SA, Son SK, Park WW, Choi SH. Clinical and radiological outcomes of unilateral biportal endoscopic lumbar interbody fusion (ULIF) compared with conventional posterior lumbar interbody fusion (PLIF): 1-year follow-up. Neurosurg Rev. 2019;42(3):753–61. https://doi.org/10.1007/s10143-019-01114-3.

71. Kim JE, Yoo HS, Choi DJ, Hwang JH, Park E, Chung S. Learning curve and clinical outcome of biportal endoscopic-assisted lumbar interbody fusion. Biomed Res Int. 2020;2020:8815432. https://doi.org/10.1155/2020/8815432.
72. Kim JE, Yoo HS, Choi DJ, Park EJ, Joe SM. Comparison of minimally invasive versus biportal endoscopic transforaminal lumbar interbody fusion for single level lumbar disease. Clin Spine Surg. 2021;34(2):E64–71. https://doi.org/10.1097/BSD.0000000000001024.
73. Quillo-Olvera J, Quillo-Reséndiz J, Quillo-Olvera D, Barrera-Arreola M, Kim JS. Ten-step biportal endoscopic transforaminal lumbar interbody fusion under computed tomography-based intraoperative navigation: technical report and preliminary outcomes in Mexico. Oper Neurosurg. 2020;19(5):608–18. https://doi.org/10.1093/ons/opaa226.
74. Kang MS, You KH, Choi JY, Heo DH, Chung HJ, Park HJ. Minimally invasive transforaminal lumbar interbody fusion using the biportal endoscopic techniques versus microscopic tubular technique. Spine J. 2021; https://doi.org/10.1016/j.spinee.2021.06.013.
75. Song KS, Lee CW, Moon JG. Biportal endoscopic spinal surgery for bilateral lumbar foraminal decompression by switching surgeon's position and primary 2 portals: a report of 2 cases with technical note. Neurospine. 2019;16(1):138–47. https://doi.org/10.14245/ns.1836330.165.
76. Park JH, Jun SG, Jung JT, et al. Posterior percutaneous endoscopic cervical foraminotomy and discectomy with unilateral biportal endoscopy. Orthopaedics. 2017;40(5):e779–83. https://doi.org/10.3928/01477447-20170531-02.
77. Song KS, Lee CW. The biportal endoscopic posterior cervical inclinatory foraminotomy for cervical radiculopathy: technical report and preliminary results. Neurospine. 2020;17(Suppl 1):S145–53.
78. Kim J, Heo DH, Lee DC, et al. Biportal endoscopic unilateral laminotomy with bilateral decompression for the treatment of cervical spondylotic myelopathy. Acta Neurochir. 2021; https://doi.org/10.1007/s00701-021-04921-0.
79. Eun SS, Eum JH, Lee SH, et al. Biportal endoscopic lumbar decompression for lumbar disk herniation and spinal canal stenosis: a technical note. J Neurol Surg A Cent Eur Neurosurg. 2017;78(4):390–6. https://doi.org/10.1055/s-0036-1592157.
80. Kim SK, Kang SS, Hong YH, et al. Clinical comparison of unilateral biportal endoscopic technique versus open microdiscectomy for single-level lumbar discectomy: a multicenter, retrospective analysis. J Orthop Surg Res. 2018;13(1):22. https://doi.org/10.1186/s13018-018-0725-1.
81. Choi DJ, Choi CM, Jung JT, et al. Learning curve associated with complications in biportal endoscopic spinal surgery: challenges and strategies. Asian Spine J. 2016;10:624–9.
82. Kang T, Park SY, Park GW, et al. Biportal endoscopic discectomy for high-grade migrated lumbar disc herniation. J Neurosurg Spine. 2020:1–6. https://doi.org/10.3171/2020.2.SPINE191452.
83. Heo DH, Lee N, Park CW, et al. Endoscopic unilateral laminectomy with bilateral discectomy using biportal endoscopic approach: technical report and preliminary clinical results. World Neurosurg. 2020;137:31–7. https://doi.org/10.1016/j.wneu.2020.01.190.
84. Park JH, Jung JT, Lee SJ. How I do it: L5/S1 foraminal stenosis and far-lateral lumbar disc herniation with unilateral bi-portal endoscopy. Acta Neurochir. 2018;160(10):1899–903.
85. Choi CM, Chung JT, Lee SJ, et al. How I do it? Biportal endoscopic spinal surgery (BESS) for treatment of lumbar spinal stenosis. Acta Neurochir. 2016;158(3):459–63. https://doi.org/10.1007/s00701-015-2670-7.
86. Hwa Eum J, Hwa Heo D, Son SK, et al. Percutaneous biportal endoscopic decompression for lumbar spinal stenosis: a technical note and preliminary clinical results. J Neurosurg Spine. 2016;24(4):602–7. https://doi.org/10.3171/2015.7.SPINE15304.
87. Kim JE, Choi DJ. Unilateral biportal endoscopic decompression by 30 degree endoscopy in lumbar spinal stenosis: technical note and preliminary report. J Orthop. 2018;15(2):366–71. https://doi.org/10.1016/j.jor.2018.01.039.

88. Kang MS, Chung HJ, Jung HJ, et al. How I do it? Extraforaminal lumbar interbody fusion assisted with biportal endoscopic technique. Acta Neurochir. 2021;163(1):295–9. https://doi.org/10.1007/s00701-020-04435-1.
89. Heo DH, Eum JH, Jo JY, et al. Modified far lateral endoscopic transforaminal lumbar interbody fusion using a biportal endoscopic approach: technical report and preliminary results. Acta Neurochir. 2021;(4):1205–9. https://doi.org/10.1007/s00701-021-04758-7.
90. Kang T, Park SY, Lee SH, et al. Spinal epidural abscess successfully treated with biportal endoscopic spinal surgery. Medicine. 2019;98(50):e18231. https://doi.org/10.1097/MD.0000000000018231.
91. Kang SS, Lee SC, Kim SK. A novel percutaneous biportal endoscopic technique for symptomatic spinal epidural lipomatosis: technical note and case presentation. World Neurosurg. 2019;129:49–54.
92. Kang MS, Heo DH, Chung HJ, et al. Biportal endoscopic posterior lumbar decompression and vertebroplasty for extremely elderly patients affected by lower lumbar delayed vertebral collapse with lumbosacral radiculopathy. J Orthop Surg Res. 2021;16:380. https://doi.org/10.1186/s13017-021-025320-0.
93. Kim KR, Park JY. The technical feasibility of unilateral biportal endoscopic decompression for the unpredicted complication following minimally invasive transforaminal lumbar interbody fusion: case report. Neurospine. 2020;17(Suppl 1):S154–9. https://doi.org/10.14245/ns.2040174.087.
94. Quillo-Olvera J, Quillo-Olvera D, Quillo-Resendiz J, et al. Unilateral biportal endoscopic-guided transcorporeal vertebroplasty with neural decompression for treating a traumatic lumbar fracture of L5. World Neurosurg. 2020;144:74–81. https://doi.org/10.1016/j.wneu.2020.08.130.
95. Ahn JS, Lee HJ, Choi DJ, et al. Extraforaminal approach of biportal endoscopic spinal surgery: a new endoscopic technique for transforaminal decompression and discectomy. J Neurosurg Spine. 2018;28(5):492–8.
96. Choi DJ, Kim JE, Jung JT, et al. Biportal endoscopic spine surgery for various foraminal lesions at the lumbosacral lesions. Asian Spine J. 2018;12(3):569–73. https://doi.org/10.4184/asj.2018.12.32.569.
97. Heo DH, Sharma S, Park CK. Endoscopic treatment of extraforaminal entrapment of L5 nerve root (far out syndrome) by unilateral biportal endoscopic approach: technical report and preliminary clinical results. Neurospine. 2019;16:130–7.
98. Sharma SB, Lin GX, Jabri H, et al. Biportal endoscopic excision of facetal cyst in the far lateral region of L5S1: 2-dimensional operative video. Oper Neurosurg. 2020;18(6):E233. https://doi.org/10.1093/ons/opz255.
99. Kim CH, Chung CK, Woo JW. Surgical outcomes of percutaneous endoscopic interlaminar lumbar discectomy for highly migrated disk herniation. Clin Spine Surg. 2016;29:E359–66.
100. Choi KC, Park CK. Percutaneous endoscopic lumbar discectomy for L5–S1 disc herniation: consideration of the relation between the iliac crest and L5–S1 disc. Pain Physician. 2016;19(2):E301–8.
101. Choi KC, Kim JS, Ryu KS, et al. Percutaneous endoscopic lumbar discectomy for L5–S1 disc herniation: transforaminal versus interlaminar approach. Pain Physician. 2013;16(6):547–56.
102. Choi KC, Shim HK, Hwang JS, et al. Comparison of surgical invasiveness between microdiscectomy and 3 different endoscopic discectomy techniques for lumbar disc herniation. World Neurosurg. 2018;116:e750–8. https://doi.org/10.1016/j.wneu.2018.05.085.
103. Ahn JS, Lee HI, Park EJ. Multifidus muscle changes after biportal endoscopic spinal surgery: magnetic resonance imaging evaluation. World Neurosurg. 2019;130:e525–34. https://doi.org/10.1016/j.wneu.2019.06.148.
104. Merter A, Kareminogullari O, Shibayama M. Comparison of radiation exposure among 3 different endoscopic discectomy techniques for lumbar disk herniation. World Neurosurg. 2020;139:e572–9. https://doi.org/10.1016/j.wneu.2020.04.079.

105. Chen T, Zhou G, Chen Z, et al. Biportal endoscopic decompression vs. microscopic decompression for lumbar canal stenosis: a systematic review and meta-analysis. Exp Ther Med. 2020;20(3):3743–51. https://doi.org/10.3892/etm.2020.9001.
106. Pranata R, Lim MA, Vania R, et al. Biportal endoscopic spinal surgery versus microscopic decompression for lumbar spinal stenosis: a systematic review and meta-analysis. World Neurosurg. 2020;138:e450–8.
107. Heo DH, Lee DC, Park CK. Comparative analysis of three types of minimally invasive decompressive surgery for lumbar central stenosis: biportal endoscopy, uniportal endoscopy, and microsurgery. Neurosurg Focus. 2019;46(5):E9. https://doi.org/10.3171/2019.2.FOCUS197.
108. Min WK, Kim JE, Choi DJ, et al. Clinical and radiological outcomes between biportal endoscopic decompression and microscopic decompression in lumbar spinal stenosis. J Orthop Sci. 2020;25(3):371–8. https://doi.org/10.1016/j.jos.2019.05.022.
109. Kim HS, Choi SH, Shim DM, et al. Advantages of new endoscopic unilateral laminectomy for bilateral decompression (ULBD) over conventional microscopic ULBD. Clin Orthop Surg. 2020;12(3):330–6. https://doi.org/10.4055/cios19136.
110. Kang T, Park SY, Kang CH, et al. Is biportal technique/endoscopic spinal surgery satisfactory for lumbar spinal stenosis patients? A prospective randomized comparative study. Medicine. 2019;98:e15451.
111. Park SM, Park J, Jang HS, et al. Biportal endoscopic versus microscopic lumbar decompressive laminectomy in patients with spinal stenosis: a randomized controlled trial. Spine J. 2020;20(2):156–65. https://doi.org/10.1016/j.spinee.2019.09.015.
112. Aygun H, Abdulshafi K. Unilateral biportal endoscopy versus tubular microendoscopy in management of single level degenerative lumbar canal stenosis: a prospective study. Clin Spine Surg. 2021;34(6):E323–8. https://doi.org/10.1097/BSD.0000000000001122.
113. Yang HS, Lee N, Park JY. Current status of biportal endoscopic decompression for lumbar foraminal stenosis: endoscopic partial facetectomy and outcome factors. J Minim Invasive Spine Surg. 2021;6(S1):S157–63.
114. Pao JL, Lin SM, Chen WC, et al. Unilateral biportal endoscopic decompression for degenerative lumbar canal stenosis. J Spine Surg. 2020;6(2):438–46. https://doi.org/10.21037/jss.2020.03.08.
115. Ito Z, Shibayamam M, Nakamura, et al. Clinical comparison of unilateral biportal endoscopic laminectomy versus microendoscopic laminectomy for single-level laminectomy: a single-center, retrospective analysis. World Neurosurg. 2021;148:e581–8. https://doi.org/10.1016/j.wneu.2021.01.031.
116. Alimi M, Hofstetter CP, Torres-Campa JM, et al. Unilateral tubular approach for bilateral laminotomy: effect on ipsilateral and contralateral buttock and leg pain. Eur Spine J. 2017;26(2):389–96. https://doi.org/10.1007/s00586-016-4594-1.
117. Kim HS, Patel R, Paudel B, et al. Early outcomes of endoscopic contralateral foraminal and lateral recess decompression via an interlaminar approach in patients with unilateral radiculopathy from unilateral foraminal stenosis. World Neurosurg. 2017;108:763–73. https://doi.org/10.1016/j.wneu.2017.09.018.
118. Park JH, Jang JW, Park WM, et al. Contralateral keyhole biportal endoscopic surgery for ruptured lumbar herniated disc: a technical feasibility and early clinical outcomes. Neurospine. 2020;17(Suppl 1):S110–9. https://doi.org/10.14245/ns.2040224.112.
119. Heo DH, Kim JS, Park CW, et al. Contralateral sublaminar endoscopic approach for removal of lumbar juxtafacet cysts using percutaneous biportal endoscopic surgery: technical reports and preliminary results. World Neurosurg. 2019;122:474–9. https://doi.org/10.1016/j.wneu.2018.11.072.
120. Akbary K, Kim JS, Park CW, et al. The feasibility and perioperative results of bi-portal endoscopic resection of a facet cyst along with minimizing facet joint resection in the degenerative lumbar spine. Oper Neurosurg. 2020;18(6):621–8. https://doi.org/10.1093/ons/opz262.

121. Kim JS, Park CW, Yeung YK, et al. Unilateral biportal endoscopic decompression via the contralateral approach in asymmetric spinal stenosis: a technical note. Asian Spine J. 2020; https://doi.org/10.31616/asj.2020.0119.
122. Akbary K, Kim JS, Park CW, et al. Biportal endoscopic decompression of exiting and traversing nerve roots through a single interlaminar window using a contralateral approach: technical feasibilities and morphometric changes of the lumbar canal and foramen. World Neurosurg. 2018;117:153–61. https://doi.org/10.1016/j.wneu.2018.05.111.
123. Park MK, Son SK. Biportal endoscopic lumbar interbody fusion: review of current evidence and the literature. J Minim Invasive Spine Surg Tech. 2021;6:S171–8. https://doi.org/10.21182/jmisst.2021.00066.
124. Heo DH, Hong YH, Lee DC, et al. Technique of biportal endoscopic transforaminal lumbar interbody fusion. Neurospine. 2020;17(Suppl 1):S129–37. https://doi.org/10.14245/ns.2040178.089.
125. Nowitzke AM. Assessment of the learning curve for lumbar microendoscopic discectomy. Neurosurgery. 2005;56(4):755–62. https://doi.org/10.1227/01.neu.0000156470.79032.7b.
126. Martin-Laez R, Martinez-Agueros JA, Suarez-Franandez D, et al. Complications of endoscopic microdiscectomy using the EASYGO! system: is there any difference with conventional discectomy during the learning-curve period? Acta Neurochir. 2012;154(6):1023–32. https://doi.org/10.1007/s00701-012-1321-5.
127. Hsu HT, Chang SJ, Yang SS, et al. Learning curve of full-endoscopic lumbar discectomy. Eur Spine J. 2013;22:727–33. https://doi.org/10.1007/s00586-012-2540-4.
128. Xu H, Liu X, Liu G, et al. Learning curve of full-endoscopic technique through interlaminar approach for L5/S1 disk herniations. Cell Biochem Biophys. 2014;70(2):1069–74.
129. Son S, Ahn Y, Lee SG, et al. Learning curve of percutaneous endoscopic interlaminar lumbar discectomy versus open lumbar microdiscectomy at the L5–S1 level. PLoS One. 2020;15(7):e0236296. https://doi.org/10.1371/journal.pone.0236296.
130. Morgenstern R, Morgenstern C, Yeung AT. The learning curve in foraminal endoscopic discectomy: experience needed to achieve a 90% success rate. SAS J. 2007;1(3):100–7. https://doi.org/10.1016/SASJ-2007-0005-RR.
131. Ahn SS, Kim SH, Kim DW. Learning curve of percutaneous endoscopic lumbar discectomy based on the period (early vs. late) and technique (in-and-out vs. in-and-out-and-in): a retrospective comparative study. J Korean Neurosurg Soc. 2015;58(6):539–9546. https://doi.org/10.3340/jkns.2015.58.6.539.
132. Ahn J, Iqbal A, Manning BT, et al. Minimally invasive lumbar decompression – the surgical learning curve. Spine J. 2016;16(8):909–16. https://doi.org/10.1016/j.spinee.2015.07.455.
133. Nomura K, Yoshida M. Assessment of the learning curve for microendoscopic decompression surgery for lumbar spinal canal stenosis through an analysis of 480 cases involving a single surgeon. Global Spine J. 2017;7(1):54–8. https://doi.org/10.1055/s-0036-1583943.
134. Park SM, Kim HJ, Kim GU, et al. Learning curve for lumbar decompressive laminectomy in biportal endoscopic spinal surgery using the cumulative summation test for learning curve. World Neurosurg. 2019;122:e1007–13. https://doi.org/10.1016/j.wneu.2018.10.197.
135. Lee CW, Yoon KJ, Kim SW. Percutaneous endoscopic decompression in lumbar canal and lateral recess stenosis – the surgical learning curve. Neurospine. 2019;16(1):63–71. https://doi.org/10.14245/ns.1938048.024.
136. Kovari VZ, Kuti A, Konya, et al. Comparison of single-level open and minimally invasive transforaminal lumbar interbody fusions presenting a learning curve. Biomed Res Int. 2020;2020:3798537. https://doi.org/10.1155/2020/3798537.
137. Neal CJ, Rosner NK. Resident learning curve for minimal-access transforaminal interbody fusion in a military training program. Neurosurg Focus. 2010;28(5):e21.
138. Lee CJ, Jang HD, Shin BJ. Learning curve and clinical outcomes of minimally invasive transforaminal lumbar interbody fusion: our experience in 86 consecutive cases. Spine. 2012;37(18):1548–57. https://doi.org/10.1097/BRS.0b013e318252d44b.

139. Lee KH, Yeo W, Soeharno H, et al. Learning curve of a complex surgical technique: minimally invasive transforaminal lumbar interbody fusion (MIS TLIF). J Spinal Disord Tech. 2014;27(7):E234–40. https://doi.org/10.1097/BSD.0000000000000089.
140. Silva PS, Pereira P, Monteiro P, et al. Learning curve and complications of minimally invasive transforaminal lumbar interbody fusion. Neurosurg Focus. 2013;35(2):E7. https://doi.org/10.3171/2013.5.FOCUS13157.
141. Kumar A, Merrill RK, Overley SC, et al. Radiation exposure in minimally invasive transforaminal lumbar interbody fusion: the effect of the learning curve. Int J Spine Surg. 2019;13(1):39–45. https://doi.org/10.14444/6006.
142. Kim JE, Yoo HS, Choi DJ, et al. Learning curve and clinical outcome of biportal endoscopic-assisted lumbar interbody fusion. Biomed Res Int. 2020;2020:8815432. https://doi.org/10.1155/2020/8815432.
143. Wu PH. Early career challenge in setting up an endoscopic spine service practice. World Neurosurg. 2020;144:264–9. https://doi.org/10.1016/j.wneu.2020.09.056.
144. Kolcun JPG, Brusko GD, Wang MY. Endoscopic transforaminal lumbar interbody fusion without general anaesthesia: technical innovations and outcomes. Ann Transl Med. 2019;7(Suppl 5):S167. https://doi.org/10.21037/atm2019.07.92.
145. Kang SY, Ksahlan ON, Singh R, et al. Advantages of the combination of conscious sedation epidural anesthesia under fluoroscopy guidance in lumbar spine surgery. J Pain Res. 2020;13:211–9.
146. Fiani B, Readron T, Selvage J, et al. Awake spine surgery: an eye-opening movement. Surg Neurol Int. 2021;12:222. https://doi.org/10.25259/SNI_153_2021.
147. Kim N, Jung SB. Percutaneous unilateral biportal endoscopic spine surgery using 30 degree arthroscope in patients with severe lumbar spinal stenosis: a technical note. Clin Spine Surg. 2019;32(8):324–239. https://doi.org/10.1097/BSD.0000000000000876.
148. Hong YH, Kim SK, Suh DW, et al. Novel instruments for percutaneous biportal endoscopic spine surgery for full decompression and dural management: a comparative analysis. Brain Sci. 2020;10(8):516. https://doi.org/10.3390/brainsci10080516.
149. Manabe H, Tezuka F, Yamashita K, et al. Operating costs of full-endoscopic lumbar spine surgery. Neurol Med Chir. 2020;60(1):26–9. https://doi.org/10.2176/nmc.oa.2019-0139.
150. Choi KC, Shim HK, Kim J, et al. Cost-effectiveness of microdiscectomy versus endoscopic discectomy for lumbar disc herniation. Spine J. 2019;19(7):1162–9. https://doi.org/10.1016/j.spinee.2019.02.003.
151. van den Akker ME, Arts MP, van den Hout WB, et al. Tubular diskectomy vs conventional microdiskectomy for the treatment of lumbar disk-related sciatica: cost utility analysis alongside a double-blind randomized controlled trial. Neurosurgery. 2011;69(4):829–35.; discussion 835–6. https://doi.org/10.1227/NEU.0b013e31822578f6.
152. Parker SL, Adogwa O, Davis BJ, et al. Cost-utility analysis of minimally invasive versus open multilevel hemilaminectomy for lumbar stenosis. J Spinal Disord Tech. 2013;26(1):42–7. https://doi.org/10.1097/BSD.0b013e318232313d.
153. Droeghaag R, Hermans SMM, Caelers IJMH, et al. Cost-effectiveness of open transforaminal lumbar interbody fusion (OTLIF) versus minimally invasive transforaminal lumbar interbody fusion (MITLIF): a systematic review and meta-analysis. Spine J. 2021;21(6):945–54. https://doi.org/10.1016/j.spinee.2021.01.018.
154. Goldstein CL, Macwan K, Sundaraajan K, et al. Perioperative outcomes and adverse events of minimally invasive versus open posterior lumbar fusion: meta-analysis and systematic review. J Neurosurg Spine. 2016;24(3):416–27. https://doi.org/10.3171/2015.2.SPINE14973.
155. Vertuani S, Nilsson J, Borgman B, et al. A cost-effectiveness analysis of minimally invasive versus open surgery techniques for lumbar spinal fusion in Italy and the United Kingdom. Value Health. 2015;18(6):810–6. https://doi.org/10.1016/j.jval.2015.05.002.
156. Witiw CD, Mansouri A, Mathieu F, et al. Exploring the expectation-actuality discrepancy: a systematic review of the impact of preoperative expectations on satisfaction and

patient reported outcomes in spinal surgery. Neurosurg Rev. 2018;41(1):19–30. https://doi.org/10.1007/s10143-016-0720-0.
157. Lattig F, Fekete TF, O'Riordan D, et al. A comparison of patient and surgeon preoperative expectations of spinal surgery. Spine. 2013;38(12):1040–8. https://doi.org/10.1097/BRS.0b013e318269c100.
158. Mancuso CA, Duculan R, Cammisa FR. Fulfilment of patients' expectations of lumbar and cervical spine surgery. Spine J. 2016;16(10):1167–74. https://doi.org/10.1016/j.spinee.2016.04.011.
159. Tong Y, Fernandez L, Bendo JA, et al. Enhanced recovery after surgery trends in adult spine surgery: a systematic review. Int J Spine Surg. 2020;14(4):623–40. https://doi.org/10.14444/7083.
160. Sugrue PA, Halpin RJ, Koski TR. Treatment algorithms and protocol practice in high-risk spine surgery. Neurosurg Clin N Am. 2013;24(2):219–30. https://doi.org/10.1016/j.nec.2012.12.012.
161. Yoo JS, Ahn J, Karmarker SS, et al. The use of tranexamic acid in spine surgery. Ann Transl Med. 2019;7(Suppl 5):S172. https://doi.org/10.21037/atm.2019.05.36.
162. Hassanzadeh H, Jain A, Tan EW, et al. Postoperative incentive spirometry use. Orthopedics. 2012;35(6):e927–31. https://doi.org/10.3928/01477447-20120525-37.
163. Elsrrage M, Soldozy S, Patel P, et al. Enhanced recovery after spine surgery: a systematic review. Neurosurg Focus. 2019;46(4):E3. https://doi.org/10.3171/2019.1.FOCUS18700.
164. Feng C, Zhang Y, Chong F, et al. Establishment and implementation of an enhanced recovery after surgery (ERAS) pathway tailored for minimally invasive transforaminal lumbar interbody fusion surgery. World Neurosurg. 2019;129:e317–23. https://doi.org/10.1016/j.wneu.2019.05.139.
165. Yang Y, Wu X, Wu W, et al. Enhanced recovery after surgery (ERAS) pathway for microendoscopy-assisted minimally invasive transforaminal lumbar interbody fusion. Clin Neurol Neurosurg. 2020;196:106003. https://doi.org/10.1016/j.clineuro.2020.106003.
166. Lewandrowski KU, Soriano-Sanchez JA, Zhang X, et al. Surgeon training and clinical implementation of spinal endoscopy in routine practice: results of a global survey. J Spine Surg. 2020;6(Suppl 1):S237–48. https://doi.org/10.21037/jss.2019.09.32.
167. Sclafani JA, Kim CW. Complications associated with the initial learning curve of minimally invasive spine surgery: a systematic review. Clin Orthop Relat Res. 2014;472:1711–7.
168. Falavigna A, Guiroy A, Taboada N. Teaching training and surgical education in minimally invasive surgery (MIS) of the spine: what are the best teaching and learning strategies for MIS? Do we have any experience and data? AOSpine. 2020;10(25):126S–9S.
169. Ransom NA, Gollogly S, Lewandrowski KU, et al. Navigating the learning curve of spinal endoscopy as an established traditionally trained spine surgeon. J Spine Surg. 2020;6(Suppl 1):S197–207. https://doi.org/10.21037/jss.2019.10.03.
170. Koehler RJ, Amsdell S, Arendt EA, et al. The Arthroscopic Surgical Skill Evaluation Tool (ASSET). Am J Sports Med. 2013;41(6):1229–37. https://doi.org/10.1177/0363546513483535.
171. Koehler RJ, Nicandri GT. Using the arthroscopic surgery skill evaluation tool as a pass-fail examination. J Bone Joint Surg Am. 2013;95(23):1–6. https://doi.org/10.2013/JBJS.M.00340.
172. Koehler RJ, Goldblatt JP, Maloney MD, et al. Assessing diagnostic arthroscopy performance in the operating room using the Arthroscopic Surgery Skill Evaluation Tool (ASSET). Arthroscopy. 2015;31(12):2314–9.e2. https://doi.org/10.1016/j.arthro.2015.06.011.
173. Martin MK, Patterson DP, Cameron KL. Arthroscopic training courses improve trainee arthroscopy skills. A stimulation-based prospective trial. Arthroscopy. 2016;32:2228–32.
174. Marcheix PS, Vergnenegre G, Dalmay F, et al. Learning the skills needed to perform shoulder arthroscopy by simulation. Orthop Traumat Surg Res. 2017;103(4):483–8.
175. Frank RM, Rego G, Grimaldi F, et al. Does arthroscopic simulation training improve triangulation and probing skills? A randomized control trial. J Surg Ed. 2019;76:1131–8.

176. Pfandler M, Lazarovici M, Stefan, et al. Virtual reality-based simulators for spine surgery: a systematic review. Spine J. 2017;17(9):1352–63. https://doi.org/10.1016/j.spinee.2017.05.016.
177. Lohre R, Wang JC, Lewandrowski, et al. Virtual reality in spinal endoscopy: a paradigm shift in education to support spine surgeons. J Spine Surg. 2020;6:S208–23. https://doi.org/10.21037/jss.2019.11.16.
178. Lin GX, Huang P, Kotheeranurak V, et al. A systematic review of unilateral biportal endoscopic spinal surgery: preliminary clinical results and complications. World Neurosurg. 2019;125:425–32. https://doi.org/10.1016/j.wneu.2019.02.038.
179. Kim W, Kim S, Kang S, et al. Pooled analysis of unsuccessful percutaneous biportal endoscopic surgery outcomes from a multi-institutional retrospective cohort of 797 cases. Acta Neurochir. 2020;162(2):279–87. https://doi.org/10.1007/s00701-019-04162-2.
180. Yan D, Zhang Z, Zhang Z. Residual leg numbness after endoscopic discectomy treatment of lumbar disc herniation. BMC Musculoskelet Disord. 2020;21(1):273. https://doi.org/10.1186/s12891-020-03302-5.
181. Lee SH, Kang BU, Ahn Y, et al. Operative failure of percutaneous endoscopic lumbar discectomy: a radiologic analysis of 55 cases. Spine. 2006;31(10):E285–90.
182. Chang HS. Influence of lumbar lordosis on the outcome of decompression surgery for lumbar canal stenosis. World Neurosurg. 2018;109:e684–90. https://doi.org/10.1016/j.wneu.2017.10.055.
183. Yamada K, Matsuda H, Nabeta M, et al. Clinical outcomes of microscopic decompression for degenerative lumbar foraminal stenosis: a comparison between patients with and without degenerative lumbar scoliosis. Eur Spine J. 2011;20(6):947–53. https://doi.org/10.1007/s00586-010-1597-1.
184. Hong YH, Kim SK, Hwang J, et al. Water dynamics in unilateral biportal endoscopic spine surgery and its related factors: an in vivo proportional regression and proficiency-matched study. World Neurosurg. 2021;149:e836–43. https://doi.org/10.1016/j.wneu.2021.01.086.
185. Kang T, Park SY, Lee SH, et al. Assessing changes in cervical epidural pressure during biportal endoscopic lumbar discectomy. J Neurosurg Spine. 2020:1–7. https://doi.org/10.3171/2020.6.SPINE20586.
186. Choi G, Kang HY, Modi HN, et al. Risk of developing seizure after percutaneous endoscopic lumbar discectomy. J Spinal Disord Tech. 2011;24(2):83–92. https://doi.org/10.1097/BSD.0b013e3181ddf124.
187. Wu J, Fang Y, Jin W. Seizures after percutaneous endoscopic lumbar discectomy: a case report. Medicine. 2020;99(47):e22470. https://doi.org/10.1097/MD.0000000000022470.
188. Joh JY, Choi G, Kong BJ, et al. Comparative study of neck pain in relation to increase of cervical epidural pressure during percutaneous endoscopic lumbar discectomy. Spine. 2009;34(19):2033–8. https://doi.org/10.1097/BRS.0b013e3181b20250.
189. Lee HG, Kang MS, Kim SY, et al. Dural injury in unilateral biportal endoscopic spinal surgery. Global Spine J. 2021;11(6):845–51. https://doi.org/10.1177/2192568220941446.
190. Hahn BS, Jang JW, Lee DG, et al. Current status of biportal endoscopic decompression for lumbar central stenosis. J Minim Invasive Spine Surg Tech. 2021;6:S164–70. https://doi.org/10.21182/jmisst.2021.00052.
191. Kullarni AG, Patel RS. Is closed-suction drainage essential after minimally invasive lumbar fusion surgery? A retrospective review of 381 cases. J Minim Invasive Spine Surg Tech. 2017;2(1):27–31. https://doi.org/10.21182/jimsst.2017.00185.
192. Hung P, Chang MC, Chou PH, et al. Is a drain necessary for minimally invasive lumbar spine fusion surgery? Eur Spine J. 2017;26(3):733–7. https://doi.org/10.1007/s00586-016-4672-4.
193. Costa F, Alves OL, Anania CD, et al. Decompressive surgery for lumbar spinal stenosis: WFNS Spine Committee Recommendations. World Neurosurg X. 2020;7:100076. https://doi.org/10.1016/j.wnsx.2020.100076.
194. Stromqvist F, Sigmundsson FG, Stromqvist B, et al. Accidental durotomy in degenerative lumbar spine surgery – a register study of 64,431 operations. Spine J. 2019;19:624–30.

195. Weiss H, Garcia RM, Hopkins B, et al. A systematic review of complications following minimally invasive spine surgery including transforaminal lumbar interbody fusion. Curr Rev Musculoskelet Med. 2019;12(3):328–39. https://doi.org/10.1007/s12178-019-09574-2.
196. Kim HS, Raorane HD, Wu PH, et al. Incidental durotomy during endoscopic stenosis lumbar decompression: incidence, classification, and proposed management strategies. World Neurosurg. 2020;139:e13–22. https://doi.org/10.1016/j.wneu.2020.01.242.
197. Lewandrowski KU, Hellinger S, de Carvalho PST, et al. Dural tears during lumbar spinal endoscopy: surgeon skill, training, incidence, risk factors, and management. Int J Spine Surg. 2021;15(2):280–91. https://doi.org/10.14444/8038.
198. Kinaci A, Moayeri N, van der Zwan A, et al. Effectiveness of sealants in prevention of cerebrospinal fluid leakage after spine surgery: a systematic review. World Neurosurg. 2019;127:597–75.
199. Robson CH, Paranathala MP, Dobson G, et al. Early mobilisation does not increase the complication rate from unintended lumbar durotomy. Br J Neurosurg. 2018:1–3. https://doi.org/10.1080/02688697.2018.1508641.
200. Farshad M, Aichmair A, Wanivenhaus F, et al. No benefit of early versus late ambulation after incidental durotomy in lumbar spine surgery: a randomized controlled trial. Eur Spine J. 2020;29(1):141–6. https://doi.org/10.1007/s00586-019-06144-5.
201. Radcliff KE, Sidhu GDS, Kepler CK, et al. Complications of flat bed rest after incidental durotomy. Clin Spine Surg. 2016;29(7):281–4. https://doi.org/10.1097/BSD.0b013e31827d7ad8.
202. Shin JK, Youn MS, Seong YJ, et al. Iatrogenic dural tear in endoscopic lumbar spinal surgery: full endoscopic dural suture repair (Youn's technique). Eur Spine J. 2018;27(Suppl 3):544–8. https://doi.org/10.1177/2192568220956606.
203. Cheng YP, Lin PY, Huang AP, et al. Durotomy repair in minimally invasive transforaminal lumbar interbody fusion by nonpenetrating clips. Surg Neurol Int. 2014;5:36.
204. Heo DH, Ha JS, Lee DC, et al. Repair of incidental durotomy using sutureless nonpenetrating clips via biportal endoscopic surgery. Global Spine J. 2020;2020:2192568220956606. https://doi.org/10.1177/2192568220956606.
205. Nam HGW, Kim HS, Park JS, et al. Double-layer TachoSil packing for management of incidental durotomy during percutaneous stenoscopic lumbar decompression. World Neurosurg. 2018;120:448–56. https://doi.org/10.1016/j.wneu.2018.09.040.
206. Nowak S, Schroeder HWS, Fleck S. Hemopatch as a new dural sealant: a clinical observation. Clin Neurol Neurosurg. 2019;176:133–7. https://doi.org/10.1016/j.clineuro.2018.12.009.
207. Park HJ, Kim SK, Lee SC, et al. Dural tear in percutaneous biportal endoscopic spine surgery: anatomic location and management. World Neurosurg. 2020;136:e578–85. https://doi.org/10.1016/j.wneu2020.01.080.
208. Anno M, Yamazaki T, Hara N, et al. The incidence, clinical features, and a comparison between early and delayed onset of postoperative spinal epidural hematoma. Spine. 2019;44(6):420–3. https://doi.org/10.1097/BRS.0000000000002838.
209. Wang L, Wang H, Zeng Y, et al. Delayed onset postoperative spinal epidural hematoma after lumbar spinal surgery: incidence, risk factors, and clinical outcomes. Biomed Res Int. 2020;2020:8827962. https://doi.org/10.1155/2020/8827962.
210. Park JH, Park S, Choi SA. Incidence and risk factors of spinal epidural hemorrhage after spine surgery: a cross-sectional retrospective analysis of a national database. BMC Musculoskelet Disord. 2020;21(1):324. https://doi.org/10.1186/s12891-020-03337-8.
211. Ahn DK, Lee JS, Shin WS, et al. Postoperative spinal epidural hematoma in a biportal endoscopic spine surgery. Medicine. 2021;100(6):e24685. https://doi.org/10.1097/MD.0000000000024685.
212. Kim JE, Choi DJ, Park EJ. Evaluation of postoperative spinal epidural hematoma after biportal endoscopic spine surgery for single-level lumbar spinal stenosis: clinical and magnetic resonance imaging study. World Neurosurg. 2019;126:e786–92. https://doi.org/10.1016/j.wneu.2019.02.150.

213. Kim JE, Choi DJ, Kim MC, et al. Risk factors of postoperative spinal epidural hematoma after biportal endoscopic spinal surgery. World Neurosurg. 2019;129:e324–9. https://doi.org/10.1016/j.wneu.2019.05.141.
214. Kim JE, Yoo HS, Choi DJ, et al. Effectiveness of gelatin-thrombin matrix sealants (Floseal®) on postoperative spinal epidural hematoma during single-level lumbar decompression using biportal endoscopic spine surgery: clinical and magnetic resonance image study. Biomed Res Int. 2020;2020:4801641. https://doi.org/10.1155/2020/4801641.

Chapter 34
Beyond the Horizon: The Future of Unilateral Biportal Endoscopic Spine Surgery

Yip-Kan Yeung, Sheung-Tung Ho, and Tsz-King Suen

Abbreviations

AR	Augmented reality
ASA	American Society of Anesthesiologists Classification
CT	Computed tomography
EMG	Electromyography
ERAS	Enhanced recovery after surgery
MEP	Motor-evoked potentials
MIS TLIF	Minimally invasive surgery transforaminal lumbar interbody fusion
MRI	Magnetic resonance imaging
NSAIDS	Nonsteroidal anti-inflammatory drugs
PLIF	Posterior lumbar interbody fusion
SSEP	Somatosensory evoked potentials
TLIF	Transforaminal lumbar interbody fusion
UBE	Unilateral biportal endoscopy
UBE-TLIF	Unilateral biportal endoscopic transforaminal lumbar interbody fusion
VAS	Visual analog scale
VR	Virtual reality
WALANT	Wide-awake local anesthesia no tourniquet

Y.-K. Yeung (✉) · S.-T. Ho
Department of Orthopaedics & Traumatology, Caritas Medical Centre, Hong Kong SAR, China
e-mail: yyk028@ha.org.hk; drhosheungtung@gmail.com

T.-K. Suen
Hong Kong Baptist Hospital, Hong Kong SAR, China
e-mail: aarsuen@gmail.com

J. Quillo-Olvera et al. (eds.), *Unilateral Biportal Endoscopy of the Spine*,
https://doi.org/10.1007/978-3-031-14736-4_34

Introduction

State of the Art and the Coming Era

Unilateral biportal endoscopic spinal surgery (UBE) has been rapidly evolving in the past years. A recent literature in 2019 mentioned 648 patients in 14 articles, with decompression or fusion performed under UBE in the PubMed database [1]. The history of spinal surgery has evolved over the generations, from open traditional to minimally invasive approaches, further to the development of microscopic, micro-endoscopic, and endoscopic surgery.

Compared with microscopic or micro-endoscopic spinal surgery, UBE preserves the advantage of being minimally invasive, at the same time demonstrating similar efficacy and safety. In the meta-analysis performed by Pranata [2], the length of hospital stay was 1.2 days in the UBE group, versus 3.5 days in the microscopy group. Two of their recruited studies showed superior results in immediate postoperative Visual Analog Scale pain score, two with less opioid consumption, and one with earlier ambulation in the UBE versus microscopy group. In the meta-analysis, the operation time, complications, and pain and Oswestry Disability Index at 2–3 months did not show statistical significance in both groups. UBE also has the advantage to zoom in close to the lesion, as well as reduce "hands-off" time from handling instruments as in microscopic surgery.

The use of flexible instruments permits higher versatility and magnification with wider access. Using two independent portals, the target lesion can be closely accessed through a panoramic view by free three-dimensional manipulation of optical and working instruments, and this does not necessitate a fixed docking [1]. The working space is not limited by the use of rigid angular or tubular retractors, and the narrow dimension of the instruments permits access to deeply seated structures, which reduces lamina resection, muscle dissection, and bone bleeding. Visual field is further improved via the use of angular devices.

Continuous saline irrigation not only improves visualization, but also prevents excessive epidural and bone bleeding, as well as limits the risk of infection. Maintaining a good water outflow helps to protect soft tissue from bone debris, and low water pressure also assists in adhesiolysis and anatomical plane dissection.

Current main obstacles hindering the development of endoscopic spinal surgery include a steep learning curve, with relative lack of knowledge and technical popularization. Surgeons unfamiliar with arthroscopic triangulation techniques may find it difficult to manipulate both the optical and working instruments with two different hands. Inadequate decompression by inexperienced surgeons has been regarded as one of the most frequently encountered complications.

It is perceived that UBE can be analogous to a new era of laparoscopic surgery replacing traditional open laparotomy in the surgical stream, or arthroscopic surgery replacing open surgery in the management of rotator cuff tears and meniscal and knee ligamentous pathologies in the orthopedic specialty. Having overcome the aforementioned obstacles, UBE may eventually become the new mainstream of spinal surgery in managing most of the spinal pathologies in the future decades.

The patients' need for early recovery, as well as return to a healthy lifestyle with a high quality of life, will increase the popularity of endoscopic spinal surgery. In managing elderly or fragile patients who cannot tolerate a prolonged general anesthesia, endoscopy under local anesthesia may provide equal or superior outcomes compared with conservative treatment.

Establishing Nomenclature in UBE Surgery

One major obstacle in the development of UBE is a relative lack of common communication language for scientific exchange. Until recently, different terminologies have been invented by different authors, even when the same surgical technique is being described. One reason is due to the rapidly emerging inspirations from surgeons specialized in various fields of interest and expertise, simultaneously exploring multiple endoscopic surgical procedures and approach corridors in different anatomical locations.

Such issue has also been raised by spinal workgroups. In 2020, an AOSpine Consensus Paper was published [3]. Endoscopic spinal surgery is classified into "full-endoscopic" and "endoscopic-assisted" surgery, depending on whether the working channel resides inside the endoscope or through a separate portal. For surgical approaches, the term "transforaminal" has more precisely replaced "posterolateral." For surgical techniques, the term "foraminotomy" has been recommended to replace "foraminoplasty." The literature concluded that posing an ideal international community aids in delivering knowledge, experience, and evidence, with the ultimate goal to improve patient care and outcomes.

With a proper nomenclature system, surgical experts can communicate efficiently, reducing confusion amongst publications, speeches, and other communication platforms. Subsequent teaching and education will be more efficient. This will promote the future development of UBE in becoming one of the mainstreams in spinal surgery.

While much contents have been described in relation to full-endoscopic surgery, the nomenclature system of endoscopic-assisted surgery has not been elaborated precisely. In their summary chart, "endoscopic-assisted surgery" is briefly categorized into decompression (UBE) and fusion (UBE fusion). Similarly, there is a current lack of MeSH terms for endoscopic spinal surgery, which also limits the ability of search engines in recognizing UBE publications. With increasing popularity in UBE surgery, similar nomenclature systems should be refined for biportal spinal operations and to be recognized internationally.

Enhanced Recovery After Surgery (ERAS) and Day Surgery

Less muscle dissection is required in UBE versus open spinal surgery. This helps to retain spinal strength and stability for early mobilization. Other factors facilitating ambulation include reduced tissue damage and blood loss, with less postoperative pain and opioid consumption [2]. Pain control and functional preservation are the key features in the prediction of early discharge.

To facilitate functional recovery and rehabilitation, UBE can be incorporated into the enhanced recovery after surgery (ERAS) program, which helps to improve surgical outcomes, patient satisfaction, and length of hospital stay. Percutaneous biportal endoscopic lumbar interbody fusion incorporated into ERAS program has been reported [4]. This includes optimizing postoperative pain management via multimodal analgesia, postoperative early mobilization and physical therapy, and a prophylactic multimodal antiemetic regimen to decrease postoperative nausea and vomiting. As a result, utility of antiemetics and opioid has declined further, facilitating early discharge [5].

First introduced in 2017, applying the principles of ERAS in lumbar spinal fusion may be important for day surgeries or operating in an outpatient surgery center [6]. Advantages include reduced bleeding and postoperative pain, as operative scars and traumatization of posterior muscular structures can be minimized. Preoperative treatment comprises preemptive analgesia, antibiotics, antiemetics, intravenous Transamin, and emotional support. Intraoperatively, the adoption of local anesthetic injection and minimally invasive spine operation, including endoscopic decompression and percutaneous pedicle screw insertion, is incorporated into the pathway. Postoperative measures include adequate pain control with patient-controlled analgesia, early oral use of gabapentin or pregabalin, nutritional support, deep vein thrombosis prevention, application of orthosis, and early ambulation. Visual Analog Scale pain score on days 1 and 2 was reported significantly lower in the ERAS versus non-ERAS group, with similar fusion rate and complications.

Amongst the protocol recommendations, the surgical method itself may be the most important factor in predicting postoperative recovery. Combining local anesthesia and conscious sedation enables outpatient surgery or even same-day surgery to be performed, which is desirable in elderly or medically compromised patients [7].

Novel Anesthesia Techniques

Currently, UBE is usually performed under general or epidural anesthesia. Local anesthesia alone may not serve the purpose of attaining adequate pain control, when the surgery involves bone resection and soft-tissue ablation in an unconfined anatomical plane. In contrast, local pain control can be achieved for surgeries at the limbs, for example, adductor canal block for knee arthroplasty and wide-awake local anesthesia no tourniquet (WALANT) for hand surgery. In future, spinal surgeons may collaborate with anesthetists to develop a novel model of anesthesia for effective local spinal pain control. This can further extend the UBE indications in elderly or poor premorbid patients, who are deemed risky to undergo prolonged general anesthesia in a prone position. Avoiding general anesthesia may also help in intraoperative assessment of neurological status, as well as permitting early postoperative rehabilitation.

The concept of "awake surgery" has extended from craniotomies to lumbar laminectomies and lumbar fusion, resulting in shorter operative time, less postoperative nausea, urinary retention, and spinal headache, with overall shorter hospital stay [8]. For laminectomies without general anesthesia, spinal or epidural anesthesia has been advocated in most studies. The success rate of epidural anesthesia can be improved by contrast dye injection under fluoroscopy, and pain relief was sustained postoperatively [9]. Local anesthesia has also been recommended for thoracic or lumbar spinal operations in ASA III or IV patients, providing equal safety and efficacy as in general anesthesia [8]. With the emerging trend towards minimally invasive spinal surgery, local or regional anesthesia will become more widely accepted in future.

In patients undergoing endoscopic TLIF using the trans-Kambin approach, local anesthesia with sedation can be used [10]. Therefore, endoscopic TLIF may reduce anesthesia-related morbidity. However, these cases were usually described in uniportal but not biportal surgeries. As the operation time of TLIF is longer than decompression alone, general endotracheal anesthesia was usually preferred. Future anticipations will be to explore the feasibility of performing UBE-TLIF under multi-modalities of local or regional anesthetic techniques, to avoid complications from general anesthesia alone. The addition of spinal anesthesia to long-acting cocktail analgesia regime may also permit a longer operation time.

Another study described the key technological innovations in "awake TLIF" surgery using endoscopic transforaminal approach [11]. This includes conscious sedation, endoscopic visualization, expandable interbody device, long-acting local analgesia, and percutaneous instrumentation. The operating time, blood loss, and length of hospital stay averaged well below conventional MIS TLIF, with a cost reduction of 15% per case. Further technical improvements have allowed operation including three spinal levels.

The use of local vasoconstrictors combined with local anesthesia for sustained postoperative pain relief can be explored. Similar to periarticular injection in knee arthroplasty, study trials on the use of long-acting liposomal bupivacaine can be performed, which may deem more effective in controlling postoperative pain and facilitating rehabilitation. However, it also depends on whether such medications will be available in the spinal center. As an alternative, 1% lidocaine can be administered, which, when combined with gabapentin or pregabalin administration, can be effective for postoperative pain control [4]. The adoption of cocktail regime, combining local anesthesia with NSAIDS, diluted adrenaline, or even steroid, may also help to concentrate the analgesia around the surgical field, leading to more efficient pain relief.

Relevant studies are lacking currently. Variability in anesthetizing experience and comfort level for awake surgery may also affect the actual clinical results. In future, spinal surgeons and pain specialists should collaborate to develop a safe and reliable mode of analgesia, to avoid complications from prolonged general anesthesia in elderly debilitated patients suffering from degenerative spinal pathology.

Advancements in Optics and Portals

Ahn summarized the development of endoscopic spinal surgery in three aspects [7]. Themes included the following: (1) for the optical channel, the advancement of endoscopes should incorporate angled or steerable optics, allowing visualization of all corners of the surgical field, and (2) for the working channel, steerable instruments in burrs, punches, and forceps will make decompression faster and safer.

An ideal optical channel should permit sufficient illumination, resolution, and magnification of the surgical site. An angled view is occasionally required for visualizing the ipsilateral lateral recess, the foraminal space, or the exiting root. The optical endoscope should not obscure the working space and working instruments. Thermal damage from the light source, and water pressure causing potential compromise to the neural structures, should be minimized. This is carried out by design improvements of the irrigation pump, optics, camera, light source, and the endoscope itself.

Compared with microscopic surgery, UBE provides a clearer operative field for ipsilateral, contralateral, and sublaminar spaces, with a high resolution and magnification [2]. The endoscope can be inserted in close proximity to the target site, unlike microscopes which work outside the patient's body with narrow visualization views. Different optical angles of arthroscopic endoscopes (e.g., 0° and 30°) are commercially available in the market. Still, these are only rigid endoscopes inserted via traditional arthroscopic portals. The use of flexible or steerable endoscopes has not been explored. Newer endoscopic designs with narrow caliber and high versatility may enable easy manipulation into the narrow sublaminar space. This helps to follow the surgical principles of being minimally invasive while allowing adequate visualization of the surgical site and facilitating target access.

Optimizing visualization is of paramount importance in endoscopic spinal surgery [12], when non-deformable bony and vulnerable neural structures are present in a confined space. Today, high-intensity light and high-resolution imaging are no longer major technological challenges. On the other hand, there are other technological innovations currently available in other specialties, which may be of value to spinal surgery. Optical chromoendoscopy, using narrowband imaging or flexible color spectrum enhancement specific for microvascular architecture, may help to differentiate dural vasculature from the surrounding soft tissue and assess the adequacy of neural decompression [12]. Tissue manipulation with light transformation via fluorescent imaging offers another potential scope for visualization enhancement. Intravenous administration of 5-aminolevulinic acid [13] and indocyanine green [14] helps to identify tumor tissues and peripheral nerves, respectively, while intrathecal fluorescein can stain cerebrospinal fluid yellow [15] and is particularly useful in detecting fistulas during dural repair surgery.

Adopting the utilization of 4K/8K endoscopes in skull base and pituitary surgeries has been published recently [16]. With these ultra-resolution endoscopes, surgical anatomies can be identified more precisely, for example the foraminal ligament in the lumbar spine. On the other hand, the availability of 3D endoscopes combined with 3D glasses or virtual reality headset also allows accurate perception of the degree of stenosis and disc protrusion. This ability of depth perception helps to estimate relative distances. Surgeons can have better tactile sensation working on a 3D interface. Adequate decompression can be achieved safely and sufficiently. A direct and detailed endplate view is also made feasible, making endoscopic fusion more accurate and successful.

The design of portals should also assist visual and working purpose. Portals should facilitate efficient irrigation fluid inflow and outflow, following the principles of "flow" operation. The length of portals is also important. A long portal tip may impinge on bony structures and limit instrument manipulation. Still, its length should be sufficient and customized to allow adequate soft-tissue retraction in patients with different body build and muscle thickness. The tip of portal design should enable anchorage to prevent repeated slip-out during manipulation, but the anchorage should not cause additional muscle injury. The material of the portal should maintain sufficient strength to withstand breakage but should not be too rigid nor bulky to avoid inadvertent muscle damage. The opening of working channels should permit easy entry and retrieval of surgical instruments.

Portals can have other special designs. Plastic cannulas with beveled ends can facilitate gentle dural retraction, without the use of additional dural retractors [17]. Similar arthroscopic metal portal designs with a beveled lip have also been described [18]. Another publication invented special portal designs that enable uniportal or biportal conversion during operation, using a magnetic connector to link up the working portal with the optical portal [19].

Novel Technological Advancements

Current endoscopic spinal surgery has several limitations, including lack of anatomical working cavity, 2D instead of 3D visualization, as well as radiation exposure. Incorporation of navigation techniques may provide real-time information of the location, orientation, and depth of surgical instruments without radiation. Incision points and optimal trajectory can be predetermined, which is essential in facilitating subsequent surgical process. Critical structures including neural, dural, vascular, and unnecessary bone resection can be avoided, which makes it particularly useful in tumor resection and minimally invasive surgery [20]. Inexperienced surgeons can also perform the procedure more safely, with less dependence on specific anatomical landmarks.

Up to present, few literatures exist describing the use of navigation in uniportal [21] and biportal [22] surgery. Intraoperative computed tomography scanning was utilized, and data was incorporated into the navigation system. Both transforaminal and interlaminar approaches have been illustrated in the lumbar spine and posterior approach in the cervical spine. The authors reported remarkable concordance of the intraoperative landmarks between the endoscopic vision and the 3D navigation system. In uniportal surgery, the scan time combined with verification time was only 11 min. Current position of the tip of the probe, needle, and working cannula could be traced, with target registration discrepancy within 0.86 mm [21]. Further studies may entail the clinical significance of adopting navigation in UBE surgery.

Future direction in navigation should focus on improved monitors for visualization, optimized operating suites for navigation, and invention of registration trackers that can provide a secure fit while not obscuring the surgical field, for example the SpineMap system of Stryker for the lumbar spine. Another innovation is the use of augmented reality headsets with real-time navigation images directly overlaid on the patient, instead of visualizing through a screen. CT-MRI co-registration can extend surgical indications to include soft-tissue pathologies without bony involvement. The incorporation of robotic surgery into navigation also appears attractive; however, its cost-effectiveness has to be ensured.

Another potential area of development is robotic-assisted endoscopic surgery. Robotic surgery shares similar features with navigation in avoiding vulnerable structures, providing accurate physical guidance and anatomical feedback while eliminating radiation exposure, making surgeons able to follow the preoperatively customized surgical plan. Robotic surgery has also been shown to be cost saving in the long run, apart from the initial hardware installation [16].

A design of a robot-assisted system for transforaminal percutaneous endoscopic lumbar surgery has been described [23]. The robot-assisted system comprises three components: preoperative planning, navigation, and foraminoplasty system. 3D visualization of the surgical segment and tissues was performed using the multimodal image fusion technique, and working channel planning was performed to avoid encountering vital structures. The entry point was dictated by patient size, dimensions of the facet joint, and desired location of the triangular working zone. The robot could achieve visual perception from a visual receptor, which could capture the patient's vertebral position in real time, automatically adjust the robotic platform and robot arm, and provide navigation using the 6-degree-of-freedom robot arm. After guiding surgeons to establish the working channel, automatic foraminoplasty would be performed using the high-speed burr, offering real-time feedback through multimode sensors such as multidimensional force, position, and acceleration.

Current available robotic systems should be more accurately termed "co-robots," as they are still relying on the interaction between computers and human operators, instead of independent functioning [24]. Either the robot facilitates instrument entry towards the target point as in navigation or the surgeons establish a trajectory for the device to align with. There is also access limitation to separate anatomical locations, as robotic models were usually constrained locally to the operative table. Currently, the use of robotics is described in screw placement, discogram, or percutaneous discectomy [16], but not for biportal spinal surgeries.

In a future vision of robotic use in UBE, robots can be equipped with tools for automated or guided portal entry. After superficial muscle dissection, lamina resection can be performed automatically according to programmed bony resection templates. During soft-tissue decompression, important structures will be protected by anatomical identification under augmented or virtual reality guidance. For further advanced envision, multiple bed-mounted robotic arms will be installed, each with two to three joints for articulation in three dimensions. Surgeons will be equipped with a headset and visor away from the operative field. The surgeon can visualize the operative site directly or from the viewpoint of the robotic arm [24]. An augmented reality display permits access to pre- and intraoperative imaging and can project target structures for recognition. Control is via sensor gloves that lend itself to natural hand motions and haptic feedback. Fail-safe mechanisms and improved maneuverability with miniaturization for efficient motions should be developed, for enhancing future robotic application in UBE spinal surgery.

Virtual reality (VR) and augmented reality (AR) have been proven useful in surgical trainings. VR offers artificially generated environment for user perception and interaction, while AR projects computer-generated virtual components onto the user's real surroundings [24]. These technologies enable remote observation and guidance by the surgical team and improve intraoperative visualization of spatial parameters and display of imaging studies. Current drawbacks include cost and lack of practical surgical application tools. Future direction should focus on the development of more immersive training scenarios and invention of wearable display systems for surgical use.

One potential adjunct aiding UBE application is the adoption of 3D printing. Its use in the field of spine surgery was first described in 1999 for complex deformity cases [25]. In the past, 3D printing was only utilized in making simple surgical instruments like retractors, forceps, and hemostats. A recent literature described using 3D printing techniques in creating customized individualized endoscopic portals [19]. 3D printing is also applicable in creating spine biomodels, hardware templates and guides, and custom implants [25]. This helps to facilitate preoperative templating and improves intraoperative accuracy and precision, making it in particular favor of complex spinal deformities, tumor surgeries, and minimally invasive surgeries. Operative time, blood loss, and transfusion rate are reduced. Future barriers to overcome include time, cost, and efficiency in practical application.

Although technological innovations are attractive, mechanical errors can still occur. Navigation markers may require additional incisions. Setting up navigation or robotic system may be time consuming and will increase overall operative time. Imaging noise can occur with vibration or changes in water flow. Additional expenses are required in the initial setting of technological devices, and initial and maintenance costs should be accounted for. The use of polarized goggles may induce dizziness and headache to surgeons due to blurry images. A standard robust surgical protocol should be reproducible with ensured safety when applying these technologies.

Intraoperative Monitoring

The practical application of neuro-monitoring in spinal surgery remains controversial. One major concern is cost-effectiveness, given the relatively low incidence of neurological deficits [26]. The use of neuro-monitoring is strongly supported in complex spinal deformity and tumor surgeries but remains controversial in routine cervical and lumbar spinal procedures.

With improvement in technologies and knowledge, there is an increasing trend towards "minimally invasive" spinal surgery. A reduced exposure corridor entails a greater risk of iatrogenic injury to neural structures [27]. Spinal cord integrity can be monitored peri-operatively with the use of electrophysiological monitoring. In general, somatosensory evoked potentials (SSEP) have high specificity in posterior decompression procedures, when sensory fibers run along the dorsal column. Motor-evoked potentials (MEP) are useful for real-time updating as prediction of temporary or permanent motor deficits. Electromyography (EMG) is more selective for monitoring of specific nerve root supplying the particular myotome, and during instrumentation to determine if the screw violates the medial cortex. However, the procedure may not be able to differentiate iatrogenic injury from chronic nerve root compression. Obtaining a baseline reading is thus recommended before the start of surgery.

The use of neuro-monitoring to prevent exiting nerve root damage by cannula insertion during transforaminal endoscopic discectomy has been reported [28]. The author concluded a threefold reduction of postoperative dysesthesia, by repositioning the inserted cannula, when more than 5% SSEP or 50% transcranial MEP amplitude reduction was detected. Similarly, the efficacy of neuro-monitoring can also be explored in biportal surgeries, when the foramen or lateral recess is being decompressed or during portal insertion.

Expanding Disease Spectrum Indications

The first described UBE procedure in 2015 entails lumbar radiculopathy, spinal stenosis, and grade I spondylolisthesis as the main indications of surgery [29]. Current indications have expanded anatomical levels to include cervical and thoracic regions [30]. One future aspect of endoscopic spinal surgery development will be exploring new spinal levels, including high cervical or craniocervical junctions, and thoracic and caudal levels [7]. Surgical indications may be extended to include motion-preserving scoliosis surgeries, tumor resections, and more complex surgical procedures [30]. Endoscopic spinal surgery can fulfill the aims of patient centricity and maintain sustainability of the healthcare system via increased cost-effectiveness, with improved patient outcomes and decreased medical costs.

Currently, disc herniation and stenosis are the two major indications for UBE. The most basic level is lumbosacral, followed by cervical and thoracic levels [7]. In disc herniation, the practical application of UBE has been extended to include migrated, recurrent, foraminal, extraforaminal, and some partially calcified discs. Disc sequestrectomy and excision of intradiscal granulations are performed via releasing annular anchorage and removing the pathological fragment. The following section illustrates some potential future surgical indications that can be considered in UBE surgery.

Target-Based Surgery

In conventional open surgery, large wound with extensive muscle stripping and bone resection is required to open up the spinal canal, even for excising small spinal lesions. UBE offers direct approach to target lesions with minimal surgical dissection. The benefits of adopting contralateral approach UBE surgery in managing small facetal cysts have been reported [31]. Using an arthroscope permits less invasive access to spinal canal or foraminal anatomies, through either the interlaminar or the transforaminal space. Our study also summarized the advantages of contralateral target-based approach in decompressing lateral recess stenosis, while the ipsilateral facet, bone, and muscle attachment can be preserved on the pathological side [17]. Our subsequent study reported more significant restoration of recess height, recess angle, and dural sac expansion, as well as better facet preservation, using contralateral versus ipsilateral approach for decompressing the lateral recess [32]. Analogous to arthroscopic loose body removal in knee, lateral recess stenosis or small spinous lesions can be more efficiently and less invasively managed by endoscopic spinal surgery, following a pre-planned trajectory.

The Unstable Spine

Currently, several approach corridors exist in managing spinal stenosis associated with spinal instability. In the case of anterior and lateral lumbar interbody fusion, indirect decompression can be achieved via restoration of disc height and sagittal balance, but the disadvantage is that stenosis caused by posterior flavum or facet hypertrophy cannot be decompressed at the same time, especially in the case of severe spinal stenosis.

Traditional TLIF enables direct posterior canal decompression, at the expense of damaging posterior muscles and ligamentous structures. TLIF performed under UBE not only reduces muscle dissection and retraction, but also enables surgeons to assess the adequacy of endplate preparation via direct visualizing of both the superior and inferior endplates. The endoscope can be inserted into the intervertebral space, and the cartilaginous endplate can be completely removed without osseous endplate injury under a magnified view [10].

In a meta-analysis study, there was no difference in the incidence of complications or fusion failure of UBE-TLIF compared with conventional PLIF or MIS-TLIF [10]. The mean length of hospital stay was significantly shorter than MIS-TLIF in two recruited studies. Postoperative pain was also lower than MIS-TLIF. In a more recent study in 2021, both hospital stay and time to ambulation were significantly reduced, and VAS-back was less in the UBE-TLIF compared with MIS-TLIF group [33]. Future TLIF instrumental designs should be modified, to facilitate UBE-fusion surgery involving insertion of screws, rods, and cages and in endplate preparation.

Spinal Infection

Few literatures described the use of biportal endoscopy in managing spinal infections, as opposed to arthroscopic debridement in joint infections. Uniportal endoscopy [34] and bilateral portal percutaneous endoscopic debridement [35] have been reported. UBE adopted for spinal infection treatment has been reported in one study in 2019 [36], which, to their belief, was the first reported series. The clinical and radiological outcome in the series of 13 patients was satisfactory, with no postoperative complications nor recurrence.

Surgeons traditionally believed that UBE was contraindicated in spinal infections [7]. Though unspecified, one may worry of infection spread accelerated by water pressure in an anatomically unconfined space. Water pressure may also induce potential damage to the neural structures previously invaded by microorganisms. Organisms retaining in dead spaces or cancellous bones may be difficult to be eradicated. The thick pus and distorted anatomy, in particular an attenuated ligamentum flavum, which potentially protects the underlying dura during bony resection, may increase the chance of iatrogenic dura injury during endoscopic debridement. Extensive and radical debridement may further destabilize the spine and accentuate spinal deformity. Irrigation before tissue sampling may also reduce the microbiological yield. For pyogenic spondylitis, it was suggested that the best indication for endoscopic debridement would be minimal or moderate destructive changes of the vertebrae in the early phase, as opposed to late extensive destruction when multiple vertebral bodies had been affected [34].

The neurological results of patients treated endoscopically appeared promising. Kang reported the neurological symptoms resolved in all eight patients after surgery [36]. Culture yield was successfully identified in 54% of cases. Manabu reported immediate postoperative pain relief in all 15 patients. In 2 patients with Frankel D neurological deficit, neurology resumed normal after endoscopic debridement [34].

Besides saline, the use of diluted povidone-iodine for irrigation in bilateral portal percutaneous endoscopic debridement has been described, in the treatment of lumbar pyogenic spondylitis [35]. Povidone-iodine not only covers a wide spectrum of organisms, but also possesses the advantage of not impeding wound healing. Although some literatures reported increased wound dehiscence with betadine, this effect was found insignificant in the Cochrane review [37]. However, there was also concern of neurotoxicity in animal studies, when the dura has been breached [38]. Although Yang [39] and Hsu [35] advocated the safety of betadine irrigation in septic spondylitis, potential negative effects may still exist in unrecognized or iatrogenic durotomy situations, which may result from severe infection and adhesion. In future, irrigation agents should be developed to attain equivalent bactericidal effects while inducing minimal adverse effects to neural structures. The effects of water pressure on the infected neural structures should also be carefully evaluated.

Cauda Equina Syndrome Due to Disc Herniation

Spinal decompression for cauda equina syndrome has been regarded as a contraindication in UBE [7]. Arguments include manipulations of already compromised neural tissues via small approach windows, leading to residual neurological deficits and potential medicolegal litigations.

On the contrary, there are studies describing the advantages of endoscopic transforaminal decompression in the management of cauda equina syndrome due to disc herniation, reporting complete bladder recovery in all 15 operated patients [40]. A majority of patients (80%) also attained motor recovery, higher than the reported 50–70% recovery in conventional open posterior surgeries. The author contributed their success to ventral access surgery that can be executed at the earliest possible instance. In addition, the procedure could be performed under local analgesia using 1:1 1% lidocaine and bupivacaine, combined with intramuscular midazolam and diclofenac, minimizing negativities of general anesthesia on the patient's visceral and cognitive function, which may also contribute to early rehabilitation and recovery.

Another study also reported the use of 0.5% lignocaine combined with intravenous sedation using midazolam and fentanyl, followed by biportal transforaminal decompression [41]. The author concluded that annulotomy was safe at the foraminal area, away from the compressed cauda equina fibers, with no risk of further neurological compromise. As the herniation has deflated the disc, approaching from the posterolateral side was unlikely to irritate the compressed neural tissue. Further studies will be required to evaluate the safety and efficacy of performing UBE decompression in patients with cauda equina syndrome.

Managing Intradural Pathologies

In the past, endoscopic management of intradural pathology was technically infeasible due to lack of appropriate surgical equipment. The endoscope may either be too large or not reliable enough for safe insertion into the intradural space. Following the invention of small and flexible endoscopes and working devices, more surgeons are exploring to manage intradural pathologies via endoscopy. For example, endoscope with external diameter less than 2 mm can safely enter and pass along the spinal cord, via the subarachnoid space of few millimeters' width. A flexible endoscope tip can move in cranial and caudal directions, to penetrate or remove a subarachnoid cyst. The filum terminale can be observed via endoscope advancement through the cauda equina, in managing cases of tethered cord syndrome. Spinal endoscopy can also provide views of ventral spinal cord without neural retraction and is effective in managing ventral spinal cord tumors or other ventral pathologies [42].

A number of novel instruments are also available. The bipolar flexible radiofrequency probe helps in the dissection and coagulation of small arteries over affected spinal nerve roots in managing intradural extramedullary tumors. Indocyanine green fluorescence endoscopy enables surgeons to appreciate the vascular anatomy and blood flow, being vital in the management of spinal cord vascular lesions like arteriovenous malformation. Development of percutaneous endoscopes also permits targeting for electrode insertion in cordotomy procedures for the management of cancer pain.

The key to success includes a meticulous surgical planning and secure watertight dural closure. The risk of bleeding and difficult hemostasis should be taken into account, and surgeons should be ready to convert to a microsurgical procedure, in managing complex dural tears or bleeding sources deemed difficult to be controlled by endoscopy alone.

Managing the Complications

Besides inadequate decompression, incidental dural tear has been regarded as one of the most common complications in UBE. Its reported incidence was 0.5–18% in lumbar spinal surgery and 2.9% in UBE [43]. Proposed factors include blurred visual field from epidural bleeding or floating bone chips. The central fold can also be easily damaged during flavectomy under the epidural fat, when the central dura was tethered to a few lines of fibrous tissue under the flavum. Dural repair or augmentation can be challenging in UBE surgery, owing to small portal access and continuous irrigation fluid inflow.

Without necessitating conversion to open surgery, the patch compression method was advocated for tears less than 1 cm [43]. TachoSil, a fibrin-based hemostat, was divided into 1 × 1 cm folds and patched over the tear site, and another 1 × 1 cm Gelfoam was added over it. The subcutaneous fascia was closed with continuous 4/0 Vicryl suture with no indwelling drain.

Endoscopic assisted durotomy repair using sutureless non-penetrating clips has also been reported [44]. The author stressed the importance of using pituitary forceps for temporary dural approximation before applying the clips, and a third portal was occasionally required. Herniated rootlets may require intradural relocation and protection with application of small Gelfoam pieces. The use of blunt titanium clips

(Anasto-Clip Vessel Closure System, LeMaitre Vascular, Inc.) could minimize the chance of rootlet injury, and metal artifacts were insignificant in postoperative MRI.

Endoscopic suturing has also been reported with a novel endoscopic knot pusher [18]. Nevertheless, authors still recommended conversion to open surgery for large defects, failed endoscopic repair, or inexperienced surgeons [44]. In future, it is suggested that rescue treatments should be readily available to facilitate endoscopic dural repair procedures.

Conclusion

Unilateral biportal endoscopic spinal surgery will be the next paradigm shift in the field of spinal surgery. Numerous potential fields of development exist with respect to classification, mode of service delivery, anesthesia, optics, portals, instruments, novel techniques, and surgical indications. Technological advancement will facilitate this new kind of minimally invasive surgery, to improve clinical results and patient outcomes, achieve satisfactory cost-effectiveness, and ensure its quality and safety within the healthcare system.

References

1. Kim JE, Choi DJ, Park EJJ, Lee HJ, Hwang JH, Kim MC, Oh JS. Biportal endoscopic spinal surgery for lumbar spinal stenosis. Asian Spine J. 2019;13(2):334–42. https://doi.org/10.31616/asj.2018.0210. Epub 2019 Apr 30. PMID: 30959588; PMCID: PMC6454273
2. Pranata R, Lim MA, Vania R, July J. Biportal endoscopic spinal surgery versus microscopic decompression for lumbar spinal stenosis: a systematic review and meta-analysis. World Neurosurg. 2020;138:e450–8. https://doi.org/10.1016/j.wneu.2020.02.151. Epub 2020 Mar 5. PMID: 32147545
3. Hofstetter CP, Ahn Y, Choi G, et al. AOSpine consensus paper on nomenclature for working-channel endoscopic spinal procedures [published correction appears in Global Spine J. 2021 Jun;11(5):819]. Global Spine J. 2020;10(2 Suppl):111S–21S. https://doi.org/10.1177/2192568219887364.
4. Heo DH, Park CK. Clinical results of percutaneous biportal endoscopic lumbar interbody fusion with application of enhanced recovery after surgery. Neurosurg Focus. 2019;46(4):E18. https://doi.org/10.3171/2019.1.FOCUS18695. PMID: 30933919
5. Smith J, Probst S, Calandra C, Davis R, Sugimoto K, Nie L, Gan TJ, Bennett-Guerrero E. Enhanced recovery after surgery (ERAS) program for lumbar spine fusion. Perioper Med (Lond). 2019;8:4. https://doi.org/10.1186/s13741-019-0114-2. PMID: 31149331; PMCID: PMC6537308
6. Michael YW, Chang PY, Grossman J. Development of an enhanced recovery after surgery (ERAS) approach for lumbar spinal fusion. J Neurosurg Spine. 2017;26(4):411–8. https://doi.org/10.3171/2016.9.SPINE16375. Epub 2016 Dec 23. PMID: 28009223
7. Ahn Y. Current techniques of endoscopic decompression in spine surgery. Ann Transl Med. 2019;7(Suppl 5):S169. https://doi.org/10.21037/atm.2019.07.98. PMID: 31624735; PMCID: PMC6778275

8. Fiani B, Reardon T, Selvage J, Dahan A, El-Farra MH, Endres P, Taka T, Suliman Y, Rose A. Awake spine surgery: an eye-opening movement. Surg Neurol Int. 2021;12:222. https://doi.org/10.25259/SNI_153_2021. PMID: 34084649; PMCID: PMC8168649
9. Kang SY, Kashlan ON, Singh R, Rane R, Adsul NM, Jung SC, Yi J, Cho HS, Kim HS, Jang IT, Oh SH. Advantages of the combination of conscious sedation epidural anesthesia under fluoroscopy guidance in lumbar spine surgery. J Pain Res. 2020;13:211–9. https://doi.org/10.2147/JPR.S227212. PMID: 32021410; PMCID: PMC6982434
10. Heo DH, Lee DC, Kim HS, Park CK, Chung H. Clinical results and complications of endoscopic lumbar interbody fusion for lumbar degenerative disease: a meta-analysis. World Neurosurg. 2021;145:396–404. https://doi.org/10.1016/j.wneu.2020.10.033. Epub 2020 Oct 13. PMID: 33065349
11. Kolcun JPG, Brusko GD, Wang MY. Endoscopic transforaminal lumbar interbody fusion without general anesthesia: technical innovations and outcomes. Ann Transl Med. 2019;7(Suppl 5):S167. https://doi.org/10.21037/atm.2019.07.92. PMID: 31624733; PMCID: PMC6778282
12. Basil GW, Kumar V, Wang MY. Optimizing visualization in endoscopic spine surgery. Oper Neurosurg (Hagerstown). 2021;21(Suppl 1):S59–66. https://doi.org/10.1093/ons/opaa382. PMID: 34128069
13. Muroi C, Fandino J, Coluccia D, Berkmann S, Fathi AR, Landolt H. 5-Aminolevulinic acid fluorescence-guided surgery for spinal meningioma. World Neurosurg. 2013;80(1–2):223.e1–3. https://doi.org/10.1016/j.wneu.2012.12.017. Epub 2012 Dec 13. PMID: 23247024
14. Kim K, Isu T, Chiba Y, Morimoto D, Ohtsubo S, Kusano M, Kobayashi S, Morita A. The usefulness of ICG video angiography in the surgical treatment of superior cluneal nerve entrapment neuropathy: technical note. J Neurosurg Spine. 2013;19(5):624–8. https://doi.org/10.3171/2013.7.SPINE1374. Epub 2013 Sep 20. PMID: 24053371
15. Seth R, Rajasekaran K, Benninger MS, Batra PS. The utility of intrathecal fluorescein in cerebrospinal fluid leak repair. Otolaryngol Head Neck Surg. 2010;143(5):626–32. https://doi.org/10.1016/j.otohns.2010.07.011. PMID: 20974330
16. Hahn BS, Park JY. Incorporating new technologies to overcome the limitations of endoscopic spine surgery: navigation, robotics, and visualization. World Neurosurg. 2021;145:712–21. https://doi.org/10.1016/j.wneu.2020.06.188. PMID: 33348526
17. Kim JS, Park CW, Yeung YK, Suen TK, Jun SG, Park JH. Unilateral bi-portal endoscopic decompression via the contralateral approach in asymmetric spinal stenosis: a technical note. Asian Spine J. 2020; https://doi.org/10.31616/asj.2020.0119. PMID: 33189115
18. Hong YH, Kim SK, Suh DW, Lee SC. Novel instruments for percutaneous biportal endoscopic spine surgery for full decompression and dural management: a comparative analysis. Brain Sci. 2020;10(8):516. https://doi.org/10.3390/brainsci10080516. PMID: 32759697; PMCID: PMC7463780
19. Yang HS, Park JY. 3D printer application for endoscope-assisted spine surgery instrument development: from prototype instruments to patient-specific 3D models. Yonsei Med J. 2020;61(1):94–9. https://doi.org/10.3349/ymj.2020.61.1.94. PMID: 31887805; PMCID: PMC6938781
20. Rawicki N, Dowdell JE, Sandhu HS. Current state of navigation in spine surgery. Ann Transl Med. 2021;9(1):85. https://doi.org/10.21037/atm-20-1335. PMID: 33553378; PMCID: PMC7859779
21. Shin Y, Sunada H, Shiraishi Y, Hosokawa M, Koh Y, Tei R, Aketa S, Motoyama Y, Yonezawa T, Nakase H. Navigation-assisted full-endoscopic spine surgery: a technical note. J Spine Surg. 2020;6(2):513–20. https://doi.org/10.21037/jss-2019-fess-19. PMID: 32656389; PMCID: PMC7340836
22. Quillo-Olvera J, Quillo-Reséndiz J, Quillo-Olvera D, Barrera-Arreola M, Kim JS. Ten-step biportal endoscopic transforaminal lumbar interbody fusion under computed tomography-based intraoperative navigation: technical report and preliminary outcomes in Mexico. Oper Neurosurg (Hagerstown). 2020;19(5):608–18. https://doi.org/10.1093/ons/opaa226. PMID: 32726423

23. Fan N, Yuan S, Du P, Zhu W, Li L, Hai Y, Ding H, Wang G, Zang L. Design of a robot-assisted system for transforaminal percutaneous endoscopic lumbar surgeries: study protocol. J Orthop Surg Res. 2020;15(1):479. https://doi.org/10.1186/s13018-020-02003-y. PMID: 33076965; PMCID: PMC7569762
24. Madhavan K, Kolcun JPG, Chieng LO, Wang MY. Augmented-reality integrated robotics in neurosurgery: are we there yet? Neurosurg Focus. 2017;42(5):E3. https://doi.org/10.3171/2017.2.FOCUS177. PMID: 28463612
25. Hsu MR, Haleem MS, Hsu W. 3D printing applications in minimally invasive spine surgery. Minim Invasive Surg. 2018;2018:4760769. https://doi.org/10.1155/2018/4760769. PMID: 29805806; PMCID: PMC5899854
26. Charalampidis A, Jiang F, Wilson JRF, Badhiwala JH, Brodke DS, Fehlings MG. The use of intraoperative neurophysiological monitoring in spine surgery. Global Spine J. 2020;10(1 Suppl):104S–14S. https://doi.org/10.1177/2192568219859314. Epub 2020 Jan 6. PMID: 31934514; PMCID: PMC6947672
27. Cofano F, Zenga F, Mammi M, Altieri R, Marengo N, Ajello M, Pacca P, Melcarne A, Junemann C, Ducati A, Garbossa D. Intraoperative neurophysiological monitoring during spinal surgery: technical review in open and minimally invasive approaches. Neurosurg Rev. 2019;42(2):297–307. https://doi.org/10.1007/s10143-017-0939-4. Epub 2018 Jan 8. PMID: 29313181
28. De Carvalho PST, Ramos MRF, da Silva Meireles AC, Peixoto A, de Carvalho P Jr, Ramírez León JF, Yeung A, Lewandrowski KU. Feasibility of using intraoperative neuromonitoring in the prophylaxis of dysesthesia in transforaminal endoscopic discectomies of the lumbar spine. Brain Sci. 2020;10(8):522. https://doi.org/10.3390/brainsci10080522. PMID: 32764525; PMCID: PMC7465602
29. Soliman HM. Irrigation endoscopic decompressive laminotomy. A new endoscopic approach for spinal stenosis decompression. Spine J. 2015;15(10):2282–9. https://doi.org/10.1016/j.spinee.2015.07.009. Epub 2015 Jul 10. PMID: 26165475
30. Moon ASM, Rajaram Manoharan SR. Endoscopic spine surgery: current state of art and the future perspective. Asian Spine J. 2018;12(1):1–2. https://doi.org/10.4184/asj.2018.12.1.1. Epub 2018 Feb 7. PMID: 29503675; PMCID: PMC5821913
31. Heo DH, Kim JS, Park CW, Quillo-Olvera J, Park CK. Contralateral sublaminar endoscopic approach for removal of lumbar juxtafacet cysts using percutaneous biportal endoscopic surgery: technical report and preliminary results. World Neurosurg. 2019;122:474–9. https://doi.org/10.1016/j.wneu.2018.11.072. Epub 2018 Nov 17. PMID: 30458327
32. Yeung YK, Park CW, Jun SG, Park JH, Tse CY. Comparative cohort study for expansion of lateral recess and facet joint injury after biportal endoscopic ipsilateral decompression and contralateral decompression. Asian Spine J. 2021; https://doi.org/10.31616/asj.2020.0656.
33. Kim JE, Yoo HS, Choi DJ, Park EJ, Jee SM. Comparison of minimal invasive versus biportal endoscopic transforaminal lumbar interbody fusion for single-level lumbar disease. Clin Spine Surg. 2021;34(2):E64–71. https://doi.org/10.1097/BSD.0000000000001024. PMID: 33633061; PMCID: PMC8035997
34. Ito M, Abumi K, Kotani Y, Kadoya K, Minami A. Clinical outcome of posterolateral endoscopic surgery for pyogenic spondylodiscitis: results of 15 patients with serious comorbid conditions. Spine (Phila Pa 1976). 2007;32(2):200–6. https://doi.org/10.1097/01.brs.0000251645.58076.96. PMID: 17224815
35. Hsu LC, Tseng TM, Yang SC, Chen HS, Yen CY, Tu YK. Bilateral portal percutaneous endoscopic debridement and lavage for lumbar pyogenic spondylitis. Orthopedics. 2015;38(10):e856–63. https://doi.org/10.3928/01477447-20151002-50. PMID: 26488778
36. Kang T, Park SY, Lee SH, Park JH, Suh SW. Spinal epidural abscess successfully treated with biportal endoscopic spinal surgery. Medicine (Baltimore). 2019;98(50):e18231. https://doi.org/10.1097/MD.0000000000018231. PMID: 31852084; PMCID: PMC6922448
37. Norman G, Atkinson RA, Smith TA, Rowlands C, Rithalia AD, Crosbie EJ, Dumville JC. Intracavity lavage and wound irrigation for prevention of surgical site infection. Cochrane

Database Syst Rev. 2017;10(10):CD012234. https://doi.org/10.1002/14651858.CD012234.pub2. PMID: 29083473; PMCID: PMC5686649

38. Akcay E, Ersahin Y, Ozer F, Duransoy YK, Camlar M, Atci I, Yagci A, Ozer O. Neurotoxic effect of povidone-iodine on the rat spine using a laminectomy-durotomy model. Childs Nerv Syst. 2012;28(12):2071–5. https://doi.org/10.1007/s00381-012-1885-7. Epub 2012 Aug 12. PMID: 22885709
39. Yang SC, Fu TS, Chen HS, Kao YH, Yu SW, Tu YK. Minimally invasive endoscopic treatment for lumbar infectious spondylitis: a retrospective study in a tertiary referral center. BMC Musculoskelet Disord. 2014;15:105. https://doi.org/10.1186/1471-2474-15-105. PMID: 24669940; PMCID: PMC3986884
40. Krishnan A, Kohli R, Degulmadi D, Mayi S, Ranjan R, Dave B. Cauda equina syndrome: a review of 15 patients who underwent percutaneous transforaminal endoscopic lumbar discectomy (PTELD) under local anaesthesia. Malays Orthop J. 2020;14(2):101–10. https://doi.org/10.5704/MOJ.2007.019. PMID: 32983384; PMCID: PMC7513651
41. Namboothiri S, Gore S, Raja P. Novel surgical technique for discogenic cauda equina syndrome - transforaminal intra discal access by annulotomy outside central spinal canal. J Spine. 2016;2016:S7. https://doi.org/10.4172/2165-7939.S7-008.
42. Endo T, Tominaga T. Use of an endoscope for spinal intradural pathology. J Spine Surg. 2020;6(2):495–501. https://doi.org/10.21037/jss.2020.01.06. PMID: 32656387; PMCID: PMC7340816
43. Kim JE, Choi DJ, Park EJ. Risk factors and options of management for an incidental dural tear in biportal endoscopic spine surgery. Asian Spine J. 2020;14(6):790–800. https://doi.org/10.31616/asj.2019.0297. Epub 2020 May 21. PMID: 32429015; PMCID: PMC7788375
44. Heo DH, Ha JS, Lee DC, Kim HS, Chung HJ. Repair of incidental durotomy using sutureless non-penetrating clips via biportal endoscopic surgery. Global Spine J. 2020;5:2192568220956606. https://doi.org/10.1177/2192568220956606. PMID: 33148035

Index

J. Quillo-Olvera et al. (eds.), *Unilateral Biportal Endoscopy of the Spine*, https://doi.org/10.1007/978-3-031-14736-4

K

L

P

R

S